Soft Tissue Tumors

Simone Mocellin

Soft Tissue Tumors

A Practical and Comprehensive Guide to Sarcomas and Benign Neoplasms

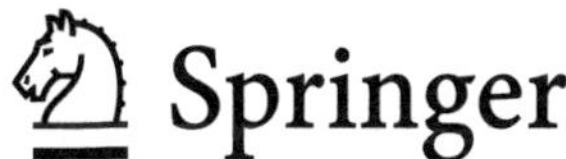

Simone Mocellin
Department of Surgery Oncology and Gastroenterology
University of Padova
Padova
Italy

Melanoma and Soft Tissue Sarcoma Unit
Istituto Oncologico Veneto (IOV-IRCCS) of Padova
Padova
Italy

ISBN 978-3-030-58712-3   ISBN 978-3-030-58710-9   (eBook)
https://doi.org/10.1007/978-3-030-58710-9

This Springer imprint is published by the registered company Springer Nature Switzerland AG
The registered company address is: Gewerbestrasse 11, 6330 Cham, Switzerland

*To my son Michele and my wife Marta, for
their infinite love and constant support*

Preface

Soft tissue tumors are a heterogeneous group of more than 200 nosological entities that include both benign neoplasms and malignant neoplasms (i.e., soft tissue sarcomas), can affect people of any age, and can arise in virtually any site of the human body. Given the number of these tumors (which is often multiplied by a variety of clinico-pathological subtypes), the epidemiological rarity of most of them, and the plethora of synonyms often utilized to refer to them, the topic of soft tissue neoplasms results complex and remembering the details on epidemiologic, clinical, pathologic, molecular, prognostic, and therapeutic details of each single entity is intrinsically challenging.

The aim of this book is to provide readers with a friendly, practical, and comprehensive guide to navigate in this complex area of oncology, bringing together the essential and most updated information on the following aspects of each tumor:

- *Definition*: Tumor name, as per World Health Organization (WHO) classification (whenever available); cell of origin of the neoplasm; biological behavior (as per WHO classification into benign, intermediate, and malignant, whenever available); list of synonyms.
- *Epidemiology and Presentation*: Essential information on epidemiological aspects and clinical presentation is provided.
- *Etiology and Predisposition*: Whenever available, data are provided on causative factors and tumor predisposition syndrome(s) the tumor is associated with.
- *Pathology*: The main histopathological features are summarized along with main issues of differential diagnosis.
- *Biomarkers*: Diagnostic, prognostic, and therapeutic biomarkers are described including proteins detectable at immunohistochemistry as well as genetic and cytogenetic alterations (e.g., mutations, chromosomal translocations, and fusion genes).
- *Prognosis*: The clinico-biological behavior of the tumor and the essential elements determining its prognosis are reported.
- *Therapy*: The therapeutic approach of each tumor is described, including surgery, chemotherapy, radiotherapy, target therapy, immunotherapy, and locoregional treatments, as appropriate.
- *References*: Key articles, books, and guidelines are listed to provide readers with authoritative, updated literature useful to deepen one's knowledge on specific topics.

The book is uniquely comprehensive not only in terms of the subjects covered for each tumor (most of the currently available publications on this topic focus mainly on the pathology features of these tumors), but also in terms of the nosological entities considered; in fact, the present publication includes not only **malignant soft tissue tumors** (most available publications are actually dedicated to sarcomas) but also **benign soft tissue tumors**. In addition, this book covers not only **somatic soft tissue tumors** (i.e., neoplasms arising from soft tissues found in extremities and thoraco-abdominal wall), but also **skin soft tissue tumors** and **visceral soft tissue tumors** (i.e., those arising in the retroperitoneum including the pelvis, mediastinum, and viscera).

In brief, the book is organized as follows:

- In the first part entitled "Basics on soft tissue tumors," the reader is provided with the general information on these neoplasms, which is of pivotal importance for the correct approach to these diseases. For example, there are principles of therapy (e.g., systemic chemotherapy for metastatic disease) that are shared across most soft tissue tumors and thus are not repeated in the sections dedicated to each tumor (where the reader can instead find data specific to a particular neoplasm); therefore, the user is encouraged to read this introductory part before going through the second part (dedicated to each single neoplasm). Importantly, all practice-changing trials (with special regard to randomized controlled trials) and their meta-analyses are mentioned and referenced so as to provide readers with the most robust evidence supporting (in particular) the therapeutic approach of patients affected with these tumors.
- In the second part entitled "List of soft tissue tumors," each nosological entity is described in detail in a dedicated section divided into paragraphs according to the topics above mentioned. The neoplasms are listed in alphabetical order for prompt identification.
- Finally, at the end of the book the reader can find an alphabetically ordered index of the names, synonyms, alternative names, and names of tumor variants of all soft tissue neoplasms described in this publication, which is a valuable resource to quickly find an item of interest.

Importantly, any indication reported in this book on the clinical management of these neoplasms is inspired by international recommendations dedicated to soft tissue sarcomas, such as the National Comprehensive Cancer Network (NCCN) and the European Society of Medical Oncology (ESMO) guidelines. In addition, if an evidence is based on the findings of randomized controlled trials, this is explicitly stated.

Overall, this publication is dedicated to health care providers (e.g., surgeons, oncologists, radiotherapists, pathologists, general practitioners, and residents in a variety of specialties), basic researchers, and policy makers interested in getting rapidly oriented in this complex field of medicine.

Contents

Part I

Basics on Soft Tissue Tumors

Definition

1

Soft tissue tumors include both benign neoplasms and malignant neoplasms (i.e., sarcomas) originating from mesenchymal cells (which derive from the mesoderm) with different types of **differentiation** such as the following: adipocytic (e.g., lipoma among benign tumors, liposarcoma among sarcomas), fibroblastic/myofibroblastic (e.g., elastofibroma, myxofibrosarcoma), fibrohistiocytic (e.g., tenosynovial giant cell tumor, malignant tenosynovial giant cell tumor), smooth muscle (e.g., leiomyoma, leiomyosarcoma), pericytic (e.g., angioleiomyoma, malignant glomus tumor), skeletal muscle (e.g., rhabdomyoma, rhabdomyosarcoma), vascular (e.g., hemangioma, angiosarcoma), and osteo-cartilagineous (e.g., soft tissue chondroma, extraskeletal osteosarcoma).

Actually the family of soft tissue tumors also includes neoplasms originating from highly specialized organ-specific mesenchymal cells (e.g., gastrointestinal stromal tumor), cells of neuroectodermal origin (e.g., schwannoma, malignant peripheral nerve sheath tumor), and undifferentiated cells (e.g., undifferentiated pleomorphic sarcoma).

Soft tissue tumors can arise virtually in any body site and are often distinguished as neoplasms originating from "somatic" soft tissues (i.e., those found in extremities and thoraco-abdominal wall) or "visceral" soft tissues (i.e., those present in the mediastinum, retroperitoneum, and viscera). Finally, with respect to the muscular sheath, these tumors are defined as superficial (above the muscle fascia) or deep (below the fascia): however, this definition has lost most of its importance since it is no longer included in the latest TNM staging system ($\rightarrow$ see section entitled "Prognosis").

The **biological behavior** is classified by the WHO into three categories: benign, intermediate (including forms that can locally recur and those at low risk of metastasis), and malignant (which are characterized by high risk of metastasis). Of note, some subtypes of soft tissue tumors classified among benign neoplasms can actually behave as tumors of intermediate malignant potential (e.g., cellular and atypical variants of benign fibrous histiocytoma).

S. Mocellin, *Soft Tissue Tumors*, https://doi.org/10.1007/978-3-030-58710-9_1

In the light of rarity and heterogeneity, collaborative international efforts (such as the European sarcoma database and tumor bank called Conticabase, https://conticabase.sarcomabcb.org/) are needed to gather together the information on pathological/molecular, clinical, and therapeutic aspects of these tumors and make significant advances at a faster pace.

Suggested Readings

Goldblum (2019) Enzinger & Weiss's soft tissue tumors, 7th edn
Lindberg (2018) Diagnostic pathology: soft tissue tumors, 2nd edn
Fletcher (2020) WHO classification of tumours of soft tissue and bone, 5th edn

Epidemiology and Presentation 2

Soft tissue tumors can arise at any age in both genders, but most of them have a predilection for specific age ranges and some are prevalent in or even specific to males or females.

Benign soft tissue tumors are about 100 times more frequent than soft tissue sarcomas: in fact, some benign soft tissue tumors (e.g., hemangiomas, lipomas, dermatofibromas) are very frequent in the population; despite their benign nature, some of these benign neoplasms—though rarely—can be life-threatening (e.g., giant hemangiomas complicated by Kasabach-Merritt syndrome or renal angiomyolipomas complicated by hemorrhage).

Soft tissue sarcomas—despite their rarity—are prognostically much more relevant since they are deadly in a significant proportion of cases (→ see section entitled "Prognosis"). In the USA, it is estimated that approximately 13,000 new cases are diagnosed each year. The majority of sarcomas arise in somatic soft tissues (about 70%), the remaining developing in viscera (about 20%, most of which being gastrointestinal stromal tumors, GISTs) and bones (about 10%; bone sarcomas are not covered in this book). Data on sarcoma epidemiology are collected by repositories such as the RARECARE in Europe (http://www.rarecare.eu/rarecancers/rarecancers.asp) and the SEER (Surveillance, Epidemiology, and End Results Program) in the USA (https://seer.cancer.gov/).

In **adults**, the annual incidence of soft tissue sarcomas is about 5 cases per 100,000 individuals, accounting for approximately 1% of all malignancies in this age population; in the light of this incidence, soft tissue sarcomas are classified among rare diseases (as defined by an incidence <6 cases/100.000 people/year). They arise in the extremities (about 50% of cases), trunk (>40%, including thoracic wall, abdominal wall, mediastinum, retroperitoneum, pelvis, and viscera), or head and neck (<10%). Of note, soft tissue sarcomas account for about 90% of all sarcomas in adults, the remaining being represented by bone sarcomas (in this book, only extraskeletal bone sarcomas are covered). For the distribution of the most frequent soft tissue sarcoma histological types, → see Fig. 2.1.

S. Mocellin, *Soft Tissue Tumors*, https://doi.org/10.1007/978-3-030-58710-9_2

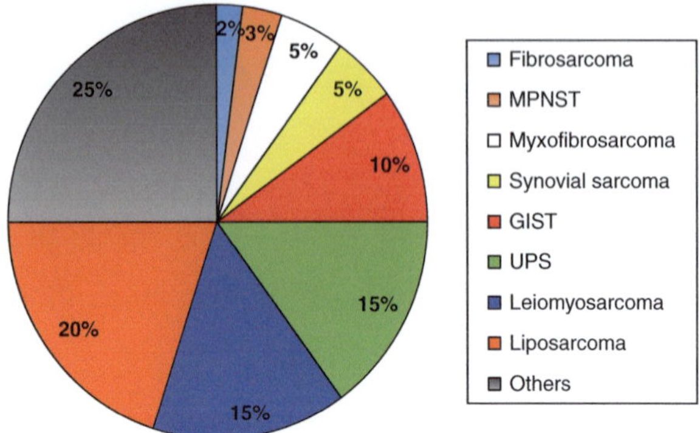

Fig. 2.1 Adult soft tissue sarcomas: distribution by histological type. *MPNST* malignant peripheral nerve sheath tumor, *GIST* gastrointestinal stromal tumor (only malignant GIST or GIST at high risk of being malignant is here considered), *UPS* undifferentiated pleomorphic sarcoma

In **children**, soft tissue sarcomas constitute about 7% of all malignancies and approximately 50% of all sarcomas (the other half being represented by bone sarcomas). The most frequent soft tissue sarcoma in this age population is rhabdomyosarcoma (with its four variants), which represents about 50% of all cases and has an annual incidence of 4.5 cases per 1,000,000 individuals aged <20 years. Overall, considering all ages, childhood cases account for approximately 10–20% of all soft tissue sarcomas.

Overall, the **clinical presentation** can be very different due to the fact that soft tissue tumors can arise from virtually any body site and thus any organ/structure can be involved by compression/infiltration. In this regard, some neoplasms are quite ubiquitous (e.g., hemangiomas), others show some predilection for specific areas (e.g., epithelioid sarcoma and extremities), and a minority are found only in specific sites/organs (e.g., gastrointestinal stromal tumor in the digestive tract). Somatic primary soft tissue tumors often present as a palpable mass, whereas visceral lesions more frequently present with compression signs/symptoms. Generally, the deeper is the lesion, the larger is the size reached by the tumor before becoming clinically symptomatic/evident. Signs and symptoms may of course depend also upon the development of metastatic disease (which most often involves lungs). Paraneoplastic syndromes are rare in patients with soft tissue sarcomas. Anyway, the clinical picture is nonspecific, and the diagnosis requires both radiological and histological assessments to be made. As regards the latter, see the below section entitled "Pathology."

As regards **imaging**, ultrasound (US) scan is useful especially for superficial lesions (e.g., it can easily suspect adipocytic tumors; it can differentiate between soft tissue masses and other masses such as lymph nodes and cysts), and its use is recommended in the UK guidelines as the first approach to superficial masses of unknown nature. Given the rarity of lymph node metastasis from sarcomas (<4%), US scan is not recommended for the routine staging of superficial regional lymph nodes.

Magnetic resonance imaging (MRI) is generally considered the best technique for the evaluation of primary soft tissue tumors (→ see an example in Fig. 2.2). MRI is recommended especially for the evaluation of primary sarcomas of the extremities, thoracic and abdominal wall, as well as head and neck.

Computed tomography (CT) scan is often considered the most suitable radiological method for the assessment of primary sarcomas of the intrathoracic and intra-abdominal cavity (e.g., those arising in the retroperitoneum and viscera)

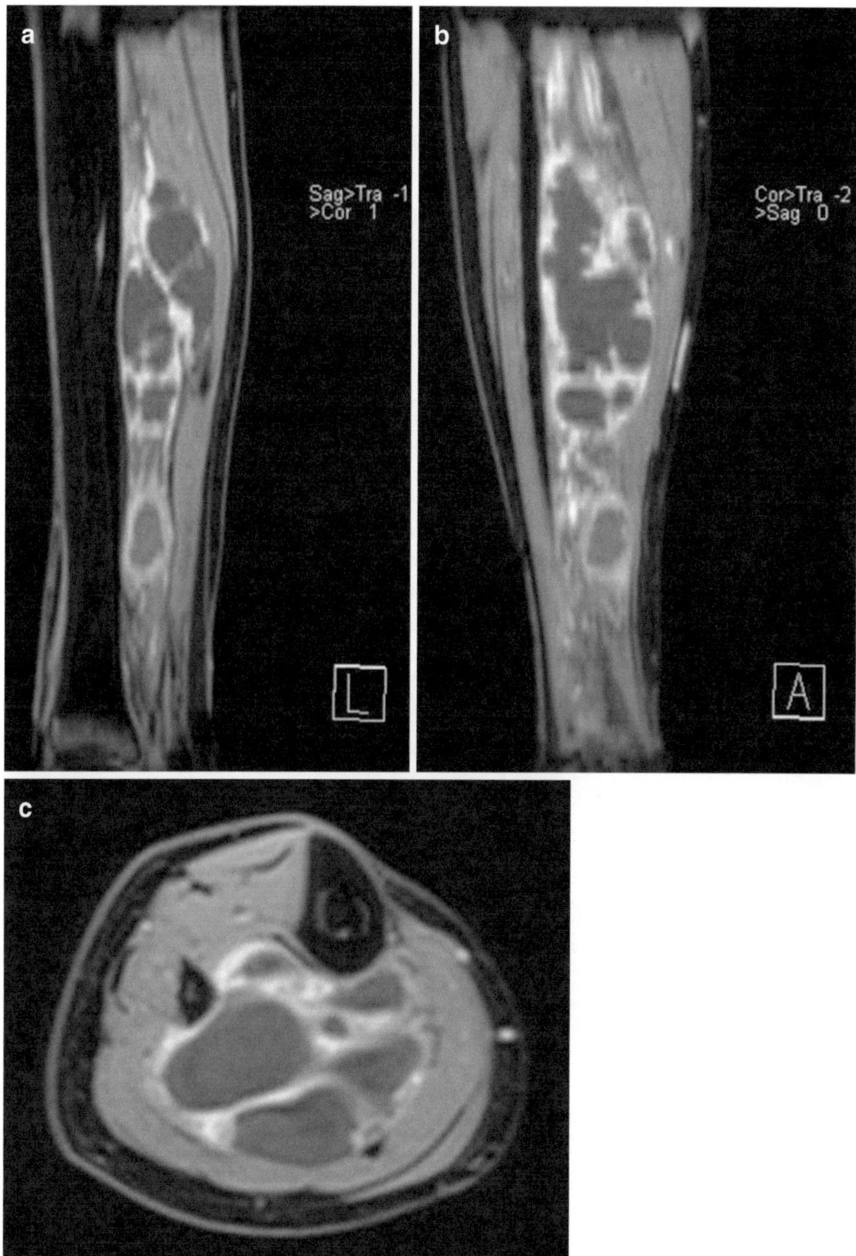

Fig. 2.2 Magnetic resonance imaging of a synovial sarcoma of the left calf in a 55-year-old female. Sagittal (**a**), coronal (**b**), and axial (**c**) planes are shown. Caudally to the main mass, a tumor satellite is visible

($\rightarrow$ see an example in Fig. 2.3). However, MRI and CT scan are considered equally accurate for retroperitoneal sarcomas. CT scan is superior to MRI for characterizing calcified tumors (e.g., myositis ossificans).

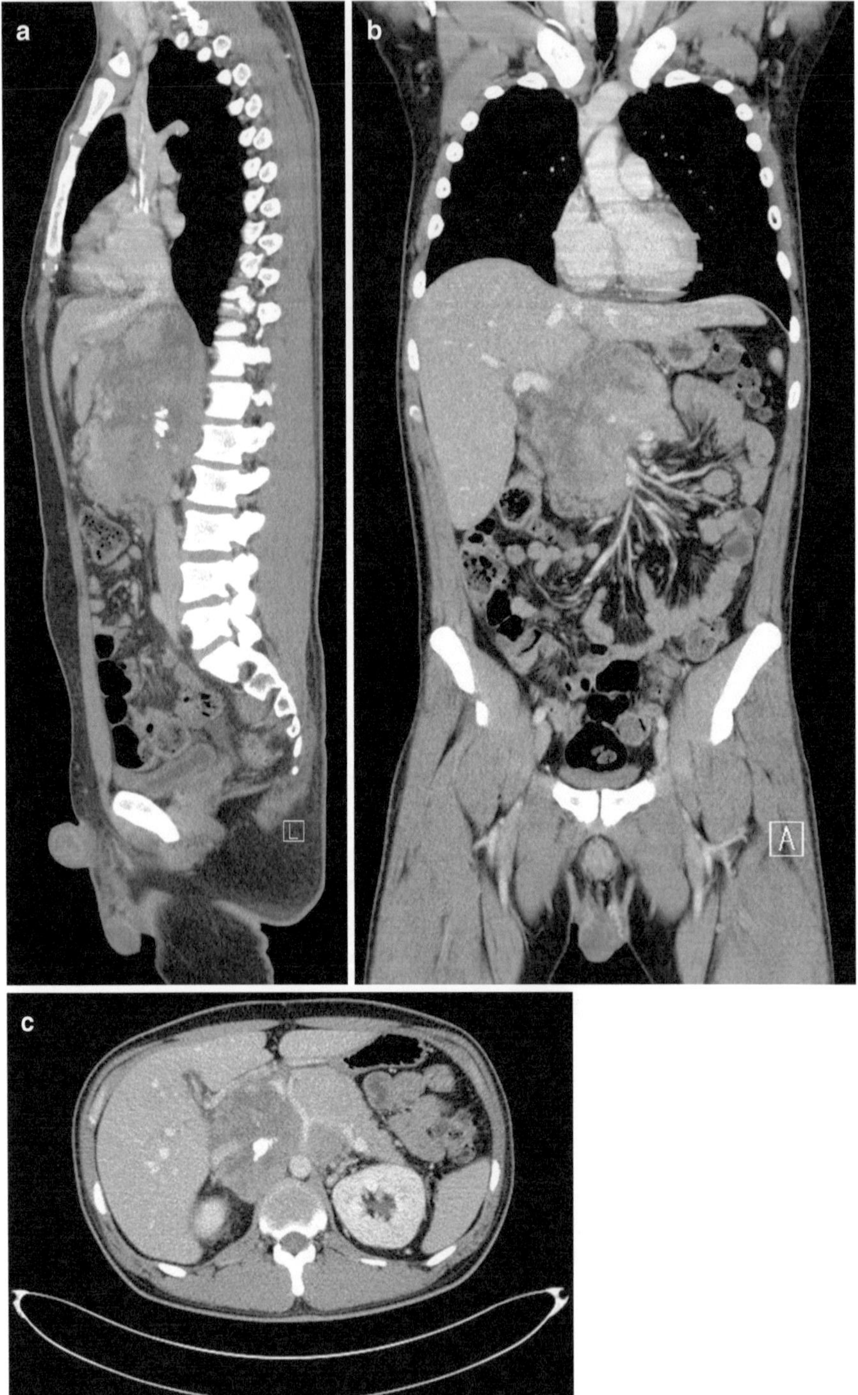

Fig. 2.3 Computed tomography scan of a retroperitoneal undifferentiated pleomorphic sarcoma in a 36-year-old male. Sagittal (**a**), coronal (**b**), and axial (**c**) planes are shown. Encasement of some major retroperitoneal vessels is evident

Disease staging includes evaluation of distant metastasis, which is best accomplished with chest CT scan (chest X-rays can be used for low-risk lesions such as low-grade sarcomas <5 cm). Abdomen CT scan, brain MRI, and total spine MRI are considered usually only in sarcomas with propensity to metastasize to the abdomen (e.g., round cell/myxoid liposarcoma, angiosarcoma, epithelioid sarcoma, and leiomyosarcoma), brain (e.g., angiosarcoma, alveolar soft part sarcoma, and clear cell sarcoma), and spine (spine bones and paraspinal tissues; e.g., round cell/myxoid liposarcoma).

For the subgroup of soft tissue sarcomas with high propensity to metastasize to lymph nodes (e.g., clear cell sarcoma, epithelioid sarcoma, synovial sarcoma, rhabdomyosarcoma), US scan (and even lymphoscintigraphy followed by sentinel node biopsy) can be taken into consideration (should the tumor arise from somatic soft tissues).

The role of positron emission tomography (PET) and PET integrated with CT scan (PET/CT) in the management of patients with soft tissue tumors is under evaluation. PET has been proposed as a tool to preoperatively determine tumor grading, to distinguish benign neoplasms (e.g., neurofibroma) from malignant ones (malignant peripheral nerve sheath tumor), to quantify tumor response to medical therapy, and to diagnose disease recurrence. However, no guideline recommends its use in the routine clinical setting.

Imaging strategies similar to those abovementioned are recommended to detect disease recurrence during patient **follow-up**, which is generally scheduled every 4–6 months for the first 2–3 years and every 6–8 months for the subsequent 2–3 years (although disease stage and biological aggressiveness are often used to modulate this schedule).

Suggested Readings

Brownstein (2020) Malignant soft-tissue sarcomas. Hematol Oncol Clin North Am 34(1):161–175

Catalano (2020) A bump: what to do next? Ultrasound imaging of superficial soft-tissue palpable lesions. J Ultrasound 23(3):287–300

Church (2017) Evaluating soft-tissue lumps and bumps. Mo Med 114(4):289–294

Gatta (2017) Burden and centralised treatment in Europe of rare tumours: results of RARECAREnet-a population-based study. Lancet Oncol 18(8):1022–1039

Lim (2019) Utility of positron emission tomography/computed tomography (PET/CT) imaging in the evaluation of sarcomas: a systematic review. Crit Rev Oncol Hematol 143:1–13

Penel (2018) Presentation and outcome of frequent and rare sarcoma histologic subtypes: a study of 10,262 patients with localized visceral/soft tissue sarcoma managed in reference centers. Cancer 124(6):1179–1187

Siegel (2020) Cancer statistics, 2020. CA Cancer J Clin 70(1):7–30

Wagner (2019) Ultrasound of soft tissue masses and fluid collections. Radiol Clin North Am 57(3):657–669

Etiology and Predisposition 3

As it occurs for most human neoplasms, the etiology of most soft tissue tumors is basically unknown, and the vast majority of them are sporadic. In a minority of cases, the following risk factors have been identified:

(a) Among **physical agents**, ionizing radiations are a well-known risk factor. For instance, radiotherapy increases by 10–50 times the risk of some soft tissue sarcomas (e.g., angiosarcoma and undifferentiated pleomorphic sarcoma) as well as the risk of osteosarcoma; of note, the interval between radiation exposure and tumor development is averagely 10–15 years; noteworthy, the combination with chemotherapy appears to shorten the time to radiation-induced sarcoma.

(b) Some **chemical agents** (e.g., herbicides such as phenoxyacetic acid, wood preservatives containing chlorophenol, contrast medium thorotrast/thorium oxide, industrial chemicals such as vinyl chloride and arsenic) are also recognized carcinogens associated with increased risk of soft tissue sarcomas (with special regard to angiosarcoma).

(c) **Biological agents** (i.e., viruses) have been linked to the development of specific soft tissue sarcomas: the best example is the tight relationship between human herpesvirus 8 (HHV8) and Kaposi sarcoma.

(d) **Chronic lymphedema** (following lymphadenectomy but also filarial infection and congenital primary lymphedema) is associated with an increased risk of lymphangiosarcoma, a condition known as Stewart-Treves syndrome.

(e) In a minority of cases, soft tissue tumors run in families where they contribute to the phenotype of **cancer predisposition syndromes**, such as hereditary retinoblastoma (associated with the development of different types of sarcomas), Li-Fraumeni syndrome (multiple types of sarcomas), Werner syndrome (undifferentiated pleomorphic sarcoma as well as other sarcomas), Gardner syndrome (desmoid tumor), Carney-Stratakis syndrome (GIST and paraganglioma), Gorlin syndrome (rhabdomyosarcoma), tuberous sclerosis (PEComas), and so on. These hereditary syndromes are generally due to germline high penetrance

S. Mocellin, *Soft Tissue Tumors*, https://doi.org/10.1007/978-3-030-58710-9_3

inactivation of tumor suppressor genes (e.g., RB1 in hereditary retinoblastoma, TP53 in Li-Fraumeni syndrome, NF1 in neurofibromatosis, and so on) or activation of oncogenes (e.g., KIT in familial GIST). The details of these as well as many other conditions predisposing to soft tissue tumor development are described in the sections dedicated to single tumors (in the second part of this book).

Due to their rarity, sarcomas have not been the target of large epidemiological studies. A recently launched multicentric population-based case-control French study (ETIOSARC) will investigate the role of lifestyle and environmental and occupational factors in the occurrence of sarcomas among adults.

As regards the molecular etiopathogenesis of **sporadic soft tissue tumors**, both germline and somatic genetic alterations have been described. Low penetrance germline polymorphisms (mainly single nucleotide polymorphisms, SNP) of genes such as TP53, ATM, ATR, BRCA2, and ERCC2 have been associated with an increased risk of tumor development, but the epidemiological rarity of these neoplasms coupled with their clinicopathological heterogeneity has so far hindered the conduction of genome-wide studies on large series of patients affected with specific tumor types, which prevents from defining the host genetic background conducive to sporadic sarcoma development.

From the viewpoint of somatic genetic alterations, soft tissue tumors (including benign and malignant neoplasms) can be divided into two main categories (each including approximately 50% of soft tissue sarcomas):

(a) Neoplasms with specific recurrent (and sometimes pathognomonic) genetic alterations such as chromosomal translocations leading to the formation of fusion genes (also known as chimeric genes and gene fusions), mutations (e.g., activating mutations of KIT oncogene in GIST), and gene amplifications (e.g., MDM2 amplification in well-differentiated and dedifferentiated liposarcoma). These tumors are also characterized by simple karyotypes, with some exceptions (e.g., dedifferentiated liposarcoma). As regards fusion genes, more than 150 such gene fusions have been so far described in approximately one third of soft tissue tumors and 20% of soft tissue sarcomas (a dedicated database of chromosome aberrations and gene fusions in human cancers is available at *https://mitelmandatabase.isb-cgc.org/*). In most cases, these chimeric genes generate transcription factors such as (e.g., EWSR1-ATF1 in clear cell sarcoma; EWSR1-FLI1 in primitive neuroectodermal tumor/Ewing sarcoma family); other fusion genes encode receptor tyrosine kinases (e.g., ETV6-NTRK3 in congenital mesoblastic nephroma; ALK-containing fusion genes in inflammatory myofibroblastic tumor), growth factors (e.g., COL1A1-PDGFB in dermatofibrosarcoma protuberans; COL6A3-CSF1 in tenosynovial giant cell tumor), chromatin regulators (e.g., BCOR-CCNB3 in undifferentiated round cell sarcoma and SS18-SSX in synovial sarcoma), or other proteins known to be involved in carcinogenesis (e.g., MIR143-NOTCH in glomus tumors). Of note, some fusion genes are present in most (if not all) cases of a given tumor type (e.g., NAB2-STAT6 in solitary fibrous tumor; EWSR1-WT1 in desmoplastic small round cell tumor), but others can be found only in a subset of cases (e.g., about 50% of inflammatory myofibroblastic tumors harbor ALK-containing fusion genes), and others can have more than just one gene partner (e.g., SS18-SSX1 and SS18-SSX2 in synovial sarcoma; FUS-DDIT3 and EWSR1-DDIT3 in myxoid liposarcoma); furthermore, in the same soft tissue tumor, different types of fusion genes can be detected, the same fusion gene can be identified in different soft tissue tumors, and some fusion genes are shared with non-soft tissue neoplasms (e.g., NTRK-containing fusion genes).

(b) Neoplasms with complex karyotypes but no specific genetic pattern (e.g., undifferentiated pleomorphic sarcoma, pleomorphic liposarcoma, leiomyosarcoma, pleomorphic rhabdomyosarcoma, and malignant peripheral nerve sheath tumor). The mutational landscape of these tumors shows that—unlike carcinomas—they are characterized mainly by copy number alterations with low mutational burden (associated with a low incidence of microsatellite instability, MSI) and only a few genes recurrently mutated across different histological types (e.g., TP53, ATRX, RB1, NF1, PIK3CA, and PTEN). For a list of most mutated genes in selected soft tissue tumors, → see Table 3.1.

Table 3.1 Top mutated genes in selected soft tissue tumors (only neoplasms with at least 100 samples available were selected). (Source: Catalogue Of Somatic Mutations In Cancer (COSMIC, *https://cancer.sanger.ac.uk/cosmic*))

Tumor	Gene	Mutated (%)
Angiosarcoma	TP53	27
	KRAS	18
	PLCG1	11
	KDR	8
	CIC	4
	NRAS	3
	PIK3CA	3
Liposarcoma NOS	PIK3CA	9
	TP53	8
	EP300	7
	KMT2D	4
	ATRX	4
	CIC	3
	CTNNB1	2
	NF1	2
	PTEN	2
	HRAS	2
	RB1	2
	KDM6A	2
	PBRM1	2
	KIT	1
	EGFR	1
	FBXW7	1
	ERBB2	1
	APC	1

(continued)

Table 3.1 (continued)

Tumor	Gene	Mutated (%)
Desmoid tumor	CTNNB1	72
	APC	18
MPNST	NF1	21
	TP53	12
	BRAF	2
	CDKN2A	2
	KRAS	1
Neurofibroma	NF1	40
Schwannoma	NF2	43
	SMARCB1	4
Leiomyoma	MED12	51
	TP53	4
Leiomyosarcoma	TP53	33
	ATRX	23
	RB1	16
	MED12	8
	PTEN	5
	CARD11	5
	KRAS	4
	ASXL1	4
	NSD1	4
	TOP1	4
	KMT2A	4
	ATM	3
	ARID1A	3
	ARID2	3
	BRCA2	3
	AR	3
	PIK3CA	2
	CDH1	2
	NF1	2
	BRAF	2
	ATM	2
Rhabdoid tumor	SMARCB1	23
Rhabdomyosarcoma (embryonal)	TP53	16
	NRAS	15
	MYOD1	11
	NF1	8
	DICER1	7
	HRAS	6
	PIK3CA	5
	PTPN11	3
	ALK	3
	CTNNB1	3
	ERBB2	3
	NOTCH1	2

Advances in the knowledge of the molecular aberrations underlying the pathogenesis of soft tissue tumors is having a major impact on the diagnostic, prognostic, and therapeutic approach to these tumors: for this reason, the most relevant genetic features are reported in the paragraph entitled "Biomarkers" within the sections dedicated to each soft tissue tumor, in the second part of the book.

Suggested Readings

Ballinger (2016) Monogenic and polygenic determinants of sarcoma risk: an international genetic study. Lancet Oncol 17(9):1261–1271

Barretina (2010) Subtype-specific genomic alterations define new targets for soft-tissue sarcoma therapy. Nat Genet 42(8):715–721

Benna (2018) Genetic susceptibility to bone and soft tissue sarcomas: a field synopsis and meta-analysis. Oncotarget 9(26):18607–18626

Cancer Genome Atlas Research Network (2017) Comprehensive and integrated genomic characterization of adult soft tissue sarcomas. Cell 171(4):950–965

Farid (2016) Sarcomas associated with genetic cancer predisposition syndromes: a review. Oncologist 21(8):1002–1013

Kim (2018) Integrated molecular characterization of adult soft tissue sarcoma for therapeutic targets. BMC Med Genet 19(Suppl 1):216

Lacourt (2019) ETIOSARC study: environmental aetiology of sarcomas from a French prospective multicentric population-based case-control study-study protocol. BMJ Open 9(6):e030013

Mariño-Enríquez (2016) Molecular pathogenesis and diagnostic, prognostic and predictive molecular markers in sarcoma. Surg Pathol Clin 9(3):457–473

Mertens (2016) Gene fusions in soft tissue tumors: recurrent and overlapping pathogenetic themes. Genes Chromosomes Cancer 55(4):291–310

Schaefer (2018) Contemporary sarcoma diagnosis, genetics, and genomics. J Clin Oncol 36(2):101–110

Suurmeijer (2019) New advances in the molecular classification of pediatric mesenchymal tumors. Genes Chromosomes Cancer 58(2):100–110

Thway (2020) Update on selected advances in the immunohistochemical and molecular genetic analysis of soft tissue tumors. Virchows Arch 476(1):3–15

Zhang (2017) Chemotherapy with radiotherapy influences time-to-development of radiation-induced sarcomas: a multicenter study. Br J Cancer 117(3):326–331

Pathology

4

Pathology assessment is necessary to make the correct diagnosis of soft tissue tumors. In particular, the correct definition of the tumor type is crucial for both prognostic evaluation and therapeutic management, which can greatly vary based on the histological classification. For the WHO classification of soft tissue tumors published in 2020, → see Table 4.1; this list does not include a number of mesenchymal tumors such as some skin and visceral neoplasms (e.g., kidney soft tissue tumors), which are covered by other WHO publications dedicated to specific organs or systems (e.g., skin neoplasms): as above mentioned, all soft tissue tumors (independently of their site of origin) are instead covered in this book.

As a general rule, any soft tissue mass larger than 3 cm, any soft tissue mass deep to the fascia, and any soft tissue mass rapidly growing should be investigated to exclude a soft tissue sarcoma.

Whenever feasible, a **core needle biopsy** (CNB) is the preferred method to obtain tumor samples; besides palpable masses of extremities and thoraco-abdominal wall, also deep lesions of the thoraco-abdominal cavities can often be sampled using CNB under the guidance of imaging techniques such as ultrasound and CT scan. Should CNB be unfeasible or fail to be diagnostic, incisional biopsy is recommended. The excision of the whole lesion should be limited to superficial small (<3 cm according to the ESMO guidelines) neoplasms or in case of failure to achieve a diagnosis with previous methods. Fine needle aspiration (FNA) is not recommended for the diagnosis of primary soft tissue tumors because cytological examination is rarely adequate to make accurate diagnosis in the field of soft tissue tumors. FNA may be useful in case of disease recurrence (especially in case of high-grade lesions). Whatever the method, the biopsy site should be carefully placed so that its track can be removed with following surgery (except for retroperitoneal sarcomas). Intraoperative frozen section technique is discouraged as it does not allow a precise diagnosis. Biopsies should be fixed in 4% buffered formalin; even better, fresh tissue can be frozen.

Currently, pathology examination of soft tissue tumors (Figs. 4.1, 4.2, and 4.3) is based not only on conventional H&E staining and immunohistochemistry (which

Table 4.1 WHO classification of soft tissue tumors

Adipocytic tumors	
Benign	Lipoma
	Lipomatosis
	Lipomatosis of nerve
	Lipoblastoma
	Angiolipoma
	Myolipoma
	Chondroid lipoma
	Spindle cell/pleomorphic lipoma
	Hibernoma
Intermediate (locally aggressive)	Atypical lipomatous tumor
Malignant	Liposarcoma, well differentiated, not otherwise specified (NOS)
	Dedifferentiated liposarcoma
	Myxoid liposarcoma
	Pleomorphic liposarcoma
Fibroblastic/myofibroblastic tumors	
Benign	Nodular fasciitis
	Proliferative fasciitis
	Proliferative myositis
	Myositis ossificans
	Fibro-osseous pseudotumor of digits
	Ischemic fasciitis
	Elastofibroma
	Fibrous hamartoma of infancy
	Fibromatosis colli
	Juvenile hyaline fibromatosis
	Inclusion body fibromatosis
	Fibroma of tendon sheath
	Desmoplastic fibroblastoma
	Mammary-type myofibroblastoma
	Calcifying aponeurotic fibroma
	Angiomyofibroblastoma
	Cellular angiofibroma
	Nuchal-type fibroma
	Gardner fibroma
	Calcifying fibrous tumor
Intermediate (locally aggressive)	Palmar/plantar fibromatosis
	Desmoid-type fibromatosis
	Abdominal (mesenteric) fibromatosis
	Lipofibromatosis
	Giant cell fibroblastoma

Table 4.1 (continued)

Adipocytic tumors	
Intermediate (rarely metastasizing)	Dermatofibrosarcoma protuberans
	Fibrosarcomatous dermatofibrosarcoma protuberans
	Pigmented dermatofibrosarcoma protuberans
	Solitary fibrous tumor
	Inflammatory myofibroblastic tumor
	Low-grade myofibroblastic sarcoma
	Myxoinflammatory fibroblastic sarcoma
	Infantile fibrosarcoma
Malignant	Adult fibrosarcoma
	Myxofibrosarcoma
	Low-grade fibromyxoid sarcoma
	Sclerosing epithelioid fibrosarcoma
So-called fibrohistiocytic tumors	
Benign	Tenosynovial giant cell tumor, localized type
	Tenosynovial giant cell tumor, diffuse type
	Deep benign fibrous histiocytoma
Intermediate (rarely metastasizing)	Plexiform fibrohistiocytic tumor
	Giant cell tumor of soft tissues
Malignant	Malignant tenosynovial giant cell tumor
Smooth muscle tumors	
Benign	Deep leiomyoma
Malignant	Leiomyosarcoma (excluding skin)
Pericytic (perivascular) tumors	
	Glomus tumor (and variants)
	Glomangiomatosis
	Malignant glomus tumor
	Myopericytoma
	Myofibroma
	Myofibromatosis
	Angioleiomyoma
Skeletal muscle tumors	
Benign	Rhabdomyoma (adult, fetal and genital types)
Malignant	Embryonal rhabdomyosarcoma
	Alveolar rhabdomyosarcoma
	Pleomorphic rhabdomyosarcoma
	Spindle cell/sclerosing rhabdomyosarcoma
Vascular tumors of soft tissue	
Benign	Hemangioma (synovial, venous, arteriovenous, and intramuscular types)
	Epithelioid hemangioma
	Angiomatosis
	Lymphangioma
Intermediate (locally aggressive)	Kaposiform hemangioendothelioma

(continued)

Table 4.1 (continued)

Adipocytic tumors	
Intermediate (rarely metastasizing)	Retiform hemangioendothelioma
	Papillary intralymphatic angioendothelioma
	Composite hemangioendothelioma
	Pseudomyogenic (epithelioid sarcoma-like) hemangioendothelioma
	Kaposi sarcoma
Malignant	Epithelioid hemangioendothelioma
	Angiosarcoma of soft tissue
Chondro-osseous tumors	
	Soft tissue chondroma
	Extraskeletal osteosarcoma
Gastrointestinal stromal tumors	
	Gastrointestinal stromal tumor
Nerve sheath tumors	
Benign	Schwannoma (including variants)
	Melanotic schwannoma
	Neurofibroma (including variants)
	Plexiform neurofibroma
	Perineurioma
	Granular cell tumor
	Dermal nerve sheath myxoma
	Solitary circumscribed neuroma
	Ectopic meningioma
	Nasal glial heterotopia
	Benign triton tumor
	Hybrid nerve sheath tumors
Malignant	Malignant peripheral nerve sheath tumor
	Epithelioid malignant peripheral nerve sheath tumor
	Malignant perineurioma
	Malignant triton tumor
	Malignant granular cell tumor
	Ectomesenchymoma (currently classified among skeletal muscle tumors)
Tumors of uncertain differentiation	
Benign	Acral fibromyxoma
	Intramuscular myxoma (including cellular variant)
	Juxta-articular myxoma
	Deep ("aggressive") angiomyxoma
	Pleomorphic hyalinizing angiectatic tumor
	Ectopic hamartomatous thymoma
Intermediate (locally aggressive)	Hemosiderotic fibrolipomatous tumor

Table 4.1 (continued)

Adipocytic tumors	
Intermediate (rarely metastasizing)	Atypical fibroxanthoma
	Angiomatoid fibrous histiocytoma
	Ossifying fibromyxoid tumor
	Ossifying fibromyxoid tumor, malignant
	Mixed tumor NOS
	Mixed tumor NOS, malignant
	Myoepithelioma
	Myoepithelial carcinoma
	Phosphaturic mesenchymal tumor, benign
	Phosphaturic mesenchymal tumor, malignant
Malignant	Synovial sarcoma NOS
	Synovial sarcoma, spindle cell
	Synovial sarcoma, biphasic
	Epithelioid sarcoma
	Alveolar soft part sarcoma
	Clear cell sarcoma of soft tissue
	Extraskeletal myxoid chondrosarcoma
	Extraskeletal Ewing sarcoma
	Desmoplastic small round cell tumor
	Extrarenal rhabdoid tumor
	Neoplasms with perivascular epithelioid cell differentiation (PEComa)
	PEComa NOS, benign
	PEComa NOS, malignant
	Intimal sarcoma
Undifferentiated/unclassified sarcomas	
	Undifferentiated spindle cell sarcoma
	Undifferentiated pleomorphic sarcoma
	Undifferentiated round cell sarcoma
	Undifferentiated epithelioid sarcoma
	Undifferentiated sarcoma NOS

Note: NOS (Not Otherwise Specified)

remains a key step especially in the definition of cell differentiation) but also on techniques such as reverse transcription-polymerase chain reaction (RT-PCR), fluorescence in situ hybridization (FISH), and DNA sequencing (including next-generation sequencing, NGS) that enables pathologists to detect genetic aberrations highly specific (and sometimes pathognomonic) for each nosological entity (see below section entitled "Biomarkers").

Differential diagnosis is often challenging across different sarcoma types as well as between benign and malignant soft tissue tumors originating from the same type of cells (e.g., lipoma versus liposarcoma; leiomyoma versus leiomyosarcoma). Differential diagnosis must also take into account other malignancies such as those secondarily located in the soft tissues (e.g., metastasis of carcinomas or melanoma

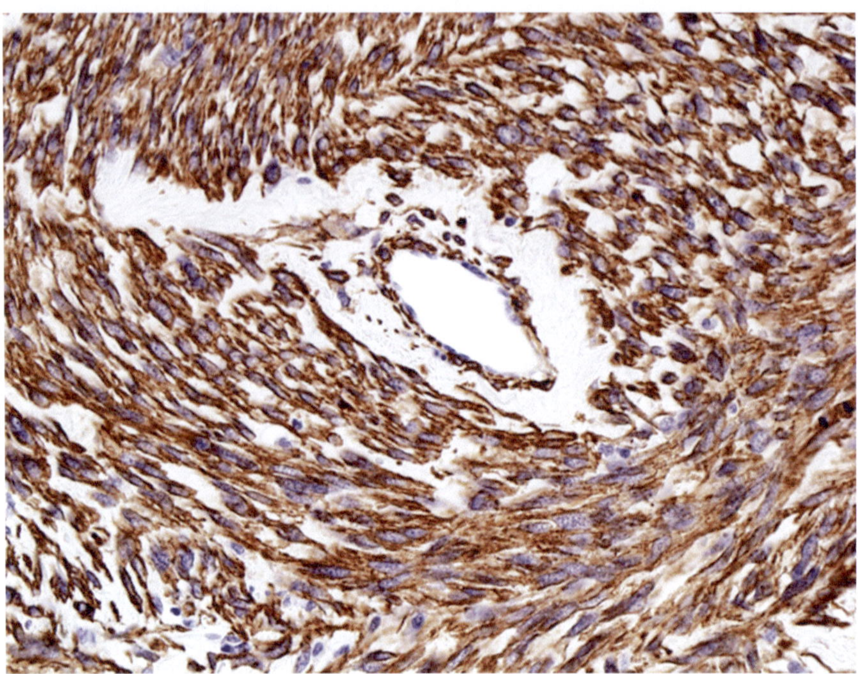

Fig. 4.1 Microscopic images of a retroperitoneal leiomyosarcoma in a 62-year-old male: hematoxylin and eosin staining (**a**) and expression of smooth muscle actin (SMA) by immunohistochemistry (**b**)

in the subcutis), tumors resembling sarcomas (e.g., carcinosarcomas and sarcomatoid carcinomas, sarcomatoid melanoma), as well as other mesenchymal neoplasms originating from hematopoietic cells (e.g., lymphomas, follicular dendritic cell sarcoma, interdigitating dendritic cell sarcoma, myeloid sarcoma, and histiocytic sarcoma) or cells present only in specific body sites (e.g., meningioma from meningothelial cells and mesothelioma from mesothelial cells).

For these reasons and due to the rarity of soft tissue sarcomas, diagnosis should be centralized in high-volume centers so that the diagnosis is made by pathologists who are expert in soft tissue tumors.

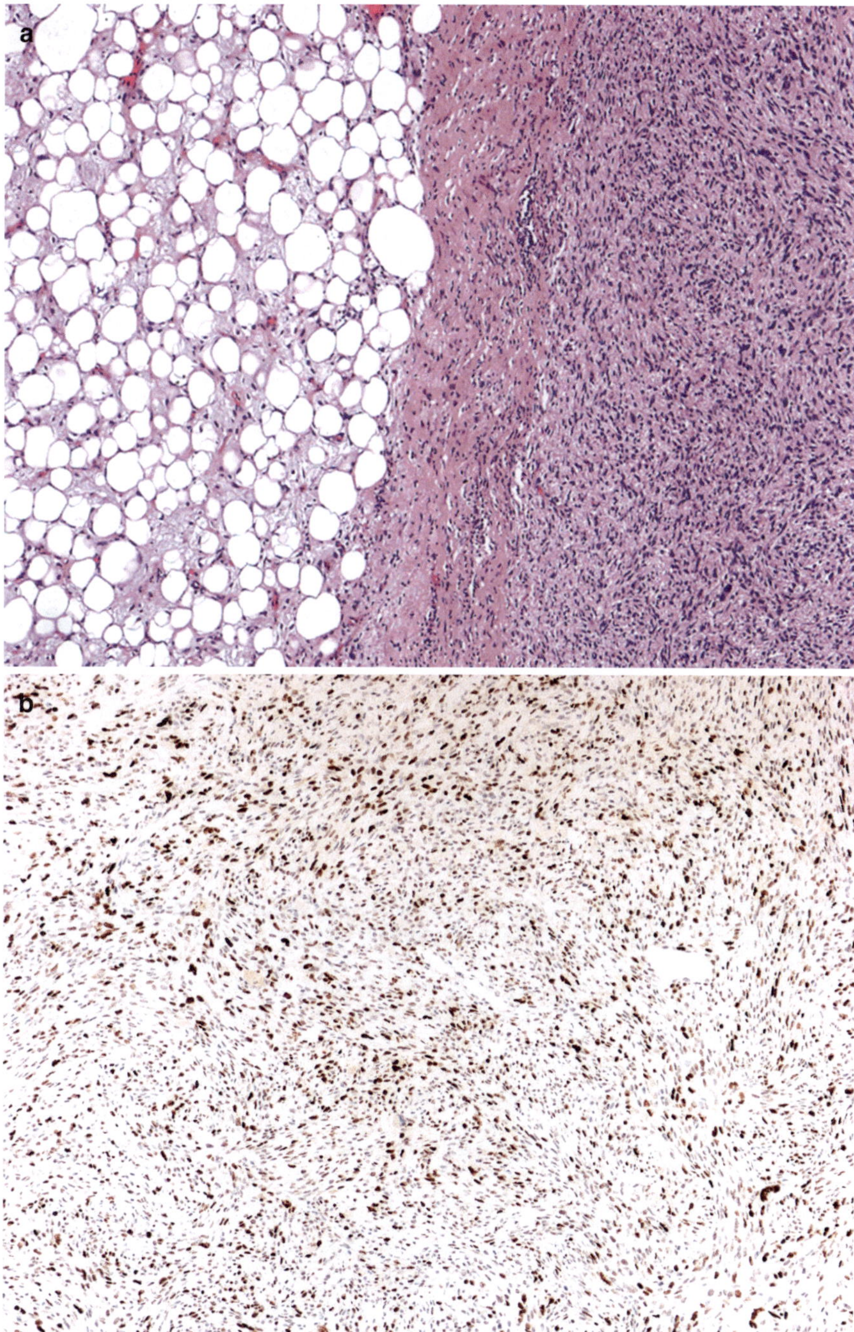

Fig. 4.2 Microscopic images of a dedifferentiated liposarcoma of the thigh in a 68-year-old female: hematoxylin and eosin staining (**a**) and expression of mouse double minute 2 (MDM2) by immunohistochemistry (**b**)

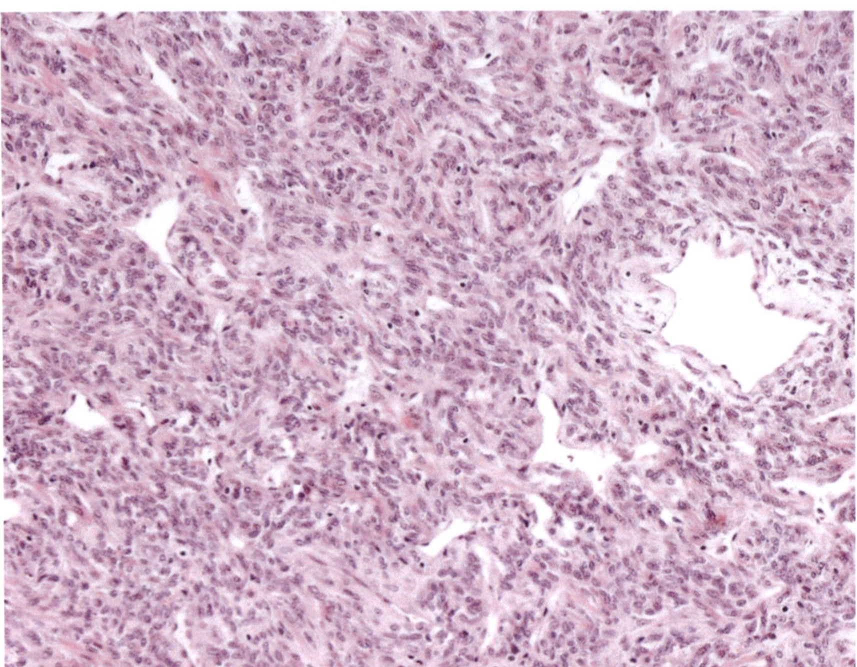

Fig. 4.3 Microscopic images of a solitary fibrous tumor of the pelvis in a 71-year-old male: hematoxylin and eosin staining (**a**) and expression of signal transducer and activator of transcription 6 (STAT6) by immunohistochemistry (**b**)

Suggested Readings

Fletcher (2020) WHO classification of tumours of soft tissue and bone, 5th edn

Goldblum (2019) Enzinger & Weiss's soft tissue tumors, 7th edn

Hornick (2019) Limited biopsies of soft tissue tumors: the contemporary role of immunohisto-chemistry and molecular diagnostics. Mod Pathol 32(Suppl 1):27–37

Jain (2010) Molecular classification of soft tissue sarcomas and its clinical applications. Int J Clin Exp Pathol 3(4):416–428

Lindberg (2018) Diagnostic pathology: soft tissue tumors, 2nd edn

Miettinen (2006) From morphological to molecular diagnosis of soft tissue tumors. Adv Exp Med Biol 587:99–113

Papke (2019) Practical application of cytology and core biopsy in the diagnosis of mesenchymal tumors. Surg Pathol Clin 12(1):227–248

Schaefer (2018) Diagnostic immunohistochemistry for soft tissue and bone tumors: an update. Adv Anat Pathol 25(6):400–412

Thway (2020) Update on selected advances in the immunohistochemical and molecular genetic analysis of soft tissue tumors. Virchows Arch 476(1):3–15

Wei (2017) Soft tissue tumor immunohistochemistry update: illustrative examples of diagnostic pearls to avoid pitfalls. Arch Pathol Lab Med 141(8):1072–1091

Yao (2020) An evidence-based guideline on the application of molecular testing in the diagnosis, prediction of prognosis, and selection of therapy in non-GIST soft tissue sarcomas. Cancer Treat Rev 85:101987

Biomarkers 5

Increased knowledge of the molecular biology of soft tissue tumors has led to the identification of a growing number of biomarkers that are useful not only for diagnostic purposes (where a single biomarker but more often a set of them are essential to make the correct diagnosis) but also to better define the biological behavior of the tumor (improving the risk stratification of patients) and to identify patients who can benefit of target therapies (drug sensitivity biomarkers).

In particular, investigators of the GENSARC study believe that molecular genetic testing should be routinely performed to improve diagnostic accuracy and appropriate clinical management of sarcomas, even when histological diagnosis is made by pathologist experts in this field.

The importance of biomarkers becomes evident as the reader goes through the second part of this book dedicated to each single soft tissue tumor.

Suggested Readings

Cancer Genome Atlas Research Network (2017) Comprehensive and integrated genomic characterization of adult soft tissue sarcomas. Cell 171(4):950–965

Italiano (2016) Clinical effect of molecular methods in sarcoma diagnosis (GENSARC): a prospective, multicentre, observational study. Lancet Oncol 17(4):532–538

Mertens (2016) Gene fusions in soft tissue tumors: recurrent and overlapping pathogenetic themes. Genes Chromosomes Cancer 55(4):291–310

Miettinen (2019) New fusion sarcomas: histopathology and clinical significance of selected entities. Hum Pathol 86:57–65

Nakano (2018) Translocation-related sarcomas. Int J Mol Sci 19(12):E3784

Oda (2017) Soft tissue sarcomas: from a morphological to a molecular biological approach. Pathol Int 67(9):435–446

Schaefer (2018) Contemporary sarcoma diagnosis, genetics, and genomics. J Clin Oncol 36(2):101–110

Taylor (2011) Advances in sarcoma genomics and new therapeutic targets. Nat Rev Cancer 11(8):541–557

S. Mocellin, *Soft Tissue Tumors*, https://doi.org/10.1007/978-3-030-58710-9_5

Xiao (2018) Advances in chromosomal translocations and fusion genes in sarcomas and potential therapeutic applications. Cancer Treat Rev 63:61–70

Yao (2020) An evidence-based guideline on the application of molecular testing in the diagnosis, prediction of prognosis, and selection of therapy in non-GIST soft tissue sarcomas. Cancer Treat Rev 85:101987

Prognosis

6

Soft tissue tumor prognosis is characterized by a wide variability, ranging from neoplasms completely indolent to those very aggressive. The biological behavior is classified by the WHO into three categories: benign, intermediate (including forms that can locally recur and those at low risk of metastasis), and malignant (which are characterized by high risk of metastasis). Of note, some subtypes of soft tissue tumors classified among benign neoplasms can actually behave as tumors of intermediate malignant potential (e.g., cellular and atypical variants of benign fibrous histiocytoma).

Considering **benign soft tissue tumors**, the overall prognosis is excellent. However, some of these neoplasms can be life-threatening because of their complications (e.g., Kasabach-Merritt syndrome in giant hemangiomas, retroperitoneal hemorrhage from renal angiomyolipoma).

Soft tissue tumors with intermediate malignant potential include forms that can locally recur and those at low risk of metastasis, while **malignant soft tissue tumors** are characterized by high risk of metastasis.

The term "sarcoma" is used for tumors with both intermediate and malignant behavior.

As regards soft tissue sarcomas, some of them may be accompanied by metastasis at presentation, the prognosis being usually dismal. Among patients without metastatic disease at presentation, about 25% will develop distant metastatic disease (after undergoing radical surgery for their primary tumor), a proportion that increases up to 50% in cases with large (>5 cm), deep-seated (underneath the fascia), intermediate-/high-grade tumors.

The lungs are the most frequent site of distant metastasis (up to 80%). Some sarcomas are characterized by metastatic spread also to other sites such as the abdomen (e.g., round cell/myxoid liposarcoma, angiosarcoma, epithelioid sarcoma, and leiomyosarcoma), brain (e.g., angiosarcoma, alveolar soft part sarcoma, and clear cell sarcoma), and spine (spine bones and paraspinal tissues; e.g., round cell/myxoid liposarcoma). Finally, soft tissue sarcomas (unlike carcinomas) rarely involve lymph nodes, though with some exception, such as rhabdomyosarcoma (10–30%),

S. Mocellin, *Soft Tissue Tumors*, https://doi.org/10.1007/978-3-030-58710-9_6

synovial sarcoma (10–20%), clear cell sarcoma (15–40%), epithelioid sarcoma (10–30%), angiosarcoma (5–10%), leiomyosarcoma (3%), and malignant peripheral nerve sheath tumor (3%).

Patient survival depends upon tumor aggressiveness, disease stage, and responsiveness to treatment: therefore, prognosis of patients with sarcoma greatly varies across different tumor types. Overall, median overall survival of patients with metastatic sarcoma is approximately 16 months. In the USA, it is estimated that approximately 5000 deaths are due to soft tissue sarcomas each year.

Soft tissue sarcoma prognosis is stratified based on the American Joint Committee on Cancer (AJCC)/Union for International Cancer Control (UICC) **TNM staging system**. Four separate TNM staging systems have been generated based on tumor anatomic location: (a) TNM for soft tissue sarcomas of the head and neck (→ see Table 6.1); (b) TNM for soft tissue sarcomas of the trunk and extremities (→ see Tables 6.2 and 6.3); (c) TNM for soft tissue sarcomas of the abdomen and thoracic visceral organs (→ see Table 6.4); and (d) TNM for soft tissue sarcomas of the retroperitoneum (→ see Tables 6.5 and 6.6). According to the latest TNM version (eighth edition, published in 2017), the notation about the depth of the tumor (above or below the muscular fascia)—which was previously associated with a worse prognosis in case of deep location—has been eliminated.

Separate TNM staging systems have been proposed for specific soft tissue sarcomas, such as rhabdomyosarcoma and gastrointestinal stromal tumor/GIST (for details → see sections dedicated to rhabdomyosarcoma and GIST in the second part of the book).

Table 6.1 TNM staging for soft tissue sarcomas of head and neck[a]

Primary tumor (T)	
Tx	T cannot be assessed
T1	Tumor ≤2 cm (greatest dimension)
T2	Tumor >2 cm to ≤4 cm (greatest dimension)
T3	Tumor >4 cm (greatest dimension)
T4	Invasion of adjacent structures
T4a	Invasion of orbit, skull base/dura, central compartment viscera, facial skeleton, or pterygoid muscles
T4b	Invasion of brain parenchyma, carotid artery, prevertebral muscles, or central nervous system via perineural spread
Regional lymph nodes (N)	
Nx	Regional lymph nodes cannot be assessed
N0	No regional lymph node metastasis
N1	Presence of regional lymph node metastasis
Distant metastasis (M)	
M0	No distant metastasis
M1	Presence of distant metastasis
Tumor grading (G)	
→ see Table 6.7	

[a]For head and neck soft tissue sarcomas, disease stages (i.e., prognostic groups) are not yet available

Table 6.2 TNM staging for soft tissue sarcomas of trunk and extremities

Primary tumor (T)	
Tx	T cannot be assessed
T1	Tumor ≤5 cm (greatest dimension)
T2	Tumor >5 cm to ≤10 cm (greatest dimension)
T3	Tumor >10 cm to ≤15 cm (greatest dimension)
T4	Tumor >15 cm (greatest dimension)
Regional lymph nodes (N)	
Nx	Regional lymph nodes cannot be assessed
N0	No regional lymph node metastasis
N1	Presence of regional lymph node metastasis
Distant metastasis (M)	
M0	No distant metastasis
M1	Presence of distant metastasis
Tumor grading (G)	
→ see Table 6.7	

Table 6.3 TNM stages for soft tissue sarcomas of trunk and extremities

Stage	T	N	M	G
IA	**T1**	N0	M0	**G1, Gx**
IB	**T2, T3, T4**	N0	M0	**G1, Gx**
II	**T1**	N0	M0	**G2, G3**
IIIA	**T2**	N0	M0	**G2, G3**
IIIB	**T3, T4**	N0	M0	**G2, G3**
IV	Any T	**N1**	M0	Any G
	Any T	Any N	**M1**	Any G

Unlike other cancers, the TNM system for soft tissue sarcomas is characterized by the inclusion of **histological grading** (also known as tumor grade, G), which adopts the system proposed by the Fédération Nationale des Centres de Lutte Contre Le Cancer (French Federation of Cancer Centers, FNCLCC) (→ see Table 6.7). For some soft tissue sarcomas, tumor grade is directly assigned based on the histological type (→ see Table 6.8). This parameter is more associated with the risk of distant metastasis and death rather than with local disease recurrence (which is mainly dictated by histological type and surgical margins); importantly, tumor grading is not recommended for the following sarcomas: malignant peripheral nerve sheath tumor, embryonal rhabdomyosarcoma, alveolar rhabdomyosarcoma, angiosarcoma, extraskeletal myxoid chondrosarcoma, alveolar soft part sarcoma, clear cell sarcoma, and epithelioid sarcoma. Of note, grading cannot be assigned after neoadjuvant (i.e., preoperative) medical treatment.

Finally, other tumor grading systems (e.g., the US National Cancer Institute grading system) have been devised and are variably utilized.

Table 6.4 TNM staging for soft tissue sarcomas of the abdomen and thoracic visceral organs[a]

Primary tumor (T)	
Tx	T cannot be assessed
T1	Tumor confined to the organ of origin
T2	Tumor extends to the tissues beyond the organ of origin
T2a	Tumor infiltrates serosa or visceral peritoneum
T2b	Tumor extends beyond serosa (e.g., mesentery)
T3	Tumor infiltrates another organ
T4	Multifocal tumor involvement
T4a	2 sites
T4b	3–5 sites
T4c	>5 sites
Regional lymph nodes (N)	
Nx	Regional lymph nodes cannot be assessed
N0	No regional lymph node metastasis
N1	Presence of regional lymph node metastasis
Distant metastasis (M)	
M0	No distant metastasis
M1	Presence of distant metastasis
Tumor grading (G)	
→ see Table 6.7	

[a]For soft tissue sarcomas of the abdomen and thoracic visceral organs, disease stages (i.e., prognostic groups) are not yet available

Table 6.5 TNM staging for soft tissue sarcomas of the retroperitoneum

Primary tumor (T)	
Tx	T cannot be assessed
T1	Tumor ≤5 cm (greatest dimension)
T2	Tumor >5 cm to ≤10 cm (greatest dimension)
T3	Tumor >10 cm to ≤15 cm (greatest dimension)
T4	Tumor >15 cm (greatest dimension)
Regional lymph nodes (N)	
Nx	Regional lymph nodes cannot be assessed
N0	No regional lymph node metastasis
N1	Presence of regional lymph node metastasis
Distant metastasis (M)	
M0	No distant metastasis
M1	Presence of distant metastasis
Tumor grading (G)	
→ see Table 6.7	

Table 6.6 TNM stages for soft tissue sarcomas of the retroperitoneum

Stage	T	N	M	G
IA	**T1**	N0	M0	**G1, Gx**
IB	**T2, T3, T4**	N0	M0	**G1, Gx**
II	**T1**	N0	M0	**G2, G3**
IIIA	**T2**	N0	M0	**G2, G3**
IIIB	**T3, T4**	N0	M0	**G2, G3**
	Any T	**N1**	M0	Any G
IV	Any T	Any N	**M1**	Any G

Table 6.7 Histological grading of soft tissue sarcomas (FNCLCC system)

Differentiation score	1	Tumor closely resembling normal tissue of origin
	2	Tumor with certain differentiation
	3	Tumor with uncertain/unknown differentiation
Mitotic score	1	Mitotic count: 0–9 per 10 HPF
	2	Mitotic count: 10–19 per 10 HPF
	3	Mitotic count: 20 or more per 10 HPF
Necrosis score	0	Absent
	1	< 50% tumor necrosis
	2	50% or more tumor necrosis
Sum up the three scores to obtain grading		
Tumor grade	Gx	Grading cannot be assessed
	G1	Total score: 2–3 (low-grade tumor)
	G2	Total score: 4–5 (intermediate-grade tumor)
	G3	Total score: 6–8 (high-grade tumor)

HPF high-power field

Table 6.8 Tumor differentiation score by histologic type

Histologic type	Differentiation score
Well-differentiated liposarcoma	1
Well-differentiated leiomyosarcoma	1
Well-differentiated fibrosarcoma	1
Myxoid liposarcoma	2
Conventional leiomyosarcoma	2
Conventional fibrosarcoma	2
Myxofibrosarcoma	2
Round cell liposarcoma	3
Pleomorphic liposarcoma	3
Dedifferentiated liposarcoma	3
Pleomorphic rhabdomyosarcoma	3
Poorly differentiated/pleomorphic leiomyosarcoma	3
Synovial sarcoma	3
Mesenchymal chondrosarcoma	3
Extraskeletal osteosarcoma	3
Extraskeletal Ewing sarcoma	3
Malignant rhabdoid tumor	3
Undifferentiated pleomorphic sarcoma	3
Undifferentiated sarcoma NOS	3

NOS not otherwise specified

Suggested Readings

AJCC Cancer Staging Manual (8th edn). Springer; 2017

Andreou (2013) Sentinel node biopsy in soft tissue sarcoma subtypes with a high propensity for regional lymphatic spread—results of a large prospective trial. Ann Oncol 24(5):1400–1405

Callegaro (2016) Development and external validation of two nomograms to predict overall survival and occurrence of distant metastases in adults after surgical resection of localized soft tissue sarcomas of the extremities: a retrospective analysis. Lancet Oncol 17:671–678

Coindre (2006) Grading of soft tissue sarcomas: review and update. Arch Pathol Lab Med 130(10):1448–1453

Ecker (2017) Implications of lymph node evaluation in the management of resectable soft tissue sarcoma. Ann Surg Oncol 24(2):425–433

Gold (2009) Development and validation of a prognostic nomogram for recurrence-free survival after complete surgical resection of localised primary gastrointestinal stromal tumour: a retrospective analysis. Lancet Oncol 10(11):1045–1052

Pasquali (2018) High-risk soft tissue sarcomas treated with perioperative chemotherapy: improving prognostic classification in a randomised clinical trial. Eur J Cancer 93:28–36

Siegel (2020) Cancer statistics, 2020. CA Cancer J Clin 70(1):7–30

Therapy

7

Given the rarity and at the same time the multiplicity of nosological entities (each one with its specific biological behavior and therapeutic sensitivity), it is universally accepted that soft tissue tumors should be referred to dedicated centers, where each case can be discussed within the frame of a multidisciplinary tumor board and all the specialists potentially involved in the management of these patients are available (e.g., pathologist, radiologist, surgical oncologist, radiotherapist, medical oncologist, orthopedic, vascular surgeon, urologist, neurosurgeon, molecular biologist). Of note, it has been demonstrated that patients treated within these specialized centers have a better survival (which is at least in part due to lack of adherence to treatment guidelines).

Benign soft tissue tumors may need treatment (mainly surgery) for diagnostic purposes, for relief of compression symptoms, or for cosmetic purposes (as requested by the patient). In contrast, the treatment of soft tissue sarcomas can be quite complex and often requires a multimodality approach: therefore, the rest of this paragraph is dedicated to the general principles of treatment for malignant soft tissue tumors (details on the therapeutic approach specific to each single tumor can be found in the second part of this book).

Surgery

Surgical radical excision remains the mainstay of treatment of all localized primary soft tissue sarcomas. The tumor often forms a pseudocapsule, but marginal resection (generally defined by less than 1 cm of surgical margin) following this anatomical "plane" often poses the patient at risk of local disease relapse due to microscopic disease extensions beyond the pseudocapsule (so-called skip metastases). Therefore, **wide excision** (i.e., removal of the neoplastic mass along with 1–2 cm of healthy margins) is the key principle in the surgical approach to these tumors. Based on the pathological examination of the surgical specimen, resections are classified into R0

S. Mocellin, *Soft Tissue Tumors*, https://doi.org/10.1007/978-3-030-58710-9_7

(microscopically negative margins), R1 (microscopically positive margins), and R2 (macroscopically positive margins).

For **sarcomas of the extremities**, wide excision may sometime require compartmental resection (i.e., removal of an entire group of muscles included in a given fascial compartment), which occurs especially in patients with large tumors: however, currently this type of surgery is utilized much less frequently than in the past.

In the extremities, the other key principle is that surgery should be function-sparing, as long as oncological radicality is guaranteed. In some cases, radical resection is not possible without a mutilating operation, that is, amputation or removal of key structures (e.g., groups of muscles, vessels, nerves) essential for limb viability and/or function. In these patients, neoadjuvant treatments (radiotherapy, chemotherapy, isolated limb perfusion, chemotherapy plus regional hyperthermia) can be utilized to downstage the tumor and possibly allow for less morbid surgery (for more information →see below paragraphs entitled "Radiotherapy" and "Chemotherapy"). Importantly, evidence from a randomized controlled trial showed that amputation (once performed in up to 50% of limb soft tissue sarcomas) is not superior to wide excision (limb-sparing surgery) plus radiotherapy in terms of overall survival (→see Table 7.1): therefore, amputation is nowadays performed rarely (5–20%), when any other types of conservative surgery are unfeasible or have failed (i.e., local disease recurrence has occurred).

In a further attempt to avoid amputation, limb-threatening sarcomas (i.e., tumors candidate for amputation due to infiltration of major neurovascular bundle of the limb, multifocal tumors, or recurrent tumors) can be treated with neoadjuvant isolated limb perfusion (ILP) followed by limb-sparing surgery (often marginal), with high rates of tumor response (≈75%) and limb salvage (≈75%) and local disease control (≈70%) reported in many series. ILP requires the complete vascular isolation of the affected limb (which is connected with an extracorporeal circuit and is generally performed with tumor necrosis factor (TNF) coupled with melphalan); of note, TNF is approved for this use in Europe but not in the USA.

In order to preserve limb function, specialists such as vascular surgeon, plastic surgeon, neurosurgeon, and orthopedic surgeon may be needed for the reconstruction of bones, major vessels and nerves, and soft tissue defects. Finally, as confirmed by a recent meta-analysis, surgery for extremity sarcomas is burdened by non-negligible rates of postoperative wound complication (30%) and reoperation (13%).

As regards **retroperitoneal sarcomas** (which represent about 15% of all soft tissue sarcomas, the most frequent histological subtypes being liposarcoma, leiomyosarcoma, and undifferentiated pleomorphic sarcoma), the optimal extent of surgery has not been evaluated in randomized trials. The anatomic constraints of the retroperitoneum make it difficult to obtain R0 resections, which is why local disease recurrence is a major issue in this group of patients (often leading patient to death despite lack of distant metastatic disease). Based on retrospective data from multiple institutions, there is a quite general consensus on the use of en bloc resection of adherent but not necessarily infiltrated organs (e.g., kidney, ascending or descending colon) in an attempt to improve local disease control.

Table 7.1 Pivotal randomized controlled trials of radiotherapy for soft tissue sarcomas

Author (year)	Disease	Comparison	Setting	Main findings	Notes
Rosemberg (1982)	Limb soft tissue sarcomas (miscellany)	Amputation vs surgery + EBRT	Localized primary tumor (adjuvant EBRT)	Overall survival: no difference	Local disease control (limb-sparing arm): 85%
Yang (1998)	Limb soft tissue sarcomas (miscellany)	Surgery + EBRT vs surgery alone	Localized primary tumor (adjuvant EBRT)	Local recurrence rate: improved by EBRT	No difference in overall survival
O'Sullivan (2002)	Limb soft tissue sarcomas (miscellany)	Adjuvant vs neoadjuvant EBRT (plus surgery)	Localized primary tumor (adjuvant/ neoadjuvant EBRT)	Higher rate of postoperative complications in neoadjuvant arm	Higher rates of late toxicities (e.g., fibrosis, joint stiffness) after postoperative EBRT
Pisters (1996)	Limb soft tissue sarcomas (miscellany)	Surgery + BRT vs surgery alone	Localized primary tumor (adjuvant BRT)	Local recurrence rate: improved by EBRT only in high-grade tumors	No difference in overall survival
Reed (2008)	Uterine sarcomas (miscellany)	Surgery + EBRT vs surgery alone	Localized primary tumor (adjuvant EBRT)	EBRT did not improve either overall or disease-free survival	Leiomyosarcomas, carcinosarcomas, and endometrial stromal sarcomas
Bonvalot (2019)	Retroperitoneal sarcomas (miscellany)	Surgery + EBRT vs surgery alone	Resectable primary tumor (neoadjuvant EBRT)	EBRT did not improve local disease control	The liposarcoma subgroup benefited from EBRT

EBRT external beam radiotherapy, *BRT* brachytherapy

Sarcomas of the thoraco-abdominal wall are generally treated with the same principles utilized for extremity sarcomas. Their wide excision may require the use of prosthetic devices as well as plastic surgery techniques in order to reconstruct the wall itself.

In general, the expertise of specialists such as plastic surgeon, vascular surgeon, orthopedic, urologist, and thoracic surgeon is required for reconstruction after surgical demolition leading to large soft tissue defects or involving large vessels, bones, bladder, or thoracic wall.

Given the low rate of spread to regional lymph nodes, prophylactic lymphadenectomy (i.e., lymph node dissection in the absence of clinically/radiologically/cytologically proven metastasis) is never indicated; radical lymphadenectomy is restricted to patients with pathologically proven metastasis. The role of sentinel node biopsy (SNB) for the staging of sarcomas with a non-negligible rate of lymph node metastasis (e.g., rhabdomyosarcoma, synovial sarcoma, clear cell sarcoma, angiosarcoma, and epithelioid sarcoma) is still debated; nevertheless, SNB is a recommended procedure for rhabdomyosarcoma (especially when located in the limbs).

In case of marginal, R1, or R2 resection, redo surgery should be the first option, whenever technically feasible (i.e., without compromising function). Adjuvant therapies should be considered when redo surgery is not performed. Mutilating surgery should be restricted to a minimum number of cases where other options are technically unfeasible or have failed. Neoadjuvant therapies should be considered when R1–R2 resection is preoperatively anticipated.

As regards local disease relapse, surgery remains the treatment of choice (when feasible): in this setting, neoadjuvant or adjuvant therapies are intensively utilized.

As regards metastatic disease, surgery should be considered for the treatment of metachronous (disease-free interval > 1 year) resectable metastatic disease (usually in the lungs); the preoperative workup should define that metastatic disease is confined to a single organ (e.g., lungs). The role of neoadjuvant and adjuvant chemotherapy in these cases is unknown. For synchronous metastasis, chemotherapy should be considered first, and then surgery might be suggested on possible residual disease (if all disease can be removed).

Finally, surgery may play a role in the palliative setting, often in combination with other therapeutic modalities.

Radiotherapy

For details on pivotal randomized controlled trials of radiotherapy, →see below Table 7.1. Information on the role of radiotherapy in specific sarcomas is reported in the second part of this book dedicated to each single tumor type.

As regards **sarcomas of the extremities**, adjuvant or neoadjuvant radiotherapy (external beam radiotherapy, EBRT, or brachytherapy, BRT) is considered for high-risk tumors, that is, high-grade (G2–G3), deep, large (>5 cm) lesions; an exception might be that of neoplasms confined to a muscular compartment and treated with a compartmental resection. Superficial or small tumors may be treated with radiotherapy based on a multidisciplinary discussion. Another indication for (adjuvant) radiotherapy is a marginal R0 or incomplete (R1–R2) resection that cannot be treated with redo surgery. It is well accepted that select tumors with favorable features (<5 cm and/or low grade) are best treated with radical surgery alone.

As regards the comparison between **EBRT** and **BRT**, no formal randomized trial is available. The advantages of BRT are the targeted dose distribution, low integral dose, and short treatment times.

As regards the comparison between **adjuvant** and **neoadjuvant radiotherapy**, local control and survival are not clinically significantly affected by treatment timing. If wound complications are foreseen to be severe, surgery followed by adjuvant radiotherapy is likely the best option; on the other side, if it is anticipated that wound complications will be manageable, neoadjuvant radiotherapy should be considered. The choice of radiotherapy timing should take into consideration also the issues linked to the need for a plastic reconstruction (e.g., skin grafts are generally damaged by postoperative radiotherapy to a larger extent as compared to cutaneous/muscular-cutaneous flaps): of note, a consensus on the best management is still lacking. With modern radiotherapy techniques (e.g., image-guided radiotherapy and intensity-modulated radiotherapy), the incidence of wound complications after preoperative radiotherapy has been reported to be lower than historically published incidence rates. The main advantage of preoperative radiotherapy is the lower rate of late morbidity (e.g., fibrosis, bone fracture): in fact, while the early wound healing complications observed with preoperative radiotherapy are usually recoverable, the late effects associated with postoperative radiotherapy are more likely to be irreversible. Another advantage of the neoadjuvant approach includes a more limited treatment volume (due to the presence of the tumor, which allows for a more targeted treatment). On the other side, postoperative radiotherapy provides physicians with important pathological considerations on the surgical specimen (such as microscopic margin status and histological tumor grading) that are unavailable with the neoadjuvant approach.

As regards **retroperitoneal sarcomas**, although some non-randomized studies reported some benefit from neoadjuvant radiotherapy, a recent randomized controlled trial (STRASS) has found no advantage in terms of local disease control in the whole cohort of patients (although a subgroup analysis has shown a benefit in patients with liposarcoma).

As regards **thoraco-abdominal wall sarcomas**, they are generally treated with the same principles utilized for extremity sarcomas.

The role of other radiotherapy modalities such as intraoperative radiation therapy (IORT) in the management of soft tissue sarcomas is being evaluated.

As regards **visceral sarcomas**, the only randomized controlled trial so far conducted regards adjuvant radiotherapy for the management of uterine sarcomas, its findings being negative.

Stereotactic body radiation therapy (SBRT) is being explored for the treatment of oligometastatic disease (as an alternative to surgery).

Radiotherapy can also be used as **definitive treatment** for tumors that are not surgically resectable (this is particularly true for Ewing sarcoma and rhabdomyosarcoma), although these cases are associated with poorer outcomes as compared to resectable sarcomas. As for other malignancies, radiotherapy can be utilized also in the **palliative setting**.

Finally, the use of radioenhancers (e.g., NBTXR3) is being tested in the clinical setting to improve the therapeutic effects of radiation therapy for sarcomas, as recently reported.

As regards **tumor response** to medical treatments, it is important to note that—unlike other malignancies—neoadjuvant radiotherapy and/or chemotherapy do not usually lead to soft tissue sarcoma shrinkage (with some exceptions such as myxoid liposarcoma and GIST); in contrast, up to 30% of sarcomas increase in size by more than 10% (especially within the first 4 weeks after neoadjuvant radiotherapy), although this is not associated with worse survival outcomes. In addition, there is no correlation between Response Evaluation Criteria in Solid Tumors (RECIST) and outcome measures: in fact, some sarcomas can show significant reductions in size despite the presence of predominantly viable tumor, whereas stable or growing tumors can show remarkable histopathological response. Reduction in contrast enhancement on magnetic resonance imaging and decreased fluorodeoxyglucose uptake on positron emission tomography are being evaluated as surrogates of tumor response, but no consensus is still available.

As opposed to radiological imaging, histological response (i.e., **tumor necrosis**), especially when equal or greater than 90% (although it is unclear if the same cutoff can be used across the many different histological subtypes of sarcomas), has been significantly associated with improved survival outcomes. To this aim, the European Organization for Research and Treatment of Cancer-Soft Tissue and Bone Sarcoma Group (EORTC-STBSG) has proposed the following classification of tumor response to neoadjuvant radiotherapy and/or chemotherapy: (a) no stainable tumor cells; (b) single stainable tumor cells or small clusters (overall below 1% of the whole specimen); (c) ≥ 1 to <10% stainable tumor cells; (d) ≥ 10 to <50% stainable tumor cells; and (e) $\geq 50\%$ stainable tumor cells.

Chemotherapy

For details of pivotal randomized controlled trials of chemotherapy, →see below Table 7.2. Chemosensitivity varies greatly across different sarcoma types; for example, rhabdomyosarcoma, Ewing sarcoma, and myxoid liposarcoma are highly chemosensitive, whereas most of the other sarcomas are either moderately or poorly chemosensitive. The following is a general description of the principles guiding chemotherapy for patients with sarcomas. Details on the role of chemotherapy in specific sarcomas are reported in the second part of this book dedicated to each single tumor type.

As regards the management of **limb and trunk soft tissue sarcomas**, the role of **adjuvant chemotherapy** (i.e., after radical surgery) is debated. In brief, a meta-analysis of randomized controlled trials published in 2008 and including 1747 patients showed a significant but small absolute risk reduction (6%) in terms of overall survival, most included studies utilizing multi-agent chemotherapy; when weighed against the toxicity of combination chemotherapy, the marginal survival improvement appeared insufficient to shift practice toward routine administration. In addition, the latest randomized controlled trial of adjuvant chemotherapy (run by the EORTC and published in 2012) failed to demonstrate a significant difference in either disease-free survival or overall survival. In the light of the conflicting available evidence, adjuvant chemotherapy is not the standard treatment in adults; however, it can be proposed (within the frame of a multidisciplinary discussion) as a therapeutic option for high-risk patients (high-grade, deep, >5 cm tumor). According to the ARST0332 study, a similar approach is recommended also for patients younger than 30 years and affected with non-rhabdomyosarcoma soft tissue sarcomas.

Mainly based on the results of two randomized controlled trials (one comparing neoadjuvant vs neoadjuvant + adjuvant chemotherapy; the other comparing

Table 7.2 Pivotal randomized controlled trials of chemotherapy for soft tissue sarcomas

Author (year)	Disease	Comparison	Setting	Main findings	Notes
Frustaci (2001)	Limb soft tissue sarcomas (high risk)	Surgery + chemotherapy vs surgery alone	Adjuvant	Chemotherapy improved both overall and disease-free survival	Chemotherapy: epirubicin + ifosfamide
Woll (2012)	Limb, trunk, and H&N soft tissue sarcomas (high risk)	Surgery + chemotherapy vs surgery alone	Adjuvant	Chemotherapy did not improve either overall or disease-free survival	Chemotherapy: doxorubicin + ifosfamide
Gronchi (2012)	Limb and trunk soft tissue sarcomas (high risk)	Neoadjuvant chemotherapy vs adjuvant + neoadjuvant chemotherapy (plus surgery)	Neoadjuvant/ Adjuvant	No overall survival difference	Chemotherapy: epirubicin + ifosfamide
Gronchi (2017)	Limb and trunk soft tissue sarcomas (high risk)	Conventional vs histology-tailored[a] chemotherapy (plus surgery)	Neoadjuvant	Conventional chemotherapy improved disease-free survival	Conventional chemotherapy: epirubicin + ifosfamide
Issels (2018)	Limb and trunk soft tissue sarcomas (high risk)	Chemotherapy + hyperthermia vs chemotherapy alone (plus surgery)	Neoadjuvant	Chemotherapy + hyperthermia improved overall and disease-free survival	Chemotherapy: doxorubicin + ifosfamide + etoposide
Gortzak (2001)	Limb and trunk soft tissue sarcomas (high risk)	Neoadjuvant chemotherapy + surgery vs surgery alone (radiotherapy was allowed)	Neoadjuvant	Neoadjuvant chemotherapy did not improve either overall or disease-free survival	Chemotherapy: doxorubicin + ifosfamide
Seddon (2017)	Soft tissue sarcomas (miscellany)	Doxorubicin vs gemcitabine + docetaxel	Metastatic (first line)	No difference in progression-free survival	–

(continued)

Table 7.2 (continued)

Author (year)	Disease	Comparison	Setting	Main findings	Notes
Tap (2017)	Soft tissue sarcomas (miscellany)	Doxorubicin vs doxorubicin + evofosfamide	Metastatic (first line)	No difference in overall survival	More adverse effects in the combo arm
Judson (2014)	Soft tissue sarcomas (miscellany)	Doxorubicin vs doxorubicin plus ifosfamide	Metastatic (first line)	No difference in overall survival	Higher response rate and toxicity rate in the combo arm
Ryan (2016)	Soft tissue sarcomas (miscellany)	Doxorubicin vs doxorubicin + palifosfamide	Metastatic (first line)	No difference in overall or progression-free survival	Palifosfamide: active metabolite of ifosfamide thus no generation of toxic metabolites
Bonvalot (2005)	Peritoneal sarcomatosis	Intraperitoneal chemotherapy + surgery vs surgery alone	Metastatic	No difference in local relapse-free, metastatic relapse-free, or overall survival	From both retroperitoneal and visceral sarcomas
Tap (2019)	Soft tissue sarcomas (miscellany)	Doxorubicin + olaratumab vs doxorubicin	Metastatic (first line)	No overall survival difference	Olaratumab: monoclonal antibody blocking the platelet-derived growth factor receptor alpha (PDGFRA)
Demetri (2016)	Liposarcoma or leiomyosarcoma	Trabectedin vs dacarbazine	Metastatic (second line)	Trabectedin improved progression-free survival	No overall survival benefit
Schöffski (2016)	Liposarcoma or leiomyosarcoma	Eribulin vs dacarbazine	Metastatic (second line)	Eribulin improved overall survival but not progression-free survival	Subgroup analysis: benefit only for liposarcoma (both overall and progression-free survival)

[a]Histology-tailored chemotherapy: trabectedin (myxoid liposarcoma), gemcitabine + dacarbazine (leiomyosarcoma), etoposide + ifosfamide (malignant peripheral nerve sheath tumor), ifosfamide (synovial sarcoma), gemcitabine + docetaxel (undifferentiated pleomorphic sarcoma)

neoadjuvant standard vs neoadjuvant histology-tailored chemotherapy), **neoadjuvant chemotherapy** is currently considered an option for patients with high-risk tumors (high-grade, large and deep lesions). This type of chemotherapy can be combined with neoadjuvant/adjuvant radiotherapy, which might improve survival according to evidence from non-randomized studies. According to a randomized controlled trial, the addition of regional hyperthermia to neoadjuvant chemotherapy improves patient survival.

The role of neoadjuvant/adjuvant chemotherapy for the management of patients with visceral and retroperitoneal sarcomas is basically unknown (with the exception of gastrointestinal stromal tumor, →see dedicated section in the second part of the book).

In the **locally advanced and metastatic setting**, systemic chemotherapy represents the first option, although the results are often unsatisfactory (with wide variation depending on histological types). Standard first-line chemotherapy is based on anthracyclines (i.e., doxorubicin, epirubicin). Combination regimens (generally with ifosfamide) are not superior to single-agent chemotherapy (with anthracycline) in terms of survival and are associated with higher toxicity rates, although a higher tumor response rate is observed (which may be useful in cases where tumor response is believed to play an important role in patient quality of life). Furthermore, attempts to improve survival rates using drugs other than anthracyclines (e.g., gemcitabine + docetaxel) have failed.

Based on evidence from non-randomized trials, the use of histology-specific chemotherapy agents has been advocated, such as trabectedin for myxoid liposarcoma, gemcitabine plus dacarbazine for leiomyosarcoma, etoposide plus ifosfamide for malignant peripheral nerve sheath tumor, ifosfamide for synovial sarcoma, and gemcitabine plus docetaxel for undifferentiated pleomorphic sarcoma. However, the results of a randomized controlled trial (ISG-STS 1001) of neoadjuvant histology-tailored chemotherapy versus conventional regimen (epirubicin + ifosfamide) have shown that survival is better in patients undergoing the latter treatment, which has tempered the enthusiasm surrounding this approach.

The addition of intraperitoneal chemotherapy (also known as early postoperative intraperitoneal chemotherapy, EPIC) to cytoreductive surgery for the treatment of peritoneal sarcomatosis has provided no survival advantage in a small randomized controlled trial. As regards hyperthermic intraperitoneal chemotherapy (HIPEC), no evidence from randomized trials is available, and its use (advocated by some investigators for sarcomas with remarkable tropism for the peritoneal surface such as desmoplastic small round cell tumor) should still be considered investigational.

As regards **second-line chemotherapy**, drugs such as ifosfamide, dacarbazine, gemcitabine, and taxanes can be utilized to treat this unfortunate subgroup of patients. More recently, trabectedin has been approved for the treatment of patients with unresectable or metastatic liposarcoma or leiomyosarcoma who received a prior anthracycline-containing regimen. Analogously, eribulin has been approved for the treatment of patients with unresectable or metastatic liposarcoma who received a prior anthracycline-containing regimen. According to a meta-analysis, second-line therapy reduces the risk of disease progression (hazard ratio = 0.51,

95% CI 0.34–0.76), although this translates into a modest absolute benefit in terms of overall (3.3 months) and progression-free (1.6 months) survival.

According to the METASARC observational study of patients with metastatic sarcomas, the role of third-line chemotherapy is limited, with the possible exception of patients with leiomyosarcoma; in particular, after failure of the second-line therapy, best supportive care should be considered, particularly in patients with non-leiomyosarcoma histology who are not eligible to participate in a clinical trial.

Chemotherapy regimens for chemosensitive sarcomas most frequently encountered in childhood such as rhabdomyosarcoma and Ewing sarcoma are discussed in the second part of this book (→see sections dedicated to each single sarcoma).

Target Therapy

The National Cancer Institute defines target therapy as the use of "drugs or other substances that block the growth and spread of cancer by interfering with specific molecules (i.e., molecular targets) that are involved in the growth, progression, and spread of cancer."

As the molecular mechanisms underlying the pathogenesis of sarcomas are elucidated, target therapy is gaining more importance in the armamentarium against these malignancies. The most striking example is that of gastrointestinal stromal tumor (GIST), where target therapy (including imatinib as well as other small molecule tyrosine kinase inhibitors) has revolutionized the management of these neoplasm both in the early and advanced disease(for details, →see the dedicated section in the second part of this book).

Another example of successful implementation of target therapy in the treatment of these tumors is pazopanib, an orally available, multitargeted, tyrosine kinase inhibitor originally approved for the treatment of renal cell carcinoma and then (based on the randomized controlled trial PALETTE) approved also for the treatment of advanced/metastatic soft tissue sarcomas in patients who underwent prior chemotherapy (excluding those with liposarcoma and GIST).

Regorafenib is also an orally available, multitargeted, tyrosine kinase inhibitor and is approved for the treatment of GIST (as well as chemotherapy-refractory advanced colorectal cancer). In a phase II randomized controlled trial (REGOSARC), investigators found that regorafenib improves progression-free survival of patients with soft tissue sarcomas (excluding liposarcoma) previously treated with anthracyclines.

Despite these and other advances (for further information, →see sections dedicated to each single sarcoma in the second part of the book), the way to a larger utilization of target therapy is highly challenging and is paved by multiple failures. Due to the objective difficulty of conducting randomized controlled trials for such rare diseases, other compounds are being considered for clinical use simply based on the favorable results observed in phase II studies (e.g., NTRK inhibitors larotrectinib and entrectinib), as described in the second part of this book.

Importantly, target therapy is revolutionizing the classical histology-based approach to drug choice: in fact, histologically different tumors may share the same pathogenic molecular derangements, which makes them potentially sensitive to the same drug targeting that specific alteration. This approach is fostering the conduction of basket trials recruiting patients with different tumor types characterized by common genetic alterations. Overall, the use of molecular tests to identify both therapeutic targets and biomarkers of drug sensitivity/resistance or prognostic significance is the basis for so-called personalized medicine or precision oncology or theragnostics.

Following these principles, most investigators suggest that patients with sarcoma (especially those with advanced/metastatic disease) should be routinely get molecular profiling of their tumor (possibly using high-throughput technologies such as next-generation sequencing, NGS), which would yield two results: to increase our knowledge on the molecular alterations underlying the pathogenesis of this heterogeneous group of malignancies (mid-/long-term aim) and to identify molecular targets for therapeutic purposes (short-term aim). Available findings on this subject are still conflicting, as the rate of druggable alterations appears to be low.

Finally, attempts are being made to combine the efficacy of chemotherapy and target therapy, although the results so far appear disappointing. Considering randomized controlled trials, the use of mTOR inhibitor ridaforolimus as maintenance treatment (after benefit from prior chemotherapy) in patients with metastatic sarcomas has led to a statistically significant (but clinically modest) improvement in progression-free survival but failed to ameliorate overall survival. Analogously, olaratumab (a monoclonal antibody blocking the platelet-derived growth factor receptor alpha, PDGFRA) was initially approved in combination with doxorubicin for the treatment of metastatic soft tissue sarcomas (based on the findings of a phase II trial), but the findings of a recent phase III randomized controlled trial (ANNOUNCE) have then confuted the previous data (and now this combination is no longer recommended in international guidelines).

Immunotherapy

Immunotherapy is revolutionizing the treatment of multiple cancer types (both in the metastatic and adjuvant setting), especially after the clinical implementation of monoclonal antibodies (e.g., pembrolizumab, nivolumab) that block immune checkpoint molecules (e.g., PD1).

As regards soft tissue sarcomas, the experience with immunotherapy is still in its infancy. Some antitumor activity of clinical relevance has been described in undifferentiated pleomorphic sarcoma and (though to a lesser degree) liposarcoma (SARC028 study), while for other sarcoma types, the evidence is basically anecdotal.

Attempts to combine different immunotherapy drugs or immunotherapy with target therapy are ongoing.

According to the scarcity of data, the role of biomarkers of immunotherapy responsiveness (e.g., PD1 expression, tumor mutational burden, B cells) is still under investigation.

Suggested Readings

Albertsmeier (2018) External beam radiation therapy for resectable soft tissue sarcoma: a systematic review and meta-analysis. Ann Surg Oncol 25(3):754–767

Andreou (2013) Sentinel node biopsy in soft tissue sarcoma subtypes with a high propensity for regional lymphatic spread—results of a large prospective trial. Ann Oncol 24(5):1400–1405

Assi (2019) Neoadjuvant isolated limb perfusion in newly diagnosed untreated patients with locally advanced soft tissue sarcomas of the extremities: the Gustave Roussy experience. Clin Transl Oncol 21(9):1135–1141

Ayodele (2020) Immunotherapy in soft-tissue sarcoma. Curr Oncol 27(Suppl 1):17–23

Baumann (2016) Efficacy and safety of stereotactic body radiation therapy for the treatment of pulmonary metastases from sarcoma: a potential alternative to resection. J Surg Oncol 114(1):65–69

Blay (2017) Improved survival using specialized multidisciplinary board in sarcoma patients. Ann Oncol 28(11):2852–2859

Blay (2019) Surgery in reference centers improves survival of sarcoma patients: a nationwide study. Ann Oncol 30(7):1143–1153

Bonvalot (2005) Randomized trial of cytoreduction followed by intraperitoneal chemotherapy versus cytoreduction alone in patients with peritoneal sarcomatosis. Eur J Surg Oncol 31(8):917–923

Bonvalot (2019a) STRASS (EORTC 62092): a phase III randomized study of preoperative radiotherapy plus surgery versus surgery alone for patients with retroperitoneal sarcoma. J Clin Oncol 37(15_suppl):11001

Bonvalot (2019b) NBTXR3, a first-in-class radioenhancer hafnium oxide nanoparticle, plus radiotherapy versus radiotherapy alone in patients with locally advanced soft-tissue sarcoma (Act.In.Sarc): a multicentre, phase 2-3, randomised, controlled trial. Lancet Oncol 20(8):1148–1159

Casali (2018) Soft tissue and visceral sarcomas: ESMO-EURACAN clinical practice guidelines for diagnosis, treatment and follow-up. Ann Oncol 29(Suppl 4):iv51–iv67

Chen (2020) Genomic-guided precision therapy for soft tissue sarcoma. ESMO Open 5(2):e000626

Chowdhary (2019) Does the addition of chemotherapy to neoadjuvant radiotherapy impact survival in high-risk extremity/trunk soft-tissue sarcoma? Cancer 125(21):3801–3809

Chudgar (2017a) Is repeat pulmonary metastasectomy indicated for soft tissue sarcoma? Ann Thorac Surg 104(6):1837–1845

Chudgar (2017b) Pulmonary metastasectomy with therapeutic intent for soft-tissue sarcoma. J Thorac Cardiovasc Surg 154(1):319–330

Comandone (2017) Salvage therapy in advanced adult soft tissue sarcoma: a systematic review and meta-analysis of randomized trials. Oncologist 22(12):1518–1527

D'Angelo (2018) Nivolumab with or without ipilimumab treatment for metastatic sarcoma (Alliance A091401): two open-label, non-comparative, randomised, phase 2 trials. Lancet Oncol 19:416–446

Dangoor (2016) UK guidelines for the management of soft tissue sarcomas. Clin Sarcoma Res 6:20. eCollection 2016

Dei Tos (2020) Evolution in the management of soft tissue sarcoma: classification, surgery and use of radiotherapy. Expert Rev Anticancer Ther 20(suppl 1):3–13

Demetri (2013) Results of an international randomized phase III trial of the mammalian target of rapamycin inhibitor ridaforolimus versus placebo to control metastatic sarcomas in patients after benefit from prior chemotherapy. J Clin Oncol 31(19):2485–2492

Demetri (2016) Efficacy and safety of trabectedin or dacarbazine for metastatic liposarcoma or leiomyosarcoma after failure of conventional chemotherapy: results of a phase III randomized multicenter clinical trial. J Clin Oncol 34(8):786–793

Drilon (2018) Efficacy of larotrectinib in TRK fusion–positive cancers in adults and children. N Engl J Med 378(8):731–739

Frustaci (2001) Adjuvant chemotherapy for adult soft tissue sarcomas of the extremities and girdles: results of the Italian randomized cooperative trial. J Clin Oncol 19(5):1238–1247

Gamboa (2020) Soft-tissue sarcoma in adults: an update on the current state of histiotype-specific management in an era of personalized medicine. CA Cancer J Clin 70(3):200–229

George (2019) Developments in systemic therapy for soft tissue and bone sarcomas. J Natl Compr Cancer Netw 17(5.5):625–628

Gortzak (2001) A randomised phase II study on neo-adjuvant chemotherapy for 'high-risk' adult soft-tissue sarcoma. Eur J Cancer 37(9):1096–1103

Gronchi (2012) Short, full-dose adjuvant chemotherapy in high-risk adult soft tissue sarcomas: a randomized clinical trial from the Italian Sarcoma Group and the Spanish Sarcoma Group. J Clin Oncol 30(8):850–856

Gronchi (2017) Histotype-tailored neoadjuvant chemotherapy versus standard chemotherapy in patients with high-risk soft-tissue sarcomas (ISG-STS 1001): an international, open-label, randomised, controlled, phase 3, multicentre trial. Lancet Oncol 18(6):812–822

Issels (2018) Effect of neoadjuvant chemotherapy plus regional hyperthermia on long-term outcomes among patients with localized high-risk soft tissue sarcoma: the EORTC 62961-ESHO 95 randomized clinical trial. JAMA Oncol 4(4):483–492

Judson (2014) Doxorubicin alone versus intensified doxorubicin plus ifosfamide for first-line treatment of advanced or metastatic soft-tissue sarcoma: a randomised controlled phase 3 trial. Lancet Oncol 15(4):415–423

Kadle (2019) Flap reconstruction of sarcoma defects in the setting of neoadjuvant and adjuvant radiation. J Reconstr Microsurg 35(4):287–293

Kelly (2020) Objective response rate among patients with locally advanced or metastatic sarcoma treated with talimogene laherparepvec in combination with pembrolizumab: a phase 2 clinical trial. JAMA Oncol 6(3):402–408

Keung (2018) Defining the incidence and clinical significance of lymph node metastasis in soft tissue sarcoma. Eur J Surg Oncol 44(1):170–177

Le Cesne (2014) Doxorubicin-based adjuvant chemotherapy in soft tissue sarcoma: pooled analysis of two STBSG-EORTC phase III clinical trials. Ann Oncol 25(12):2425–2432

Loi (2018) Stereotactic body radiotherapy for oligometastatic soft tissue sarcoma. Radiol Med 123(11):871–878

MacNeill (2017) Randomized controlled trials in soft tissue sarcoma: we are getting there! Surg Oncol Clin N Am 26(4):531–544

Mahmoud (2017) Overall survival advantage of chemotherapy and radiotherapy in the perioperative management of large extremity and trunk soft tissue sarcoma; a large database analysis. Radiother Oncol 124(2):277–284

Mir (2016) Safety and efficacy of regorafenib in patients with advanced soft tissue sarcoma (REGOSARC): a randomised, double-blind, placebo-controlled, phase 2 trial. Lancet Oncol 17(12):1732–1742

Nakano (2018) Current molecular targeted therapies for bone and soft tissue sarcomas. Int J Mol Sci 19(3):E739

Nakano (2020) Precision medicine in soft tissue sarcoma treatment. Cancers (Basel) 12(1):221

Neuwirth (2017) Isolated limb perfusion and infusion for extremity soft tissue sarcoma: a contemporary systematic review and meta-analysis. Ann Surg Oncol 24(13):3803–3810

O'Sullivan (2002) Preoperative versus postoperative radiotherapy in soft-tissue sarcoma of the limbs: a randomised trial. Lancet 359(9325):2235–2241

Osgood (2017) FDA approval summary: eribulin for patients with unresectable or metastatic liposarcoma who have received a prior anthracycline-containing regimen. Clin Cancer Res 23(21):6384–6389

Pang (2016) Contemporary therapy for advanced soft-tissue sarcomas in adults: a review. JAMA Oncol 2(7):941–947

Patel (2019) Overall survival and histology-specific subgroup analyses from a phase 3, randomized controlled study of trabectedin or dacarbazine in patients with advanced liposarcoma or leiomyosarcoma. Cancer 125(15):2610–2620

Pervaiz (2008) A systematic meta-analysis of randomized controlled trials of adjuvant chemotherapy for localized resectable soft-tissue sarcoma. Cancer 113(3):573–581

Petitprez (2020) B cells are associated with survival and immunotherapy response in sarcoma. Nature 577(7791):556–560

Pisters (1996) Long-term results of a prospective randomized trial of adjuvant brachytherapy in soft tissue sarcoma. J Clin Oncol 14(3):859–868

Pisters (2007) Long-term results of prospective trial of surgery alone with selective use of radiation for patients with T1 extremity and trunk soft tissue sarcomas. Ann Surg 246(4):675–681

Pollack (2018) Emerging targeted and immune-based therapies in sarcoma. J Clin Oncol 36(2):125–135

Quiroga (2020) Activity of PD1 inhibitor therapy in advanced sarcoma: a single-center retrospective analysis. BMC Cancer 20(1):527

Reed (2008) Phase III randomised study to evaluate the role of adjuvant pelvic radiotherapy in the treatment of uterine sarcomas stages I and II: an European Organisation for Research and Treatment of Cancer Gynaecological Cancer Group Study (protocol 55874). Eur J Cancer 44(6):808–818

Rehmani (2020) Adjuvant radiation therapy for thoracic soft tissue sarcomas: a population-based analysis. Ann Thorac Surg 109(1):203–210

Roeder (2017) Intraoperative radiation therapy (IORT) in soft-tissue sarcoma. Radiat Oncol 12(1):20

Rosenberg (1982) The treatment of soft-tissue sarcomas of the extremities: prospective randomized evaluations of limb-sparing surgery plus radiation therapy compared with amputation and the role of adjuvant chemotherapy. Ann Surg 196(3):305–315

Rosenthal (2020) Nodal metastases of soft tissue sarcomas: risk factors, imaging findings, and implications. Skeletal Radiol 49(2):221–229

Rossi (2013). Adherence to treatment guidelines for primary sarcomas affects patient survival: a side study of the European CONnective TIssue CAncer NETwork (CONTICANET). Ann Oncol 2013;24(6):1685-1691

Ryan (2016) PICASSO III: a phase III, placebo-controlled study of doxorubicin with or without palifosfamide in patients with metastatic soft tissue sarcoma. J Clin Oncol 34(32):3898–3905

Salah (2018) Tumor necrosis and clinical outcomes following neoadjuvant therapy in soft tissue sarcoma: a systematic review and meta-analysis. Cancer Treat Rev 69:1–10

Savina (2017) Patterns of care and outcomes of patients with METAstatic soft tissue SARComa in a real-life setting: the METASARC observational study. BMC Med 15(1):78

Schöffski (2016) Eribulin versus dacarbazine in previously treated patients with advanced liposarcoma or leiomyosarcoma: a randomised, open-label, multicentre, phase 3 trial. Lancet 387(10028):1629–1637

Seddon (2017) Gemcitabine and docetaxel versus doxorubicin as first-line treatment in previously untreated advanced unresectable or metastatic soft-tissue sarcomas (GeDDiS): a randomised controlled phase 3 trial. Lancet Oncol 18(10):1397–1410

Slump (2019) Risk factors for postoperative wound complications after extremity soft tissue sarcoma resection: a systematic review and meta-analyses. J Plast Reconstr Aesthet Surg 72(9):1449–1464

Smrke (2020) Update on systemic therapy for advanced soft-tissue sarcoma. Curr Oncol 27(Suppl 1):25–33

Spunt (2020) A risk-based treatment strategy for non-rhabdomyosarcoma soft-tissue sarcomas in patients younger than 30 years (ARST0332): a Children's Oncology Group prospective study. Lancet Oncol 21(1):145–161

Subbiah (2018) Multimodality treatment of desmoplastic small round cell tumor: chemotherapy and complete cytoreductive surgery improve patient survival. Clin Cancer Res 24(19):4865–4873

Tap (2017) Doxorubicin plus evofosfamide versus doxorubicin alone in locally advanced, unresectable or metastatic soft-tissue sarcoma (TH CR-406/SARC021): an international, multicentre, open-label, randomised phase 3 trial. Lancet Oncol 18(8):1089–1103

Tap (2019) ANNOUNCE: a randomized, placebo (PBO)-controlled, double-blind, phase (Ph) III trial of doxorubicin (dox) + olaratumab versus dox + PBO in patients (pts) with advanced soft tissue sarcomas (STS). J Clin Oncol 37(18_suppl):LBA3

Tawbi (2017) Pembrolizumab in advanced soft-tissue sarcoma and bone sarcoma (sarc028): a multicentre, two-cohort, single-arm, open-label, phase 2 trial. Lancet Oncol 18:1493–1501

Trédan (2019) Molecular screening program to select molecular-based recommended therapies for metastatic cancer patients: analysis from the ProfiLER trial. Ann Oncol 30(5):757–765

van der Graaf Winette (2012) Pazopanib for metastatic soft-tissue sarcoma (PALETTE): a randomised, double-blind, placebo-controlled phase 3 trial. Lancet 379:1879–1886

van Houdt (2017) Treatment of retroperitoneal sarcoma: current standards and new developments. Curr Opin Oncol 29(4):260–267

Vieira (2020) Response to anti-PD1 immunotherapy in patients with metastatic cutaneous sarcoma: case reports and literature review. Oxf Med Case Reports 2020(1):omz138

von Mehren (2018) Soft tissue sarcoma, version 2.2018, NCCN clinical practice guidelines in oncology. J Natl Compr Cancer Netw 16(5):536–563

Voss (2017) Adherence to national comprehensive cancer network guidelines is associated with improved survival for patients with stage 2A and stages 2B and 3 extremity and superficial trunk soft tissue sarcoma. Ann Surg Oncol 24(11):3271–3278

Wagner (2017) Detection of lymph node metastases in pediatric and adolescent/young adult sarcoma: sentinel lymph node biopsy versus fludeoxyglucose positron emission tomography imaging-A prospective trial. Cancer 123(1):155–160

Wang (2015) Significant reduction of late toxicities in patients with extremity sarcoma treated with image-guided radiation therapy to a reduced target volume: results of Radiation Therapy Oncology Group RTOG-0630 trial. J Clin Oncol 33(20):2231–2238

Wardelmann (2016) Evaluation of response after neoadjuvant treatment in soft tissue sarcomas; the European Organization for Research and Treatment of Cancer-Soft Tissue and Bone Sarcoma Group (EORTC-STBSG) recommendations for pathological examination and reporting. Eur J Cancer 53:84–95

Wilding (2019) The landscape of tyrosine kinase inhibitors in sarcomas: looking beyond pazopanib. Expert Rev Anticancer Ther 19(11):971–991

Wilky (2019) Axitinib plus pembrolizumab in patients with advanced sarcomas including alveolar soft-part sarcoma: a single-centre, single-arm, phase 2 trial. Lancet Oncol 20:837–848

Wisdom (2018) Rationale and emerging strategies for immune checkpoint blockade in soft tissue sarcoma. Cancer 124(19):3819–3829

Woll (2012) Adjuvant chemotherapy with doxorubicin, ifosfamide, and lenograstim for resected soft-tissue sarcoma (EORTC 62931): a multicentre randomised controlled trial. Lancet Oncol 13(10):1045–1054

Wright (2012) The role of sentinel lymph node biopsy in select sarcoma patients: a meta-analysis. Am J Surg 204(4):428–433

Yang (1998) Randomized prospective study of the benefit of adjuvant radiation therapy in the treatment of soft tissue sarcomas of the extremity. J Clin Oncol 16(1):197–203

Part II

Soft Tissue Tumors

8

Acoustic Neuroma

Definition

Acoustic neuroma is a benign peripheral nerve sheath tumor of the eighth cranial nerve arising from Schwann cells (→ see also section entitled "Schwannoma"). Although commonly used, the term "acoustic neuroma" is inaccurate because this neoplasm does not derive from the acoustic branch of the VIII cranial nerve (but rather from the vestibular branch) and is not a neuroma (→ see section entitled "Neuroma").

It is also known as acoustic neurinoma, vestibular schwannoma (which would probably be the best term), vestibular neuroma, and vestibular neurilemmoma.

Epidemiology and Presentation

Acoustic neuroma accounts for approximately 10% of intracranial neoplasms and 80–90% of tumors at the cerebellopontine angle. It occurs mainly in adults (mainly between 30 and 60 years), although it can rarely affect children. A moderate female prevalence is observed. The tumor typically arises from the vestibular branch of the vestibulocochlear nerve and thus tends to occupy the cerebellopontine angle.

The clinical presentation depends on the involvement of the eighth cranial nerve as well as the compression of surrounding structures such as other cranial nerves, the cerebellum, and the brain stem. Most patients complain unilateral hearing loss (slowly progressive), other symptoms being tinnitus, vertigo, headache, and facial numbness. As the mass grows (up to 5 cm), the brain stem can be compressed, which can lead to gait abnormalities. During pregnancy, symptoms may become worse.

Diagnosis is made with a contrast-enhanced magnetic resonance imaging or contrast-enhanced computed tomography scan.

The preoperative distinction between acoustic neuroma and other cerebellopontine angle lesions (e.g., meningioma, which accounts for 5–10% of neoplasms in this location) is important for technical and prognostic reasons.

Etiology and Predisposition

Exposure to ionizing radiations has been associated with increased risk of developing acoustic neuroma. Analogously, exposure to radiofrequency electromagnetic fields (due to the use of mobile phone) has been associated with an increased risk of developing this tumor, although the issue is debated.

Although most acoustic neuromas are unilateral and sporadic, a minority develops within the frame of the following syndromes:

1. **Neurofibromatosis type 2**: this condition is caused by inactivating mutations of the NF2 tumor suppressor gene[1], which encodes a protein called merlin (also known as schwannomin), which is expressed particularly in Schwann cells. This syndrome has an estimated incidence of 1 in 33,000 people and is considered to have an autosomal dominant pattern of inheritance. Patients with neurofibromatosis type 2 carry a germline mutation of a copy of the NF2 tumor suppressor gene: in about 50% of cases, the altered gene is inherited from an affected parent, while the remaining cases result from new mutations in the NF2 gene (i.e., occur in patients without a family history of the disease). The biallelic inactivation of the NF2 gene is then acquired through a somatic mutation. These patients usually develop multiple schwannomas before the age of 30 years: in particular, bilateral vestibular schwannoma is the hallmark of neurofibromatosis type 2 (which is also known as bilateral acoustic neuroma, BAN) and accounts for about 8% of all acoustic neuromas. Individuals with neurofibromatosis type 2 develop acoustic neuroma earlier in life as compared to sporadic cases (peak incidence around the third decade of life); moreover, syndromic acoustic neuroma occurs in neurofibromatosis type 2 much more often than in neurofibromatosis type 1, although the latter is much more common. Patients may also develop meningioma (50% of patients; often multiple) and glioma (most frequently ependymoma of the cervical spinal cord).
2. **Neurofibromatosis type 1**: also called von Recklinghausen disease, this condition is characterized by skin pigmentation and the growth of different tumor types (mainly neurofibromas). Unilateral acoustic neuroma has been reported in up to 20% of individuals with this syndrome. The incidence of neurofibromatosis

---

[1] NF2: this gene encodes neurofibromin 2, a protein that is similar to some members of the ERM (ezrin, radixin, moesin) family of proteins that are thought to link cytoskeletal components with proteins in the cell membrane.

type 1 is about 1 in 3000 people worldwide. Inactivating mutations in the NF1 tumor suppressor gene[2] are the cause of neurofibromatosis type 1, which has an autosomal dominant pattern of inheritance. In about 50% of cases, the germline mutation is inherited from an affected parent; the remaining cases result from new mutations in the NF1 gene and occur in people without a family history of the syndrome. For more details on this syndrome, → see the section entitled "Neurofibroma."

Pathology

Macroscopically, the neoplasm is rubbery-firm and has a well-defined capsule. Evidence of cystic degeneration or hemorrhage may be present in large lesions. Microscopically, the tumor is composed of spindle cells arranged in a biphasic mode: Antoni A pattern (cellular) and Antoni B pattern (hypocellular, myxoid), with Verocay bodies (whorling or palisading of nuclei) being typically observed. Regressive ("ancient") changes (cellular pleomorphism with hyperchromasia, cystic degeneration, necrosis, calcification, hemorrhage) are common. Some cases are highly cellular (cellular schwannoma). Mitotic figures are absent or rare. Electron microscopy shows the characteristic features of the Schwann cells.

Biomarkers

The tumor is diffusely and strongly positive for S100. It stains negative for cytokeratins, chromogranin, and synaptophysin.

Prognosis

Acoustic neuroma is a benign tumor. Exceptionally, de novo malignancies of the vestibulocochlear nerve have been reported; even rarer is the malignant transformation of a previously histologically diagnosed benign vestibular schwannoma.

---

[2]NF1: this gene encodes neurofibromin 1, a negative regulator of the RAS signal transduction pathway. Neurofibromin acts by accelerating the conversion of active GTP-bound RAS to its inactive GDP-bound form. The RAS signaling can be activated by receptor tyrosine kinases following the binding of growth factors, which results in increased AKT and/or MEK activity. In addition, RAS controls the generation of cyclic AMP (cAMP) through protein kinase C (PKC) following the activation of a G protein-coupled receptor (GPCR).

Therapy

Neurosurgery (microsurgical resection) is the conventional treatment. After surgery, magnetic resonance imaging is required within 6–12 months to document the completeness of tumor removal. The most common complications of surgery include hearing loss (the most common), injury to the anterior inferior cerebral artery, hemorrhage, cerebellar trauma, facial paralysis, and hydrocephalus.

Stereotactic **radiotherapy** is a valuable alternative to surgery and is gaining momentum (although no formal comparison between the two treatments is available).

Observation can be considered in case of small lesions and in elderly patients with numerous comorbidities.

As regards **targeted therapy**, bevacizumab[3] improves hearing in approximately 35–40% of patients with neurofibromatosis type 2 and progressive vestibular schwannomas.

Suggested Readings

Goshtasbi (2020) The changing landscape of vestibular schwannoma diagnosis and management: a cross-sectional study. Laryngoscope 130(2):482–486

Lu (2019) Efficacy and safety of bevacizumab for vestibular schwannoma in neurofibromatosis type 2: a systematic review and meta-analysis of treatment outcomes. J Neurooncol 144(2):239–248

Miller (2018) Cancer epidemiology update, following the 2011 IARC evaluation of radiofrequency electromagnetic fields (Monograph 102). Environ Res 167:673–683

Momoli (2017) Probabilistic multiple-bias modeling applied to the Canadian data from the interphone study of mobile phone use and risk of glioma, meningioma, acoustic neuroma, and parotid gland tumors. Am J Epidemiol 186(7):885–893

Pettersson (2014) Long-term mobile phone use and acoustic neuroma risk. Epidemiology 25(2):233–241

Plotkin (2019) Multicenter, prospective, phase II and biomarker study of high-dose bevacizumab as induction therapy in patients with neurofibromatosis type 2 and progressive vestibular schwannoma. J Clin Oncol 37(35):3446–3454

Tucker (2019) Long-term tumor control rates following gamma knife radiosurgery for acoustic neuroma. World Neurosurg 122:366–371

---

[3] Bevacizumab: monoclonal antibody blocking VEGFA (vascular endothelial growth factor A).

Definition

Acquired digital fibrokeratoma (ADFK) is a benign, fibrous tumor of the skin. ADFK is not included in the World Health Organization (WHO) classification of skin tumors. It is also known as acral fibrokeratoma and acquired periungual fibrokeratoma.

Epidemiology and Presentation

ADFK is a relatively rare lesion originally described in the fingers (hence the name); actually it can occasionally occur on the lower lip, nose, elbow, pre-patellar area, nail bed, and heel (therefore, the term "acral fibrokeratoma" would probably be more accurate). This neoplasm arises more frequently in middle-aged adults. Typically, it presents as a small solitary asymptomatic papule (generally less than 1 cm in size) surrounded by a characteristic hyperkeratotic collarette.

Pathology

The lesion presents with hyperkeratotic and acanthotic epidermis with thick collagen bundles oriented along the vertical axis in the dermis. The dermal component shows one of three histological variants: type 1 is the most common variant and presents as a dome-shaped lesion consisting of a dermal core of thick, densely packed collagen bundles with fine elastic fibers; type 2 is a mainly tall and hyperkeratotic lesion with more fibroblasts arranged in the cutis than type 1, along with reduced elastic fibers; and type 3 is the least common variant and presents as a flat to the dome-shaped lesion with poorly cellular dermal core, edematous structures, and no elastic fibers.

S. Mocellin, *Soft Tissue Tumors*, https://doi.org/10.1007/978-3-030-58710-9_9

Differential diagnosis may be needed with the following: common wart (verruca vulgaris, the most frequent neoplasm of the hand and fingers, it is caused by human papillomavirus types 1, 2, 4, and 29); cutaneous horn (a clinical diagnosis referring to an exophytic and hyperkeratotic growth that contains a column of keratin; histological examination may show a premalignant or malignant underlying lesion); neurofibroma (→ see dedicated section); pyogenic granuloma (→ see dedicated section); and acrochordon (also known as skin tag, soft fibroma, cutaneous papilloma, cutaneous tag, fibroma pendulum, and fibroma molluscum; non-acral location, pedunculated, less hyperkeratotic, less dense connective tissue).

Biomarkers

Immunostaining is not contributory.

Prognosis

ADFK is a benign lesion without risk of malignant transformation.

Therapy

Surgical excision is the treatment of choice.

Suggested Readings

Longhurst (2015) An unknown mass: the differential diagnosis of digit tumors. Int J Dermatol 54(11):1214–1225

Shih (2019) Acquired digital fibrokeratoma: review of its clinical and dermoscopic features and differential diagnosis. Int J Dermatol 58(2):151–158

Acral Fibromyxoma

Definition

Acral fibromyxoma is a benign tumor of uncertain differentiation. It is also known as superficial acral fibromyxoma, digital fibromyxoma, and cellular digital fibroma.

Epidemiology and Presentation

This rare dermal-based tumor is typically located in the hands or feet (hence the term "acral") and especially the digits (with particular regard to the subungual and periungual space). It can occur at any age although most patients are aged 40 years or older, with a slight male predominance. The dome-shaped, polypoid or verrucoid slow-growing nodule can be asymptomatic or painful.

Pathology

The tumor, which is well circumscribed and centered in the dermis, is made of a moderately cellular proliferation of spindled and stellate-shaped fibroblasts arranged in a storiform or fasciculated pattern and included in a myxoid or collagenous matrix with prominent vessels and mast cells. Mitotic figures are usually rare (<1 per 10 HPF); rare multinucleate cells are found in approximately 50% of cases. Usually, nuclear atypia and pleomorphism are minimal, and atypical mitotic figures are absent.

Differential diagnosis may be needed with the following: acquired digital fibrokeratoma (paucicellular, can be CD34 negative); cutaneous myxoma (also known as superficial angiomyxoma; lobulated pattern, poorly demarcated; it may contain an epithelial component; it may be associated with Carney complex); dermatofibrosarcoma protuberans (hands and feet are unusual sites; tight storiform pattern at least focally; infiltrative); benign fibrous histiocytoma (not well circumscribed; typically

S. Mocellin, *Soft Tissue Tumors*, https://doi.org/10.1007/978-3-030-58710-9_10

it does not involve fingers, palms, or soles; CD34 negative); myxoid neurofibroma (no increased vasculature, S100 positive); myxoinflammatory fibroblastic sarcoma (inflammatory myxohyaline tumor of distal extremities; virocyte-like and lipoblast-like bizarre cells, prominent inflammation); sclerosing perineurioma (cells are arranged in corded, trabecular, and onion-skinned whorling patterns; usually CD34 negative and claudin positive); and glomus tumor (it contains smooth muscle cells which are SMA[1] and MSA[2] positive).

Biomarkers

Acral fibromyxoma typically stains positive for CD34, vimentin, and CD99 and negative for S100, desmin, MUC4, STAT6, and cytokeratins. Unlike intramuscular or cellular myxomas, GNAS mutations are not present.

Most tested lesions show loss of RB1 expression.

Prognosis

It is a benign tumor, although local recurrences are reported in up to 20% of cases.

Therapy

Surgical excision.

Suggested Readings

Agaimy (2017) Superficial acral fibromyxoma: clinicopathological, immunohistochemical, and molecular study of 11 cases highlighting frequent Rb1 loss/deletions. Hum Pathol 60:192–198
Fletcher (2020) WHO classification of tumours of soft tissue and bone, 5th edn
Paral (2017) Acral manifestations of soft tissue tumors. Clin Dermatol 35(1):85–98

---

[1] SMA: smooth muscle actin.

[2] MSA: muscle-specific actin.

Definition

Adult fibrosarcoma (AFS) is a (usually) high-grade malignancy arising from fibroblasts. It is also known as adult-type fibrosarcoma.

Epidemiology and Presentation

In the past, AFS was considered one of the most common soft tissue sarcomas in adults. In contrast, currently it is believed to represent only 1–3% of adult sarcomas due to the fact that most previously diagnosed fibrosarcomas are now classified otherwise, such as dedifferentiated liposarcoma, fibromatosis, fibrosarcomatous dermatofibrosarcoma protuberans (DFSP), low-grade fibromyxoid sarcoma, malignant peripheral nerve sheath tumor (MPNST), synovial sarcoma, or undifferentiated pleomorphic sarcoma (UPS) (→ see dedicated sections).

AFS is most common in middle-aged and older adults (median age: 50 years), and most cases arise in the deep soft tissues of the extremities, trunk, and head and neck. Those in the skin and subcutis are more likely to represent fibrosarcomatous change in DFSP (→ see dedicated section). The diagnosis of fibrosarcoma in visceral organs is questionable. Retroperitoneal fibrosarcoma is very rare and is likely to represent low-grade dedifferentiated liposarcoma in most instances.

Pathology

Fibrosarcoma is composed of relatively monomorphic spindled cells (characteristically arranged in a herringbone pattern with variable collagen deposition) showing no or moderate pleomorphism. Lesions showing a greater degree of pleomorphism should be better classified as undifferentiated pleomorphic sarcoma (→ see

© The Editor(s) (if applicable) and The Author(s), under exclusive license to
Springer Nature Switzerland AG 2021
S. Mocellin, *Soft Tissue Tumors*, https://doi.org/10.1007/978-3-030-58710-9_11

dedicated section). Hemorrhage and necrosis can be seen in high-grade tumors. Generally, it is a diagnosis of exclusion.

Differential diagnosis may be needed with the following: low-grade fibromyxoid sarcoma (also known as Evans tumor), dedifferentiated liposarcoma, synovial sarcoma, sclerosing epithelioid fibrosarcoma, myxofibrosarcoma, undifferentiated pleomorphic sarcoma (more pronounced pleomorphism), MPNST, solitary fibrous tumor, aggressive fibromatosis (less cellular, less hyperchromasia, no atypia; <1 mitotic figure per HPF[1]), angiosarcoma (spindle cell type), rhabdomyosarcoma, leiomyosarcoma, and epithelioid sarcoma. When AFS arises close to the skin, fibrosarcomatous DFSP, spindle cell malignant melanoma, and sarcomatoid carcinoma should be excluded.

Biomarkers

Vimentin is often the only positive biomarker. CD34-positive tumors showing fibrosarcoma morphology probably represent a fibrosarcomatous progression of a DFSP or that of a solitary fibrous tumor. Staining for S100, cytokeratins, and smooth muscle biomarkers is typically negative.

AFS has been reported to show multiple numerical and structural chromosomal abnormalities (aneuploidy), without involvement of a specific locus (complex karyotype sarcoma).

Prognosis

More than 80% of AFS are high grade (FNCLCC[2] grade II or III); low-grade lesions can progress to high-grade sarcoma when the neoplasm recurs. AFS is an aggressive malignant neoplasm, with multiple local recurrences and parenchymal metastases, the 5-year overall survival rate being about 50%. The probability of local recurrence relates to completeness of excision and ranges between 15 and 70%. Averagely, 50% of cases relapse and 25% metastasize (mainly to lungs and bone, rarely to lymph nodes).

Therapy

Surgery is the mainstay of primary tumor treatment. AFS is characterized by its low sensitivity toward radiotherapy and chemotherapy.

---

[1] HPF: high-power field.

[2] FNCLCC: Fédération Nationale des Centres de Lutte Contre Le Cancer.

Suggested Readings

Augsburger (2017) Current diagnostics and treatment of fibrosarcoma—perspectives for future therapeutic targets and strategies. Oncotarget 8(61):104638–104653

Fletcher (2020) WHO classification of tumours of soft tissue and bone, 5th edn

Folpe (2020) "Hey!—Whatever happened to hemangiopericytoma and fibrosarcoma?" an update on selected conceptual advances in soft tissue pathology which have occurred over the past 50 years. Hum Pathol 95:113–136

Sheng (2001) Expression of COL1A1-PDGFB fusion transcripts in superficial adult fibrosarcoma suggests a close relationship to dermatofibrosarcoma protuberans. J Pathol 194(1):88–94

Definition

Adult rhabdomyoma is a benign tumor showing mature skeletal (striated) muscle differentiation. It is also known as adult extra-cardiac rhabdomyoma, rhabdomyomatous hamartoma, and rhabdomyoma purum.

Along with fetal rhabdomyoma and genital rhabdomyoma ($\rightarrow$ see dedicated sections), it belongs to the extra-cardiac subgroup of rhabdomyomas ($\rightarrow$ see also the section entitled "Rhabdomyoma").

Epidemiology and Presentation

It is a very rare neoplasm representing <2% of all muscular tumors. Most cases develop in the head and neck (parapharyngeal space, salivary glands, larynx, mouth, and soft tissue of the neck). Very rarely it has been described in other sites such as the mediastinum. The lesion occurs mainly in men (M:F = 3:1), the median age being 60 years (range: 30–80 years). The tumor commonly presents as a slow-growing, painless mass (median diameter: 3 cm) which can cause compression of adjacent structures. The tumor is multifocal in 25% of cases.

Unlike cardiac rhabdomyoma and fetal rhabdomyoma ($\rightarrow$ see dedicated sections), adult rhabdomyoma is not associated with either basal cell nevus syndrome (Gorlin syndrome) or with tuberous sclerosis complex (TSC).

Pathology

Tumor cells are large and polygonal with abundant granular eosinophilic cytoplasm and small round vesicular nuclei; the cytoplasm may be vacuolated ("spider cells") or contain rod-like inclusions or cross striations (well-differentiated skeletal muscle cells). Neither mitotic activity nor atypia are encountered.

© The Editor(s) (if applicable) and The Author(s), under exclusive license to
Springer Nature Switzerland AG 2021
S. Mocellin, *Soft Tissue Tumors*, https://doi.org/10.1007/978-3-030-58710-9_12

Differential diagnosis may be needed with the following: alveolar soft part sarcoma, granular cell tumor (no skeletal muscle differentiation, smaller cells with poorly defined cell borders, often overlying pseudoepitheliomatous hyperplasia, S100 positive); hibernoma (no skeletal muscle differentiation); paraganglioma (positive for NSE,[1] synaptophysin, and chromogranin); and well-differentiated rhabdomyosarcoma.

Biomarkers

Adult rhabdomyoma stains positive for MSA,[2] desmin, and myogenin, whereas it stains negative for EMA[3] and CD68.

Prognosis

Adult rhabdomyoma is a benign tumor, but it often recurs. However, it does not infiltrate contiguous structures or metastasize.

Therapy

Surgical excision is the treatment of choice.

---

[1] NSE: neuron-specific enolase.
[2] MSA: muscle-specific actin.
[3] EMA: epithelial membrane antigen.

Definition

Alveolar rhabdomyosarcoma (ARMS) is a malignant tumor with skeletal muscle cell differentiation. It is also known as monomorphous round cell rhabdomyosarcoma.

It is one of the four subtypes of rhabdomyosarcoma ($\rightarrow$ see section entitled "Rhabdomyosarcoma") along with embryonal (ERMS), pleomorphic (PRMS), and spindle cell/sclerosing (SRMS) rhabdomyosarcoma ($\rightarrow$ see dedicated sections).

Epidemiology and Presentation

ARMS occurs less frequently than embryonal RMS (ERMS) and comprises about 20% of all pediatric RMS (roughly 1% of malignancies found in children and adolescents). It develops more often in adolescents and young adults (i.e., later in life as compared to ERMS), but it may occur at any age (median age: 8 years).

ARMS most commonly arises in the extremities although it can be found in other body sites (e.g., paraspinal and perineal regions, paranasal sinuses, breast). ARMS typically presents as a rapidly growing mass; symptoms depend upon tumor site (and thus compression of neighborhood structures).

Etiology and Predisposition

For details on the risk of rhabdomyosarcoma associated with some cancer predisposition syndromes, $\rightarrow$ see section entitled "Rhabdomyosarcoma."

© The Editor(s) (if applicable) and The Author(s), under exclusive license to
Springer Nature Switzerland AG 2021
S. Mocellin, *Soft Tissue Tumors*, https://doi.org/10.1007/978-3-030-58710-9_13

Pathology

ARMS is a highly cellular neoplasm containing a monomorphous population of primitive cells with round nuclei and features of arrested myogenesis. Typically, nests of neoplastic cells are arranged in alveolar spaces (like lung alveoli, hence the name). The solid variant of ARMS lacks the fibrovascular stromal septa separating tumor cells into discrete nests and forms sheets of round cells with variable rhabdomyoblastic differentiation.

Differential diagnosis may be needed with the following: alveolar soft part sarcoma (PAS-positive[1] intracytoplasmic crystalline rods and granules); Merkel cell carcinoma (negative for desmin, myogenin, and MyoD1; it lacks the characteristic fusion gene); and metastatic neuroendocrine carcinoma (positive for cytokeratins, synaptophysin, S100, and EMA[2]; desmin negative; it lacks the characteristic fusion gene).

Biomarkers

ARMS typically stains positive for myogenin (strong and homogeneous), desmin, and MyoD1.

Most ARMS cases (about 80%) carry either the t(2;13)(q35;q14) chromosomal translocation, which is the most frequent (60%) and leads to the formation of the **PAX3-FOXO1 fusion gene**,[3] or the t(1;13)(p36;q14) chromosomal translocation, which is present in a minority of cases (20%) and leads to the formation of the **PAX7-FOXO1 fusion gene** (see Footnote 3). The resulting chimeric protein products are believed to play a key role in ARMS pathogenesis.

Amplification of NMYC[4] is observed in 50% and is associated with more aggressive behavior.

---

[1] PAS: periodic acid Schiff.

[2] EMA: epithelial membrane antigen.

[3] PAX3 and PAX7 encode members of the paired box transcription factor family, which are expressed in skeletal muscle progenitors, whereas FOXO1 encodes a widely expressed member of the forkhead transcription factor family. These fusion genes encode chimeric transcription factors containing an amino-terminal PAX3 or PAX7 region with an intact DNA-binding domain and a carboxy-terminal FOXO1 region containing an intact transcriptional activation domain. In contrast to wild-type PAX3 and PAX7 proteins, the PAX3-FOXO1 and PAX7-FOXO1 fusion proteins have enhanced transcriptional activity. PAX3-FOXO1 binds to DNA regions containing E-box DNA-binding motifs as well as PAX3-binding sites along with the E-box-specific transcription factor N-Myc (encoded by MYCN) and myogenic basic helix-loop-helix transcription factors MYOD1 and myogenin (encoded by MYOD1 and MYOG, respectively) and generates super-enhancers near a subset of target genes, including ALK (encoding anaplastic lymphoma kinase), FGFR4 (encoding fibroblast growth factor receptor 4), as well as MYCN, MYOD1, and MYOG. In addition, PAX3-FOXO1 also interacts directly or indirectly with chromatin-related proteins, including chromatin remodeling protein bromodomain-containing protein 4 (BRD4).

[4] NMYC: this gene is a member of the MYC family and encodes a protein with a basic helix-loop-helix (bHLH) domain. The encoded protein is located in the nucleus and must dimerize with another bHLH protein in order to bind DNA. Amplification of this gene is associated with a variety of tumors, most notably neuroblastoma.

Prognosis

ARMS is a high-grade malignant neoplasm that is intrinsically more aggressive than ERMS and tends to be of high stage at presentation (metastatic disease is present at first diagnosis in 20–30% of cases).

Patients with fusion-negative ARMS have a better prognosis; among patients with translocation-positive tumor, patients with PAX3 fusion-positive ARMS have been reported to have reduced survival compared with that of patients with PAX7 fusion-positive ARMS.

For more details on staging and prognosis, → see the "Rhabdomyosarcoma" section.

Therapy

Currently, risk-adapted multimodality treatment (personalized therapy) is the standard of care. For details → see the section entitled "Rhabdomyosarcoma."

Following the role of PAX-FOXO1 chimeric protein in ARMS pathogenesis (see Footnote 3), efforts are underway to modulate the activity of disease-specific chimeric proteins, such as the use of inhibitors of the bromodomain and extra-terminal domain (BET) family proteins (based on the dependency of EWS/ETS transcription factors on BET epigenetic reader proteins).

Suggested Readings

Cameron (2019) Adult-type rhabdomyoma of the omohyoid muscle. Case Rep Otolaryngol 2019:4706582

Cochran (2019) Bromodomains: a new target class for drug development. Nat Rev Drug Discov 18(8):609–628

Drabbe (2020) Embryonal and alveolar rhabdomyosarcoma in adults: real-life data from a Tertiary Sarcoma Centre. Clin Oncol (R Coll Radiol) 32(1):e27–e35

Fletcher (2020) WHO classification of tumours of soft tissue and bone, 5th edn

Gryder (2017) PAX3-FOXO1 establishes myogenic super enhancers and confers BET bromodomain vulnerability. Cancer Discov 7(8):884–899

Pappo (2018) Rhabdomyosarcoma, Ewing sarcoma, and other round cell sarcomas. J Clin Oncol 36(2):168–179

Skapek (2019) Rhabdomyosarcoma. Nat Rev Dis Primers 5(1):1

Alveolar Soft Part Sarcoma

14

Definition

Alveolar soft part sarcoma (ASPS) is a malignant tumor of uncertain differentiation. It was previously referred to as malignant myoblastoma, granular cell myoblastoma, and malignant granular cell myoblastoma.

Epidemiology and Presentation

ASPS is a rare malignancy representing less than 1% of all soft tissue sarcomas. Although it may occur at any age, it is most common between 15 and 35 years. Of note, a female predominance is observed until the age of 30 years, whereas males are more frequently affected after this age.

ASPS develops most frequently in the deep soft tissues of the thigh or buttock, although in children and infants the head and neck region (e.g., tongue and orbit) is the most typical affected site. Very rare cases have been described almost anywhere in the body (including viscera).

Clinically, the lesion generally presents as a slow-growing, painless mass (size range: 2–15 cm). Metastatic disease to the lungs or brain may be the first disease manifestation. Symptoms depend on the site of origin. Hypervascularization is usually observed by contrast-enhanced computed tomography scan and magnetic resonance imaging.

Pathology

ASPS presents as a poorly circumscribed mass with a soft consistency; areas of necrosis and hemorrhage can be found. Microscopically, it is composed of large, uniform, epithelioid cells (round or polygonal in shape, with abundant, eosinophilic, granular cytoplasm) arranged in solid nests and/or alveolar structures (hence the

S. Mocellin, *Soft Tissue Tumors*, https://doi.org/10.1007/978-3-030-58710-9_14

name). The distinctively organoid or nesting pattern is sometimes absent, particularly in younger patients. The nests are separated by septa of connective tissue containing sinusoidal vascular channels. Loss of cellular adhesion coupled with necrosis of the centrally located cells in the nests leads to the commonly observed pseudoalveolar pattern. Multinucleation, nuclear atypia, and mitotic figures are uncommon, while vascular invasion is frequently detected. The cells often (but not always) contain highly characteristic rhomboid or rod-shaped intracytoplasmic inclusions (better observed upon PAS[1] staining after diastase digestion).

Differential diagnosis may be needed with the following: renal cell carcinoma (cytokeratin positive, no PAS-positive intracytoplasmic inclusions); paraganglioma (positive for chromogranin and synaptophysin, negative for desmin); granular cell tumor (presence of numerous lysosomes with particulate content; absence of PAS-positive crystals); and melanoma (positive for melanocytic biomarkers; absence of PAS-positive crystals). In all cases, detection of disease specific chromosomal translocation (see below) is helpful.

Biomarkers

The most typical immunohistochemistry finding is the strong nuclear staining for TFE3 (resulting from the chromosomal translocation below described), which contrasts with the weak or absent expression in most normal cells; of note, strong nuclear immunoreactivity for TFE3 can also be observed in some granular cell tumors. Staining for desmin and S100 may be positive, but no expression of HMB45 is detected (unlike PEComa). ASPS results negative also for synaptophysin, chromogranin, neurofilament proteins, cytokeratins, and EMA.

ASPS is characterized by the presence of the chromosomal translocation t(X;17) (p11;q25) which leads to the formation of the **ASPSCR1-TFE3 fusion gene**.[2] This gene rearrangement is highly specific and sensitive for ASPS among sarcomas, while the same genetic alteration is found also in a small subgroup of patients with renal cell carcinoma.

Prognosis

ASPS is a high-grade malignancy although the course is often indolent. The tumor is characterized by a relatively low rate of local recurrence after radical surgery (about 10%) and a high rate of distant metastasis (up to 80% of cases); the latter can

---

[1] PAS: periodic acid Schiff.

[2] The ASPSCR1-TFE3 fusion protein localizes to the nucleus where it acts as a transcription factor causing activation of the MET signaling pathway (which might make ASPS sensitive to MET inhibitors). TFE3 belongs to the microphthalmia family of bHLH-LZ transcription factors (MiT/TFE) which is composed of four members: MITF, TFEB, TFE3, and TFEC; neoplasms with alterations in these genes are also called MiT family tumors.

occur at presentation (about 50%), early in the course of the disease, but also many years after first diagnosis (which calls for long term follow up).

Prognostic factors are tumor size and stage (with special regard to the presence of metastatic disease). Of note, histological features have no prognostic significance (the use of the FNCLCC[3] grading system is not indicated for ASPS). In patients with non-metastatic disease at presentation, survival rates have been reported to be 60% at 5 years, 38% at 10 years, and 15% at 20 years. A 5-year disease-free survival rate of 71% has been reported in patients presenting with distant metastasis, but with longer follow-up, the rates drop remarkably.

Distant metastasis occurs more frequently in the lung, bone, and brain; lymph node metastasis is infrequent.

Therapy

Surgery is the mainstay of treatment for primary disease. **Radiotherapy** has been utilized for the treatment of high-risk (margin positive) resected primary ASPS in an EpSSG[4] prospective trial and has been associated with improved local disease control in a multivariate analysis of a SEER[5] series of ASPS; however, data are scarce, and no international guideline recommends its use in patients with ASPS.

For metastatic disease, conventional **chemotherapy** (anthracycline-based) is largely ineffective (tumor response rates <10%): along with other tumors such as well-differentiated liposarcoma and clear cell sarcoma, ASPS is considered one of the most chemoresistant soft tissue sarcomas.

Target therapy (e.g., sunitinib,[6] pazopanib,[7] cediranib[8]) appears more effective than chemotherapy, with clinical benefit (tumor response + disease stabilization) being observed in up to 50% of patients. In particular, the NCCN[9] and ESMO[10] guidelines mention sunitinib and cediranib as systemic therapy drugs for ASPS. Immunotherapy alone (with immune checkpoint inhibitors) and a combination of target therapy (axitinib[11]) plus immunotherapy (pembrolizumab[12]) are also being tested.

---

[3] FNCLCC: Fédération Nationale des Centres de Lutte Contre Le Cancer.

[4] EpSSG: European paediatric Soft tissue sarcoma Study Group.

[5] SEER: Surveillance Epidemiology and End Results program.

[6] Sunitinib: tyrosine kinase inhibitor targeting the following: PDGFR, VEGFR, KIT, FLT3, CSF1R, RET.

[7] Pazopanib: tyrosine kinase inhibitor targeting the following: VEGFR, PDGFR, KIT.

[8] Cediranib: tyrosine kinase inhibitor targeting the following: VEGFR.

[9] NCCN: National Comprehensive Cancer Network.

[10] ESMO: European Society for Medical Oncology.

[11] Axitinib: tyrosine kinase inhibitor targeting the following: VEGFR.

[12] Pembrolizumab: monoclonal antibody blocking the following: PD1.

Suggested Readings

Brennan (2018) Alveolar soft part sarcoma in children and adolescents: the European paediatric soft tissue sarcoma study group prospective trial (EpSSG NRSTS 2005). Pediatr Blood Cancer 65(4):e26942

Conry (2020) Complete response to dual immunotherapy in a young adult with metastatic alveolar soft part sarcoma enabled by a drug recovery program in a community practice. J Adolesc Young Adult Oncol 9(3):449–452

Dickson (2020) Genetic diversity in alveolar soft part sarcoma: a subset contain variant fusion genes, highlighting broader molecular kinship with other MiT family tumors. Genes Chromosomes Cancer 59:23–29

Fletcher (2020) WHO classification of tumours of soft tissue and bone, 5th edn

Flores (2018) Alveolar soft part sarcoma in children and young adults: a report of 69 cases. Pediatr Blood Cancer 65(5):e26953

George (2019) Developments in systemic therapy for soft tissue and bone sarcomas. J Natl Compr Cancer Netw 17(5.5):625–628

Judson (2019) Cediranib in patients with alveolar soft-part sarcoma (CASPS): a double-blind, placebo-controlled, randomised, phase 2 trial. Lancet Oncol 20(7):1023–1034

Paoluzzi (2019) Diagnosis, prognosis, and treatment of alveolar soft-part sarcoma: a review. JAMA Oncol 5(2):254–260

Portera (2001) Alveolar soft part sarcoma: clinical course and patterns of metastasis in 70 patients treated at a single institution. Cancer 91(3):585–591

Schöffski (2018) Activity and safety of crizotinib in patients with alveolar soft part sarcoma with rearrangement of TFE3: European Organization for Research and Treatment of Cancer (EORTC) phase II trial 90101 'CREATE'. Ann Oncol 29(3):758–765

Soheilifar (2018) Molecular landscape in alveolar soft part sarcoma: implications for molecular targeted therapy. Biomed Pharmacother 103:889–896

Stacchiotti (2011) Sunitinib in advanced alveolar soft part sarcoma: evidence of a direct antitumor effect. Ann Oncol 22(7):1682–1690

Stacchiotti (2018) Activity of Pazopanib and Trabectedin in advanced alveolar soft part sarcoma. Oncologist 23(1):62–70

Wang (2016) Prognostic factors in alveolar soft part sarcoma: a SEER analysis. J Surg Oncol 113(5):581–586

Wilky (2019) Axitinib plus pembrolizumab in patients with advanced sarcomas including alveolar soft-part sarcoma: a single-centre, single-arm, phase 2 trial. Lancet Oncol 20(6):837–848

Yang (2018) Emerging roles and regulation of MiT/TFE transcriptional factors. Cell Commun Signal 16(1):31

Definition

Anastomosing hemangioma is a benign tumor of vascular origin.

Epidemiology and Presentation

This rare tumor, originally described in the genitourinary tract, can occur also in other viscera (gastrointestinal tract, liver) as well as somatic soft tissues (with a predilection for paraspinal areas).

Pathology

The lesion is composed of anastomosing sinusoidal capillary-sized vessels (hence the name) with mild endothelial nuclear variability and scattered hobnailed endothelial cells. The mitotic activity is scarce or absent. Fibrin thrombi are typically present, while extramedullary hematopoiesis and mature fat are observed in approximately 50% of cases. Overall, this benign vascular tumor displays overlapping features with well-differentiated forms of angiosarcoma.

Differential diagnosis may be needed with the following: angiosarcoma (diffusely infiltrative growth pattern; prominent cytological alterations, including high-grade cytological atypia, multilayering of endothelial cells and high mitotic activity); retiform hemangioendothelioma (predilection for the distal extremities; usually it involves the skin; similar appearance to normal rete testis); hobnail hemangioma (usually involves the skin; wedge-shaped vascular proliferation with dilated vascular channels superficially and less conspicuous vessels in the deep aspect of the lesion); and accessory spleen (encapsulated).

S. Mocellin, *Soft Tissue Tumors*, https://doi.org/10.1007/978-3-030-58710-9_15

Biomarkers

It stains positive for endothelial biomarkers (e.g., CD31, CD34, ERG). It stains negative for HHV8 (human herpes virus 8).

Recurrent somatic mutations of genes GNA11, GNAQ, and GNA14[1] have been reported and are believed to be driver alterations in the pathogenesis of this tumor.

Prognosis

Anastomosing hemangioma is a benign tumor.

Therapy

Surgical excision is the treatment of choice.

Suggested Readings

Cheon (2018) Anastomosing hemangioma of the kidney: radiologic and pathologic distinctions of a kidney cancer mimic. Curr Oncol 25(3):e220–e223

John (2016) Anastomosing hemangiomas arising in unusual locations: a clinicopathologic study of 17 soft tissue cases showing a predilection for the paraspinal region. Am J Surg Pathol 40(8):1084–1089

Lappa (2020) Anastomosing hemangioma: short review of a benign mimicker of angiosarcoma. Arch Pathol Lab Med 144(2):240–244

Liau (2020) GNA11 joins GNAQ and GNA14 as a recurrently mutated gene in anastomosing hemangioma. Virchows Arch 476(3):475–481

Merritt (2019) Anastomosing hemangioma of liver. J Radiol Case Rep 13(6):32–39

---

[1] GNAQ, GNA11, GNA14: these locuses encode guanine nucleotide-binding proteins (G-proteins), which modulate the activity of G protein-coupled receptors (GPCR) that are involved in a variety of cell signaling transduction pathways.

Definition

Aneurysmal fibrous histiocytoma (AnFH) is a low-grade fibrohistiocytic tumor. It is considered an uncommon variant of benign fibrous histiocytoma (→ see dedicated section).

Epidemiology and Presentation

AnFH usually presents as a solitary, pigmented (blue-black, yellow, red) or skin-colored cutaneous nodule which can reach a diameter of some centimeters. Most frequently involved sites are limbs and trunk of middle-aged adults.

Pathology

AnFH is a cellular, poorly demarcated dermal proliferation composed of bland fusiform to rounded mononuclear as well as multinucleated giant cells distributed haphazardly and in storiform areas with characteristic prominent cleft-like or cavernous blood-filled pseudovascular spaces (no endothelial cell lining), hemosiderin deposits, and abundant hemosiderin-rich macrophages. Mitotic activity is frequently observed.

Differential diagnosis may be needed with the following: pigmented dermatofibrosarcoma protuberans (it occurs in subcutis and stains positive for CD34); melanoma (positive for melanocytic biomarkers); Kaposi sarcoma (it presents as violaceous papules in older individuals; endothelial lining of the enlarged clefts is present; positive for HHV8 and CD34); spindle cell hemangioma (it is located in the subcutis, is poorly circumscribed, and consists of true vascular capsules lined with endothelium); angiomatoid fibrous histiocytoma (it occurs mostly on extremities of younger people; presence of myxoid structure fibrous pseudocapsule and marked chronic inflammatory infiltrate); and angiosarcoma (it occurs more frequently on the face and scalp of elderly and in those with a history of radiation therapy; lined by endothelial cells, variable atypia; CD31 and CD34 positive).

Biomarkers

AnFH usually stains negative for CD34, CD31, CD68, and desmin but positive for vimentin.

The chromosomal translocation t(3;11)(p21;q13) leading to the formation of the **LAMTOR1-PRKCD fusion gene**[1] has been reported to recurrently occur in AnFH.

Prognosis

Like other variants of benign fibrous histiocytoma (i.e., cellular and atypical fibrous histiocytoma), AnFH can recur locally (in about 20% of cases, especially if incompletely excised). Very rare cases of metastasis have been reported.

Therapy

Surgical excision (possibly wide) is the treatment of choice.

Suggested Readings

Antony (2017) Aneurysmal variant of fibrous histiocytoma—a rare entity known for recurrence. J Clin Diagn Res 11(6):ED08–ED09

Doyle (2013) Metastasizing "benign" cutaneous fibrous histiocytoma: a clinicopathologic analysis of 16 cases. Am J Surg Pathol 37(4):484–495

Jedrych (2018) Aneurysmal fibrous histiocytomas with recurrent rearrangement of the PRKCD gene and LAMTOR1-PRKCD fusions. J Cutan Pathol 45(12):966–968

---

[1] LAMTOR1 (late endosomal/lysosomal adaptor, MAPK and MTOR activator 1) encodes a protein involved in amino acid sensing and activation of mTORC1, a signaling complex promoting cell growth in response to growth factors, energy levels, and amino acids. PRKCD encodes a member of the protein kinase C family of serine- and threonine-specific protein kinases (involved in a range of cell functions).

Angiofibroma 17

The angiofibroma family is composed of the following (→ see dedicated sections for more information on single tumors):

- Cellular angiofibroma
- Cutaneous angiofibroma
- Angiofibroma of soft tissue
- Nasopharyngeal angiofibroma
- Giant cell angiofibroma (→ see section entitled "Solitary Fibrous Tumor")

S. Mocellin, *Soft Tissue Tumors*, https://doi.org/10.1007/978-3-030-58710-9_17

Definition

Angiofibroma of soft tissue (AST) is a benign mesenchymal tumor which belongs to the angiofibroma family ($\rightarrow$ see section entitled "Angiofibroma").

Epidemiology and Presentation

AST can be observed in both sexes and in a broad age range. It presents as a slow-growing mass, most often in the deep tissues of the upper and lower extremities but occasionally in a superficial (cutaneous) location.

Pathology

AST is neoplasm with fibroblastic and vascular components. It presents as a vaguely lobular, variably cellular proliferation of bland, uniform spindle cells in an abundant, variably myxoid or collagenous extracellular matrix with numerous small, thin-walled, branching blood vessels. The tumor has a prominent vasculature and may have an infiltrative growth pattern: these features could lead to a misdiagnosis, such as malignant vascular tumor.

Differential diagnosis may be needed with the following: cellular angiofibroma (usually in genital region, more cellular, usually positive for estrogen receptor and progesterone receptor); low-grade fibromyxoid sarcoma (often >6 cm and infiltrative; 45% of cases have epithelioid areas; 40% of cases contain poorly formed but large collagen rosettes); low-grade myxofibrosarcoma (infiltrative borders, more solid areas are often observed similar to typical undifferentiated pleomorphic sarcoma; it has curvilinear vessels thick wall and condensation of cells around vessels); myxoid liposarcoma (prominent chicken wire vasculature, numerous signet ring lipoblasts particularly at periphery of lobules, mucoid matrix rich in

S. Mocellin, *Soft Tissue Tumors*, https://doi.org/10.1007/978-3-030-58710-9_18

hyaluronidase sensitive acid mucopolysaccharides; it may have large mucoid pools; S100 positive); and solitary fibrous tumor (fibroblast-like cells with patternless pattern, thick bands of collagen, and prominent branching, hyalinized vessels; positive for STAT6, CD34, and CD99).

Biomarkers

AST typically tests positive for nuclear expression of NCOA2: however, this is not specific since other spindle cell neoplasms also express this biomarker. AST stains variably positive for EMA,[1] SMA,[2] desmin, and CD34, while STAT6 is not expressed.

The chromosomal translocation t(5;8)(p15;q13) leading to the formation of the **AHRR-NCOA2 fusion gene**[3] is a frequent finding in AST; rarely, GTF2I-NCOA2 fusion gene and GAB1-ABL1 fusion gene have also been described in this tumor.

Prognosis

It has a benign clinical course with a very low probability of recurrence after complete excision.

Therapy

Surgical excision is the treatment of choice.

---

[1] EMA: epithelial membrane antigen.

[2] SMA: smooth muscle actin.

[3] AHRR-NCOA2 fusion gene: the protein encoded by AHRR participates in the aryl hydrocarbon receptor (AhR) signaling cascade, which is involved in regulation of cell growth and differentiation. It functions as a feedback modulator by repressing AhR-dependent gene expression. Of note, the AHRR-NCOA2 chimeric protein leads to upregulation of aryl hydrocarbon receptor target genes. The protein encoded by NCOA2 functions as a transcriptional coactivator for nuclear hormone receptors (e.g., steroid, thyroid, retinoid, and vitamin D receptors); this protein acts as an intermediary factor for the ligand-dependent activity of these nuclear receptors, which regulate their target genes upon binding of cognate response elements. The NCOA2 gene has been found to be involved in translocations that result in fusions with other genes in various cancers, such as the lysine acetyltransferase 6A (KAT6A) gene in acute myeloid leukemia, the ETS variant 6 (ETV6) gene in acute lymphoblastic leukemia, and the HES-related family bHLH transcription factor with YRPW motif 1 (HEY1) gene in mesenchymal chondrosarcoma.

Suggested Readings

Bekers (2017) Soft tissue angiofibroma: clinicopathologic, immunohistochemical and molecular analysis of 14 cases. Genes Chromosomes Cancer 56(10):750–757

Jin (2012) Fusion of the AHRR and NCOA2 genes through a recurrent translocation t(5;8) (p15;q13) in soft tissue angiofibroma results in upregulation of aryl hydrocarbon receptor target genes. Genes Chromosomes Cancer 51(5):510–520

Mindiola-Romero (2020) A concise review of angiofibroma of soft tissue: a rare newly-described entity that can be encountered by dermatopathologists. J Cutan Pathol 47(2):179–185

Definition

Angiokeratoma is a benign vascular tumor of the skin.

Epidemiology and Presentation

Angiokeratoma presents as a small red to brown/black papule or nodule with verrucous surface (multiple papules/nodules can cluster to form a lesion).

Five subtypes with similar histology can be distinguished: (1) angiokeratoma of Mibelli (observed in children and adolescents on dorsum of toes and fingers); (2) angiokeratoma of Fordyce (scrotal skin of elderly people); (3) angiokeratoma corporis diffusum (clustered papules in a bathing suit distribution; associated with Anderson-Fabry disease, an X-linked recessive lysosomal storage disease); (4) angiokeratoma circumscriptum (the rarest subtype, usually congenital, associated with nevus flammeus, cavernous hemangioma, Klippel-Trenaunay syndrome, Cobb syndrome); and (5) idiopathic solitary or multiple angiokeratomas.

Pathology

The lesion is characterized by superficial vascular ectasia (often with thrombosis) in the papillary dermis and overlying epidermal hyperplasia (acanthosis or hyperkeratosis). Lesions may be solitary or multiple/diffuse.

Differential diagnosis may be needed with the following: hemangioma, lymphangioma, and pigmented/melanocytic lesions (thrombosis can mimic pigment).

© The Editor(s) (if applicable) and The Author(s), under exclusive license to
Springer Nature Switzerland AG 2021
S. Mocellin, *Soft Tissue Tumors*, https://doi.org/10.1007/978-3-030-58710-9_19

Biomarkers

Non-specific

Prognosis

Angiokeratoma is a benign lesion.

Therapy

Exeresis (with surgery or other ablative techniques such as cryotherapy and laser) is the treatment of choice.

Suggested Readings

Basu (2018) Penile angiokeratoma (Peaker): a distinctive subtype of genital angiokeratoma. Cureus 10(12):e3793

Zampetti (2012) Angiokeratoma: decision-making aid for the diagnosis of Fabry disease. Br J Dermatol 166(4):712–720

Zeng (2016) Angiokeratoma of Fordyce response to long pulsed Nd:YAG laser treatment. Dermatol Ther 29(1):48–51

Definition

Angioleiomyoma (ALM) is a benign neoplasm classified among pericytic (perivascular) tumors (along with glomus tumor, myopericytoma, and myofibroma). Alternative names are angiomyoma and vascular leiomyoma.

Epidemiology and Presentation

ALM is a relatively common tumor which accounts for about 5% of all benign soft tissue tumors. Lesions in the lower limbs occur in females more frequently than in males, while lesions in the upper extremities or head are more frequent in males. ALM occurs at any age, although it is commonest in the fourth to sixth decade of life. This tumor may arise anywhere in the body, but it is most frequently observed in the extremities, followed by the head and trunk. The lesion is typically centered in the subcutis and less often in the dermis. Clinically, ALM presents as a solitary, small (usually <2 cm), slow-growing firm nodule, with pain being present in more than half of patients (often provoked by exposure to cold or pressure, pregnancy, or menses). Other painful superficial nodules are glomus tumor, traumatic neuroma, eccrine spiradenoma, and angiolipoma.

Magnetic resonance imaging shows mixed hyperintense and isointense areas on T2-weighted images, the hyperintense areas being significantly enhanced after intravenous contrast administration.

Etiology and Predisposition

Epstein-Barr virus (EBV) infection in immunocompromised patients has been associated with ALM.

Pathology

ALM is composed of well-differentiated smooth muscle cells arranged around many vascular channels. Mitotic figures are usually absent or very scarce. Histological variants include solid ALM (about two thirds of cases, with closely packed smooth muscle cells), venous ALM (about one fourth of cases, with variably gaping venous lumina surrounded by thick muscular coats), and cavernous ALM (about 10% of cases, with dilated vascular channels with thin or thick walls between septa composed of smooth muscle, somewhat simulating cavernous hemangioma).

Of note, a morphological continuum exists between ALM and myopericytoma (→ see dedicated section).

Differential diagnosis may be needed with the following: angiomyolipoma (prominent adipose tissue component; HMB45 positive) and leiomyoma (no prominent vascular component).

Biomarkers

Tumor cells are consistently positive for SMA,[1] MSA,[2] and calponin and variably positive for h-caldesmon, desmin, and vimentin. ALM stains negative for HMB45 and estrogen receptor.

Genetic analysis has demonstrated that most ALM cases are diploid.

Prognosis

ALM is a benign tumor.

Therapy

Surgical excision is the treatment of choice.

Suggested Readings

Chang (2019) Pericytes in sarcomas and other mesenchymal tumors. Adv Exp Med Biol 1147:109–124
Fletcher (2013) WHO classification of tumours of soft tissue and bone, 4th edn
Hong (2017) A case report of angioleiomyoma of uterus. Obstet Gynecol Sci 60(5):494–497
Rawal (2018) Angioleiomyoma (vascular leiomyoma) of the oral cavity. Head Neck Pathol 12(1):123–126

---

[1] SMA: smooth muscle actin.

[2] MSA: muscle-specific actin.

Definition

This is a benign neoplasm of adipocytic origin. An intramuscular or parenchymal/visceral lesion (previously known as infiltrating angiolipoma) is a different neoplasm composed of larger vessels and is more appropriately considered to be a hemangioma (→ see dedicated section).

Epidemiology and Presentation

Angiolipoma is a common soft tissue tumor that most frequently occurs in the late teens or early adulthood. It is more common in males than in females. The typical site is the subcutis of the extremities, but the trunk can also be involved. Visceral and spinal cases have been reported. Superficial lesions can be painful.

Etiology and Predisposition

Although multiple angiolipomas most often occur sporadically, a family history can be identified in a minority of cases (approximately 5%). **Familial angiolipomatosis** (also known as familial multiple angiolipomatosis) is a rare condition with an autosomal dominant transmission pattern that is characterized by multiple subcutaneous tumors and a family history of similar lesions, which are not associated with malignant neoplasms. Familial angiolipomatosis might be regarded as a subtype of familial multiple lipomatosis (→ see section entitled "Lipomatosis"). Familial angiolipomatosis may need to be differentiated from neurofibromatosis type 1 (→ see section entitled "Neurofibroma"): thus, in cases of multiple subcutaneous tumors and a family history of similar lesions, histologic examination is important to establish the correct diagnosis.

Pathology

Angiolipoma typically consists of mature adipocytes and thin-walled capillary-sized vessels, which often contain fibrin thrombi.

Differential diagnosis may be needed with Kaposi sarcoma and angiosarcoma (not circumscribed, usually not subcutaneous, atypia present, no scattered adipocytes).

Biomarkers

No informative immunostaining pattern is available. Angiolipoma is characterized by a normal karyotype.

Prognosis

It is a benign lesion with no tendency to recur. Malignant transformation has not been reported.

Therapy

Surgical excision is the treatment of choice.

Suggested Readings

Abbasi (2007) Familial multiple angiolipomatosis. Dermatol Online J 13(1):3
Cohen (2019) Painful tumors of the skin: "calm hog fled pen and gets back". Clin Cosmet Investig Dermatol 12:123–132
Fletcher (2013) WHO classification of tumours of soft tissue and bone, 4th edn
Garib (2015) Autosomal-dominant familial angiolipomatosis. Cutis 95(1):E26–E29
Kamata (2019) Bronchial angiolipoma successfully treated by sleeve resection of the right bronchus intermedius: a case report. BMC Surg 9(1):13
Kumar (1989) Autosomal dominant inheritance in familial angiolipomatosis. Clin Genet 35(3):202–204
Shen (2019) PET/CT and MR features of infiltrating spinal angiolipoma. Clin Nucl Med 44(3):e148–e150
Yasuda (2020) String-like symptomatic angiolipoma of the esophagus. Dig Endosc 32(3):437

Definition

Angiomatoid fibrous histiocytoma (AFH) is a soft tissue tumor of uncertain differentiation and intermediate malignant potential. It is also referred to as angiomatoid malignant fibrous histiocytoma.

Epidemiology and Presentation

Incidence peaks in the first two decades of life, with no gender differences. AFH locates in the subcutis, extremities being the most common sites. Many cases occur in regions where lymph nodes are normally sited, such as antecubital fossa, popliteal fossa, axilla, inguinal area, and neck.

It typically presents as a painless superficial soft tissue lump (median diameter: 2 cm), sometimes mimicking a hematoma or a hemangioma. It has been very rarely reported in deep sites (e.g., retroperitoneum, mediastinum, omentum). Systemic symptoms, such as fever, anemia, and weight loss, occasionally occur and appear to be mediated by overexpression of cytokine interleukin-6 (IL-6).

An AFH-like lesion has been (very rarely) reported to occur intracranially: this tumor shows low proliferation indices, frequently has a connection with the dura, and bears recurrent EWSR1 rearrangements; some investigators have recently proposed to term this lesion "intracranial myxoid mesenchymal tumor with EWSR1-CREB family gene fusions."

Pathology

Four morphological features (which can be present in varying proportions) characterize AFH: (1) nodules of either spindle or more histiocytoid cells, with a distinctive syncytial growth (most consistent feature); (2) pseudoangiomatous spaces filled

© The Editor(s) (if applicable) and The Author(s), under exclusive license to
Springer Nature Switzerland AG 2021
S. Mocellin, *Soft Tissue Tumors*, https://doi.org/10.1007/978-3-030-58710-9_22

with blood and surrounded by neoplastic cells; (3) thick fibrous pseudocapsule with significant hemosiderin deposition; and (4) pericapsular rim of lymphoplasmacytic cells with occasional germinal centers (resembling a lymph node metastasis).

Tumor cells may have moderate pleomorphism and mitotic activity.

Differential diagnosis may be needed with the following: inflammatory granuloma (no vascular spaces); aneurysmal fibrous histiocytoma (no pseudocapsule, no inflammatory cells, desmin negative); spindle cell hemangioma (poorly circumscribed); Kaposi sarcoma (slit-like blood-filled spaces, positive for CD34 and HHV8 positive); follicular dendritic cell sarcoma (positive for CD21 and CD35); Ewing sarcoma (although the classic form is morphologically distinct from AFH, atypical variants can resemble AFH, and biomarkers such as CD99 and EWSR1 fusion genes are not useful as they are shared by both diseases); rhabdomyosarcoma (it occurs deeply; infiltrative growth, no peripheral lymphoid cuff, rhabdomyoblasts in embryonal RMS, alveolar architecture in alveolar RMS, positive for myogenin and MyoD1); angiosarcoma (endothelial tufting present, positive for CD31 and CD34, negative for desmin); malignant extrarenal rhabdoid tumor (younger age, sheets of large polygonal cells, poorly circumscribed and infiltrative growth, cytokeratin positive, INI1/SMARCB1 loss); undifferentiated pleomorphic sarcoma (it occurs deeply in older patients; no fusion genes); metastatic lymph node (true lymph node architecture, atypical tumor cells, history of primary malignancy, positive for primary malignancy biomarkers such as cytokeratins); and myoepithelial tumors of soft tissues (often positive for EMA, coexistence of S100 and cytokeratins; EWSR1 rearrangements can be shared).

Biomarkers

AFH stains positive for desmin, EMA,[1] CD68, and CD99 in about 50% of cases. Tumor cells can also express IL-6. AFH stains consistently negative for S100 protein, CD21, CD35, CD34, and cytokeratins.

AFH is characterized by the presence of the chromosomal translocation t(2;22) (q33;q12), resulting in the **EWSR1-CREB1 fusion gene**[2] in more than 90% of cases. Rarely, other gene rearrangements have been described, such as FUS-ATF1

---

[1] EMA: epithelial membrane antigen.

[2] EWSR1-CREB1 fusion gene: EWSR1 encodes for an RNA-binding protein and is involved in the recurrent translocations associated with a number of soft tissue tumors other than angiomatoid fibrous histiocytoma such as the Ewing family of tumors, desmoplastic small round cell tumor, extraskeletal myxoid chondrosarcoma, myxoid liposarcoma (rarely), and clear cell sarcoma. CREB1 (cyclic AMP responsive-binding protein) encodes a basic leucine zipper transcription factor that is involved in cAMP and calcium-induced transcriptional activation. The EWSR1-CREB1 chimeric protein is believed to play a key role in oncogenesis. In particular, the formation of the EWSR1-CREB1 fusion gene leads to continuous activation of CREB1 and IL-6 production, because the promoter region of IL-6 has a CREB binding site. IL-6 might be responsible of both paraneoplastic syndrome and tumor growth (by means of an autocrine loop).

fusion gene and EWSR1-ATF1 fusion gene (from t(12;22)(q13;q12)). Detection of these fusion genes can be useful for differential diagnosis purposes.

Prognosis

AFH can recur locally in up to 10–20% of cases; lymph node metastasis has been reported in 2–4% of cases, whereas deaths attributable to distant metastases have been only very rarely reported (the outcome of patients with distant metastasis is generally fatal). No clinical or pathological prognostic factors have been so far identified.

Therapy

Surgery (wide excision) is the treatment of choice for primary tumor. **Target therapy** with tocilizumab[3] has been utilized in a couple of patients with promising results in terms of control of both paraneoplastic syndrome and tumor growth.

Suggested Readings

Akiyama (2015) Paraneoplastic syndrome of angiomatoid fibrous histiocytoma may be caused by EWSR1-CREB1 fusion-induced excessive interleukin-6 production. J Pediatr Hematol Oncol 37(7):554–559

Bale (2018) Intracranial myxoid mesenchymal tumors with EWSR1-CREB family gene fusions: myxoid variant of angiomatoid fibrous histiocytoma or novel entity? Brain Pathol 28(2):183–191

Ballester (2020) Intracranial myxoid mesenchymal tumor with EWSR1-ATF1 fusion. J Neuropathol Exp Neurol 79(3):347–351

Fletcher (2013) WHO classification of tumours of soft tissue and bone, 4th edn

Khan (2019) Primary adrenal angiomatoid fibrous histiocytoma with novel EWSR1-ATF1 gene fusion exon-exon breakpoint. Pediatr Dev Pathol 22(5):472–474

Potter (2018) Therapeutic response of metastatic angiomatoid fibrous histiocytoma carrying EWSR1-CREB1 fusion to the interleukin-6 receptor antibody tocilizumab. Pediatr Blood Cancer 65(10):e27291

Thway (2015) Angiomatoid fibrous histiocytoma: the current status of pathology and genetics. Arch Pathol Lab Med 139(5):674–682

Villiger (2014) A simple Baker's cyst? Tocilizumab remits paraneoplastic signs and controls growth of IL-6-producing angiomatoid malignant fibrous histiocytoma. Rheumatology (Oxford) 53(7):1350–1352

Yoshida (2019) Expanding the phenotypic spectrum of mesenchymal tumors harboring the EWSR1-CREM fusion. Am J Surg Pathol 43(12):1622–1630

---

[3] Tocilizumab: monoclonal antibody blocking IL6R (interleukin-6 receptor).

Definition

Angiomyofibroblastoma (AMF) is a benign tumor classified among the fibroblastic-myofibroblastic tumors.

Epidemiology and Presentation

AMF is an uncommon lesion (the incidence is estimated to equal that of aggressive angiomyxoma) arising mainly in women between menarche and menopause. Almost all cases develop in the perineal subcutaneous tissue (the majority in the vulva; only 10% of cases in the vagina). The lesion presents as a slow-growing, painless and well-circumscribed nodule (usually <5 cm), often erroneously confused with cyst of the Bartholin's gland in the vulvar location.

Pathology

The lesion displays prominent small, thin-walled and ectatic vessels located in abundant loose stroma. Tumor cells are round to spindled and are characteristically located around the vessels. Mitoses are rare; necrosis and atypia are absent. Multinucleate tumor cells are common. Rare cases display a morphological appearance mimicking aggressive angiomyxoma.

Differential diagnosis may be needed with the following: aggressive angiomyxoma (not circumscribed, >5 cm, less cellular, less vascular, but vessels are large and thick walled; stromal mucin and red blood cells extravasation are present; infrequent plump stromal cells); cellular angiofibroma (more cellular uniformly, perivascular hyalinization and large, thick-walled vessels; usually desmin negative); and epithelioid leiomyoma (more cellular, no biphasic pattern, usually no binucleation).

© The Editor(s) (if applicable) and The Author(s), under exclusive license to
Springer Nature Switzerland AG 2021

S. Mocellin, *Soft Tissue Tumors*, https://doi.org/10.1007/978-3-030-58710-9_23

Biomarkers

Tumor cells are positive for desmin, estrogen receptor, and progesterone receptor, while they usually stain negative (sometimes focally positive) for SMA[1] and MSA.[2] Of note, desmin staining may be weak or absent in postmenopausal cases.

Prognosis

AMF is a benign tumor with excellent prognosis.

Therapy

Surgical excision is the treatment of choice.

Suggested Readings

Eckhardt (2018) Vaginal angiomyofibroblastoma: a case report and review of diagnostic imaging. Case Rep Obstet Gynecol 2018:7397121
Fletcher (2013) WHO classification of tumours of soft tissue and bone, 4th edn
Monib (2019) Massive angiomyofibroblastoma of the glans penis. BMJ Case Rep 12(6):e229486

---

[1] SMA: smooth muscle actin.
[2] MSA: muscle-specific actin.

Definition

Angiomyolipoma (AML) is a benign neoplasm and is a member of the perivascular epithelioid cell tumor (PEComa) family (for details → see section entitled "PEComa").

Epidemiology and Presentation

AML most frequently occurs in the kidney (where it is the most common benign tumor), the most frequent extrarenal site being the adrenals (other sites: liver and lymph nodes, ovary). Sporadic cases are generally diagnosed in middle age adults, with a female prevalence. It accounts for about 1% of all resected renal tumors. The neoplasm is generally asymptomatic (it is often discovered as an incidentaloma); flank pain and hematuria may be present. AML may coexist with renal cell carcinoma (especially clear cell carcinoma); the tumor diameter ranges from 1 to 25 cm (mean: 6 cm). AML is usually unilateral and unifocal: multiple or bilateral tumors suggest underlying tuberous sclerosis.

Radiological imaging (magnetic resonance and computed tomography) is often sufficient to make the diagnosis (with special regard to the characteristic appearance with fat content in the classic variant), although definitive diagnosis may require pathology assessment (with special regard to the rare epithelioid variant).

Etiology and Predisposition

Although most AMLs occur sporadically, approximately 20% of patients with AML have tuberous sclerosis complex (TSC), a hereditary syndrome caused by germline variation in the TSC1 or TSC2 genes. For more details on TSC, → see section entitled "PEComa." TSC-related AML occurs in younger patients (without gender predilection) and grows at a faster pace as compared to sporadic AML. Moreover, TSC-associated AML is more likely to have an epithelioid component than sporadic AML. Beginning in childhood, up to 80% of TSC patients develop renal angiomyolipoma. In adult TSC patients, renal complications are the leading cause of death.

Pathology

Macroscopically, the lesion is circumscribed but not encapsulated with a pushing border; the cut surface can have red (vascular component), gray-white (smooth muscle component), or yellow (adipose component) appearance; despite the benign nature, AML may involve the intrarenal venous system, the renal vein, or the vena cava.

Microscopically, the classic triphasic variant is composed of thick dysmorphic blood vessels, smooth muscle, and adipose tissue (the amount of each component is variable). The smooth muscle component may be hypercellular, atypical, pleomorphic, or epithelioid; the vascular component is made of thick-walled hyalinized vessels; the fat component is made of mature adipose tissue and is found in more than 90% of cases. The so-called epithelioid angiomyolipoma is characterized by a pure or predominant population of polygonal cell with clear or densely eosinophilic cytoplasm and large hyperchromatic bizarre nuclei, multinucleation hemorrhage mitotic figures, and necrosis being common.

Differential diagnosis may be needed with the following: renal cell carcinoma, clear cell type (positive for cytokeratins, PAX8, and CAIX; negative for SMA and usually negative for melanocytic biomarkers); well-differentiated liposarcoma (no vascular component, negative for melanocytic markers and SMA; MDM2 amplification); leiomyoma (no vascular or adipose component, negative for melanocytic biomarkers); leiomyosarcoma (prominent atypia, infiltrative, usually no vascular or adipose component; negative for melanocytic biomarkers); pleomorphic rhabdomyosarcoma (smooth muscle component is markedly atypical, tumor is infiltrative, no vascular or adipose component; negative for melanocytic biomarkers); melanoma (marked atypia, no adipose or vascular component; negative for SMA); and adrenal cortical carcinoma (usually abundant mitotic figures and marked pleomorphism; it may be positive for Melan-A but is positive also for inhibin and calretinin and negative for S100, HMB45, and SMA).

Biomarkers

AML is characterized by the coexpression of melanocytic (HMB45, MART1/Melan-A) and smooth muscle (MSA, SMA) biomarkers; S100 is positive in the fat component. It negatively stains for cytokeratins, PAX8, CAIX, GATA3, and inhibin.

Prognosis

AML is considered a benign neoplasm. However, retroperitoneal hemorrhage is an important complication which can be deadly (the risk of bleeding is proportional to the lesion size). Moreover, epithelioid AML (though rare) may show an aggressive behavior with distant metastasis and mortality.

Therapy

Active surveillance is the suggested management for small AML. Clinical intervention is mainly indicated when there is a substantial risk of rupture. Minimally invasive therapies including **surgery** (partial nephrectomy) and transcatheter **arterial embolization**, as well as **target therapy** with mammalian target of rapamycin (mTOR) inhibitors (e.g., everolimus), are employed for patients who require treatment.

Neoadjuvant treatment with mTOR inhibitors may be utilized to make partial nephrectomy feasible.

Especially in TSC patients, treatment with mTOR inhibitors has become the key strategy to reduce the need of preventive embolization or even partial nephrectomy and ultimately to preserve kidney function.

Different algorithms have been proposed to select patients who should go intervention: generally, treatment intervention is recommended (even in asymptomatic cases) for TSC-associated AML greater than 3 cm and in sporadic AML greater than 4–5 cm in size.

Suggested Readings

Anis (2020) Selective arterial embolization for large or symptomatic renal angiomyolipoma: 10 years of follow-up. Urology 135:82–87

Brakemeier (2017) Treatment of renal angiomyolipoma in tuberous sclerosis complex (TSC) patients. Pediatr Nephrol 32(7):1137–1144

Cao (2020) The independent indicators for differentiating renal cell carcinoma from renal angiomyolipoma by contrast-enhanced ultrasound. BMC Med Imaging 20(1):32

Flum (2016) Update on the diagnosis and management of renal angiomyolipoma. J Urol 195(4 Pt 1):834–846

Guo (2019) Application of everolimus in preoperative neoadjuvant therapy of tuberous sclerosis complex associated with renal angiomyolipoma: a single-center report of 5 cases. Clin Genitourin Cancer 17(6):e1099–e1103

Naito (2020) Identification of a specific ultrasonographic finding for differentiating hepatic angiomyolipoma from hepatocellular carcinoma. Clin Imaging 59(2):104–108

Swärd (2020) Renal angiomyolipoma-patient characteristics and treatment with focus on active surveillance. Scand J Urol 54(2):141–146

Wu (2020) Fate of pediatric renal angiomyolipoma during mTOR inhibitor treatment in tuberous sclerosis complex. Urology 139:161–167

Ye (2020) Differentiation between fat-poor angiomyolipoma and clear cell renal cell carcinoma: qualitative and quantitative analysis using arterial spin labeling MR imaging. Abdom Radiol 45(2):512–519

Definition

Angiosarcoma (AS) is a malignant tumor of vascular origin. It is also known as hemangiosarcoma, malignant hemangioendothelioma, malignant angioendothelioma, lymphedema-associated angiosarcoma, and lymphangiosarcoma.

Epidemiology and Presentation

AS accounts for 1–3% of all soft tissue sarcomas and can affect patients of all ages although the incidence peak in the seventh decade of life, with a male predominance. Its annual incidence has been estimated to be one case for every million people.

The primary sites of angiosarcoma include the skin (the most frequent site, the head and neck being the most common cutaneous site), breast (→ see section entitled "Breast Angiosarcoma"), soft tissue, viscera (especially liver and spleen; → see section entitled "Hepatic Angiosarcoma"), and bone. Clinical presentation varies considerably depending on the primary site: cutaneous AS presents as bruise-like patches, violaceous nodules, or plaques, whereas AS of soft tissue presents as an enlarged painful mass of deep muscles of the lower extremities (approximately 40% of cases) or as a mass of retroperitoneum, mediastinum, or mesentery; the clinical presentation of visceral AS is variable depending on the organ involved. Since extensive hemorrhage is commonly present, the lesion can be confused with a hematoma.

Etiology and Predisposition

Although its etiology is unknown in most cases (**primary angiosarcoma**), a subset of AS is associated with specific risk factors (**secondary angiosarcoma**). In particular, secondary AS is associated with exposure to ionizing radiation (mainly

S. Mocellin, *Soft Tissue Tumors*, https://doi.org/10.1007/978-3-030-58710-9_25

breast AS after radiotherapy for breast carcinoma, which has been reported to occur in approximately 1 out of 1000 cases even 20 years after exposure), ultraviolet radiation (occurs mainly on the scalp of elderly men), chronic lymphedema (due to lymphadenectomy or lymphatic diseases such as filariasis; the AS lymphedema association is known as Stewart-Treves syndrome), and chemicals such as vinyl chloride (utilized in the production of PVC; it has been associated with the development of hepatic AS) and thorotrast (utilized as contrast agent in radiology, it has been associated with hepatic AS).

Li-Fraumeni syndrome (LFS) has been associated with an increased risk of angiosarcoma in multiple locations such as the liver, spleen, breast, head and neck, and (rarely) heart. In most cases (80%), LFS is triggered by the germline mutations in the TP53 tumor suppressor gene (encoding the p53 protein). The estimated prevalence of causal deleterious germline TP53 mutations is approximately 1/20,000. The lifetime risk of cancer in LFS is about 70% for men and close to 100% for women. Typical cancers observed in LFS include early-onset breast cancer, adrenal cortical carcinoma, soft tissue and bone sarcomas (especially rhabdomyosarcoma and osteosarcoma), and brain tumors (choroid plexus carcinoma, astrocytoma, medulloblastoma, and glioblastoma). LFS is inherited in an autosomal dominant pattern; most patients with LFS inherit an altered copy of the gene from an affected parent: In 7–20% of cases, however, the altered gene is the result of a new mutation in the gene that occurred during the formation of reproductive cells or very early in development. For a cancer to develop in LFS, a somatic mutation involving the other copy of the TP53 gene must occur, according to the classical Knudson two-hit hypothesis.

Recently, a germline missense variant (p.R117C) in the POT1 gene (encoding protection of telomeres 1, a protein involved in telomere maintenance) has been proven to be responsible for cardiac angiosarcoma, a very rare malignant tumor that represents <10% of cardiac malignancies.

Pathology

Macroscopically it usually presents as multinodular hemorrhagic and necrotic nodules. Microscopically AS shows a variety morphological appearances ranging from areas of well-formed anastomosing vessels with limited cell atypia to solid sheets of high-grade epithelioid or spindled cells without clear formation of vessels composed of high-grade spindled and epithelioid cells (multiple patterns may be present in the same lesion, which calls for accurate tumor sampling). An AS with predominant epithelioid cells is called epithelioid angiosarcoma, which can be misdiagnosed as a carcinoma because of morphological and immunophenotypical commonalities. Most AS are high-grade tumors with brisk mitotic activity, coagulative necrosis, and marked nuclear atypia.

Differential diagnosis may be needed with other vascular lesions such as atypical post-radiation vascular proliferations (relatively common in radiated skin, can form an erythematous lesion, consists of dilated round or angulated vessels in the dermis lined by a single layer of endothelium that shows mild/absent cytological atypia without mitoses), Kaposi sarcoma (HHV8 positive), and papillary endothelial hyperplasia (also known as Masson tumor, a non-neoplastic benign intravascular lesion only, with papillary formations with hyaline or fibrous stalks, anastomosing vascular channels, plump endothelial cells; no necrosis, no atypia, no atypical mitotic figures).

Biomarkers

AS expresses typical vascular biomarkers (e.g., CD34, CD31, ERG, FLI1) and occasionally lymphatic biomarkers (e.g., podoplanin). Epithelioid AS can coexpress epithelial antigens (e.g., cytokeratins, EMA), which should be kept in mind for differential diagnosis with carcinomas. Immunostaining for HHV8 is negative (which is helpful to differentiate AS from Kaposi sarcoma).

AS has not been associated with specific genetic alterations except for high-level **MYC gene amplification** (chromosome 8q24),[1] which is a consistent hallmark of radiation-induced and lymphedema-associated AS.

Prognosis

AS is a high-grade malignancy associated with high rates of disease recurrence (70%) and mortality (50%), representing the most aggressive type of all vascular malignancies (once metastasized the median survival is 4–12 months). Negative prognostic factors are the following: older age, retroperitoneal location, large size, high mitotic rate, necrosis, and epithelioid subtype. In the light of the high metastatic potential, thoraco-abdominal computed tomography scan coupled with central nervous system magnetic resonance imaging is suggested for staging purposes.

Therapy

Surgery (wide excision) is the mainstay of treatment for localized primary AS, although ill-defined margins can make radical surgery a challenging task; in order to maximize the curative intent, large skin removal may be needed, which may require plastic surgery techniques to repair cutaneous defects. In order to improve local disease control, adjuvant **radiotherapy** is often delivered. Definitive

---

[1] MYC: this is a proto-oncogene and encodes a nuclear phosphoprotein (c-Myc) that plays a key role in cell cycle progression, apoptosis, and cellular transformation. The encoded protein forms a heterodimer with the related transcription factor MAX: then, this complex binds to the E-box DNA consensus sequence and regulates the transcription of specific target genes. Amplification of this gene is frequently observed in numerous human cancers, including radiation-induced angiosarcoma. Translocations involving this gene are associated with Burkitt lymphoma and multiple myeloma.

radiotherapy has been also utilized as the only treatment for patients unsuitable for surgery; the combination of radiotherapy plus chemotherapy has been proposed as an alternative to surgery. Other **locoregional treatments** such as electrochemotherapy and isolated limb perfusion are available for the control of localized disease not amenable to surgery.

Patients with locally advanced or metastatic disease are treated with systemic **chemotherapy**; beside the "pan-sarcoma" doxorubicin (which—however—has not been evaluated in prospective studies dedicated to AS), there is prospective non-randomized evidence supporting the use of paclitaxel (often considered as first-line treatment). **Targeted therapy** with multikinase small molecule inhibitors such as sunitinib[2] and sorafenib[3] has been tested in the clinical setting with some benefit. Despite some promising results in non-randomized studies of bevacizumab[4] as a single agent, a randomized trial of paclitaxel with or without bevacizumab showed no difference between the study arms. Pazopanib[5] is approved for the second-line treatment of metastatic soft tissue sarcomas based on the results of the PALETTE randomized controlled trial that included patients with AS. Attempts to identify biomarkers predictive of response to target therapy are underway. PIK3CA-activating mutations[6] have been recently reported in AS, which suggests a therapeutic rationale for the use of PI3K inhibitors already available in the clinical setting (e.g., alpelisib, currently approved for breast cancer treatment). Also in the light of the high tumor mutation burden that can be found in this tumor, **immunotherapy** with anti-PD1 checkpoint inhibitors is being tested in patients with AS, with some encouraging results.

Suggested Readings

Agulnik (2013) An open-label, multicenter, phase II study of bevacizumab for the treatment of angiosarcoma and epithelioid hemangioendotheliomas. Ann Oncol 24(1):257–263

Calvete (2015) A mutation in the POT1 gene is responsible for cardiac angiosarcoma in TP53-negative Li-Fraumeni-like families. Nat Commun 6:8383

---

[2] Sunitinib: tyrosine kinase inhibitor targeting the following: PDGFR, VEGFR, KIT, FLT3, CSF1R, RET.

[3] Sorafenib: tyrosine kinase inhibitor targeting the following: BRAF, KIT, RET, FGFR1, FLT3, VEGFR1, VEGFR2, VEGFR3, PDGFRB.

[4] Bevacizumab: monoclonal antibody blocking VEGFA (vascular endothelial growth factor A).

[5] Pazopanib: tyrosine kinase inhibitor targeting the following: VEGFR, PDGFR, KIT.

[6] PIK3CA: this gene encodes for phosphatidylinositol-4,5-bisphosphate 3-kinase catalytic subunit alpha, the catalytic subunit of phosphatidylinositol 3-kinase (PI3K) that phosphorylates phosphatidylinositol to generate phosphatidylinositol 3,4,5-trisphosphate (PIP3), which is dephosphorylated by the protein product of tumor suppressor gene PTEN (a negative regulator of the PI3K-AKT pathway). PIP3 plays a key role by recruiting PH domain-containing proteins to the membrane, including AKT1 and PDPK1, activating signaling cascades involved in cell growth, survival, proliferation, motility, and morphology in response to various growth factors (e.g., EGF, insulin, IGF1, VEGFA, and PDGF). PIK3CA is the most recurrently mutated gene in breast cancer and has been found to important in a number of cancer types (PIK3CA is considered an oncogene).

Campana (2016) Angiosarcoma on lymphedema (Stewart-Treves syndrome): a 12-year follow-up after isolated limb perfusion, limb infusion, and electrochemotherapy. J Vasc Interv Radiol 27(3):444–446

Campana (2019) Electrochemotherapy for advanced cutaneous angiosarcoma: a European register-based cohort study from the International Network for Sharing Practices of electrochemotherapy (InspECT). Int J Surg 72:34–42

Fletcher (2020) WHO classification of tumours of soft tissue and bone, 5th edn

Florou (2019) Angiosarcoma patients treated with immune checkpoint inhibitors: a case series of seven patients from a single institution. J Immunother Cancer 7(1):213

Fujisawa (2014) Chemoradiotherapy with taxane is superior to conventional surgery and radiotherapy in the management of cutaneous angiosarcoma: a multicentre, retrospective study. Br J Dermatol 171(6):1493–1500

Guida (2016) Local treatment with electrochemotherapy of superficial angiosarcomas: efficacy and safety results from a multi-institutional retrospective study. J Surg Oncol 114(2):246–253

Habeeb (2019) The molecular diagnostics of vascular neoplasms. Surg Pathol Clin 12(1):35–49

Italiano (2012) Comparison of doxorubicin and weekly paclitaxel efficacy in metastatic angiosarcomas. Cancer 118(13):3330–3336

Kollár (2017) Pazopanib in advanced vascular sarcomas: an EORTC soft tissue and bone sarcoma group (STBSG) retrospective analysis. Acta Oncol 56(1):88–92

Mito (2019) Radiation-associated sarcomas: an update on clinical, histologic, and molecular features. Surg Pathol Clin 12(1):139–148

Momen (2019) Dramatic response of metastatic cutaneous angiosarcoma to an immune checkpoint inhibitor in a patient with xeroderma pigmentosum: whole-genome sequencing aids treatment decision in end-stage disease. Cold Spring Harb Mol Case Stud 5(5):a004408

Painter (2020) The angiosarcoma project: enabling genomic and clinical discoveries in a rare cancer through patient-partnered research. Nat Med 26(2):181–187

Papke (2020) What is new in endothelial neoplasia? Virchows Arch 476(1):17–28

Penel (2008) Phase II trial of weekly paclitaxel for unresectable angiosarcoma: the ANGIOTAX study. J Clin Oncol 26(32):5269–5274

Radaelli (2014) Emerging therapies for adult soft tissue sarcoma. Expert Rev Anticancer Ther 14(6):689–704

Ravi (2016) Antitumor response of VEGFR2- and VEGFR3-amplified angiosarcoma to Pazopanib. J Natl Compr Cancer Netw 14(5):499–502

Ray-Coquard (2015) Paclitaxel given once per week with or without bevacizumab in patients with advanced angiosarcoma: a randomized phase II trial. J Clin Oncol 33(25):2797–2802

Rombouts (2019) Assessment of radiotherapy-associated angiosarcoma after breast cancer treatment in a Dutch population-based study. JAMA Oncol 5(2):267–269

Shon (2019) Epithelioid vascular tumors: a review. Adv Anat Pathol 26(3):186–197

Steininger (2019) Masson's tumor of the breast: rare differential for new or recurrent breast cancer-case report, pathology, and review of the literature. Breast J 26(4):752–754

van der Graaf (2012) Pazopanib for metastatic soft-tissue sarcoma (PALETTE): a randomised, double-blind, placebo-controlled phase 3 trial. Lancet 379(9829):1879–1886

Weidema (2019) Targeting angiosarcomas of the soft tissues: a challenging effort in a heterogeneous and rare disease. Crit Rev Oncol Hematol 138:120–131

Yamamoto (2010) Histological type of thorotrast-induced liver tumors associated with the translocation of deposited radionuclides. Cancer Sci 101(2):336–340

Definition

Angiomatosis is a benign lesion of vascular origin. Although included in the World Health Organization (WHO) classification of benign tumors, it is unclear whether it should be considered a neoplasm or a malformation. It is also known as soft tissue angiomatosis and angiomatosis of soft tissue. It can be considered a subtype of hemangioma (→ see dedicated section) of the soft tissues extended to large segments of body.

Angiomatosis is considered as a "provisionally unclassified" vascular anomaly by the International Society for the Study of Vascular Anomalies (ISSVA).

Epidemiology and Presentation

Angiomatosis is a rare condition affecting a large segment (many centimeters) of the body and involving (multiple) muscles and (generally secondarily) the skin/subcutis. About two thirds of cases present in the first two decades of life with no significant gender differences. More than 50% of cases occur in the lower extremity, followed by the chest wall, abdomen, and upper extremity. Most lesions are likely congenital but, due to their deep location, they become apparent later on during adolescence or adulthood. Patients typically complain about swelling of the affected part, which can vary in size and especially during exercise.

The arterial component may be evidenced by images on Doppler ultrasound: high-flow hemodynamic features can rule out slow-flow intramuscular vascular anomalies such as venous malformations and fibro-adipose vascular anomaly (FAVA, a condition known to be related to somatic variations in the PIK3CA gene), although can be confused with other high-flow lesions (e.g., arteriovenous malformations).

Magnetic resonance imaging generally shows an ill-defined T2-hyperintense infiltrative lesion with adipocytic component.

© The Editor(s) (if applicable) and The Author(s), under exclusive license to
Springer Nature Switzerland AG 2021
S. Mocellin, *Soft Tissue Tumors*, https://doi.org/10.1007/978-3-030-58710-9_26

Etiology and Predisposition

Angiomatosis corresponds to PTEN hamartoma of soft tissue (PHOST) in the context of **PTEN hamartoma tumor syndrome** (PHTS), a disease inherited in an autosomal dominant pattern that gathers together several related conditions caused by mutations in the PTEN gene[1] (e.g., **Bannayan-Riley-Ruvalcaba syndrome** and **Cowden syndrome**) and is characterized by the growth of multiple hamartomas and an increased risk of developing certain malignancies (e.g., breast, thyroid, and endometrial cancer). However, angiomatosis can be observed in patients who do not display the clinical features of PHTS: non-PHTS cases of angiomatosis are likely to be caused by somatic mutations in the PIK3CA gene. Interestingly, somatic activating variations of the PIK3CA gene have been described in CLOVES syndrome (characterized by overgrowth of adipose tissue in the abdomen that is often associated with a reddish birthmark on the skin over it, in addition to blood vessel, skin, and bone abnormalities), Klippel-Trenaunay syndrome (characterized by red birthmark called "port-wine stain," abnormal overgrowth of soft tissues such as skin and muscles, as well as bones and vein malformations), and various vascular anomalies, where they resulted in a broad spectrum of tissue abnormalities referred to as "PIK3CA-related overgrowth syndromes," including venous malformations, FAVA, and (rarely) arteovenous malformations.

Pathology

Histologically, angiomatosis is an ill-defined lesion presenting as an admixture of fibro-adipose tissue and a vascular component characterized by a diffuse proliferation of benign, architecturally well developed and mitotically quiescent blood vessels (a mixture of large arteries, veins, and small capillaries).

Due to the deep location, large size, ill-defined limits, and non-homogeneous composition with areas suggestive of an adipose component, clinical (radiological) and pathological **differential diagnosis** may be needed with the following: intramuscular vascular anomalies, infiltrating lipoma, myxolipoma, angiomyxolipoma, angiolipoma, intramuscular angioma, liposarcoma, and low-grade myxofibrosarcoma.

---

[1] PIK3CA encodes for phosphatidylinositol-4,5-bisphosphate 3-kinase catalytic subunit alpha, the catalytic subunit of phosphatidylinositol 3-kinase (PI3K) that phosphorylates phosphatidylinositol to generate phosphatidylinositol 3,4,5-trisphosphate (PIP3), which is dephosphorylated by the protein product of tumor suppressor gene PTEN (a negative regulator of the PI3K-AKT pathway). PIP3 plays a key role by recruiting PH domain-containing proteins to the membrane, including AKT1 and PDPK1, activating signaling cascades involved in cell growth, survival, proliferation, motility, and morphology in response to various growth factors (e.g., EGF, insulin, IGF1, VEGFA, and PDGF). PIK3CA is the most recurrently mutated gene in breast cancer and has been found to important in a number of cancer types (PIK3CA is considered an oncogene).

Biomarkers

Angiomatosis stains negative for GLUT1 (which is instead typically positive in infantile hemangioma, → see dedicated section).

Prognosis

Angiomatosis is biologically benign and does not spontaneously regress. Most lesions persist after surgical excision (due to their ill-defined limits which hamper a radical resection), and 50% of cases recur even multiple times.

Therapy

Surgical excision is the treatment of choice (when deemed necessary), but it is not always feasible in a conservative (function sparing) manner.

Suggested Readings

Aronniemi (2017) Angiomatosis of soft tissue as an important differential diagnosis for intramuscular venous malformations. Phlebology 32(7):474–481

Boccara (2020) Soft tissue angiomatosis: another PIK3CA-related disorder. Histopathology 76(4):540–549

Chism (2017) PTEN hamartoma of the soft tissue: the initial manifestation of an underlying PTEN hamartoma tumor syndrome in a 4-year-old female. Skeletal Radiol 46(11):1591–1595

Fletcher (2013) WHO classification of tumours of soft tissue and bone

Flors (2019) Soft-tissue vascular malformations and tumors. Part 1: classification, role of imaging and high-flow lesions. Radiologia 61(1):4–15

Kurek (2012) PTEN hamartoma of soft tissue: a distinctive lesion in PTEN syndromes. Am J Surg Pathol 36(5):671–687

Val-Bernal (2005) Soft-tissue angiomatosis in adulthood: a case in the forearm showing a prominent myxoid adipose tissue component mimicking liposarcoma. Pathol Int 55(3):155–159

Angiomyxoma is a benign soft tissue tumor. There are two types of angiomyxoma:

- Superficial angiomyxoma (also known as cutaneous angiomyxoma): → see dedicated section for more information.
- Deep angiomyxoma (also known as aggressive angiomyxoma): → see dedicated section for more information.

S. Mocellin, *Soft Tissue Tumors*, https://doi.org/10.1007/978-3-030-58710-9_27

Arteriovenous Malformation Hemangioma

28

Definition

Arteriovenous malformation hemangioma (AVMH) is a benign vascular lesion. This entity is recognized by the World Health Organization (WHO) but not by the International Society for the Study of Vascular Anomalies (ISSVA), which prefers to keep distinguished the arteriovenous malformations (characterized by the presence of arteriovenous shunts) from hemangiomas (where the shunts are absent). It is also known as arteriovenous hemangioma.

There are two AVMH variants: deep AVMH and superficial AVMH (also known as cutaneous AVMH, cirsoid aneurysm, and acral arteriovenous tumor). When this lesion involves multiple tissue planes, it is also referred to as "angiomatosis." Superficial AVMH resembling clinically and histologically Kaposi sarcoma is also known as pseudo-Kaposi sarcoma or acroangiodermatitis.

Epidemiology and Presentation

AVMH represent about 14% of all vascular anomalies in children. Although a large proportion of AVMH (especially deep AVMH) are congenital, acquired AVMH have been reported. Deep AVMH is less frequent than superficial AVMH and affects children and young adults. AVMH arises most commonly in the head and neck (including the brain), followed by the limbs. Other internal organs (e.g., lungs, uterus) may be involved. Patients with scalp AVMH often present with a slow-growing pulsatile nodule/papule/mass and may experience bleeding, tinnitus, and headache.

The presence of arteriovenous shunting is essential for the diagnosis and can be confirmed clinically by auscultation; however, angiography is usually needed to confirm the clinical suspicion.

Unlike infantile hemangioma (→ see dedicated section), AVMH does not regress spontaneously.

Etiology and Predisposition

AVMH is common in the lungs and brain of patients with **hereditary hemorrhagic telangiectasia** (HHT, also known as **Osler-Weber-Rendu syndrome**), a rare autosomal dominant genetic disorder characterized by vessel anomalies (i.e., telangiectasias, arteriovenous malformations) formation in the skin, mucous membranes (nasal, oral, gastrointestinal), and viscera (e.g., lungs, liver, and brain); more than 80% of all cases of HHT are due to mutations in one of two genes, ENG and ACVRL1.

Pathology

AVMH is characterized by large numbers of vessels of different sizes, including veins (more abundantly) and arteries. Areas mimicking a cavernous or capillary hemangioma can be present, as well as thrombosis and calcification. Recognition of arteriovenous shunts is difficult (elastin stains are helpful to distinguish arteries from veins), which is why radiological imaging remains a key diagnostic step.

Differential diagnosis may be needed with the following: Kaposi sarcoma (CD34 and HHV8 positive), venous hemangioma (venous vessels only), and infantile hemangioma (GLUT1 positive).

Biomarkers

No specific biomarkers are currently available.

Prognosis

Although AVMH is a benign condition, lesions large enough can lead to limb hypertrophy, heart failure, and consumption coagulopathy (Kasabach-Merritt syndrome). Moreover, both superficial and deep lesions may complicate with bleeding.

Therapy

Surgical excision may be difficult because of the extent of the lesion, which should be determined by angiographic imaging. Local recurrence is common just because of the difficulty to yield complete excision.

Suggested Readings

Adegboyega (2005) Hemangioma versus vascular malformation: presence of nerve bundle is a diagnostic clue for vascular malformation. Arch Pathol Lab Med 129(6):772–775

Chea (2019) Acroangiodermatitis of Mali and Stewart-Bluefarb syndrome. Cutis 103(6):336–339

Fletcher (2013). WHO classification of tumours of soft tissue and bone (4th edition)

Definition

Atypical fibrous histiocytoma (AFH) is an uncommon variant of benign fibrous histiocytoma of the skin ($\rightarrow$ see section entitled "Benign Fibrous Histiocytoma). It has been also named dermatofibroma with monster cells.

Epidemiology and Presentation

AFH affects people with a wide age range (5 to 90 years; median age: 38 years), without gender preference. The most commonly affected locations are the extremities, followed by trunk, head, neck, and genital areas. The lesion—located on the skin—ranges from 0.5 to 12 cm in greatest dimension.

Pathology

AFH presents as a dermis-centered proliferation of pleomorphic, spindle, and/or polyhedral cells with mainly large, hyperchromatic, irregular, or bizarre nuclei, set in a background of classic features of fibrous histiocytoma. Multinucleated giant cells (monster cells), pleomorphism, mitotic activity (from 1 to 15 per 10 HPF[1]), and atypical mitoses can be also variably present. Lesions with marked atypical features represent potential pitfalls for overinterpretation as pleomorphic sarcoma. Neither necrosis nor vascular invasion is observed.

Differential diagnosis may be necessary with the following: atypical fibroxanthoma (sun damaged areas of head and neck in elderly, no classic features of fibrous histiocytoma); dermatofibrosarcoma protuberans (strongly positive for CD34, no

---

[1] HPF: high-power field

S. Mocellin, *Soft Tissue Tumors*, https://doi.org/10.1007/978-3-030-58710-9_29

pleomorphism); pleomorphic sarcomas (infiltrative, marked atypia, brisk mitotic activity, necrosis, no classic features of fibrous histiocytoma); nodular melanoma (strongly positive for S100); and spindle cell squamous cell carcinoma (strongly positive for cytokeratins).

Biomarkers

AFH may stain positive for vimentin, factor XIII, and CD34. It stains negative for CD68, S100, desmin, cytokeratins, and EMA[2].

Prognosis

A benign outcome is expected in most cases. However, similar to the cellular and aneurysmal variants of fibrous histiocytoma, atypical fibrous histiocytoma shows a higher tendency to recur locally than ordinary fibrous histiocytoma (14% vs. 1–2%). AFH may rarely metastasize.

Therapy

Surgical wide excision is the treatment of choice.

Suggested Readings

Kaddu (2002) Atypical fibrous histiocytoma of the skin: clinicopathologic analysis of 59 cases with evidence of infrequent metastasis. Am J Surg Pathol 26(1):35–46
Wang (2014) Atypical fibrous histiocytoma arising in the perianal area: a case report and review of the literature. Am J Dermatopathol 36(2):171–173

---

[2] EMA: epithelial membrane antigen

Definition

Atypical fibroxanthoma (AFX) is a tumor of intermediate malignant potential classified among the soft tissue tumors of uncertain differentiation. The term "superficial malignant fibrous histiocytoma" should no longer be utilized.

It belongs to a group of atypical cutaneous spindle cell neoplasms referred to as the *SLAM*, which stands for *s*pindled squamous cell carcinoma, *l*eiomyosarcoma, AFX, and spindled *m*elanoma.

Epidemiology and Presentation

AFX is a dermal-based lesion that typically presents as a red or pink rapid-growing nodule or papule (sometimes ulcerated) or plaque arising on sun-damaged skin of elderly patients (men are affected much more frequently than women), with special regard to head and neck region (90% of cases). Usually the nodule measures less than two centimeters and is asymptomatic.

Dermoscopy reveals polymorphic vessels (linear, dotted, hairpin, arborescent, and/or highly tortuous vessels) radiating to the center of the lesion with intervening white areas.

The differential diagnosis includes basal cell carcinoma, squamous cell carcinoma, Merkel cell carcinoma, amelanotic melanoma, leiomyosarcoma, atypical dermatofibroma, pleomorphic dermal sarcoma, and metastasis from other malignancies.

S. Mocellin, *Soft Tissue Tumors*, https://doi.org/10.1007/978-3-030-58710-9_30

Etiology and Predisposition

AFX etiology is poorly understood. Ultraviolet light is believed to play an important role since most lesions appear on the sun-exposed head and neck area of Caucasian patients. The incidence is increased in immunosuppressed populations.

Pathology

AFX presents as a circumscribed dermal nodule usually within sun-damaged skin (elastosis). It is composed of spindled to round or epithelioid tumor cells organized in a fascicular pattern. Bizarre multinucleated pleomorphic cells are present. High mitotic rate and many atypical mitotic figures are also present. It closely resembles undifferentiated pleomorphic sarcoma (which is also called pleomorphic dermal sarcoma when arising from the dermis, → see dedicated section) but centered in dermis.

The tumor should not extensively involve the subcutaneous tissue or deeper structures (i.e., muscle or fascia): if so, the lesion may represent a pleomorphic dermal sarcoma.

Several variants have been described, such as the following: angiomatoid, chondroid, clear cell, granular cell, keloidal, myxoid, osteoclastic, osteoid, and pigmented AFX.

Differential diagnosis may be needed with the following: angiosarcoma spindle cell variant (prominent vascular spaces; positive for vascular biomarkers such as CD31 and ERG); atypical fibrous histiocytoma (→ see dedicated section); leiomyosarcoma pleomorphic type (usually more fascicular growth pattern, desmin positive); pleomorphic dermal sarcoma (though morphologically very similar, more deeply infiltrative lesion with a worse prognosis; complete excision may be needed to correctly classify the neoplasm as superficial biopsy of both tumors may look histologically identical); spindled or desmoplastic melanoma (S100 positive); and squamous cell carcinoma spindle cell type (cytokeratin positive).

Biomarkers

The staining pattern of AFX is nonspecific, and the diagnosis is largely made by exclusion, also based on the negative staining for markers such as S100, cytokeratins, CD31, ERG, CD34, desmin, and h-caldesmon.

Prognosis

Overall, AFX has a good prognosis after complete excision: its outcome has been compared to that of cutaneous leiomyosarcoma, while it is much better than that of pleomorphic dermal sarcoma. However, it can recur (in about 10% of cases) and rarely metastasize. Metastatic cases have been mainly observed in tumors with necrosis, invasion into deep subcutis and beyond, as well as lymphovascular invasion and perineural infiltration: actually these features should cast doubts on the diagnosis of AFX and rather lead to the diagnosis of pleomorphic dermal sarcoma.

Therapy

Surgery (wide excision) is the treatment of choice.

Suggested Readings

Chapman (2019) Atypical Fibroxanthoma. Semin Cutan Med Surg 38(1):E65–E66

Phan (2019) Time to recurrence after surgical excision of atypical fibroxanthoma-updated systematic review and meta-analysis. Australas J Dermatol 60(3):e220–e222

Sandhu (2019) Cutaneous Leiomyosarcoma: A SEER Database Analysis. Dermatol Surg [Epub ahead of print]

Soleeymani (2019) Atypical Fibroxanthoma and Pleomorphic Dermal Sarcoma: Updates on Classification and Management. Dermatol Clin 37(3):253–259

Kohlmeyer (2017) Cutaneous sarcomas. J Dtsch Dermatol Ges 15(6):630–648

Mentzel (2017) Atypical Fibroxanthoma Revisited. Surg Pathol Clin 10(2):319–335

Fletcher (2013). WHO classification of tumours of soft tissue and bone (4th edition)

Atypical Lipomatous Tumor

Atypical lipomatous tumor is an alternative name of well-differentiated liposarcoma: → see dedicated section for details on this neoplasm.

Definition

Atypical vascular lesion (AVL) is a benign proliferative skin lesion. It is also known as atypical vascular proliferation.

Epidemiology and Presentation

AVL presents as one or more circumscribed papules, bluish purple nodules, small vesicles, or erythematous plaques (within the irradiated field), the median lesion diameter being 0.5 cm.

Etiology and Predisposition

AVL is due to the exposure to radiation. It typically develops on the skin of the breast after radiotherapy. It occurs 1–12 years (mean 6 years) after therapy, within the irradiated field.

Pathology

AVL is composed of an atypical proliferation of vessels: according to the type of vessels involved, two AVL types are recognized: (1) lymphatic type and (2) vascular type.

The lesion is relatively well-circumscribed, with anastomosing growth pattern of irregular slit-like vascular spaces dissecting dermal collagen but not extending into subcutis. Vessels are lined by single layer of endothelial cells without atypia, micropapillary tufts being often encountered. Overall, it resembles benign lymphangioendothelioma or patch-stage Kaposi sarcoma.

© The Editor(s) (if applicable) and The Author(s), under exclusive license to
Springer Nature Switzerland AG 2021
S. Mocellin, *Soft Tissue Tumors*, https://doi.org/10.1007/978-3-030-58710-9_32

Differential diagnosis is of special importance with angiosarcoma (→ see dedicated section): AVL differs from angiosarcoma for the well-circumscribed nature, lack of multilayering, lack of mitosis, lack of hemorrhage, no extension into the subcutaneous tissue, and lack of MYC amplification/expression.

Other lesions that should be differentiated from AVL are hobnail hemangioma (smaller, more superficial, and more localized) and lymphangioendothelioma (it has intravascular papillary stromal projections that resemble papillary endothelial hyperplasia).

Biomarkers

AVL stains typically positive for CD31 (variably for CD34), whereas it stains negative for MYC[1] protein product (c-Myc). No MYC amplification is present.

Prognosis

AVL is a benign lesion. Its relevance lies in the differential diagnosis with angiosarcoma and in its potential evolution into angiosarcoma: as regards the latter, vascular-type AVL is at higher risk for subsequent development of angiosarcoma.

Therapy

Surgical excision is the approach of choice (mainly to make differential diagnosis with angiosarcoma).

Suggested Readings

Cornejo (2015) The utility of MYC and FLT4 in the diagnosis and treatment of postradiation atypical vascular lesion and angiosarcoma of the breast. Hum Pathol 46(6):868–875

Fraga-Guedes (2015) Angiosarcoma and atypical vascular lesions of the breast: diagnostic and prognostic role of MYC gene amplification and protein expression. Breast Cancer Res Treat 151(1):131–140

Ronen (2019) Postradiation vascular lesions of the breast. J Cutan Pathol 46(1):52–58

---

[1] MYC: this is a proto-oncogene and encodes a nuclear phosphoprotein (c-Myc) that plays a key role in cell cycle progression, apoptosis, and cellular transformation. The encoded protein forms a heterodimer with the related transcription factor MAX: then, this complex binds to the E-box DNA consensus sequence and regulates the transcription of specific target genes. Amplification of this gene is frequently observed in numerous human cancers, including radiation-induced angiosarcoma. Translocations involving this gene are associated with Burkitt lymphoma and multiple myeloma.

This is a recently recognized type of sarcoma molecularly characterized by the rearrangement of the BCOR gene.

For details → see the section entitled "Ewing-like sarcomas."

Definition

Benign fibrous histiocytoma (BFH), which is among the most common soft tissue neoplasms, is a morphologically benign fibrohistiocytic tumor. Despite the name, cells of origin are not histiocytes. There are two BFH subtypes:

- Superficial BFH (the most frequent subtype, also known as dermatofibroma, cutaneous fibrous histiocytoma, common fibrous histiocytoma, and superficial fibrous histiocytoma)
- Deep BFH (also known as soft tissue fibrous histiocytoma and deep fibrous histiocytoma).

Malignant fibrous histiocytoma ($\rightarrow$ see dedicated section), which might be intended as the malignant counterpart of BFH, is a nosological entity that is currently replaced by other types of sarcomas (e.g., undifferentiated pleomorphic sarcoma).

For general information on different types of fibrous histiocytomas $\rightarrow$ see section entitled "Fibrous Histiocytoma."

Epidemiology and Presentation

Dermatofibroma is a frequent cutaneous lesion (the most frequent mesenchymal skin tumor) that can occur at all ages but is more common between 20 and 50 years; it is more frequently located in lower limbs of women. It is unclear whether it is a reactive or neoplastic process (frequently appears after minor injuries to the skin). Its typical appearance is that of a slow-growing dome-shaped, firm in consistency, pigmented at the periphery, asymptomatic, and small (< 1 centimeter in diameter, although giant lesions have been reported) lesion, but many variants have been described.

127

S. Mocellin, *Soft Tissue Tumors*, https://doi.org/10.1007/978-3-030-58710-9_34

Deep fibrous histiocytoma is rare, as it accounts for < 1% of fibrohistiocytic tumors; its most common location is the extremities, followed by the head and neck region. Most deep BFHs are subcutaneous, whereas approximately 10% originate from visceral soft tissues (e.g., retroperitoneum, mediastinum, pelvis); intramuscular site is uncommon, and visceral organs are exceedingly rare sites of occurrence.

Pathology

Composed of a mixture of fibroblastic and histiocytic cells, collagen, and blood vessels, the deep lesions are more cellular than typical cutaneous fibrous histiocytomas but share a storiform architecture.

BFH shows a branching, hemangiopericytoma-like vascular pattern, which can make difficult the differential diagnosis with solitary fibrous tumor (particularly when CD34 is expressed).

There is generally no nuclear pleomorphism, except for rare variants such as the well-defined atypical fibrous histiocytoma (AFH, → see dedicated section).

Mitoses are typically < 5 per 10 HPF[1] but may be numerous (> 10 per 10 HPF).

Several variants have been described (e.g., epithelioid fibrous histiocytoma, aneurysmal fibrous histiocytoma, cellular fibrous histiocytoma, AFH, angiomatoid fibrous histiocytoma). For general information on different types of fibrous histiocytomas → see section entitled "Fibrous Histiocytoma."

Differential diagnosis may be needed with the following: atypical fibroxanthoma (characteristic gross appearance and storiform pattern); basal cell carcinoma (positive for BerEP4); dermatofibrosarcoma protuberans (infiltrative; CD34 positive); Kaposi sarcoma (vascular tumor with red blood cell extravasation and HHV8[2] positivity); low-grade myofibroblastic sarcoma (ill-defined fascicles, infiltrative growth, desmin positive); neurofibroma (S100 positive cells and serpentine nuclei); nodular fasciitis (red blood cells extravasation and loosely arranged bundles of fibroblasts); Rosai-Dorfman disease (CD68-positive histocytes); sclerosing leiomyoma (positivity for smooth muscle biomarkers); and storiform collagenoma (CD34 positive).

Biomarkers

Expression of CD34 is far more common (about 40%) in deep fibrous histiocytoma than in dermatofibroma (where CD34 is used to differentiate CD34-negative BFH from dermatofibrosarcoma protuberans which is typically CD34 positive). In deep lesions, CD34 expression calls for differential diagnosis with solitary fibrous tumor (→ see dedicated section). In general, biomarker expression may be difficult to interpret because of the presence of entrapped reactive cells.

---

[1] HPF: high power field

[2] HHV8: human herpes virus 8

Immunohistochemical expression of HMGA2 is present in about 90% of cases and is considered a useful biomarker.

Because of its relative monomorphism and frequent fascicularity, cellular fibrous histiocytoma (→ see dedicated section) can easily be mistaken for a malignancy: in particular, CD34—which is often used to distinguish it from dermatofibrosarcoma protuberans—is positive in one third of cases.

Epithelioid fibrous histiocytoma is characterized by rearrangements of the ALK gene (→ see section entitled "Epithelioid Fibrous Histiocytoma").

Angiomatoid fibrous histiocytoma is characterized by rearrangement of the CREB1 as well as other genes (→ see section entitled "Angiomatoid Fibrous Histiocytoma").

Prognosis

Despite the benign histological appearance, this tumor has been reported to rarely relapse (<5%) and (even more rarely) metastasize. In particular, similarly to AFH (→ see dedicated section), cellular and aneurysmal variants of BFH show a higher tendency (about 20%) to recur locally than ordinary fibrous histiocytoma and may very rarely metastasize. Angiomatoid fibrous histiocytoma can locally relapse (10–15%), occasionally metastasize to lymph nodes (2%), and exceptionally give rise to distant metastasis (lungs).

Therapy

Surgical excision is the treatment of choice. Follow-up is necessary due to the above mentioned possibility of disease recurrence.

Suggested Readings

Alves (2014) Variants of dermatofibroma--a histopathological study. An Bras Dermato 89(3):472–477

Dreux (2010) Value and limitation of immunohistochemical expression of HMGA2 in mesenchymal tumors: about a series of 1052 cases. Mod Pathol 23(12):1657–1666

Felty (2019) Epithelioid Fibrous Histiocytoma: A Concise Review. Am J Dermatopatho 41(12):879–883

Fletcher (2020). WHO classification of tumours of soft tissue and bone (5th edition)

Hornick (2019) Cutaneous soft tissue tumors: how do we make sense of fibrous and "fibrohistiocytic" tumors with confusing names and similar appearances? Mod Pathol Epub ahead of print]

Khan (2019) Primary Adrenal Angiomatoid Fibrous Histiocytoma With Novel EWSR1-ATF1 Gene Fusion Exon-Exon Breakpoint. Pediatr Dev Pathol 22(5):472–474

Lodewick (2014) Fatal case of metastatic cellular fibrous histiocytoma: case report and review of literature. Am J Dermatopathol 36(9):e156–e162

Mentzel (2013) Malignant dermatofibroma: clinicopathological, immunohistochemical, and molecular analysis of seven cases. Mod Pathol 26(2):256–267

Nabatanzi (2019) Aneurysmal Fibrous Histiocytoma: Clinicopathology Analysis of 30 Cases of a Rare Variant of Cutaneous Fibrohistiocytoma. Curr Med Sci 39(1):134–137

Volpicelli (2012) Desmin and CD34 positivity in cellular fibrous histiocytoma: an immunohistochemical analysis of 100 cases. J Cutan Pathol 39(8):747–752

Definition

Benign metastasizing leiomyoma (BML) is a benign appearing smooth muscle tumor which presents as metastatic disease (usually in the lungs) in women with a history of uterine leiomyoma (→ see dedicated section).

Epidemiology and Presentation

BML is an exceedingly rare nosological entity. It typically affects women during their reproductive age or older (range, 35–65 years; mean, 45 years) with a personal history of uterine leiomyoma: BML can be either synchronous or metachronous with respect to uterine leiomyoma (for metachronous lesions, the onset time can be as long as 20 years).

The lung is most common site, although other sites have been described (e.g., lymph nodes, retroperitoneum, skin, and bone). BML can present with multiple nodules and measure from few millimeters to few centimeters in size. Most cases are asymptomatic; otherwise, dyspnea, cough, hemoptysis, and chest pain can occur.

Diagnosis derives from the combination of biopsy plus personal history of uterine leiomyoma. Upon computed tomography, the disease usually presents as multiple, diffuse, well-defined, nodular, non-enhancing soft tissue lesions. Positron emission tomography is typically negative.

Etiology and Predisposition

BML is believed to originate from the hematogenous spread of uterine leiomyoma; alternatively, it might represent the metastatic phase of a well-differentiated uterine leiomyosarcoma (mistakenly diagnosed as leiomyoma).

S. Mocellin, *Soft Tissue Tumors*, https://doi.org/10.1007/978-3-030-58710-9_35

Pathology

BML presents as well-circumscribed, solitary or multiple nodules of smooth muscle, mimicking the uterine counterpart: the tumor is composed of whorled to intersecting fascicles of ovoid to elongated spindled cells with eosinophilic cytoplasm and oval to cigar-like nuclei; large, irregular, thick-walled vessels are usually present. Of note, atypia, necrosis, vascular invasion, and mitotic figures are absent.

Differential diagnosis may be needed with the following: leiomyomatous hamartoma, low-grade leiomyosarcoma, and lymphangioleiomyomatosis (less well-circumscribed, it may display mitoses and necrosis; HMB45 positive).

Biomarkers

BML stains positive for desmin, SMA, caldesmon, estrogen receptor, and progesterone receptor. It stains negative for TTF1, S100, EMA, CK7, CK20, chromogranin, synaptophysin, HMB45, and CD10.

From the cytogenetics viewpoint, BML shows findings similar to those of uterine leiomyoma ($\rightarrow$ see dedicated section).

Prognosis

Usually the clinical course is benign. Only bulky disease can lead to massive hemoptysis and/or respiratory failure.

Therapy

Due to the rarity of the disease, no consensus exists. Surveillance is acceptable for indolent, asymptomatic disease. Medical therapy (e.g., GnRH agonists and aromatase inhibitors) may be considered as the disease is hormone-sensitive. Surgery (hysterectomy, bilateral oophorectomy) may also be taken into consideration.

Suggested Readings

Barnaś (2017) Benign metastasizing leiomyoma: A review of current literature in respect to the time and type of previous gynecological surgery. PLoS One 12(4):e0175875

Bowen (2012) Genomic imbalances in benign metastasizing leiomyoma: characterization by conventional karyotypic, fluorescence in situ hybridization, and whole genome SNP array analysis. Cancer Gene 205(5):249–254

Huang (2019) Pulmonary and mediastinum metastasis of uterine leiomyoma: A case report. Medicine (Baltimore) 98(49):e18276

Ofori (2019) Benign metastasizing leiomyoma presenting with miliary pattern and fatal outcome: Case report with molecular analysis & review of the literature. Respir Med Case Rep 27:100831

Yuan (2019) Multiple organ benign metastasizing leiomyoma: A case report and literature review. J Obstet Gynaecol Res 45(10):2132–2136

Definition

Benign Triton tumor is a neoplasm classified among nerve sheath tumors. It is also known as neuromuscular choristoma,[1] neuromuscular hamartoma,[1] and nerve rhabdomyoma.

For information on malignant Triton tumor → see dedicated section.

Epidemiology and Presentation

It is an extremely rare lesion mainly arising in infancy or childhood, without gender differences. Typically, it involves large nerves or plexi (mainly sciatic nerve and the brachial plexus). Clinically, the neoplasm presents with signs/symptoms related to peripheral neuropathy or plexopathy. Of note, intraoperative stimulation of the affected nerve leads to contraction not only of the innervated muscle but also the abnormal nerve (due to the presence of skeletal muscle fibers within the nerve).

Pathology

Benign Triton tumor presents as an expansile intraneural mass characterized by the intimate interposition of haphazardly arranged bundles of mature skeletal muscle fibers between clusters of nerve fibers.

---

[1] Choristoma is a form of heterotopia (normal tissue found in abnormal locations) and is not a neoplasm (unlike tumors, the growth of a choristoma is normally regulated). Choristoma differs from hamartoma: while the former consisits of normal tissue growing in an abnormal location (e.g., gastric mucosa located in a Meckel diverticulum of the distal ileum), the latter is a disorganized (but non neoplastic) overgrowth of tissues in their normal location (e.g., Peutz-Jeghers polyps in the intestine).

S. Mocellin, *Soft Tissue Tumors*, https://doi.org/10.1007/978-3-030-58710-9_36

Prognosis

This neoplasm is benign.

Therapy

Surgical excision is the treatment of choice. As the lesion is benign, preoperative diagnosis is critical to prevent overtreatment and consequent nerve damage due to surgical excision.

Suggested Readings

Castro (2005) Benign triton tumor of the trigeminal nerve. AJNR Am J Neuroradiol 26(4):967–969
Fletcher (2013) WHO classification of tumours of soft tissue and bone (4th edition)
Thakrar (2014) Benign triton tumor: multidisciplinary approach to diagnosis and treatment. Pediatr Dev Pathol 17(5):400–405

Definition

Biphenotypic sinonasal sarcoma (BSS) is a malignant tumor recently recognized by the World Health Organization.

Epidemiology and Presentation

BSS is an exceedingly rare neoplasm that appears to arise uniquely in the sinonasal tract. Most cases occur in adults (mean age: 50 years), with women being affected more frequently than men.

BSS is infiltrative, often involves multiple sites within the sinonasal tract, and frequently extends to the orbit and/or the cribriform plate.

Pathology

BSS is characterized by both myogenic and neural differentiation (hence the name), which can be demonstrated by immunohistochemistry. BSS displays a fascicular growth pattern of uniform and mildly atypical spindle cells, with entrapped hyperplastic surface epithelium being a frequent finding. The stroma is generally characterized by hemangiopericytoma-like vessels. Occasionally, tumors may display rhabdomyoblastic differentiation.

Differential diagnosis may be needed with other highly cellular spindle cell neoplasms that may arise in the sinonasal tract, such as glomangiopericytoma (no herringbone pattern, no S100 positivity); solitary fibrous tumor (ectatic staghorn vasculature; thick bands of stromal collagen; strong CD34 and STAT6 positivity); schwannoma (presence of hyper- and hypocellular areas and nuclear palisading; no actin expression; diffuse S100 but also SOX10 positivity); malignant peripheral nerve sheath tumor (spindled cells arranged in herringbone-like fascicles;

S. Mocellin, *Soft Tissue Tumors*, https://doi.org/10.1007/978-3-030-58710-9_37

hyperchromatic and pleomorphic nuclei with frequent mitoses; tumor necrosis; weak S100 positivity; at least focal SOX10 expression); leiomyoma and leiomyosarcoma (cigar shaped nuclei; positive for SMA and desmin but no S100 expression); spindle cell rhabdomyosarcoma (variable number of rhabdomyoblasts; diffuse positivity for desmin, myogenin and MyoD1); and monophasic synovial sarcoma (variable positivity for cytokeratins and TLE1; no expression of SMA and MSA; characteristic SS18-SSX1/2 gene fusions).

Biomarkers

Myogenic (e.g., SMA, MSA, desmin) and neural (e.g., S100) differentiation can be demonstrated by immunohistochemistry, but this biomarker pattern is relatively nonspecific. PAX3[1] expression (due to the below reported chromosomal rearrangements) is considered highly accurate. BSS stains negative for CD34, cytokeratins, STAT6, SOX10, and synaptophysin.

BSS is characterized by recurrent **chromosomal translocations** present in most lesions and leading to the formation of PAX3-containing fusion genes, MAML3[2] being the most frequent fusion partner (rare partners: NCOA2 and FOXO1).

Prognosis

BSS is a low-grade malignancy: about half patients experience local disease recurrence, although distant metastasis has not yet been reported.

Therapy

Surgery is the treatment of choice, although clear margins are difficult to obtain in the sinonasal tract.

The role of radiotherapy and chemotherapy is unclear.

Suggested Readings

Andreasen (2018) Biphenotypic sinonasal sarcoma: demographics, clinicopathological characteristics, molecular features, and prognosis of a recently described entity. Virchows Arch 473(5):615–626

---

[1] PAX3 (paired box 3) encodes a member of the paired box transcription factor family (which plays a critical role in fetal development). PAX3 rearrangements are found also in alveolar rhabdomyosarcoma

[2] MAML3 (Mastermind Like Transcriptional Coactivator 3) encodes a protein with transcription coactivator activity

Gross (2020) Soft Tissue Special Issue: Biphenotypic Sinonasal Sarcoma: A Review with Emphasis on Differential Diagnosis. Head Neck Pathol 14(1):33–42

Jo (2018) Expression of PAX3 Distinguishes Biphenotypic Sinonasal Sarcoma From Histologic Mimics. Am J Surg Pathol 42(10):1275–1285

Thompson (2018) New tumor entities in the 4th edition of the World Health Organization classification of head and neck tumors: Nasal cavity, paranasal sinuses and skull base. Virchows Arch 472(3):315–330

Wang (2014) Recurrent PAX3-MAML3 fusion in biphenotypic sinonasal sarcoma. Nat Genet 46:666–668

The following are the soft tissue tumors of the bladder according to the World Health Organization Classification of Tumours of the Urinary System and Male Genital Organs (Part B: Prostate and Bladder Tumors). Of note, other soft tissue tumors afftecting the bladder are described in the literature.

For details on each single neoplasm → see dedicated sections.

Tumor	Notes
Angiosarcoma	-
Granular cell tumor	-
Hemangioma	-
Inflammatory myofibroblastic tumor	-
Leiomyoma	-
Leiomyosarcoma	-
Neurofibroma	-
Perivascular epithelioid cell tumor	PEComa
Rhabdomyosarcoma	-
Solitary fibrous tumor	-

Definition

Breast angiosarcoma is a malignant tumor of vascular origin ($\rightarrow$ see the section entitled "Angiosarcoma" for general information on this sarcoma).

Epidemiology and Presentation

Angiosarcoma of the breast accounts for 0.05% of all primary breast malignancies and < 1% of all of soft tissue tumors but represents the most frequent type of breast sarcoma.

The tumor (average size: 5 cm) can present as a purple to bluish (possibly ulcerated) nodule or (more insidiously) as a lesion mimicking a skin ecchymosis (which must always be biopsied, especially in women who underwent breast radiotherapy).

Etiology and Predisposition

Two subtypes of breast angiosarcoma are usually recognized: primary (without known causative exposure) and secondary breast angiosarcoma (when the tumor occurs in patients previously exposed to radiation). Primary tumors occur earlier (mean age: 45–50 years) as compared to secondary tumors (mean age: 70). Secondary lesions develop on average 8 years after radiotherapy (range: 4 to 12 years). It is estimated that after radiotherapy for breast cancer, approximately one in 1000 women will develop radiation-induced angiosarcoma.

S. Mocellin, *Soft Tissue Tumors*, https://doi.org/10.1007/978-3-030-58710-9_39

Pathology

For general description → see the section entitled "Angiosarcoma."

The tumor can present with different grades of differentiation, which can coexist.

Well-differentiated tumors/areas resemble benign vascular lesions with anastomosing/branching, often dilated vascular channels lined by minimally atypical endothelial cells. Mitoses are rare or absent, as well as tufting of endothelial cells; in these cases, the key distinguishing feature from benign vascular lesions is an infiltrative growth pattern.

Moderately differentiated tumors/areas are similar to low-grade tumors but with increased mitoses, endothelial tufting, and foci of solid growth pattern.

Poorly differentiated tumors/areas show marked pleomorphism, mitoses, necrosis, solid growth, and extravasation of blood from malignant vessels forming blood lakes; moreover, these high-grade cases may show epithelioid and spindled cytology with no obvious vasoformative morphology.

Especially in irradiated breasts, angiosarcoma should be differentiated from atypical vascular lesions.

Biomarkers

Angiosarcoma stains positive for vascular markers (ERG, CD31, CD34, factor VIII) and negative for cytokeratins, estrogen receptor, and progesterone receptor. Typically, secondary angiosarcoma shows **MYC gene amplification**[1] and c-Myc expression.

Prognosis

Breast angiosarcoma is an aggressive malignancy with an overall poor prognosis associated with high rates of both local recurrences and distant metastases. The prognosis of primary angiosarcoma does not significantly differ from that of secondary angiosarcoma (reported differences in terms of overall survival probably reflect different age onsets).

Although the role of tumor grading is uncertain and its use is often discouraged, some investigators have reported worse outcomes for higher grade lesions.

---

[1] MYC: this is a proto-oncogene and encodes a nuclear phosphoprotein (c-Myc) that plays a key role in cell cycle progression, apoptosis, and cellular transformation. The encoded protein forms a heterodimer with the related transcription factor MAX: then, this complex binds to the E-box DNA consensus sequence and regulates the transcription of specific target genes. Amplification of this gene is frequently observed in numerous human cancers, including radiation-induced angiosarcoma. Translocations involving this gene are associated with Burkitt lymphoma and multiple myeloma

Therapy

For general information on angiosarcoma therapy → see section entitled "Angiosarcoma."

Surgery represents the mainstay of treatment for localized lesions. Mastectomy does not appear to add any additional benefit to breast conserving surgery. Mastectomy is preferred by some authors because of the macroscopically ill-defined margins of the tumor, which makes it more uncertain to obtain disease-free margins with breast conserving surgery.

Adjuvant radiotherapy is often used and might improve disease-free survival, while the role of adjuvant chemotherapy is even more uncertain.

Although lymph node metastasis is possible, breast angiosarcoma has most often a hematogenous spread, so that lymph node evaluation is not part of routine treatment or staging (unless lymph node involvement is clinically suspected).

Metastatic disease is treated with systemic chemotherapy, usually based on anthracyclines or taxanes.

Suggested Readings

Abdou (2019) Primary and secondary breast angiosarcoma: single center report and a meta-analysis. Breast Cancer Res Treat 178(3):523–533

Duncan (2018) Sarcomas of the Breast. Surg Clin North Am 98(4):869–876

Morgan (2012) Cutaneous radiation-associated angiosarcoma of the breast: poor prognosis in a rare secondary malignancy. Ann Surg Oncol 19(12):3801–3808

Painter (2020) The Angiosarcoma Project: enabling genomic and clinical discoveries in a rare cancer through patient-partnered research. Nat Med 26(2):181–187

Rombouts (2019) Assessment of Radiotherapy-Associated Angiosarcoma After Breast Cancer Treatment in a Dutch Population-Based Study. JAMA Oncol 5(2):267–269

Salminen (2019) Treatment and Prognosis of Radiation-Associated Breast Angiosarcoma in a Nationwide Population. Ann Surg Oncol [Epub ahead of print]

Yin (2017) Prognosis and treatment of non-metastatic primary and secondary breast angiosarcoma: a comparative study. BMC Cancer 17(1):295

Definition

Breast phyllodes tumor (BPT) is a biphasic fibroepithelial tumor with biological behavior ranging from benign to borderline to malignant. It is also known as cystosarcoma phyllodes and phyllodes tumor. Although classified by the World Health Organization among fibroepithelial tumors (and not among mesenchymal neoplasms), BPT is here considered because the malignant version is due to the mesenchymal component (hence the name cystosarcoma phyllodes).

Epidemiology and Presentation

BPT accounts for about 1% of breast neoplasms. The mean age at presentation is 45 years. The lesion can present either as a discrete palpable mass that rapidly enlarges or as a non-palpable nodule identified on screening mammogram. Axillary nodal enlargement is present in 15% of cases, but it is often reactive and not due to metastatic disease. Rarely, BPT secretes IGF2[1] causing paraneoplastic hypoglycemia.

Three subtypes of BPT are recognized: benign (60–80% of all cases), borderline (10%), and malignant (10–30%), on the basis of histological characteristics of the stromal elements. Clinically it can be difficult to distinguish BPT from fibroadenoma.

Pathology

Phyllodes tumors are composed of both epithelial elements and connective tissue stroma with spindled cells (resembling fibroblasts and myofibroblasts).

---

[1] IGF2: insulin-like growth factor 2

Histopathologically, these lesions consist of epithelium-lined cysts with a hypercellular stroma. The diagnosis of BPT is dependent upon this histopathological appearance, and, therefore, preoperative diagnosis with fine needle aspiration (FNA) is difficult. The majority of phyllodes tumors can be diagnosed preoperatively using a combination of imaging and preoperative core biopsy, while diagnostic excision biopsy is used for uncertain cases.

Distinction between benign vs borderline vs malignant BPT is based on the presence of cellular pleomorphism, nuclear atypia, mitotic activity, overgrowth of the stroma, and infiltrative borders.

Differential diagnosis may be needed with fibroadenoma, which shows neither tissue fragmentation, increased stromal cellularity around glands, atypia, or stromal overgrowth and presents with fewer mitoses.

Biomarkers

The stromal component of BPT stains positive for vimentin, desmin, and actin and negative for cytokeratins, EMA,[2] and S100.

Prognosis

While benign BPT behaves similarly to fibroadenoma, malignant BPT carries a significant risk of recurrence and metastasis. Approximately 10% of patients with BPT develop distant metastases, a rate that can increase up to 20% in patients with histologically malignant BPT. The commonest sites for distant metastases are the lung, bone, and abdominal viscera.

In contrast to epithelial breast cancer, it is uncommon to have axillary nodal metastases, and when there are enlarged nodes, they may be reactive.

Positive surgical margin is significantly associated with disease recurrence.

Therapy

The treatment of choice is **surgical excision** with a clear margin. Breast conservation surgery has been practiced, particularly if the lesion-to-breast size ratio allows excision with reasonable cosmesis. In malignant tumors, and when the lesion is large and/or the surgical margins close, **radiotherapy** has been added as an adjuvant treatment. However, breast conservation without radiotherapy has also been reported to provide adequate local control, particularly for smaller tumors (<2 cm). More recently, local recurrence rates in the range of 10% to 20% have been reported, with no difference in the survival between patients managed with breast conservation or mastectomy. For metastatic disease, doxorubicin-based regimens typical for most soft tissue sarcomas are utilized.

---

[2] EMA: epithelial membrane antigen

Suggested Readings

Chao (2019) Adjuvant radiotherapy and chemotherapy for patients with breast phyllodes tumors: a systematic review and meta-analysis. BMC Cancer 19(1):372

Lu (2019) Local Recurrence of Benign, Borderline, and Malignant Phyllodes Tumors of the Breast: A Systematic Review and Meta-analysis. Ann Surg Oncol 26(5):1263–1275

Mitus (2019) Phyllodes tumors of the breast. The treatment results for 340 patients from a single cancer centre. Breast 43:85–90

Papas (2019) Malignant phyllodes tumors of the breast: A comprehensive literature review. Breast J Epub ahead of print]

Yamamoto (2019) Effective Treatment of a Malignant Breast Phyllodes Tumor with Doxorubicin-Ifosfamide Therapy. Case Rep Oncol Med 2019:2759650

Spitaleri (2013) Breast phyllodes tumor: a review of literature and a single center retrospective series analysis. Crit Rev Oncol Hematol 88(2):427–436

41

Many primary benign and malignant soft tissue tumors can affect the breast (for more details on soft tissue tumors of the skin → see section entitled "Skin Soft Tissue Tumors"). The most common breast soft tissue sarcoma is angiosarcoma. Primary breast sarcoma accounts for about 1% of all breast malignancies and less than 5% of all soft tissue sarcomas; estimated annual incidence is five new cases per million women.

The following is the list of primary soft tissue tumors of the breast, according to the World Health Organization classification published in 2019.

Other entities (e.g., breast phyllodes tumor, myoepithelioma) not included in this list are described in this book.

For details on single tumors → see sections dedicated to each neoplasm.

Tumor
Angiolipoma
Angiomatosis
Angiosarcoma
Atypical vascular lesion
Desmoid-type fibromatosis
Granular cell tumor
Hemangioma
Inflammatory myofibroblastic tumor
Leiomyoma
Leiomyosarcoma
Lipoma
Liposarcoma
Myofibroblastoma
Neurofibroma
Nodular fasciitis
Pseudoangiomatous stromal hyperplasia
Schwannoma

© The Editor(s) (if applicable) and The Author(s), under exclusive license to
Springer Nature Switzerland AG 2021
S. Mocellin, *Soft Tissue Tumors*, https://doi.org/10.1007/978-3-030-58710-9_41

Definition

Calcifying aponeurotic fibroma (CAF) is a benign neoplasm classified among fibroblastic-myofibroblastic tumors. It is also known as juvenile aponeurotic fibroma and aponeurotic fibroma.

Epidemiology and Presentation

CAF is an exceedingly rare tumor affecting mainly childhood and adolescence, which is usually found on the hands or feet. It presents as a small (1–3 cm), slow-growing and ill-defined soft tissue mass infiltrating adjacent soft tissues and is typically associated with tendons and aponeuroses. Standard X-rays may show calcifications.

Pathology

CAF is a biphasic neoplasm composed of moderately cellular and infiltrative, fibromatosis-like areas and nodules of calcification associated with more rounded epithelioid cells often radiating from the center of the calcifications. Tumor cells lack significant atypia and show only rare mitotic figures. Multinucleated osteoclast-like giant cells are frequently found. The background stroma, particularly in the calcified areas, varies from hyalinized to chondroid.

Differential diagnosis may be needed with the following: chondroma of soft parts (it may involve hands, but it is usually well circumscribed with more well developed chondroid differentiation; no infiltration of adjacent tissue; no surrounding epithelioid cells); fibrous hamartoma of infancy (immature mesenchyme, fibroblasts are arranged in trabeculae but no palisading, no cartilage or calcification, no hands or feet); infantile fibromatosis (it usually involves head and neck and

S. Mocellin, *Soft Tissue Tumors*, https://doi.org/10.1007/978-3-030-58710-9_42

proximal extremities in infants, not hands and feet of children or young adults, background is more myxoid than chondroid, calcification is rare); and superficial and desmoid fibromatosis (usually no calcification or chondroid differentiation, nuclear expression of beta-catenin).

Biomarkers

Tumor cells are usually SMA[1] positive and desmin negative (supporting a fibroblastic-myofibroblastic origin). Nuclear expression of beta-catenin is lacking.

A chromosomal translocation between chromosomes 2 and 4 leads to the generation of the **FN1-EGF fusion gene**[2] in most cases and could be the main driver mutation in CAF.

Prognosis

Although benign, CAF is characterized by high rates of local recurrence (up to 50%).

Therapy

Surgical excision is the treatment of choice.

Suggested Readings

Fletcher (2020) WHO classification of tumours of soft tissue and bone (5th edition)
Puls (2016) FN1-EGF gene fusions are recurrent in calcifying aponeurotic fibroma. J Pathol 238(4):502–507
Romano (2017) Masson's tumor and calcifying aponeurotic fibroma: two rare soft tissue lesions in the same finger. High-resolution ultrasound features with histopathological correlations. Med Ultrason 19(4):457–461

---

[1] SMA: smooth muscle actin

[2] FN1-EGF fusion gene: FN1 encodes fibronectin, a glycoprotein present in a soluble dimeric form in plasma and in a dimeric or multimeric form at the cell surface and in extracellular matrix; fibronectin is involved in cell adhesion and migration processes including embryogenesis, wound healing, blood coagulation, host defense, and metastasis. EGF encodes a member of the epidermal growth factor superfamily; by binding with high affinity to cell surface the epidermal growth factor receptor (EGFR), this protein acts a potent mitogenic factor that plays an important role in the growth, proliferation, and differentiation of numerous cell types

Calcifying Fibrous Tumor

43

Definition

Calcifying fibrous tumor (CFT) is a benign neoplasm classified among fibroblastic-myofibroblastic tumors.

It is also known as childhood fibrous tumor with psammoma bodies and calcifying fibrous pseudotumor.

Epidemiology and Presentation

CFT is a rare lesion affecting patients in a wide range of age and no gender preference. The lesion presents as a painless and well circumscribed with a diameter that can reach several centimeters. CFT can arise virtually anywhere: superficial and deep somatic soft tissues (e.g., limbs, neck, scrotum, back, and abdominal wall), viscera (e.g., gastrointestinal tract including the mesentery), mediastinum, omentum, peritoneum, and pleura. The mass can cause compression of adjacent structures. Tumors of somatic tissues occur more often in children, whereas visceral tumors occur more frequently in adults.

Etiology and Predisposition

CFT has been associated with trauma as well as Castleman disease (a benign lymphoproliferative disorder that may present as a localized or multicentric form; the clinical manifestations are heterogeneous, ranging from asymptomatic discrete lymphadenopathy to recurrent episodes of diffuse lymphadenopathy with severe systemic symptoms).

© The Editor(s) (if applicable) and The Author(s), under exclusive license to 153
Springer Nature Switzerland AG 2021
S. Mocellin, *Soft Tissue Tumors*, https://doi.org/10.1007/978-3-030-58710-9_43

Pathology

CFT is a hypocellular fibroblastic proliferation associated with chronic inflammation (scattered lymphocytes and plasma cells with/without the formation of follicles with germinal centers) and prominent calcification (dystrophic or psammomatous).

Differential diagnosis may be needed with the following: calcifying aponeurotic fibroma (more cellular, usually distal location, usually smaller lesion); desmoplastic fibroblastoma (older patients, low cellularity, larger prominent fibroblasts, no microcalcifications, no prominent inflammatory infiltrate); idiopathic retroperitoneal fibrosis and related sclerosing fibroinflammatory lesions (more inflammation, especially plasma cells and eosinophils); and inflammatory myofibroblastic tumor (more cellular, no calcifications, ALK rearrangement in half cases, often actin positive).

Biomarkers

Tumor cells are positive for CD34 and vimentin, whereas they are negative for SMA,[1] MSA,[2] ALK,[3] desmin, S100, and cytokeratins.

Prognosis

CFT is a benign lesion and local recurrence is rare.

Therapy

Surgical excision is the treatment of choice.

Suggested Readings

Marbaniang (2019) Castleman's disease associated with calcifying fibrous tumor: A rare association with review of literature. J Lab Physicians 11(2):171–173

Pezhouh (2017) Clinicopathologic study of calcifying fibrous tumor of the gastrointestinal tract: a case series. Hum Pathol 62:199–205

Chorti (2016) Calcifying Fibrous Tumor: Review of 157 Patients Reported in International Literature. Medicine (Baltimore) 95(20):e3690

Prochaska (2016) Retroperitoneal calcifying fibrous tumor mimicking an adrenal tumor. J Surg Case Rep 2016(6):rjw049

Fletcher (2013) WHO classification of tumours of soft tissue and bone (4th edition)

---

[1] SMA: smooth muscle actin

[2] MSA: muscle specific actin

[3] ALK: Anaplastic lymphoma (receptor tyrosine) kinase

Cardiac tumors, benign or malignant, are rare (most of them being benign). The most common benign tumor is cardiac myxoma, whereas sarcomas are the most common malignant lesions.

Heart soft tissue tumors are rare neoplasms but represent the most frequent type of heart primary tumor. These tumors often are not diagnosed until autopsy due to rarity and nonspecificity of signs and symptoms.

Tumors that metastasize to the heart from other organs occur 100–1000-folds more commonly than primary cardiac neoplasms: therefore, primary soft tissue tumors must be differentiated from secondary heart neoplasms.

Heart sarcomas have a dismal prognosis due to their aggressive biological behavior, but benign cardiac soft tissue tumors may also be associated with significant mortality due to their negative hemodynamic effects.

The following are the most common types of cardiac soft tissue tumors reported in the literature:

Tumor	Notes
Angiosarcoma	Most frequent malignant heart tumor. The incidence of primary cardiac tumors is estimated to be between 0.001 and 0.003% in general population. A mutation in the POT1 gene is responsible for cardiac angiosarcoma in TP53-negative Li-Fraumeni-like families For general information on angiosarcoma → see dedicated section
Fibroma	This benign tumor is rare but common among cardiac tumors in children. It is found in 10% of Gorlin syndrome patients (nevoid basal cell carcinoma syndrome)
Hemangioma	This benign tumor is rare, accounting for < 5% of benign cardiac tumors. It occurs at all ages and is multiple in 30% of cases. Usually asymptomatic, it may cause sudden death or significant cardiac dysfunction by displacing large portions of atria and ventricles For general information on lipoma → see dedicated section
Leiomyosarcoma	It accounts for about 8% of cardiac sarcomas

S. Mocellin, *Soft Tissue Tumors*, https://doi.org/10.1007/978-3-030-58710-9_44

Tumor	Notes
Lipoma	Represents about 10% of primary cardiac tumors For general information on lipoma → see dedicated section
Myxoma	Most frequent benign heart tumor For more details on cardiac myxoma → see dedicated section
Osteosarcoma	It represents 3–9% of cardiac sarcomas
Papillary fibroelastoma	Benign tumor that typically involves one of the heart valves. Accounts for approximately 10% of all primary tumors of the heart (third most common type of primary tumor of the heart behind cardiac myxoma and cardiac lipoma)
Rhabdomyoma	This benign neoplasm accounts for 50–90% of primary heart tumors in children. It is usually discovered within the first year of life. It may obstruct valvular orifice or cardiac chamber and may present with sudden cardiac death. 50% of patients have tuberous sclerosis; sporadic cases are occasionally associated with congenital heart disease. Of note, many tumors regress spontaneously, whereas excision is necessary in case of left ventricular outflow tract obstruction or refractory arrhythmia For more details → see section entitled "Cardiac Rhabdomyoma"
Rhabdomyosarcoma	This sarcoma is rare (4–7% of cardiac sarcomas) but most common cardiac malignancy in infants and children, where it occurs more frequently For general information on rhabdomyosarcoma → see dedicated section

Cardiac Myxoma 45

Definition

Heart myxoma is an endocardial-based benign tumor which is thought to originate from mesenchymal cells.

Epidemiology and Presentation

It is the most frequent type of cardiac neoplasm (about 40% of all primary tumors of the heart), which occurs more commonly in women (mean age: 50 years) and affects mainly the left atrium (90% occur in atria, 80% on left side).

Symptoms are related to hemodynamic effects (e.g., "wrecking ball effect" for pedunculated myxoma, mitral stenosis effect) and embolism (peripheral or pulmonary, depending on the tumor site). Usually the tumor must reach several centimeters in diameter before becoming symptomatic. Ultrasonography (echocardiography), computed tomography scan, and magnetic resonance imaging are useful to suspect the diagnosis.

Etiology and Predisposition

Most myxomas (90%) arise sporadically (90%), while a minority (10%) occurs within the frame of a hereditary syndrome (familial myxoma).

The so-called **Carney syndrome** is a rare tumor predisposition disease inherited in an autosomal dominant manner and characterized by cardiac myxoma (in this syndrome the myxoma tends to occur more often in males, to arise in more than one heart chamber, and often causes symptoms earlier than non-syndromic myxoma), skin angiomyxoma (typically multiple), spotty skin pigmentation, endocrine hyperactivity, schwannoma, and epithelioid blue nevi.

© The Editor(s) (if applicable) and The Author(s), under exclusive license to
Springer Nature Switzerland AG 2021
S. Mocellin, *Soft Tissue Tumors*, https://doi.org/10.1007/978-3-030-58710-9_45

Germline mutations in protein kinase A regulatory subunit 1 alpha (PRKAR1A, a tumor suppressor gene) have been identified as the genetic cause of this syndrome (somatic mutations of this gene appear to play a role also in the development of non-syndromic cardiac myxomas).

Pathology

Macroscopically the lesion presents as a soft, polypoid, pale, lobulated mass. Microscopically the tumor is composed of complex structures resembling cords, nests, rings, or poorly formed glands, often surrounding blood vessels. Cells are stellate or globular with abundant eosinophilic cytoplasm. No atypia is present; mitoses are rare. Typical is the presence of abundant mucopolysaccharide (myxoid) ground substance containing chondroitin sulfate and hyaluronic acid.

Differential diagnosis may be needed with the following: left atrial thrombus; metastatic carcinoma (in case of myxoma with glandular structures; carcinoma has atypia and mitotic activity); myxoid sarcoma; and papillary fibroelastoma (on valve cusps, avascular papillary fronds).

Biomarkers

Cardiac myxoma stains positive for CD31, CD34, and calretinin; it stains negative for CD68 and cytokeratins (except for glandular elements which may stain positive).

Prognosis

Although cardiac myxoma is a benign tumor, its prognosis can be dismal due to the hemodynamic and embolic complications.

Therapy

Surgical exeresis is the only effective treatment. Though rare, disease recurrence is possible if surgery is not radical.

Suggested Readings

Colin (2018) Cardiac myxoma: a contemporary multimodality imaging review. Int J Cardiovasc Imaging 34(11):1789–1808

Kirsechner (2000) Mutations of the gene encoding the protein kinase A type I-alpha regulatory subunit in patients with the Carney complex. Nat Genet 26(1):89–92

Maleszewski (2014) PRKAR1A in the development of cardiac myxoma: a study of 110 cases including isolated and syndromic tumors. Am J Surg Pathol 38(8):1079–1087

Wei (2019) Clinical features and surgical results of cardiac myxoma in Carney complex. J Card Surg 34(1):14–19

Cardiac Rhabdomyoma

46

Definition

Cardiac rhabdomyoma is a benign tumor originating from striated muscle cells. Along with extra-cardiac rhabdomyomas (which include adult, fetal, and genital rhabdomyoma; for details → see dedicated sections), it belongs to the rhabdomyoma family (→ see also the section entitled "Rhabdomyoma").

Epidemiology and Presentation

It represents 50–90% of primary heart tumors in children. It is usually discovered in patients during the first year of life. It may obstruct valvular orifice or cardiac chamber causing hemodynamic effects and may present with sudden cardiac death. It is believed to be caused by inactivating mutations in TSC1 and TSC2 tumor suppressor genes.

It can be sporadic or syndromic (→ see below paragraph).

Etiology and Predisposition

About 50% of patients have **tuberous sclerosis complex** (TSC), a genetic syndrome inherited in an autosomal dominant manner and caused by inactivating mutations in TSC1 (9q34) and TSC2 (16p13.3) tumor suppressor genes (which encode proteins inhibiting the mTOR pathway). TSC is characterized by multisystem hamartomas/tumors, most frequently observed in the skin, brain, kidney, lung, and heart. Skin involvement includes the following: hypomelanotic macules (ash leaf, within the first years of life), angiofibromas (appear at the age of 3–4 years as erythematous and papulo-nodular lesions; → see dedicated section), ungual fibromas, cephalic and lumbar fibrous plaques (shagreen patch), and "confetti" skin lesions (childhood to adolescence). The brain is involved in almost all cases of TSC in particular with

© The Editor(s) (if applicable) and The Author(s), under exclusive license to   159
Springer Nature Switzerland AG 2021
S. Mocellin, *Soft Tissue Tumors*, https://doi.org/10.1007/978-3-030-58710-9_46

cortico/subcortical tubers and subependymal giant cell astrocytoma (SEGA, which can cause hydrocephalus). Early-onset epilepsy is present in 85% of patients. Neuropsychiatric features have also been reported. Renal angiomyolipoma ($\rightarrow$ see dedicated section) develops during childhood and presents with pain, hematuria, retroperitoneal hemorrhage, abdominal masses, hypertension, and renal failure. Lymphangioleiomyomatosis ($\rightarrow$ see dedicated section), multifocal micronodular pneumocyte hyperplasia (MMPH) and pulmonary cysts develop during adulthood and manifest with dyspnea, pneumothorax, or chylothorax. Cardiac rhabdomyoma can appear during the fetal period and may become symptomatic (outflow tract obstruction or by interfering with valvular function) during infancy and childhood.

Pathology

Macroscopically, the lesion presents as a small, firm, gray to white, well-circumscribed myocardial mass (often multiple) that protrudes into ventricles (average size: 3–4 cm).

Microscopically, the tumor is composed of clear cells and large, rounded, polygonal cells ("spider cells") with glycogen vacuoles separated by strands of cytoplasm extending between cell membrane and nucleus. No mitotic activity is usually detected.

Differential diagnosis may be needed with the following: glycogen storage disease (no well-formed nodules, cells have intercalated disks at poles by electron microscopy); granular cell tumor (epicardial, no vacuoles, no myofibers, S100 positive, desmin and myoglobin negative); and lipoma (usually epicardial, no myofibers, no glycogen).

Biomarkers

Cardiac rhabdomyoma stains positive for myoglobin, actin, desmin, and vimentin, whereas it stains negative for S100.

Prognosis

Cardiac rhabdomyoma is a benign tumor, but hemodynamic effects (outflow tract obstruction or refractory arrhythmia) can be fatal. Of note, many tumors regress spontaneously.

Therapy

Surgery may be necessary in case of lack of spontaneous regression of a hemodynamically symptomatic lesion, especially if located in the left ventricle.

As regards **target therapy**, mTOR inhibitors (e.g., sirolimus, everolimus) have been reported to be effective in treating symptomatic cardiac rhabdomyomas.

Suggested Readings

Chaurasia (2013) Cardiac rhabdomyoma in familial tuberous sclerosis. J Cardiovasc Thorac Res 5(2):71–72

Davis (2019) Use of Cardiac MRI to Assess Antitumor Efficacy of Everolimus in Sporadic Cardiac Rhabdomyoma. Pediatrics 143(6):e20182495

Dhulipudi (2019) Symptomatic improvement using everolimus in infants with cardiac rhabdomyoma. Ann Pediatr Cardiol 12(1):45–48

Park (2019) Sirolimus therapy for fetal cardiac rhabdomyoma in a pregnant woman with tuberous sclerosis. Obstet Gynecol Sci 62(4):280–284

Song (2018) Spontaneous Regression of Cardiac Rhabdomyoma Presenting as Severe Left Ventricular Inlet Obstruction in a Neonate with Tuberous Sclerosis. Case Rep Cardiol 2018:8395260

Definition

Cellular angiofibroma (CAF) is a benign tumor classified among the fibroblastic-myofibroblastic tumors.

It is also known as male angiomyofibroblastoma-like tumor. For other types of angiofibromas, → see section entitled "Angiofibroma."

Epidemiology and Presentation

CAF is a rare tumor developing in adults (peak incidence: 50 years in females, 70 years in males) with equal gender distribution. Most cases have been reported to arise in the superficial soft tissues of the vulvovaginal region and the inguinoscrotal or paratesticular region; rare cases have been described in the retroperitoneum, trunk, iliac spine, oral mucosa, and knee. The lesion typically presents as a slow-growing well-circumscribed painless mass (ranging from 1 to 20 cm in diameter), which can be mistaken with Bartholin's cyst (in females) or a hernia (in males).

Pathology

CAF is a cellular and highly vascularized fibroblastic tumor closely related to spindle cell lipoma and myofibroblastoma.

The neoplasm is composed of uniform, spindled cells in a loosely fibrous stroma containing numerous small to medium-sized thick-walled ectatic or branching vessels. The number of mitoses varies (up to 10 per 10 HPF[1]). Mast cells are frequent. Small aggregates of adipocytes can be found in half cases.

---

[1] HPF: high power field

© The Editor(s) (if applicable) and The Author(s), under exclusive license to
Springer Nature Switzerland AG 2021
S. Mocellin, *Soft Tissue Tumors*, https://doi.org/10.1007/978-3-030-58710-9_47

Cellular angiofibroma with sarcomatous transformation (vacuolated lipoblasts or pleomorphic spindle cells showing features either of pleomorphic liposarcoma, atypical lipomatous tumor, or pleomorphic spindle cell sarcoma) has been rarely reported, mainly in vulvar cases. Another rare variant with worrisome features is known as atypical cellular angiofibroma.

Differential diagnosis may be needed with the following: aggressive angiomyxoma (usually large and deep, hypocellular, infiltrative margin, desmin positive); angiomyofibroblastoma (less uniform cellularity, smaller vessels, usually desmin positive); leiomyoma (positive for SMA and desmin); pleomorphic hyalinizing angiectatic tumor (usually on lower extremity, presence of TGFBR3-MGEA5 fusion gene); solitary fibrous tumor (hypercellular and hypocellular areas, prominent staghorn vessels, hyalinized collagen, CD34 positive).

Biomarkers

Tumor cells are generally positive for estrogen receptor and progesterone receptor (both in males and females) and negative for desmin, S100, and cytokeratins. CD34 and SMA[2] are variably expressed. CAF typically carries a genetic deletion involving the RB1 gene in chromosome 13q14 region.

Prognosis

CAF is a benign tumor and local recurrence is very rare. Even cases with atypia or sarcomatous transformation have been reported to have a benign behavior.

Therapy

Surgical excision is the treatment of choice.

Suggested Readings

Chien (2020) First Glance of Molecular Profile of Atypical Cellular Angiofibroma/Cellular Angiofibroma with Sarcomatous Transformation by Next Generation Sequencing. Diagnostics (Basel) 10(1):E35

Creytens (2016) Cellular Angiofibroma With Sarcomatous Transformation Showing Pleomorphic Liposarcoma-Like and Atypical Lipomatous Tumor-Like Features. Am J Dermatopathol 38(9):712–714

Fletcher (2020) WHO classification of tumours of soft tissue and bone (5th edition)

Khmou (2016) Cellular angiofibroma of the vulva: a poorly known entity, a case report and literature review. BMC Clin Pathol 16:8

---

[2] SMA: smooth muscle actin

Definition

Cellular fibrous histiocytoma (CFH) is a variant of benign fibrous histiocytoma ($\rightarrow$ see dedicated section). It is also known as cellular dermatofibroma and cellular benign fibrous histiocytoma. For other types of fibrous histiocytomas, $\rightarrow$ see section entitled "Fibrous Histiocytoma."

Epidemiology and Presentation

CFH accounts for about 5% of all benign fibrous histiocytoma cases. It can occur at any age (mean age: 40 years), with no gender difference. It develops in the skin, most frequently of the extremities (about two thirds of all cases). It presents as a skin colored cutaneous lesion up to 3 cm in diameter.

Pathology

CFH is characterized by high cellularity, monomorphism, and a mixed fascicular and storiform growth pattern of spindle cells. At the periphery of the tumor, hyalinized collagen bundles surrounded by tumor cells are a consistent finding. Mitotic activity (mean: 3 mitotic figures per 10 HPF[1], but it may be > 10) is present in virtually all cases and correlates with cellularity, but no atypia or pleomorphism are detected.

Differential diagnosis may be needed with the following: benign fibrous histiocytoma (less cellularity); dermatofibrosarcoma protuberans (usually presents as larger and multinodular lesion; typically CD34 positive; chromosomal translocation leading to COL1A1-PDGFB fusion gene); and leiomyosarcoma (smooth muscle

---

[1] HPF: high power field

S. Mocellin, *Soft Tissue Tumors*, https://doi.org/10.1007/978-3-030-58710-9_48

morphology with cigar shaped nuclei, pleomorphism, infiltrative dermal growth, positive for multiple muscle biomarkers).

Biomarkers

CFH often stains positive for vimentin, CD163, CD68, and SMA[2]. It may stain positive for desmin and rarely for CD34. It stains negative for CD117, S100, HMB45, and cytokeratins.

Prognosis

CFH has a significant risk of local recurrence (approximately 25%). Metastasis has been reported in rare cases.

Therapy

Surgical excision (possibly wide) is the treatment of choice.

Suggested Readings

Doyle (2013) Metastasizing "benign" cutaneous fibrous histiocytoma: a clinicopathologic analysis of 16 cases. Am J Surg Pathol 37(4):484–495
Lodewick (2014) Fatal case of metastatic cellular fibrous histiocytoma: case report and review of literature. Am J Dermatopathol 36(9):e156–e162
Volpicelli (2012) Desmin and CD34 positivity in cellular fibrous histiocytoma: an immunohistochemical analysis of 100 cases. J Cutan Pathol 39(8):747–752

---

[2] SMA: smooth muscle actin

Definition

Cherry hemangioma is acquired tumor of vascular origin. It is also known as cherry angioma, senile angioma, senile hemangioma, and Campbell de Morgan spot.

Epidemiology and Presentation

Cherry hemangioma is a very common skin lesion. Its incidence increases with the age; although it can be found in up to 5% of adolescents, in most cases cherry hemangioma starts developing after the third decade of life, and it affects 75% of adults over the age of 75 years. It presents as an asymptomatic, well-circumscribed, flat erythematous macule or as a dome-shaped, bright red papule of few millimeters in size. It is usually located on upper extremities and trunk and rarely on face, hands, and feet. Bleeding can occur after trauma.

Pathology

Cherry hemangioma is a proliferation of newly formed dilated capillaries and post-capillary venules in the superficial dermis, with a lobular pattern.

Biomarkers

Cherry hemangioma is characterized by a high frequency (80%) of mutually exclusive mutations in GNA14, GNAQ, and GNA11 genes (which establishes its neoplastic nature).

© The Editor(s) (if applicable) and The Author(s), under exclusive license to
Springer Nature Switzerland AG 2021
S. Mocellin, *Soft Tissue Tumors*, https://doi.org/10.1007/978-3-030-58710-9_49

Prognosis

Excellent.

Therapy

Treatment is unnecessary, unless for cosmetic reasons.

Suggested Reading

Liau (2019) High frequency of GNA14, GNAQ, and GNA11 mutations in cherry hemangioma: a histopathological and molecular study of 85 cases indicating GNA14 as the most commonly mutated gene in vascular neoplasms. Mod Pathol 32(11):1657–1665

Definition

Chondroid lipoma is a benign adipocytic tumor. For general details on different types of lipomas, → see section entitled "Lipoma."

Epidemiology and Presentation

It is very rare and affects mainly young women (median age, 35 years; range, 15 to 70 years). Lesions are typically deep, deep subcutaneous fat or skeletal muscle. Most cases are located in the proximal extremities and limb girdles. Clinically, it presents as a slow-growing, painless nodule/mass up to 10 cm in diameter.

Pathology

Chondroid lipoma is characterized by features of both embryonal fat and embryonal cartilage: it is made of lipoblasts in a myxoid-chondroid matrix that intermingle with mature adipocytes. It lacks pleomorphism, atypia, mitotic activity, and mature cartilage.

Differential diagnosis may be needed with the following: chondrolipoma (also known as lipoma with chondroid metaplasia; true cartilage is present); extraskeletal chondroma (distal extremities, mature hyaline cartilage, no fat); extraskeletal myxoid chondrosarcoma (prominent fibrous septa; chondroblasts typically lack intracytoplasmic vacuoles, no mature fat; frequently has mitotic figures and necrosis; typical chromosomal translocations); myxoid liposarcoma (different sites, usually no prominent cords or clusters of cells; delicate plexiform capillary matrix; no chondroid matrix; it carries a typical chromosomal translocation); and lipoblastoma (restricted to children; uniform population of lipoblasts; typical chromosomal translocations).

© The Editor(s) (if applicable) and The Author(s), under exclusive license to
Springer Nature Switzerland AG 2021
S. Mocellin, *Soft Tissue Tumors*, https://doi.org/10.1007/978-3-030-58710-9_50

Biomarkers

The tumor stains positive for S100 (strongly in the mature fatty component, weak in the lipoblastic elements) and vimentin. It stains negative for EMA,[1] HMB45,[2] and SMA[3].

Chondroid lipoma has been repeatedly reported to harbor a t(11;16)(q13;p13) chromosomal translocation resulting in the **C11orf95-MKL2 fusion gene**[4].

Prognosis

Chondroid lipoma is a benign tumor, recurrences being very rare.

Therapy

Surgical excision is the treatment of choice.

Suggested Readings

Escobar (2014) PET/CT and MRI of chondroid lipoma of the deltoid muscle. Clin Nucl Med 39(11):984–987
Fletcher (2020) WHO classification of tumours of soft tissue and bone (5th edition)
Huang (2019) Characteristics of chondroid lipoma: A case report and literature review. Medicine (Baltimore) 98(19):e15587
Thway (2012) Chondroid lipoma: an update and review. Ann Diagn Pathol 16(3):230–234

---

[1] EMA: epithelial membrane antigen

[2] HMB45: monoclonal antibody recognizing melanosomal glycoprotein gp100

[3] SMA: smooth muscle actin

[4] C11orf95-MKL2 fusion gene: chromosome 11 open reading frame 95 is a protein coding gene (diseases associated with C11orf95 include RELA fusion-positive ependymoma and cellular ependymoma). MKL2 (myocardin-like protein 2, also known as MRTFB: myocardin-related transcription factor B) acts as a transcriptional coactivator of serum response factor (SRF); it is required for skeletal myogenic differentiation, and its alterations are associated with chondroid lipoma and extraskeletal chondroma.

This is a recently recognized type of sarcoma molecularly characterized by the rearrangement of the CIC gene.

For details → see the section entitled "Ewing-Like Sarcomas,"

Definition

Clear cell sarcoma (CCS) is a malignant tumor of uncertain differentiation. It is also known as melanoma of soft parts. For kidney clear cell sarcoma → see dedicated section.

Epidemiology and Presentation

CCS is a rare tumor typically occurring in young adults (peak incidence, third–fourth decade of life; age range, 15–75 years), without gender difference. The neoplasm affects almost always the extremities, with the foot/ankle region accounting for 40% of all cases. It develops in the deep soft tissues, frequently in close relationship with tendons and aponeuroses. Rarely CCS occurs in the head and neck, trunk, retroperitoneum, viscera (e.g., gastrointestinal tract), or bone. Clinically, the lesion generally presents as a slow-growing mass (usually < 5 cm, although lesions > 10 cm can be observed) being present for months or years. Pain and/or tenderness may be present. Of note, CCS is one of the soft tissue sarcomas with the highest rate of metastasis to regional lymph nodes.

Pathology

Microscopically, one distinctive feature is the nested growth pattern (collagenous bands separate the neoplasm into compartments). Tumor cells show an epithelioid morphology, although areas with spindled cells can be present. Despite the name, CCS cells most frequently show scarcely eosinophilic or amphophilic cytoplasm, clear cells representing only a minority of tumor cells. Nuclear pleomorphism and

© The Editor(s) (if applicable) and The Author(s), under exclusive license to
Springer Nature Switzerland AG 2021
S. Mocellin, *Soft Tissue Tumors*, https://doi.org/10.1007/978-3-030-58710-9_52

mitotic activity (mean: 4 mitoses per 10 HPF[1]) can be observed but are less prominent than in melanoma. Floret-like giant cells are frequently found useful diagnostic clue. Using Fontana stain, melanin can be detected in two thirds of cases (which is consistent with the finding of melanosomes upon ultrastructural analysis).

Differential diagnosis may be needed with melanoma (negative for EWSR1-ATF1 fusion gene); in the gastrointestinal tract, CCS should be differentiated from malignant gastrointestinal neuroectodermal tumor (GNET; for more details → see section entitled "Gastrointestinal Clear Cell Sarcoma").

Biomarkers

A consistent melanocytic differentiation (i.e., positivity for S100, HMB45 and MITF) is a characteristic feature of CCS (hence the name melanoma of soft parts). The tumor stains negative for SMA and desmin.

The genetic hallmark of CCS is the presence of the chromosomal translocation t(12;22)(q13;q12) which leads to the formation of the **EWSR1-ATF1 fusion gene**[2] in more than 90% of cases. Rarely, the chromosomal translocation t(2;22)(q33;q12) leads to the formation of the **EWSR1-CREB1 fusion gene**. ATF1 and CREB1 are members of the CREB basic leucine zipper transcription factor family and bind to cAMP-inducible promoters. The EWSR1-ATF1 chimeric protein is believed to play a key role in CCS pathogenesis, likely by targeting the MITF promoter (which would lead to melanocyte differentiation) and MET promoter.

Prognosis

Despite the usually slow progression, CCS is a malignancy characterized by a poor prognosis with 5-year, 10-year and 20-year survival rates of 67%, 33%, and 10%, respectively, underscoring the fact that many patients develop disease recurrence even more than 10 years after the initial diagnosis (which calls for long-term follow-up). Negative prognostic factors are tumor size (>3–5 cm), necrosis, and local disease relapse. Gastrointestinal CCS is associated with even worse prognosis than somatic soft tissue CCS.

---

[1] HPF: high power field

[2] EWSR1-ATF1 fusion gene: EWSR1 encodes for an RNA-binding protein and is involved in the recurrent translocations associated with a number of soft tissue tumors other than clear cell sarcoma such as the Ewing family of tumors, desmoplastic small round cell tumor, extraskeletal myxoid chondrosarcoma, myxoid liposarcoma (rarely), and angiomatoid fibrous histiocytoma. ATF1 gene encodes an activating transcription factor, which belongs to the ATF subfamily and bZIP (basic-region leucine zipper) family. It influences cellular physiologic processes by regulating the expression of downstream target genes, which are related to growth, survival, and other cellular activities; this protein is phosphorylated at serine 63 in its kinase-inducible domain by serine/threonine kinases, cAMP-dependent protein kinase A, calmodulin-dependent protein kinase I/II, mitogen- and stress-activated protein kinase, and cyclin-dependent kinase 3 (CDK-3).

Therapy

Surgery is the mainstay of treatment; sentinel node biopsy has been proposed for improving disease staging.

Locoregional treatments such as radiotherapy and isolated limb perfusion can be used to avoid amputation.

Chemotherapy is scarcely effective for metastatic disease.

As regards **target therapy**, attempts to exploit the rearrangement of the EWSR1 gene (which leads to overexpression of MET) to treat CCS with crizotinib[3] have yielded scarce results. Clinical experience with **immunotherapy** is in its infancy.

Suggested Readings

Akkooi v (2006) Sentinel node biopsy for clear cell sarcoma. Eur J Surg Oncol 32(9):996–999

Andreou (2013) Sentinel node biopsy in soft tissue sarcoma subtypes with a high propensity for regional lymphatic spread--results of a large prospective trial. Ann Oncol 24(5):1400–1405

Aw (2019) Clear Cell Sarcoma of the Kidney. Arch Pathol Lab Med 143(8):1022–1026

Cellier (2018) Cutaneous Melanocytoma With CRTC1-TRIM11 Fusion: Report of 5 Cases Resembling Clear Cell Sarcoma. Am J Surg Pathol 42(3):382–391

Cornillie (2016) Biology and management of clear cell sarcoma: state of the art and future perspectives. Expert Rev Anticancer Ther 16(8):839–845

Fletcher (2020). WHO classification of tumours of soft tissue and bone (5th edition)

Gonzaga (2018) The epidemiology and survivorship of clear cell sarcoma: a National Cancer Database (NCDB) review. J Cancer Res Clin Oncol 144(9):1711–1716

Green (2018) Clear cell sarcoma of the gastrointestinal tract and malignant gastrointestinal neuroectodermal tumour: distinct or related entities? A review. Pathology 50(5):490–498

Hantsechke (2010) Cutaneous clear cell sarcoma: a clinicopathologic, immunohistochemical, and molecular analysis of 12 cases emphasizing its distinction from dermal melanoma. Am J Surg Pathol 34(2):216–222

Joo (2009) Primary gastrointestinal clear cell sarcoma: report of 2 cases, one case associated with IgG4-related sclerosing disease, and review of literature. Ann Diagn Pathol 13(1):30–35

Keung (2018) Defining the incidence and clinical significance of lymph node metastasis in soft tissue sarcoma. Eur J Surg Oncol 44(1):170–177

Li (2019) Prognostic Factors for Survival in Patients with Clear Cell Sarcoma: An Analysis of the Surveillance, Epidemiology, and End Results (SEER) Database. Med Sci Monit 25:6950–6956

Maduekwe (2009) Role of sentinel lymph node biopsy in the staging of synovial, epithelioid, and clear cell sarcomas. Ann Surg Oncol 16(5):1356–1363

Marcrom (2017) Complete response of mediastinal clear cell sarcoma to pembrolizumab with radiotherapy. Clin Sarcoma Res 7:14

Nawrocki (2020) A rare case of primary dermal clear cell sarcoma with focal epidermotropism: An entity difficult to distinguish from melanoma. J Cutan Pathol [Epub ahead of print]

Pletneva (2014) Clear cell melanoma: a cutaneous clear cell malignancy. Arch Pathol Lab Med 138(10):1328–1336

Schoffski (2017) Activity and safety of crizotinib in patients with advanced clear-cell sarcoma with MET alterations: European Organization for Research and Treatment of Cancer phase II trial 90101 'CREATE'. Ann Oncol 28(12):3000–3008

---

[3] Crizotinib: small molecule tyrosine kinase inhibitor targeting the following: ALK, MET

Wolak (2018) Malignant gastrointestinal neuroectodermal tumor (clear cell sarcoma-like tumor of the gastrointestinal tract) of the small intestine in a 12-year-old boy. Dev Period Med 22(4):358–363

Wright (2012) The role of sentinel lymph node biopsy in select sarcoma patients: a meta-analysis. Am J Surg 204(4):428–433

Definition

Clear cell sugar tumor (CCST) is a (generally) benign neoplasm belonging to the PEComa family (→ see section entitled "Perivascular Epithelioid Cell Tumor"). It is also known as clear cell tumor of the lung.

Epidemiology and Presentation

CCST is a very rare neoplasm mainly affecting adults over 40 years, without gender predilection. It typically localizes in the lungs (generally in periphery, rarely in trachea or bronchi), although it can arise in extrapulmonary sites (e.g., breast).

CCST generally presents as an asymptomatic lesion (often it is found incidentally upon radiological imaging performed for other reasons) with maximum diameter smaller than 5 cm; otherwise it can present with nonspecific symptoms.

Computed tomography and magnetic resonance imaging can detect hypervascularization, and positron emission tomography may reveal fluorodeoxyglucose uptake, but they cannot be accurate and diagnosis requires tumor biopsy and histological evaluation.

Etiology and Predisposition

Rarely, CCST develops within the frame of **tuberous sclerosis** (sometimes in association with lymphangioleiomyomatosis and micronodular pneumocyte hyperplasia). For more details on tuberous sclerosis → see section entitled "Perivascular Epithelioid Cell Tumor."

CCST has been reported to be associated also with the **Birt-Hogg-Dubé syndrome,** a rare genodermatosis inherited in an autosomal dominant pattern and caused by germline mutations tof the folliculin (FLCN) gene, a tumor suppressor

S. Mocellin, *Soft Tissue Tumors*, https://doi.org/10.1007/978-3-030-58710-9_53

gene whose protein product is involved in mTOR signaling pathway regulating cell growth and metabolism. Clinically, the Birt-Hogg-Dubé syndrome is characterized by fibrofolliculomas of the skin, pulmonary cysts (which can lead to pneumothorax), and renal neoplasms.

Pathology

CCST is composed of sheets of large cells with clear to eosinophilic granular cytoplasm and PAS-positive glycogen granules (it strikingly resembles renal cell carcinoma). A sclerotic (variably prominent) vasculature is present. Mitoses are rare or absent.

Differential diagnosis may be needed with the following: primary or metastatic carcinomas with clear cell pattern (e.g., renal cell carcinoma); metastatic clear cell sarcoma; metastatic melanoma; and paraganglioma.

Biomarkers

CCST stains positive for melanocytic (HMB45, MART1/Melan-A, MITF; variably positive or negative for S100) and smooth muscle biomarkers (SMA, desmin). It does not express cytokeratins or EMA.

Prognosis

CCST behaves usually a benign tumor, although rare cases of metastatic disease have been described. Malignant features may include lesion size greater than 5 cm, nuclear pleomorphism, increased mitoses, and necrosis.

Therapy

Surgery is the treatment of choice.

Suggested Readings

Chang (2018) Clear cell "sugar" tumor of the lung: a case report and review of the literature. AME Case Rep 2:40

Flieder (1997) Clear cell "sugar" tumor of the lung: association with lymphangioleiomyomatosis and multifocal micronodular pneumocyte hyperplasia in a patient with tuberous sclerosis. Am J Surg Pathol 21(10):1242–1247

Gunji-Niitsu (2016) Benign clear cell "sugar" tumor of the lung in a patient with Birt-Hogg-Dubé syndrome: a case report. BMC Med Genet 17(1):85

Tsilimigras (2017) Clear cell "sugar tumor" of the lung: Diagnostic features of a rare pulmonary tumor. Respir Med Case Rep 23:52–54

54

Definition

Composite hemangioendothelioma (CHE) is a vascular tumor of intermediate aggressiveness.

Epidemiology and Presentation

CHE is a very rare tumor usually developing in adults (with female predominance). It affects the skin of distal extremities, although some cases arising in other sites have been described. An association with chronic lymphedema has been reported. Lesions are generally nodular (up to several centimeters in size), red-blue in color, and long-standing (many years).

Pathology

CHE is made of histologically benign and malignant vascular components (in various proportions) which include epithelioid hemangioendothelioma, retiform hemangioendothelioma, spindle cell hemangioma, angiosarcoma (with low-grade angiosarcomatous appearance), and benign vascular lesions (lymphangioma, angiomatosis, arteriovenous malformation, cavernous hemangioma).

Prognosis

CHE is a locally aggressive, rarely metastasizing vascular neoplasm. Local recurrence can occur after many years, and the rare metastatic disease mainly localizes in lymph nodes.

© The Editor(s) (if applicable) and The Author(s), under exclusive license to Springer Nature Switzerland AG 2021
S. Mocellin, *Soft Tissue Tumors*, https://doi.org/10.1007/978-3-030-58710-9_54

Therapy

Surgical excision is the treatment of choice.

Suggested Readings

Fletcher (2020) WHO classification of tumours of soft tissue and bone (5th edition)
Papke (2020) What is new in endothelial neoplasia? Virchows Arch 476(1):17–28
Shon (2019) Epithelioid vascular tumors: a review. Adv Anat Pathol 26(3):186–197

Definition

Congenital hemangioma (CHA) is a benign tumor of vascular origin. For further details on the hemangioma family → see section entitled "hemangioma".

Epidemiology and Presentation

CHA incidence is unclear, an estimate being 1% of all newborns. As compared to infantile hemangioma (→ see dedicated section), CHA is significantly less frequent: in a retrospective review of 6459 children with vascular anomalies observed in a specialized Chinese center, infantile hemangioma, CHA, and vascular malformations were diagnosed in 43%, 14%, and 43% of patients, respectively.

CHA has similar distribution in males and females. It can occur anywhere in the skin, but most frequently arises in the extremities and retroauricular area. CHA is fully developed at birth and then, either rapidly involutes during the first year of life or may never show involution. The tumor, which is not painful, can reach several centimeters in diameter (average: 5 cm).

According to the evolution, three types of CHA are defined:

1. *Rapidly involuting congenital hemangioma* (RICH) presents at birth either as a red-purple color plaque with gross telangiectasia, or as a flat violaceous lesion, or as a raised greyish tumor surrounded by a pale halo with multiple small telangiectasias. RICH undergoes a rapid regression phase and completely disappears by 12–18 months of age.
2. *Non-involuting congenital hemangioma* (NICH) presents at birth as a pink or purple-colored plaque-like lesions with prominent overlying gross telangiectasia and peripheral blanching. NICH does not show a regression phase and may grow proportionately with the child growth.

© The Editor(s) (if applicable) and The Author(s), under exclusive license to
Springer Nature Switzerland AG 2021
S. Mocellin, *Soft Tissue Tumors*, https://doi.org/10.1007/978-3-030-58710-9_55

3. *Partially involuting congenital hemangioma* (PICH) resembles RICH but shows only partial involution.

Of note, although CHA typically affects the skin, it may occasionally develop in the liver ($\rightarrow$ see Chap. 123).

Diagnosis is usually clinical; however, ultrasound and magnetic resonance imaging may be useful to confirm diagnosis of cutaneous CHA. Radiological imaging is necessary for the diagnosis of the (rare) cases developing in the liver.

Pathology

Pathological assessment may be needed, especially to differentiate CHA from malignant neoplasms. Microscopically, lobules of small endothelial cells are accompanied by large malformed (dysplastic) muscular vessels and smaller, thin-walled dilated vessels. The lobular (proliferative) areas include tufts of endothelium, similar to those seen in innate hemangioma or tufted angioma. Only rare mitotic figures can be found within vascular lobules.

Biomarkers

Unlike infantile hemangioma, CHA stains negative for GLUT1.[1] Like infantile hemangioma, CHA stains positive for CD31, CD34, and WT1.[2]

CHA is characterized by mutually exclusive missense mutations that alter glutamine at amino acid 209 (Glu209) in GNAQ[3] or GNA11[4] in all tested samples.

Prognosis

CHA is a benign tumor and complete involution occurs in RICH cases. Nonetheless, the following complications can occur: (1) ulceration, which may lead to severe bleeding and superinfection; (2) transient thrombocytopenia and coagulopathy with hypofibrinogenemia and anemia are potential complications of RICH, especially in

---

[1] GLUT1: this gene (also known as SLC2A1, solute carrier family 2 member 1) encodes a major glucose transporter in the mammalian blood-brain barrier.

[2] WT1: the Wilms tumor 1 gene encodes a transcription factor with an essential role in the normal development of the urogenital system. It is mutated in a small subset of patients with Wilms tumor.

[3] GNAQ: the G protein subunit alpha Q gene encodes a guanine nucleotide-binding protein. The encoded protein, an alpha subunit in the Gq class, couples a seven-transmembrane domain receptor to activation of phospholipase C-beta.

[4] GNA11: the G protein subunit alpha 11 gene encodes a protein belonging to the family of guanine nucleotide-binding proteins (G proteins), which function as modulators or transducers in various transmembrane signaling systems. G proteins are composed of three units: alpha, beta, and gamma. This gene encodes one of the alpha subunits (subunit alpha 11).

liver lesions; the clinical picture may resemble the Kasabach-Merritt syndrome, a life-threatening complication typical of other rare congenital vascular tumors (e.g., tufted angioma, hemangioendothelioma), but it never reaches the profound and protracted thrombocytopenia and disseminated intravascular coagulation proper of that condition; (3) high-output heart failure from arteriovenous shunting and cardiac overload has been reported in a small number of infants with large CHA (>7 cm); (4) cosmetic disfigurement.

Therapy

The therapeutic indication must be individualized based upon the tumor size and location, tendency to spontaneous involution, and presence of complications. Unlike infantile hemangioma, CHA is not responsive to medications, and surgery remains the mainstay of treatment. For uncomplicated lesions, the recommendation is to wait until the second year of age in order to confirm that the tumor is a NICH: once this diagnosis is certain, surgery of uncomplicated lesions can be posticipated until otherwise decided by the patient/family since there is no risk of malignant transformation.

Suggested Readings

Ayturk (2016) Somatic activating mutations in GNAQ and GNA11 are associated with congenital hemangioma. Am J Hum Genet 98(4):789–795

Johnson (2018) Vascular tumors in infants: case report and review of clinical, histopathologic, and immunohistochemical characteristics of infantile hemangioma, pyogenic granuloma, noninvoluting congenital hemangioma, tufted angioma, and kaposiform hemangioendothelioma. Am J Dermatopathol 40(4):231–239

Wildgruber (2019) Vascular tumors in infants and adolescents. Insights Imaging 10(1):30

Yang (2015) Clinical characteristics and treatment options of infantile vascular anomalies. Medicine (Baltimore) 94(40):e1717

Definition

Congenital mesoblastic nephroma (CMN) is a kidney tumor with potentially malignant behavior originating from spindled mesenchymal cells. It is also known as mesoblastic nephroma (previously named fetal renal hamartoma leiomyomatous renal hamartoma).

Epidemiology and Presentation

CMN is the most common kidney tumor found in infants younger than 6 months and accounts for about 4% of childhood kidney neoplasms. The median age of diagnosis is 1–2 months, males being affected more frequently (M/F = 2:1); more than 90% of cases arise within the first year of life, and more than 15% of the cases are diagnosed prenatally (the diagnosis should be questioned when suspected in individuals older than 2 years).

CMN typically presents as an abdominal mass detected by ultrasound scan. Concurrent findings may include hypertension (20% of cases), polyhydramnios (15%), hematuria (10%), hypercalcemia (5%), and elevated serum levels of renin (1%). Most patients present with localized (i.e., non-metastatic) disease. In most patients, disease is classified at presentation as stage I or II (i.e., localized), few patients present with stage III (i.e., locally advanced/infiltrating), and very rarely patients present with stage IV (presence of metastasis) or V (i.e., tumors in both kidneys) disease.

Pathology

Mesoblastic nephroma can be divided into the following three histologic subtypes:

(a) Classic mesoblastic nephroma (about 24% of cases): resembles leiomyoma with whorled cut surface; it may be cystic; hemorrhage and necrosis are unusual; microscopically, the tumor is composed of bland spindled myofibroblasts and thin collagen fibers; mitoses are rare; and necrosis/desmoplasia are not present.
(b) Cellular mesoblastic nephroma (66%): it is very similar to infantile fibrosarcoma; necrosis and large cystic areas and hemorrhage are frequently encountered; the tumor is composed of sheetlike proliferation of plump, atypical spindle cells; and mitotic figures (25–30/10 HPF) and necrosis are frequent.
(c) Mixed mesoblastic nephroma (10%): a mixture of classic and cellular patterns.

Differential diagnosis may be needed with the following: clear cell sarcoma (predominantly in children from 2 to 3 years of age; clear cells and chicken wire vasculature, low mitotic rate; negative for smooth muscle biomarkers); rhabdoid tumor (more invasive margins, generally epithelioid cells with cytoplasmic inclusions and prominent nucleoli, it often presents with metastasis; INI1 negative); Wilms tumor (the most common childhood kidney neoplasm, older age, blastema, and nephrogenic rests are present; bilateral kidney tumors, concurrent birth defects and/or metastatic disease at presentation favor the diagnosis of Wilms tumor); infantile sarcoma (aggressive sarcoma typically presenting in the lower extremities, head and neck of infants during their first year of life; it may be impossible to differentiate these two nosological entities, which are believed to be correlated).

Biomarkers

CMN stains positive for smooth muscle actin (SMA) and vimentin (occasionally WT1). It stains negative for cytokeratins (except for entrapped epithelium), laminin, desmin, and CD34.

The **chromosomal translocation** t(12;15)(q13;q25) leads to the formation of the ETV6-NTRK3 fusion gene[1] and occurs almost exclusively in the cellular and mixed

---

[1] ETV6-NTRK3 fusion gene: ETV6 encodes an ETS family transcription factor associated with leukemia and congenital fibrosarcoma. NTRK3 encodes neurotrophic receptor tyrosine kinase 3 and belongs to the tropomyosin receptor kinases (TRK) family which also includes NTRK1 (encoding neurotrophic receptor tyrosine kinase 1) and NTRK2 (neurotrophic receptor tyrosine kinase 2). The encoded proteins elicit activities that regulate the natural growth, differentiation, and survival of neurons when they interact with endogenous neutrotrophin ligands. Chromosomal rearrangements involving in-frame fusions of these genes with various partners, translocations in the TRK kinase domains, mutations in the TRK ligand-binding site, amplifications of NTRK, or the expression of TRK splice variants can result in constitutively activated chimeric TRK fusion proteins that can act as oncogenic drivers that promote cell proliferation and survival in tumor cell lines.

mesoblastic nephroma subtypes. This chromosomal rearrangement is also typical of other tumors such as infantile fibrosarcoma, salivary mammary analogue secretory carcinoma, and breast secretory carcinoma. Other NTRK-based gene fusions have been described, such as EML4-NTRK3. NTRK-based fusion genes can be identified by DNA-based or RNA-based sequencing (e.g., NGS) or other assays such as fluorescence in situ hybridization (FISH) or immunohistochemistry.

Prognosis

Overall, the prognosis is good (5-year survival: 95%). In 5–10% of cases, the disease recurs or metastasizes (usually cellular type) to the lung, brain, or rarely bone (generally by age 1 year). Poor prognostic factors include cellular variant and advanced stage.

Therapy

Surgery (nephrectomy) is the mainstay of treatment. Adjuvant **chemotherapy** (primarily dactinomycin/vincristine and sometimes doxorubicin) may be suggested for patients with stage III cellular subtype mesoblastic nephromas who are aged 3 months or older at diagnosis.

Disease recurrence is usually treated with a combination of chemotherapy, **radiotherapy**, and surgery.

As regards **target therapy**, NTRK inhibitors such as either larotrectinib[2] or entrectinib[3] are indicated for the treatment of advanced/metastatic CMN. In particular, larotrectinib has been the first tyrosine kinase inhibitor to be granted approval by the Food and Drug Administration (FDA) for a tumor-agnostic indication (i.e., the treatment of adult and pediatric patients with advanced solid tumors harboring an NTRK gene fusion); analogously, entrectinib has been subsequently FDA approved for patients with any solid tumor bearing NTRK fusions.

Suggested Readings

AACR (2020) Entrectinib OK'd for cancers with NTRK fusions, NSCLC. Cancer Discov 9(10):OF2

Albert (2019) TRK fusion cancers in children: a clinical review and recommendations for screening. J Clin Oncol 37(6):513–524

Al-Salama (2019) Entrectinib: first global approval. Drugs 79(13):1477–1483

Church (2018) Recurrent EML4-NTRK3 fusions in infantile fibrosarcoma and congenital mesoblastic nephroma suggest a revised testing strategy. Mod Pathol 31(3):463–473

---

[2] Larotrectinib: tyrosine kinase inhibitor targeting the following—NTRK1, NTRK2, NTRK3.

[3] Entrectinib: tyrosine kinase inhibitor targeting the following—NTRK1, NTRK2, NTRK3, ROS1, ALK.

El Demellawy (2016) Congenital mesoblastic nephroma: a study of 19 cases using immunohisto-chemistry and ETV6-NTRK3 fusion gene rearrangement. Pathology 48(1):47–50

Farago (2020) Larotrectinib, a selective tropomyosin receptor kinase inhibitor for adult and pediatric tropomyosin receptor kinase fusion cancers. Future Oncol 16(9):417–425

Gooskens (2017) Congenital mesoblastic nephroma 50 years after its recognition: a narrative review. Pediatric Blood Cancer 64(7):e26437

Halalsheh (2018) Dramatic bone remodeling following larotrectinib administration for bone metastasis in a patient with TRK fusion congenital mesoblastic nephroma. Pediatr Blood Cancer 65(10):e27271

Hong (2020) Larotrectinib in patients with TRK fusion-positive solid tumours: a pooled analysis of three phase 1/2 clinical trials. Lancet Oncol [Epub ahead of print]. https://doi.org/10.1016/S1470-2045(19)30856-3

Definition

Cutaneous angiofibroma (CAF) is a benign tumor classified among the fibrohistio-cytic neoplasms. It is also known as fibrous papule (when located on the face), pearly penile papule (on the penis), periungual angiofibroma or Koenen tumor or periungual fibroma (underneath the nails), or oral fibroma (in the mouth).

Epidemiology and Presentation

CAF usually locates in the skin of middle-aged persons with special regard to the skin of the face (and the nose in particular). Other (rare) locations are the penis, periungual skin, and oral mucosa.

Fibrous papule presents as an indolent, single, dome-shaped, sessile, skin-colored, or slightly erythematous papule ranging from 3 to 6 mm in diameter.

It is important to distinguish between ordinary CAF (also referred to as sporadic angiofibroma) and multiple facial CAF (also known as syndromic angiofibroma) associated with tuberous sclerosis complex (TSC) and, less frequently, Birt-Hogg-Dubé syndrome and multiple endocrine neoplasia type 1 (MEN1) ($\rightarrow$ see below paragraph for more details). Clinically, differential diagnosis for CAF of the face may be needed with acne, acrochordon, intradermal melanocytic nevus, basal cell carcinoma, and adnexal tumors; periungual angiofibroma can mimic a verruca vulgaris and subungual exostosis, whereas pearly penile papules can be confused with condyloma acuminatum and molluscum contagiosum.

Etiology and Predisposition

1. Facial angiofibroma is considered one of the most typical clinical features of **tuberous sclerosis complex** (TSC), a genetic neurocutaneous disease inherited in an autosomal dominant pattern and caused by inactivating mutations of TSC1 (chromosome 9q34) and TSC2 (16p13.3), two tumor suppressor genes whose protein products indirectly inhibit mTOR. TSC is characterized by multiple hamartomas and neoplasms affecting the skin (e.g., hypomelanotic macules called ash leaf present within the first years of life; CAF appearing at age 3–4 years), kidneys (e.g., angiomyolipoma), heart (cardiac rhabdomyoma), brain (where tubers and other lesions lead to early-onset epilepsy in 85% of patients and other neuropsychiatric features—such as intellectual disability, attention-deficit/hyperactivity disorder, autism spectrum disorders—can occur), and lungs (e.g., lymphangioleiomyomatosis, pulmonary cysts causing pneumothorax). Within TSC, angiofibroma (where CAF is also known as adenoma sebaceum) typically arises on the face in childhood and early adulthood; both facial CAF (three or more are needed) and periungual CAF (two or more are needed) are two of the major criteria for TSC.

2. Multiple facial CAF can also be found in **Birt-Hogg-Dubé syndrome**, a hereditary condition associated with multiple benign skin tumors (such as fibrofolliculomas—which are pathognomonic for this syndrome; trichodiscomas and fibroepithelial polyp), lung cysts (which can cause pneumothorax), and an increased risk of both benign kidney tumors and kidney cancer. Symptoms of Birt-Hogg-Dubé syndrome generally do not appear until adulthood. This syndrome is inherited with an autosomal dominant pattern and is due to an inactivating mutation of FLCN, a tumor suppressor gene encoding a protein called folliculin, an inhibitor of the mTOR pathway.

3. Analogously, multiple facial CAF can also be found in **multiple endocrine neoplasia type 1** (MEN1), a cancer predisposition syndrome inherited with an autosomal dominant pattern and characterized by the development of hormonally active parathyroid tumors (95% of patients), pancreatic islet tumors (40%), and anterior pituitary tumors (30%). 95% of patients develop clinical symptoms by the fifth decade. Non-endocrine tumors found in patients with MEN1 include angiofibroma (88%), collagenoma (72%), adrenocortical tumor (35%), lipoma (33%), carcinoid tumor and carcinoid syndrome (10%), and meningioma. MEN1 is caused by inactivating mutations in MEN1 (11q13), a tumor suppressor gene encoding the menin protein.

Pathology

CAF is a fibrous neoplasm composed by a proliferation of stellate and spindled cells, thin-walled blood vessels with dilated lumina in the dermis, and a collagenized stroma. Multinucleated fibroblasts are often present and mitotic figures are rare. CAF differs from an angioma as the latter does not contain stellate cells or cellular stroma.

Besides the classic form, seven histologic variants of fibrous papule have been described:

1. Hypercellular fibrous papule is characterized by markedly dense infiltrate of spindle-shaped and round proliferating fibroblasts. It may be mistaken for atypical fibroxanthoma, which presents clinically as a rapidly growing ulcerated exophytic tumor, featuring strong positivity for CD10.
2. Pigmented fibrous papule is a lesion where the junctional melanocytic proliferation is particularly prominent or/and associated with a large number of dermal melanophages. Differential diagnosis with benign nevus or malignant melanoma is aided by immunoreactivity for melanocyte biomarkers (e.g., S100).
3. Inflammatory fibrous papule is characterized by a dense, diffuse dermal infiltrate of lymphocytes with plasma cells, histiocytes, and sometimes neutrophils. The differential diagnosis with an infectious process or (more rarely) a lymphoma may be needed.
4. Pleomorphic fibrous papule features bizarre, stellate fibroblasts within the angiofibromatous stroma. Histologically, it may mimic a pleomorphic fibroma, which can be easily differentiated clinically by larger size and different location (i.e., trunk or proximal extremities). Given the pleomorphic aspect of the fibroblasts, a range of malignant neoplasms with scattered pleomorphic tumor cells in the dermis may also need to be considered for differential diagnosis.
5. Clear cell fibrous papule is characterized by a proliferation of single or small clusters of cells with vacuolated or finely granular cytoplasm. The differential diagnosis includes a range of dermal clear cell tumors such as balloon cell nevus (S100 positive), xanthoma (foamy cells arranged in aggregates and CD68 positive), sebaceous carcinoma (cytokeratin and EMA positive), and metastatic renal cell carcinoma (PAX8 positive).
6. Granular cell fibrous papule is characterized by stromal cells containing abundant cytoplasm made up of periodic acid Schiff positive but diastase-resistant granules. These cells express CD68 but are always S100 negative. Differential diagnosis may be needed with granular cell tumor, which features S100 positivity.
7. Epithelioid cell fibrous papule features a proliferation of large cells organized as small nests or sheets and needs to be distinguished from melanocytic (Spitz nevus, malignant melanoma) and fibrohistiocytic (dermatofibroma, epithelioid fibrous histiocytoma, and xanthogranuloma) neoplasms. The presence of a junctional component, melanin pigment, and immunoreactivity with S100 and Melan-A is a useful clue for a nevus/melanoma; dermatofibroma shows entrapment of collagen toward the periphery and does not tend to involve the face.

Biomarkers

Spindled and stellate cells are positive for Factor XIIIa and negative for cytokeratins and S100.

Prognosis

This is a benign tumor without any malignant potential.

Therapy

Treatment is usually unnecessary in sporadic CAF (unless for esthetic reasons). Most patients with tuberous sclerosis complex experience disfigurement caused by multiple CAF (especially on the face): these subjects can require surgery or laser treatment, but this approach can leave scars on the affected skin. Beta-blockers have been used for long time in the treatment of vascular lesions: while oral propranolol can be effective but is burdened by side effects, topical timolol 0.5% solution or gel has proven to be very successful in the treatment of superficial hemangiomas.

Recently, a randomized controlled trial has demonstrated that local **target therapy** with mTOR inhibitors (e.g., sirolimus gel 0.2%) provides an effective alternative to **surgery** or **laser therapy**.

Suggested Readings

Damman (2018) Fibrous papule: a histopathologic review. Am J Dermatopathol 40(8):551–560
Nguyen (2018) The cutaneous manifestations of tuberous sclerosis complex. Am J Med Genet C Semin Med Genet 178(3):321–325
Wataya-Kaneda (2018) Sirolimus gel treatment vs placebo for facial angiofibromas in patients with tuberous sclerosis complex: a randomized clinical trial. JAMA Dermatol 154(7):781–788

Cutaneous Angiosarcoma

58

The skin is the most frequent site of involvement for angiosarcoma.

For details → see sections entitled "Angiosarcoma" and "Breast angiosarcoma".

Suggested Readings

Conic (2020) Incidence and outcomes of cutaneous angiosarcoma: a SEER population-based study. J Am Acad Dermatol 83:809–816 [Epub ahead of print]

Ishida (2018) Cutaneous angiosarcoma: update on biology and latest treatment. Curr Opin Oncol 30(2):107–112

Mitteldorf (2018) Deceptively bland cutaneous angiosarcoma on the nose mimicking hemangioma—a clinicopathologic and immunohistochemical analysis. J Cutan Pathol [Epub ahead of print]. https://doi.org/10.1111/cup.13275

Shustef (2017) Cutaneous angiosarcoma: a current update. J Clin Pathol 70(11):917–925

S. Mocellin, *Soft Tissue Tumors*, https://doi.org/10.1007/978-3-030-58710-9_58

59

Cutaneous Epithelioid Angiomatous Nodule

Definition

Cutaneous epithelioid angiomatous nodule (CEAN) is a benign lesion of the skin in the morphological spectrum of epithelioid vascular tumors. The pathogenesis of CEAN is unclear (reactive process similar to pyogenic granuloma versus hamartoma versus neoplastic origin).

Epidemiology and Presentation

CEAN is a very rare lesion occurring in a wide age range (15–80 years) but most frequently in young adults, without significant gender difference. It usually presents as a single papule or nodule red to blue in color, with rare reports of multiple lesions. The lesion is usually small (mean diameter: 5 mm). Most lesions develop on the trunk, extremities, and head and neck.

Pathology

CEAN presents as an unilobular lesion with dominantly solid areas. The cells in the solid areas show an epithelioid morphology with scattered blister cells (cells containing intracellular lumina). Overlying epidermis can be thin (due to stretching) or is hyperplastic and acanthotic. The periphery of the lesion usually contains scattered inflammatory cells. The vascular nature of the lesion can be documented by vascular markers such as CD31, CD34, and Factor VIII. Low mitotic activity is observed.

Differential diagnosis may be needed with multiple skin lesions such as the following: pyogenic granuloma (dominantly occurs in the trauma-predisposed sites, but it is known to occur in other locations as well; however, it usually shows a multilobular and a vascular growth pattern with relative paucity of the solid areas and epithelioid cells; in contrast, CEAN shows a dominantly solid and epithelioid morphology); epithelioid hemangioma (it usually shows multilobular vascular proliferations without a solid component, and it usually extends into the deep dermis and subcutis with intralesional fibrosis; in contrast, CEAN is usually a unilobular lesion confined to the dermis and is predominantly composed of solid component with a minor vascular component and perilesional fibrosis; moreover, epithelioid hemangioma shows a significant lymphoid component in the form of lymphoid aggregate or follicle along with numerous interspersed eosinophils); bacillary angiomatosis (it can be distinguished from CEAN by its usual occurrence in the immunosuppressed individuals and by the presence of neutrophils, basophilic material, and occasional demonstration of the causative organism *Bartonella henselae* in the Warthin-Starry stain); epithelioid hemangioendothelioma (this is a low-grade malignant vascular tumor occurring in young females and shows angiocentric lesion in 30–50% of cases; however, other cases of epithelioid hemangioendothelioma lack angiocentricity and instead show tumor cells invading the native tissue in infiltrating cords and trabeculae; the individual cells are relatively monomorphic and show characteristic blister cell morphology; nonetheless, it can be distinguished from CEAN by its tissue infiltrating nature, trabecular pattern, angiocentricity when present, presence of cellular atypia, and brisk mitotic activity); epithelioid angiosarcoma (the tumor cells usually are arranged in diffuse sheets and irregular vascular pattern; in contrast, CEAN lacks the infiltrative growth pattern, deep soft tissue involvement, leaky vascular channels lined by atypical endothelial cells with multilayering, frequent mitoses and atypical mitotic figures and occasional areas of necrosis); nevus and melanoma (they can show epithelioid morphology: whereas nevus shows a benign morphology, melanoma is its malignant counterpart typified by prominent nucleoli, atypia, and mitoses; both nevus and melanoma cells show positivity for S100, Melan-A, and HMB45 on immunohistochemistry); and epithelioid rhabdomyosarcoma (presence of both mitoses and atypia; expression of markers of skeletal muscle differentiation such as desmin, myogenin, and myoD1).

Biomarkers

The epithelioid cells show positivity for CD34, CD31, and Factor VIII. Staining for cytokeratins, CD163, and estrogen receptor is negative.

Prognosis

CEAN is a benign lesion.

Therapy

Surgical excision is needed mainly for diagnostic purposes.

Suggested Readings

Brenn (2004) Cutaneous epithelioid angiomatous nodule: a distinct lesion in the morphologic spectrum of epithelioid vascular tumors. Am J Dermatopathol 26(1):14–21
Chetty (2018) Cutaneous epithelioid angiomatous nodule: a report of a series including a case with moderate cytologic atypia and immunosuppression. Diagn Pathol 13(1):50
Ko (2015) Diagnostically challenging epithelioid vascular tumors. Surg Pathol Clin 8(3):331–351
Sorrells (2019) Granular cell cutaneous epithelioid angiomatous nodule. J Cutan Pathol 46(11):864–866

60

Cutaneous Fibroepithelial Polyp

Definition

Cutaneous fibroepithelial polyp is a benign lesion classified among fibrous, fibro-histiocytic, and myofibroblastic skin neoplasms. It is also known as acrochordon, skin tag, skin fibroma, soft fibroma, cutaneous papilloma, cutaneous tag, fibroma pendulum, and fibroma molluscum.

Epidemiology and Presentation

It is a very common cutaneous lesion occurring in adults, especially on intertriginous areas (i.e., axilla, groin), face (especially eyelids), and neck. Rarely, fibroepithelial polyps have been described in the mucosa of the genital, urinary, and respiratory areas.

Fibroepithelial polyp presents as a soft papilloma, flesh-colored to dark brown, mainly pedunculated; it ranges from a few millimeters to (rarely) some centimeters in size.

It may be associated with diabetes, obesity, and metabolic syndrome.

It may bother patients because it may be associated with symptoms such as itching, pain, and rubbing against clothes or simply because of their appearance.

Etiology and Predisposition

Multiple lesions can be observed in **Birt-Hogg-Dubé syndrome**, a hereditary condition associated with multiple benign skin tumors (such as fibrofolliculomas—which are pathognomonic for this syndrome; trichodiscomas; and fibroepithelial polyp), lung cysts (which can cause pneumothorax), and an increased risk of both benign kidney tumors and kidney cancer. Symptoms of Birt-Hogg-Dubé syndrome generally do not appear until adulthood. This syndrome is inherited with an

© The Editor(s) (if applicable) and The Author(s), under exclusive license to
Springer Nature Switzerland AG 2021
S. Mocellin, *Soft Tissue Tumors*, https://doi.org/10.1007/978-3-030-58710-9_60

autosomal dominant pattern and is due to an inactivating mutation of FLCN, a tumor suppressor gene encoding a protein called folliculin; the pathogenesis of this syndrome follows the classic two-hit hypothesis originally described for retinoblastoma.

Pathology

Microscopically, it is composed of a fibrovascular core covered by squamous epithelium. Ischemic necrosis may be present due to spontaneous torsion.

Prognosis

Cutaneous fibroepithelial polyp is an innocuous benign lesion.

Therapy

Surgical excision.

Suggested Readings

Akpinar (2012) Association between acrochordons and the components of metabolic syndrome. Eur J Dermatol 22(1):106–110

Gollow (2019) Large pedunculated vulval fibroepithelial polyp. BMJ Case Rep 12(7):e230449

Hajji (2019) A rare case of successful endoscopic management of a fibroepithelial polyp with intussusception of the ureter and periodic prolapse into bladder. Ann R Coll Surg Engl 101(2):e66–e70

Hong (2019) Modified laparoscopic partial ureterectomy for adult ureteral fibroepithelial polyp: technique and initial experience. Urol Int 102(1):13–19

Jabbour (2019) Glottic obstruction from fibroepithelial polyp. Am J Case Rep 20:219–223

Lozano-Peña (2019) Giant fibroepithelial polyp of the vulva. Australas J Dermatol 60(1):70–71

Ushiki (2008) A rare case of a tracheal fibroepithelial polyp treated by an endobronchial resection. Intern Med 47(19):1723–1726

Cutaneous Leiomyoma

61

Definition

Cutaneous leiomyoma (CLM) is a benign skin tumor arising from smooth muscle cells. Based on the site of origin, CLM is also called piloleiomyoma (arising from the erector pili musculature of the hair follicle) and genital leiomyoma (arising from the smooth muscle found in the scrotum, labia, or nipple). When multiple lesions are present, the condition is also known as cutaneous leiomyomatosis.

Some investigators include angioleiomyoma ($\rightarrow$ see dedicated section) among cutaneous leiomyomas.

Epidemiology and Presentation

Piloleiomyoma occurs more frequently in adults than children, without significant differences between males and females. Most patients begin to develop these lesions between 20 and 40 years of age. Angioleiomyoma occurs more frequently than piloleiomyoma, which in turn is more common than genital leiomyoma.

Piloleiomyoma characteristically present as either a solitary dermal nodule or multiple dermal nodules in a clustered, linear, dermatomal, or scattered distribution. The nodules range in size from 2 to 20 mm and may be skin-colored, pink, red, or red-brown. Solitary piloleiomyoma is more frequent on the lower extremity, while multiple piloleiomyomas frequently present on the extensor surface of extremities and trunk. The most common presenting complaint among patients with multiple piloleiomyomas is pain, which may occur spontaneously or may be provoked by pressure, cold temperatures, strong emotion, or light touch.

Genital leiomyoma typically develops on the genitals, including the scrotum, penis, and vulva, but it may also arise on the nipple-areolar complex. The lesion generally presents as an asymptomatic, solitary nodule.

Angioleiomyoma generally presents in females in their 40s to 60s as a firm, often painful, subcutaneous nodule on the lower extremity.

S. Mocellin, *Soft Tissue Tumors*, https://doi.org/10.1007/978-3-030-58710-9_61

Macroscopically, the **differential diagnosis** may be extensive given the nonspecific appearance of solitary lesions. Painful skin lesions that should be differentiated include blue rubber bleb nevus, angiolipoma, neuroma, glomus tumor, neurilemmoma, endometrioma, granular cell tumor, and eccrine spiradenoma. Dermatofibroma may also be considered in the differential diagnosis. Multiple cutaneous leiomyomas (piloleiomyomas) tend instead to have a distinctive clinical appearance.

Etiology and Predisposition

Piloleiomyoma can arise either sporadically or as part of an autosomal dominant genetic syndrome called **multiple cutaneous and uterine leiomyomatosis** (MCUL). This condition, also known as Reed syndrome and **hereditary leiomyomatosis with renal cell carcinoma** (HLRCC), typically occurs as a result of a heterozygous germline mutation of the FH (fumarate hydratase) gene, which is involved in the Krebs cycle and could act as a tumor suppressor gene. Approximately 90% of patients with multiple cutaneous leiomyomas harbor a heterozygous germline mutation in the FH gene. Female patients with FH mutations commonly display both piloleiomyomas (85%) and symptomatic uterine leiomyomas (>90%). Uterine leiomyomas associated with FH mutation tend to be larger (up to 10 cm), more numerous, develop at a younger age, and more frequently require hysterectomy in comparison to non-hereditary uterine leiomyomas. However, the most concerning feature of an FH mutation is the association with an aggressive variant of renal cell carcinoma (type II papillary renal cell carcinoma) which develops in approximately 15% of patients: of note, in this subgroup of patients developing renal cell carcinoma, the malignancy is metastatic at presentation in about 50% of cases.

Pathology

Piloleiomyoma—which is found in the reticular dermis close to a hair follicle—is composed of interweaving bundles of smooth muscle cells with typical "blunt-ended cigar-shaped nuclei" and eosinophilic cytoplasm in a background of collagen bundles. Mitotic figures are rarely observed (if present, they should raise suspicion for leiomyosarcoma).

Genital leiomyoma (especially scrotal lesions) tends to have a more spindle cell appearance, while vulvar lesions display more epithelioid cells.

Angioleiomyoma is a deeper, well-circumscribed neoplasm, mostly located in the upper subcutaneous tissues. Pathology evaluation reveals tightly compact myocytes in a world pattern around vascular channels.

Biomarkers

CLM stains positive for smooth muscle markers and desmin.

Prognosis

Although CLM is a benign tumor, patients with multiple cutaneous leiomyomas (piloleiomyomas) may be affected with MCUL/HLRCC, which increases their susceptibility to developing renal cell carcinoma.

Therapy

Surgical excision may be needed for both diagnostic purposes and for pain relief. CLM is characterized by a high rate of local recurrence after surgery (even a few weeks after surgery). Cryotherapy and laser therapy can also be utilized as ablative treatments.

Medical therapy may be indicated for patients with painful lesions who are not considered to be surgical candidates (e.g., extensive forms of cutaneous leiomyomatosis). To this aim, several drugs have been proposed, such as nifedipine, nitroglycerin, doxazosin, gabapentin, pregabalin, and duloxetine. Injection of botulinum toxin into the lesions is associated with mixed results for symptomatic relief.

Suggested Readings

Alam (2005) Clinical features of multiple cutaneous and uterine leiomyomatosis: an underdiagnosed tumor syndrome. Arch Dermatol 141(2):199–206

Bhola (2018) A retrospective review of 48 individuals, including 12 families, molecularly diagnosed with hereditary leiomyomatosis and renal cell cancer (HLRCC). Familial Cancer 17(4):615–620

Hammer (2019) Nipple leiomyoma: a rare neoplasm with a broad spectrum of histologic appearances. J Cutan Pathol 46(5):343–346

Rieder (2015) Piloleiomyomas in multiple cutaneous and uterine leiomyoma syndrome (hereditary leiomyomatosis and renal cell cancer or Reed syndrome). Dermatol Online J 21(12). pii: 13030/qt16s9k7bv

62

Definition

Cutaneous leiomyosarcoma (CLMS) is a primary skin malignancy originating from smooth muscle cells. Two subtypes can be identified: (1) dermal leiomyosarcoma and (2) subcutaneous leiomyosarcoma. CLMS is also known as superficial leiomyosarcoma to differentiate it from deep leiomyosarcoma (which occurs in deep soft tissues, retroperitoneum, viscera; → see Chap. 148). Of note, the skin is a relatively frequent site of metastatic leiomyosarcoma.

Epidemiology and Presentation

The mean age of presentation is 50–70 years. As regards dermal leiomyosarcoma, men are typically overrepresented (ratio of approximately 3:1); no gender differences have been reported for subcutaneous leiomyosarcoma. CLMS usually measures up to 3 cm in size (on average, dermal lesions are smaller than subcutaneous lesions) and is found most often in the extremities; it presents most commonly as a slowly growing, tender, or painful nodule (skin-colored or reddish).

Metastatic lesions from CLMS typically affect the lungs. However, CLMS characteristically metastasizes also to other skin sites; moreover, a unique feature of DLMS is the disproportionately high rate of metastases to the scalp.

Pathology

Microscopically, CLMS presents as a proliferation of atypical smooth muscle cells. The lesion can demonstrate a spectrum of findings ranging from well-differentiated interlacing bundles of spindled tumor cells with elongated cigar-shaped nuclei, to moderately differentiated tumors with atypical nuclei and amphophilic nucleoli, to poorly differentiated tumors composed of anaplastic spindle cells. Malignant features are highly cellular masses with nuclear pleomorphism and increased mitoses.

Differential diagnosis may be needed with the following: cutaneous leiomyoma (no atypia, no mitoses); atypical fibroxanthoma (desmin negative, CD10 positive); achromic melanoma (S100 positive); Kaposi sarcoma (HHV8 positive); spindle cell squamous carcinoma (cytokeratin positive); epithelioid angiosarcoma; and malignant peripheral nerve sheath tumor (S100 positive).

Biomarkers

CLMS stains positive for HHF35 (90%), SMA (90%), vimentin, and desmin (75%).

Prognosis

Overall, CLMS (superficial leiomyosarcoma) has a better prognosis than deep leiomyosarcoma. Among CLMS subtypes, dermal leiomyosarcoma is associated with a better prognosis as compared to subcutaneous leiomyosarcoma. In particular, dermal leiomyosarcoma has been reported to locally recur in up to 35% of cases and to metastasize in up to 14% of cases; in contrast, subcutaneous leiomyosarcoma locally recurs in up to 62% of cases, whereas it metastasizes in up to 61% of cases. Recent reports suggest that dermal leiomyosarcoma is associated with a more indolent course than it was believed in the past, with a 24% local recurrence rate and a 4% metastasis rate (its prognosis appears to equal that of atypical fibroxanthoma with a 5-year disease-specific survival rate of 98% and an overall survival rate of 85%); accordingly, the names "atypical intradermal smooth muscle neoplasm" and "atypical smooth muscle tumor" have been proposed.

Tumor size is an important prognostic factor: the survival rate for CLMS smaller than 2 cm is reported to be about 95%, but it drastically decreases to 30% for lesions greater than 5 cm. In this regard, the AJCC TNM staging system, which is prognostically useful for deep leiomyosarcoma, does not appear to be equally effective to stratify the risk of superficial leiomyosarcoma, which is rarely greater than 5 cm.

Histologic grading according to the FNCLCC[1] system has been reported to correlate with risk of recurrence and metastasis.

Therapy

Surgery is the standard treatment (wide excision with 1–2 cm margins). Re-excision is recommended in cases of local relapse.

---

[1] FNCLCC: Fédération Nationale des Centres de Lutte Contre Le Cancer.

Radiotherapy can be considered as an adjuvant treatment for tumors with close margins, high-grade lesions, or tumors where additional surgery would compromise function.

Chemotherapy is rarely used for the management of non-metastatic disease.

Suggested Readings

Kohlmeyer (2017) Cutaneous sarcomas. J Dtsch Dermatol Ges 15(6):630–648

Kuflik (2003) Dermal leiomyosarcoma. J Am Acad Dermatol 48:S51–S53

Llombart (2019) Leiomyosarcoma and pleomorphic dermal sarcoma: guidelines for diagnosis and treatment. Actas Dermosifiliogr 110(1):4–11

Patt (2016) Soft tissue sarcomas in skin: presentations and management. Semin Oncol 43(3):413–418

Sandhu (2020) Cutaneous leiomyosarcoma: a SEER database analysis. Dermatol Surg 46:159–164 [Epub ahead of print]

Winchester (2014) Leiomyosarcoma of the skin: clinical, histopathologic, and prognostic factors that influence outcomes. J Am Acad Dermatol 71(5):919–925

Definition

Dedifferentiated liposarcoma (DDLS) is a malignant tumor (usually non-lipogenic) deriving from the dedifferentiation of a primary or recurrent well-differentiated liposarcoma (WDLS, → see dedicated section). Dedifferentiation occurs in up to 20% of WDLS, although the risk is higher for deep-seated locations (especially retroperitoneum) as compared to superficial sites. For general information on liposarcomas → see Chap. 155. As regards the other types of liposarcomas (i.e., well-differentiated liposarcoma, myxoid/round cell liposarcoma, pleomorphic liposarcoma) → see dedicated sections.

Epidemiology and Presentation

DDLS represents about 15–20% of all liposarcomas. It generally affects adult people (incidence peak: 50–60 years). DDLS accounts for most pleomorphic sarcomas in the retroperitoneum.

Retroperitoneum is the most common site; other locations include extremities, spermatic cord, and, more rarely, head and neck, mediastinum, and trunk. Cases occurring in subcutaneous tissue are very rare.

Computed tomography and magnetic resonance imaging can usually identify areas of WDLS admixed with areas of DDLS, which can be especially useful to guide a core needle biopsy into the dedifferentiated component.

Pathology

DDLS generally consists of large multinodular yellow masses containing solid, grey non-lipomatous areas (corresponding to the dedifferentiation areas, which often show necrosis). The abrupt transition from WDLS to a non-lipogenic sarcoma

© The Editor(s) (if applicable) and The Author(s), under exclusive license to
Springer Nature Switzerland AG 2021
S. Mocellin, *Soft Tissue Tumors*, https://doi.org/10.1007/978-3-030-58710-9_63

(usually high-grade) is the hallmark of DDLS; however, a well-differentiated component may not always be identifiable.

Typically, dedifferentiated areas resemble undifferentiated pleomorphic sarcoma or intermediate to high-grade myxofibrosarcoma. However, cases with low-grade dedifferentiation can occur: in these cases, dedifferentiation is characterized by the presence of uniform fibroblastic spindle cells with mild nuclear atypia. Low-grade DDLS can be confused with spindle cell WDLS, which contains atypical adipocytes or lipoblasts, while dedifferentiated areas (both low-grade and high-grade) are usually non-lipogenic. Low-grade DDLS is virtually indistinguishable from cellular WDLS.

Differential diagnosis may be needed also with the following: leiomyosarcoma (even in pleomorphic cases there are usually areas with morphology distinctive of well-differentiated leiomyosarcoma, whereas there is no WDLS component and no MDM2 amplification); malignant peripheral nerve sheath tumor (no WDLS component, history of neurofibromatosis may be present, MDM2 may be amplified in 20% of cases, more commonly located in the deep soft tissues of the extremities than in the retroperitoneum); pleomorphic liposarcoma (lipoblasts in the background of a pleomorphic sarcoma, no WDLS component, MDM2 negative); rhabdomyosarcoma (no WDLS component, no MDM2 amplification); sarcomatoid carcinoma (cytokeratin positive, clinical history of a primary epithelial malignancy, no WDLS component, no MDM2 amplification); sarcomatoid mesothelioma (clinical history of asbestos exposure, cytokeratin positive, no WDLS component, no MDM2 amplification); and undifferentiated pleomorphic sarcoma (retroperitoneal tumors are DDLS until proven otherwise; no MDM2 amplification).

Biomarkers

Diffuse nuclear expression of MDM2[1] and/or CDK4[2] is virtually always present, in line with **MDM2 amplification** as well as **CDK4 amplification** (12q13-15 chromosomal region). MDM2 amplification is widely used to differentiate DDLS from other resembling tumors.

---

[1] MDM2: This oncogene (mouse double minute 2, also known as HMD2) encodes a nuclear-localized E3 ubiquitin ligase. The encoded protein can promote tumor formation by targeting tumor suppressor proteins, such as p53, for proteasomal degradation. MDM2 is inhibited by the tumor suppressor protein p14/ARF (one of the two products of CDKN2A).

[2] CDK4: Cyclin-dependent kinase 4 encodes a member of the Ser/Thr protein kinase family. This protein is a catalytic subunit of the protein kinase complex that is important for cell cycle G1 phase progression. The activity of this kinase is restricted to the G1-S phase, which is controlled by the regulatory subunits D-type cyclins and by the CDK inhibitor p16/INK4a (one of the two products of CDKN2A). CDK4 is responsible for the phosphorylation (and thus inhibition) of retinoblastoma gene (RB) product. Mutations in CDK4 as well as in its related genes including D-type cyclins, CDKN2A, and RB are be associated with tumorigenesis of a variety of cancers.

Prognosis

DDLS can metastasize in approximately 20–30% of cases. Moreover, DDLS is characterized by high local recurrence rates (>50%). In particular, virtually all retroperitoneal lesions recur locally if patients are followed up for a sufficient time span. Analogously, mortality rates—which are about 30% at 5 years—are much higher after 10–20 years of follow-up.

The extent or morphological pattern of dedifferentiated areas does not predict outcome. The most important prognostic factor is anatomical location, with retroperitoneal lesions being associated with the worst clinical course. On average, despite its high-grade morphology, DDLS has a less aggressive clinical course than other types of high-grade sarcomas: the relative lack of complex karyotypic aberrations coupled with the rarity of TP53 gene alterations (which are instead frequently found in other high-grade pleomorphic sarcomas) might underlie the relative discrepancy between morphology and clinical outcome.

Therapy

Surgery is the mainstay of treatment: this therapeutic approach can be curative for cases originating from the extremities but rarely for retroperitoneal tumors due to the difficulty to achieve a complete resection in this body compartment. There is some retrospective evidence that resection of retroperitoneal sarcomas along with adjacent organs (e.g., kidney, colon) might be beneficial in terms of survival (even when the organs are not infiltrated), probably because of the higher chance to be oncologically radical. DDLS of the extremities (or the thoraco-abdominal wall) can be treated with 1 cm margin of healthy tissue (whenever feasible without compromising function), and vascular resection may be an option for lesions encasing a vascular bundle; for extremity DDLS greater than 5 cm in size or with close margins, adjuvant **radiotherapy** is recommended (neoadjuvant radiotherapy can also be planned preoperatively).

The only randomized controlled trial (STRASS) so far available on neoadjuvant radiotherapy for retroperitoneal sarcomas has not demonstrated an abdominal recurrence-free survival advantage over surgery alone in patients with histologically proven localized and resectable primary soft tissue malignancies (although subgroup analysis shows a significant benefit for the liposarcoma subset).

For locally recurrent disease, surgery remains the best option (when feasible), but the prognosis is dismal (especially for retroperitoneal disease).

DDLS is considered a chemoresistant neoplasm. For patients with locally advanced/unresectable or metastatic disease, anthracycline-based **chemotherapy** remains the standard first-line treatment. As second-line treatment, gemcitabine plus docetaxel and high-dose ifosfamide monotherapy can be used. More recently, trabectedin and eribulin have been approved for the treatment of patients with metastatic liposarcoma who failed anthracycline-based first-line chemotherapy. As regards **target therapy**, based on the characteristic CDK4/MDM2 amplification, both CDK inhibitors (e.g., palbociclib, which is currently approved for the treatment of other malignancies such as breast cancer) and MDM2 inhibitors are under investigation. **Immunotherapy** (e.g., anti-PD1 monoclonal antibody pembrolizumab) is also being tested in the clinical setting with some promising results.

Suggested Readings

Bonvalot (2009) Primary retroperitoneal sarcomas: a multivariate analysis of surgical factors associated with local control. J Clin Oncol 27:31–37

Bonvalot (2019) STRASS (EORTC 62092): a phase III randomized study of preoperative radiotherapy plus surgery versus surgery alone for patients with retroperitoneal sarcoma. J Clin Oncol 37(15_Suppl):11001

Crago (2016) Liposarcoma: multimodality management and future targeted therapies. Surg Oncol Clin N Am 25(4):761–773

Demetri (2016) Efficacy and safety of trabectedin or dacarbazine for metastatic liposarcoma or leiomyosarcoma after failure of conventional chemotherapy: results of a phase III randomized multicenter clinical trial. J Clin Oncol 34(8):786–793

Dickson (2016) Progression-free survival among patients with well-differentiated or dedifferentiated liposarcoma treated with CDK4 inhibitor palbociclib: a phase 2 clinical trial. JAMA Oncol 2(7):937–940

Fletcher (2020) WHO classification of tumours of soft tissue and bone (5th edition)

Gahvari (2020) Dedifferentiated liposarcoma: systemic therapy options. Curr Treat Options Oncol 21(2):15

Gronchi (2009) Aggressive surgical policies in a retrospectively reviewed single-institution case series of retroperitoneal soft tissue sarcoma patients. J Clin Oncol 27:24–30

Hirata (2019) Integrated exome and RNA sequencing of dedifferentiated liposarcoma. Nat Commun 10(1):5683

Lee (2017) Clinical and molecular spectrum of liposarcoma. J Clin Oncol 36:151–159

Schöffski (2016) Eribulin versus dacarbazine in previously treated patients with advanced liposarcoma or leiomyosarcoma: a randomised, open-label, multicentre, phase 3 trial. Lancet 387(10028):1629–1637

Tawbi (2017) Pembrolizumab in advanced soft-tissue sarcoma and bone sarcoma (SARC028): a multicentre, two-cohort, single-arm, open-label, phase 2 trial. Lancet Oncol 18(11):1493–1501

Thway (2019) Well-differentiated liposarcoma and dedifferentiated liposarcoma: an updated review. Semin Diagn Pathol 36(2):112–121

Definition

Deep angiomyxoma (DAM) is a benign mesenchymal tumor of uncertain differentiation and represents the deep variant of angiomyxoma ($\rightarrow$ see Chap. 239). DAM is also known as aggressive angiomyxoma.

Epidemiology and Presentation

DAM develops in the pelvis or in the perineum. It generally affects adult females aged 30–70 years (it never occurs before puberty). Although some cases actually arise in men, careful pathology review should be obtained before diagnosing DAM in males. The mass (which can reach several centimeters in diameter) is initially asymptomatic and then can cause quite generic symptoms due to compression of adjacent structures.

Pathology

The tumor is characterized by abundant myxoid matrix (containing scattered vessels of varying caliber) and a dominant population of stellate and spindle cells (low to moderate cellularity). No significant atypia or pleomorphism are present, and mitotic figures are rare.

Differential diagnosis may be needed with the following: myxoma; myxoid liposarcoma; myxofibrosarcoma; nerve sheath myxoma; and other soft tissue tumors with secondary myxoid change.

S. Mocellin, *Soft Tissue Tumors*, https://doi.org/10.1007/978-3-030-58710-9_64

Biomarkers

Neoplastic cells often stain positive for estrogen receptor, progesterone receptor, and desmin. Expression of CD34, vimentin, and SMA[1] is variable. DAM stains negative for S100, EMA,[2] cytokeratins, CD117, beta-catenin, and caldesmon.

Karyotypic aberrations involving chromosome 12 lead to rearrangements of the HMGA2 locus (12q14.3) in about one third of cases, and HMGA2 overexpression can be found in about 90% of cases (HMGA2 is a sensitive but nonspecific biomarker). For instance, chromosomal translocation t(11;12)(q22.1;q14.3) leads to the formation of **HMGA2-YAP1** fusion gene.[3]

Prognosis

DAM is a benign tumor, but disease relapses are reported in more than one third of cases after surgery.

Therapy

Surgery is the mainstay of treatment. When tumor excision requires mutilating surgery or general conditions contraindicate surgery, promising results have been reported with hormonal therapy (gonadotropin-releasing hormone agonists, antiestrogens and aromatase inhibitors).

Suggested Readings

Dreux (2010) Value and limitation of immunohistochemical expression of HMGA2 in mesenchymal tumors: about a series of 1052 cases. Mod Pathol 23(12):1657–1666
Fletcher (2020) WHO classification of tumours of soft tissue and bone, 5th edn. IARC Press, Lyon
Fucà (2019) Treatment outcomes and sensitivity to hormone therapy of aggressive angiomyxoma: a multicenter, international, retrospective study. Oncologist 24(7):e536–e541

---

[1] SMA: smooth muscle actin.

[2] EMA: epithelial membrane antigen.

[3] HMGA2-YAP1 fusion gene: HMGA2 (high-mobility group AT-hook 2) encodes a protein that belongs to the nonhistone chromosomal high-mobility group (HMG) protein family. HMG proteins function as architectural factors and are essential components of the enhanceosome; HMGA2 contains structural DNA-binding domains and may act as a transcriptional regulating factor; rearrangements of this gene that have been associated with myxoid liposarcoma suggests a role in adipogenesis and mesenchymal differentiation. YAP1 encodes yes-associated protein 1, a downstream nuclear effector of the Hippo signaling pathway (which is involved in development, growth, repair, and homeostasis); YAP1 is known to play a role in the development and progression of multiple cancers as a transcriptional regulator of this signaling pathway.

Lee (2019) Novel HMGA2-YAP1 fusion gene in aggressive angiomyxoma. BMJ Case Rep 12(5):e227475

Pannier (2019) Hormonal therapies in uterine sarcomas, aggressive angiomyxoma, and desmoid-type fibromatosis. Crit Rev Oncol Hematol 143:62–66

Sutton (2012) Aggressive angiomyxoma. Arch Pathol Lab Med 136(2):217–221

Definition

Dermal nerve sheath myxoma (DNSM; also simply called nerve sheath myxoma) is a benign peripheral nerve sheath tumor. It is also known as myxoid neurothekeoma or classic neurothekeoma, although DNSM is currently considered a distinct nosological entity.

Epidemiology and Presentation

DNSM is a rare tumor occurring in a wide age range (8–80 years) but mainly in young adults, without gender differences. Most cases (85%) arise in the extremities, fingers being the commonest site (one third of cases). Clinically, it presents typically as a small, superficial, flesh-colored, slow-growing nodule (0.5–5 cm) which is usually asymptomatic. The lesion, which is dermal-centered, often shows a multinodular growth pattern.

Pathology

DNSM is an unencapsulated lesion composed of small epithelioid ring-like and spindled Schwann cells (arranged in cords, nests, and syncytial-like aggregates) embedded in an abundant myxoid matrix. Nuclear atypia may be present but is mild, and mitoses are uncommon. Scattered vessels of small caliber are present.

Differential diagnosis may be needed with the following: neurothekeoma (→ see below Table 65.1); plexiform neurofibroma (associated with neurofibromatosis type 1; stroma contains collagen fibers with shredded carrot appearance; fibroblasts stain positive for CD34, Schwann cells for S100); myxoid schwannoma (usually encapsulated, alternating Antoni A and Antoni B areas, nuclear palisading/Verocay bodies, hyalinized vessels); cutaneous myoepithelioma (it may show a lobular,

S. Mocellin, *Soft Tissue Tumors*, https://doi.org/10.1007/978-3-030-58710-9_65

Table 65.1 Differential diagnosis between DNSM and neurothekeoma: clinicopathological features

	DNSM	Neurothekeoma
Incidence	Fivefold less frequent	Fivefold more frequent
Age	Older	Younger
Gender	M = F	F > M
Site of involvement	Mainly extremities	Mainly head and neck
Disease recurrence	Frequent	Rare
Molecular profile	Similar to schwannoma	Similar to fibrous histiocytoma
Immunohistochemistry	S100 positive CD10 negative	S100 negative CD10 positive

reticular, or syncytial growth pattern with myxoid stroma; poorly circumscribed, often with an overlying hyperplastic epidermis; positive for S100 and GFAP, but also cytokeratins or EMA); superficial acral fibromyxoma (or digital fibromyxoma; almost always adjacent to the nail bed of fingers and toes, typically well circumscribed; positive for CD34, variably positive for CD10, CD99, and SMA; displays loss of RB1; negative for S100 and desmin); cutaneous myxoma (superficial angiomyxoma; associated with Carney complex in 50% of cases; most common in head and neck and trunk; well-circumscribed, vaguely lobulated tumor with prominent mucinous matrix and vascularity, contains variably shaped fibroblasts but is less cellular with accompanying inflammatory infiltrate containing neutrophils; up to 25% of cases have entrapped epithelial structures; positive for CD34 but negative for S100).

Biomarkers

Neoplastic Schwann cells are diffusely positive for S100 and moderately to diffusely reactive for GFAP,[1] NSE,[2] and CD57. Strong positivity for collagen IV is present around neoplastic tumor cells. DNSM stains negative for CD10, HMB45, CD63, and SMA.[3]

Prognosis

DNSM is a benign tumor but is associated with a high rate of local relapse (up to 45%).

---

[1] GFAP: glial fibrillary acidic protein.

[2] NSE: neuron specific enolase.

[3] SMA: smooth muscle actin.

Therapy

Surgery is the treatment of choice.

Suggested Readings

Behera (2019) Clinical, dermoscopic and histopathological features of a rare cutaneous neural tumour. Clin Exp Dermatol 44(2):206–209

Fetsch (2005) Nerve sheath myxoma: a clinicopathologic and immunohistochemical analysis of 57 morphologically distinctive, S-100 protein- and GFAP-positive, myxoid peripheral nerve sheath tumors with a predilection for the extremities and a high local recurrence rate. Am J Surg Pathol 29(12):1615–1624

Fletcher (2020) WHO classification of tumours of soft tissue and bone, 5th edn. IARC Press, Lyon

Vered (2011) Classic neurothekeoma (nerve sheath myxoma) and cellular neurothekeoma of the oral mucosa: immunohistochemical profiles. J Oral Pathol Med 40(2):174–180

Dermatofibroma

66

Dermatofibroma is a benign skin neoplasm also known as cutaneous fibrous histiocytoma. It is a subtype of benign fibrous histiocytoma.

For additional information → see Chap. 34.

S. Mocellin, *Soft Tissue Tumors*, https://doi.org/10.1007/978-3-030-58710-9_66

Definition

Dermatofibrosarcoma protuberans (DFSP) is a superficial malignancy (included among skin sarcomas). The cellular origin of DFSP is unknown, potential cell candidates being histiocytes, fibroblasts, and dendritic cells (it is currently classified among fibroblastic-myofibroblastic soft tissue tumors).

Epidemiology and Presentation

DFSP usually develops in young to middle-aged adult patients, although any age can be affected. It is a rare tumor (<1 per 100,000 people per year), but is the second most frequent skin sarcoma (after Kaposi sarcoma). It accounts for approximately 5% of all soft tissue sarcomas. According to a Surveillance, Epidemiology, and End Results (SEER) analysis, DFSP is the second most frequent skin sarcoma accounting for approximately 18% of all cases (preceded only by Kaposi sarcoma, which accounts for about 70% of cases).

DFSP generally presents as a painless nodular or multinodular cutaneous lesion, often with a long history of slow growth. Early lesions may show plaque-like growth with peripheral red discoloration (clinically similar to morphea). The tumor may rapidly grow due to transformation into fibrosarcomatous DFSP.

DFSP develops most commonly on the trunk and the proximal extremities (very rarely feet/hands), followed by the head and neck region.

The very early clinical stage of DFSP is considered to be that of a non-protuberant (flat) lesion (usually pink or violet), which eventually (and slowly) develops into the typical protuberant form. But in some cases, the lesion retains the non-protuberant feature and is called plaque-like DFSP or atrophic DFSP. Clinically, these tumors often mimic benign lesions, such as morphea, atrophoderma, atrophic scars, anetoderma, lipoatrophy, or medallion-like dermal dendrocyte hamartoma.

S. Mocellin, *Soft Tissue Tumors*, https://doi.org/10.1007/978-3-030-58710-9_67

Etiology and Predisposition

Most cases of DFSP occur sporadically. However, a high incidence of DFSP with unique characteristics (e.g., multicentricity, early onset) is observed in children affected with adenosine deaminase-deficient severe combined immunodeficiency (ADA-SCID), a syndrome characterized by immunodeficiency and defective DNA repair machinery.

Pathology

Classical DFSP is a low-grade malignancy that typically diffusely infiltrates the dermis and subcutis. The tumor cells grow along the fibrous septa of the subcutaneous tissue and intercalate with fat lobules, which leads to a honeycomb (or storiform) pattern. DFSP is composed of cytologically uniform spindled cells. Cytological atypia is minimal and mitotic activity is usually low. Rarely, DFSP infiltrates deep soft tissues.

Differential diagnosis may be necessary with the following: dermatofibroma (also storiform pattern but non-infiltrative, less cellular than DFSP, factor XIIIa positive, CD34 negative); undifferentiated pleomorphic sarcoma/atypical fibroxanthoma (storiform pattern but also moderate/marked pleomorphism and nuclear atypia); desmoplastic melanoma; Kaposi sarcoma; solitary fibrous tumor (spindle cells with a patternless distribution; prominent branching vasculature, keloid-like collagen bundles, positive for STAT6); and cutaneous leiomyosarcoma (plump spindle cells with a fascicular architecture; ovoid/cigar-shaped nuclei; atypical mitoses usually present; typically positive for desmin and h-caldesmon and negative for CD34).

Several DFSP variants have been described:

- **Fibrosarcomatous DFSP** is a DFSP variant (10–15% of all cases) that is characterized by high-grade malignant potential and represents a morphological progression of classical DFSP to a usually fascicular pattern which is associated with an increased biological aggressiveness culminating in the capability of metastasizing. This form can arise de novo or after local recurrence of a conventional DFSP. The fibrosarcomatous component often shows a nodular growth and is composed of cellular spindle cell fascicles with a herringbone pattern; the tumor cells in fibrosarcomatous areas are characterized by increased atypia and proliferative activity. This variant may mimic other spindle cell sarcomas such as malignant peripheral nerve sheath tumor, synovial sarcoma (which has specific fusion genes such as SS18-SSX1 or SS18-SSX2), and leiomyosarcoma (which shows consistent expression of smooth muscle markers such as desmin and h-caldesmon).
- **Sclerosing DFSP** or sclerotic DFSP is characterized by the existence of paucicellular or hypocellular collagen accounting for at least 50% of the tumor; this lesion can be misdiagnosed as other benign sclerosing lesions and mesenchymal

neoplasms, such as sclerosing epithelioid fibrosarcoma, sclerotic or desmoplastic leiomyosarcoma, and desmoplastic melanoma.

- **Pigmented DFSP** (also known as Bednar tumor) is a rare variant that contains pigmented dendritic melanocytic cells and occurs predominantly in persons of African heritage (it includes 1–5% of all DFSP cases); the differential diagnosis of Bednar tumor includes fibrous histiocytoma, neurofibroma, malignant melanoma, and cellular blue nevus.
- **Myxoid DFSP** is a rare variant that shows prominent myxoid stroma (comprising at least 50% of the tumor) with a more nodular growth and numerous vessels often producing a more variable architecture, which may need differential diagnosis with benign tumors with myxoid stroma, such as spindle cell lipoma.
- **Myoid DFSP** is a rare variant that contains bundles and nests of spindled, myofibroblastic tumor cells; immunohistochemically, myoid tumor areas are CD34 negative, desmin negative, and smooth muscle actin positive.
- **Plaque-like DFSP** is a rare variant that displays a flat growth resembling benign plaque-like CD34-positive dermal fibroma.
- **Giant cell fibroblastoma** (→ see dedicated section) is considered by some investigators the juvenile variant of DFSP as it has the same translocation (→ see below paragraph).

Biomarkers

Malignant cells stain strongly positive for CD34 (which can also be observed in other sarcomas, such as myofibrosarcoma, epithelioid sarcoma, and angiosarcoma). Remarkably, fibrosarcomatous DFSP may lose CD34 expression in about 50% of the cases. DFSP stains negative for desmin, S100, CD117 (KIT), and cytokeratins.

DFSP is characterized (>95% of cases) by the chromosomal translocation t(17,22)(q21;q13), which generates the **COL1A1-PDGFB fusion gene**.[1] This chimeric gene can be detected by RT-PCR[2] or preferably by FISH[3] in DFSP as well as in related neoplasms (e.g., giant cell fibroblastoma → see dedicated section). The COL1A1-PDGFB fusion gene codes for a protein that is proteolytically processed to a biologically active PDGFB ligand. As malignant cells express the PDGFB

---

[1] COL1A1-PDGFB fusion gene: COL1A1 (collagen type I alpha 1 chain) encodes the pro-alpha1 chains of type I collagen whose triple helix comprises two alpha1 chains and one alpha2 chain. Type I is a fibril-forming collagen found in most connective tissues and is abundant in the bone, cornea, dermis, and tendon. PDGFB encodes platelet-derived growth factor subunit B, a member of the protein family comprised of both platelet-derived growth factors (PDGF) and vascular endothelial growth factors (VEGF); the encoded preproprotein is proteolytically processed to generate platelet-derived growth factor subunit B, which can homodimerize, or, alternatively, heterodimerize with the related platelet-derived growth factor subunit A: ultimately, these proteins bind and activate PDGF receptor (PDGFR) tyrosine kinases, which play a role in a wide range of cell activities.

[2] RT-PCR: reverse transcriptase-polymerase chain reaction.

[3] FISH: fluorescence in situ hybridization.

receptor on their cell surfaces, an autocrine stimulation is believed to drive DFSP carcinogenesis.

Prognosis

Conventional DFSP is a low-grade sarcoma that shows a locally aggressive growth with a high rate (20–50%) of local recurrences, unless widely excised. Conventional DFSP almost never metastasizes, and when it does, this usually occurs after multiple local relapses. Accordingly, the 10-year survival rate for patients with conventional DFSP is about 99%.

Fibrosarcomatous DFSP is a high-grade sarcoma that shows a rate of local recurrence similar to that of conventional DFSP, but distant metastasis occurs in up to 50% of cases, and prognosis is consequently worse; progression to fibrosarcomatous DFSP is observed in 10–15% of cases.

The incidence of local recurrence from Bednar tumor is 11–13%, which is lower than that from conventional DFSP; furthermore, metastasis from Bednar tumor is extremely rare.

Therapy

Surgery is the mainstay of treatment (a cuff of 2–3 cm of healthy tissue surrounding the lesion should be obtained). DFSP responds poorly to chemotherapy and radiotherapy. In the rare cases where obtaining clear margins is unfeasible, **radiotherapy** has been suggested.

Based on the rational that COL1A1-PDGFB fusion leads to upregulation of PDGFB signaling through an autocrine activation loop, **targeted therapy** has shown significant antitumor activity. In particular, tyrosine kinase inhibitor imatinib[4] is currently FDA-approved for unresectable recurrent and metastatic DFSP. Imatinib has also been proposed for the neoadjuvant treatment of large primary lesions in the light of its 50% overall tumor response rate (which favors less demolitive surgery).

Sunitinib,[5] another PDGFR[6] inhibitor with a higher affinity for this target receptor, has shown favorable results in patients with DFSP after imatinib failure.

---

[4] Imatinib: tyrosine kinase inhibitor targeting the following—KIT, RET, BCR, PDGFRA.

[5] Sunitinib: tyrosine kinase inhibitor targeting the following—PDGFR, VEGFR, KIT, FLT3, CSF1R, RET.

[6] PDGFR: platelet-derived growth factor receptor is a family of tyrosine kinase receptors including PDGFR alpha (PDGFRA) and beta (PDGFRB). The receptor is activated by binding to its ligands, which belong to the PDGF family, PDGFA, PDGFB, PDGFC, and PDGFD, which form either homodimers or heterodimers (PDGF-AA, -AB, -BB, -CC, -DD). Depending on which growth factor is bound, PDGFR homo- or heterodimerizes. These growth factors are mitogens for cells of mesenchymal origin and play an important role in organ development, wound healing, and tumor progression.

Suggested Readings

Allen (2019) Dermatofibrosarcoma protuberans. Dermatol Clin 37(4):483–488

Fletcher (2020) WHO classification of tumours of soft tissue and bone, 5th edn. IARC Press, Lyon

Hornick (2020) Cutaneous soft tissue tumors: how do we make sense of fibrous and "fibrohistio-cytic" tumors with confusing names and similar appearances? Mod Pathol 33:56–65 [Epub ahead of print]

Iwasaki (2019) Current update on the molecular biology of cutaneous sarcoma: dermatofibrosar-coma protuberans. Curr Treat Options Oncol 20(4):29

Köster (2020) Genomic and transcriptomic features of dermatofibrosarcoma protuberans: Unusual chromosomal origin of the COL1A1-PDGFB fusion gene and synergistic effects of amplified regions in tumor development. Cancer Genet 241:34–41

Malhotra (2012) Dermatofibrosarcoma protruberans treatment with platelet-derived growth factor receptor inhibitor: a review of clinical trial results. Curr Opin Oncol 24(4):419–424

Navarrete-Dechent (2019) Imatinib treatment for locally advanced or metastatic dermatofibrosar-coma protuberans: a systematic review. JAMA Dermatol 155(3):361–369

Rouhani (2008) Cutaneous soft tissue sarcoma incidence patterns in the U.S.: an analysis of 12,114 cases. Cancer 113(3):616–627

Snow (2020) Conservative re-excision is a safe and simple alternative to radical resection in revision surgery for dermatofibrosarcoma protuberans. Ann Surg Oncol 27(3):919–923

Ugurel (2014) Neoadjuvant imatinib in advanced primary or locally recurrent dermatofibrosar-coma protuberans: a multicenter phase II DeCOG trial with long-term follow-up. Clin Cancer Res 20(2):499–510

Definition

Dermatomyofibroma (DMF) is a benign mesenchymal skin tumor of myofibroblastic origin. It is also known as cutaneous myofibroma.

Epidemiology and Presentation

DMF is a rare cutaneous tumor that affects mainly young adults, with female prevalence. The neoplasm appears as a plaque-like (less frequently as a nodular) dermal lesion, the shoulder region being the most common anatomic site (other sites: the axilla, neck, and upper trunk; pediatric cases occur more often in the neck). Clinically, it presents as an asymptomatic lesion (typically solitary; cases with multiple lesions are very rare) that usually measures between 1 and 5 cm in diameter, its color varying from skin color to red-brown.

Pathology

DMF consists of well-defined diffuse proliferation of monomorphic spindle cells (oriented parallel to the surface of the epidermis) separated by collagen fibers and located on the reticular dermis. The lesion lacks cellular atypia and proliferative activity; it respects skin appendages and does not affect the subcutaneous adipose tissue. The overlying epidermis is normal.

The importance in establishing the diagnosis of DMF is to distinguish it from invasive tumors such as dermatofibrosarcoma protuberans (DFSP) and piloleiomyoma (desmin positive).

Differential diagnosis. The major differential diagnosis is dermatofibrosarcoma protuberans (DFSP): both lesions are composed of spindle-shaped cells which are CD34 positive; in contrast to DFSP, tumor cells in DMF do not carry the

S. Mocellin, *Soft Tissue Tumors*, https://doi.org/10.1007/978-3-030-58710-9_68

COL1A1-PDGFB fusion gene. Cutaneous leiomyoma (also known as piloleiomyoma) is desmin positive (and may be painful). Neurofibroma is S100 positive and supplants skin appendages. Neurothekeoma (which may be painful) stains positive for vimentin, SMA, MITF1, CD10, and NKI-C3 but stains negative for S100. DMF can also be mistaken by a hypertrophic scar: the differentiation between the two lesions may be aided by the presence of elastic fibers, which is preserved in DMF and are usually reduced or lost in hypertrophic scar; moreover, DMF is not caused by trauma.

Biomarkers

The tumor lacks S100 and desmin expression but may express SMA and vimentin. Staining for CD34 is variable. Unlike DFSP, no translocation leading to the formation of the COL1A1-PDGFB fusion gene has been found in DMF.

Prognosis

DMF is a benign tumor.

Therapy

Surgical excision is the treatment of choice.

Suggested Readings

Campagnolo (2017) Dermatomyofibroma. An Bras Dermatol 92(1):101–103
Wollina (2019) Dermatomyofibroma—a rare mesenchymal tumor with maintained horripilation. Dermatol Ther 32(4):e12967

Desmoid-Type Fibromatosis

Definition

Desmoid-type fibromatosis (DTF) is a neoplasm with intermediate biological aggressiveness classified among fibroblastic-myofibroblastic tumors. It is also known as aggressive fibromatosis, deep fibromatosis, musculoaponeurotic fibromatosis, desmoid tumor, desmoid fibromatosis, and also simply desmoid. Along with superficial fibromatosis (→ see dedicated section), DTF belongs to the family of fibromatoses.

Epidemiology and Presentation

DTF is rarer than superficial fibromatosis, with an incidence of 3–5 cases per million per year. It is estimated that DTF accounts for approximately 0.03% of all neoplasms and 3% of all soft tissue tumors. As below explained, DTF has been associated with genetic traits, endocrine factors, and trauma (including surgical trauma such as surgery for prophylactic colectomy in patients with Gardner syndrome).

Traditionally, deep fibromatosis is classified into three subtypes, based on the localization:

1. Extra-abdominal DTF: it represents about 45% of all cases; virtually any site can be affected, with the shoulder, chest wall, back, thigh, and head and neck region being the most frequently involved.
2. Abdominal wall DTF: it represents about 45% of all cases; musculoaponeurotic components of the wall are involved.
3. Intra-abdominal DTF: it accounts for about 10% of all cases; the mesentery, pelvis, or retroperitoneum can be involved.

S. Mocellin, *Soft Tissue Tumors*, https://doi.org/10.1007/978-3-030-58710-9_69

In children there is no gender difference, and most cases are extra-abdominal. Between puberty and young adults, a female prevalence is observed, the abdominal wall being the most frequent localization. Later in life, DTF is again equally distributed between genders, and the most frequent localizations are abdominal and extra-abdominal.

Extra-abdominal DTF presents usually as a solitary lesion (usually 5–10 cm in diameter), but synchronous multicentric lesions are observed in 5–15% of cases, often in the same extremity (75–100%); moreover, a soft tissue mass in the extremity of a previously diagnosed DTF should be regarded as a second desmoid tumor until proven otherwise; lesions in the head and neck often behave more aggressively and may surround the axillary vessels, trachea, and brachial plexus, limiting the curative potential of surgical resection. The lesion can extend a great distance from the dominant mass, which makes it difficult to obtain microscopically free surgical margins. Magnetic resonance imaging is the radiological tool of choice as it shows characteristic low signal intensity bands on all pulse sequences (corresponding to hypocellular areas which do not show signal enhancement following gadolinium administration) and linear fascial extensions ("fascial tail" sign).

Abdominal wall DTF is the most common soft tissue tumor of the abdominal wall and affects women in about 90% of cases, with 95% of these patients having had at least one child. It presents usually as a solitary lesion (usually 3–7 cm in diameter) of the abdominal wall, typically occurring in women of childbearing age (usually 20–30 years of age) during or more frequently within the first year following a pregnancy and in women who use oral contraceptives; these findings, along with the observation of tumor progression during pregnancy and regression upon menopause, suggest an endocrine role in the pathogenesis of this DTF subtype. However, in analogy to extra-abdominal fibromatosis, abdominal wall fibromatosis may occur secondary to trauma: these lesions arise following a surgical procedure in 20% of cases, with 50% of these occurring within 4 years from surgery. Magnetic resonance imaging shows the same features above described for extra-abdominal DTF.

Intra-abdominal DTF of the pelvis (pelvic fibromatosis) presents as a slow-growing usually asymptomatic mass (which can be mistaken for an ovarian tumor) occurring most frequently in women aged 20–35 years. DTF of the small bowel mesentery (mesenteric fibromatosis) is the most common location for intra-abdominal fibromatosis, is the most common primary tumor of the mesentery, and (unlike pelvic fibromatosis, which shows a female predilection) shows a slight male predominance. Mesenteric fibromatosis can arise between 14 and 75 years of age (average age: 40 years). Due to the deep location, intra-abdominal fibromatosis may reach a large diameter (equal to or greater than 10 cm) before diagnosis.

This DTF subtype presents with abdominal pain or as a palpable abdominal mass; complications such as gastrointestinal bleeding, small bowel obstruction, fistula formation, bowel perforation, or hydronephrosis can occur. A differential diagnosis may be needed with lymphoma, metastatic disease, carcinoid, sclerosing mesenteritis, gastrointestinal stromal tumor (GIST), mesenteric lipodystrophy, and idiopathic retroperitoneal fibrosis. Computed tomography scan is frequently the modality of choice for detection and follow-up of intra-abdominal fibromatosis, which shows a soft tissue density with radiating strands projecting into the adjacent mesenteric fat. Magnetic resonance imaging appears to be diagnostically equivalent to computed tomography with the advantage of avoiding radiation exposure.

Etiology and Predisposition

DTF pathogenesis is still largely unknown, although genetic, endocrine (→ see above paragraph on abdominal DTF), and physical factors (trauma, including surgery) appear to be involved.

DTF is usually sporadic, but its incidence is remarkably increased (about 100-fold) in patients with hereditary disorders such as familial adenomatous polyposis (FAP) and its variant called Gardner syndrome (or Gardner-type FAP).

Classic FAP is inherited in an autosomal dominant manner and is due to inactivating germline mutations of the APC tumor suppressor gene, whose protein product promotes rapid degradation of CTNNB1 (encoding beta-catenin) and thus negatively regulates the Wnt signaling pathway. FAP has a birth incidence of about 1/8300 and manifests equally in both sexes. The disease causes the formation of hundreds of colorectal adenomatous polyps, with a lifetime risk of developing colorectal carcinoma greater than 90% (FAP accounts for about 1% of all colorectal cancer cases).

FAP may present some extraintestinal manifestations such as osteoma, dental abnormalities, congenital hypertrophy of the retinal pigment epithelium (CHRPE), desmoid tumor, and extracolonic cancers (thyroid, liver, bile ducts, and central nervous system); some lesions (extracolonic polyps, skull and mandible osteoma, dental abnormalities, epidermoid cysts, and fibroma) are indicative of the Gardner syndrome (intra-abdominal fibromatosis is the subtype most commonly associated with this syndrome), whereas the association of FAP with medulloblastoma is referred to as the Turcot syndrome.

It is estimated that 5–10% of all DTF cases arise in the context of FAP, that 10–30% of FAP patients develop DTF, and that 8–16% of patients with DTF have FAP.

Pathology

Pathological diagnosis is mandatory and should be obtained on a core needle biopsy. DTF arises in deep soft tissues, is characterized by infiltrative growth (with infiltration of the surrounding soft tissue structures), and is poorly circumscribed. DTF shows a proliferation of spindled cells of uniform appearance and arranged in long sweeping bundles, set in a collagenous stroma containing variably prominent blood vessels. Cytological atypia is absent, and mitotic rate is variable (as with superficial fibromatoses). Keloid-like collagen or extensive hyalinization may be found.

Differential diagnosis may be needed with the following: scar tissue (very hypocellular with a non-infiltrative growth pattern; typically it has a history of trauma or surgical procedure at the site; beta-catenin negative); Gardner fibroma (smaller and more hypocellular lesion with dense collagen bundles, most commonly associated with Gardner syndrome; beta-catenin nuclear expression is positive but the lesion results negative for CTNNB1 somatic mutations); palmar/plantar fibromatosis (only on the hands or feet, no CTNNB1 or APC mutations); nodular fasciitis (nodular architecture with areas of more loosely arranged stellate and "tissue culture-like" cells; mitotic activity is more common; beta-catenin negative, USP6 gene rearrangement is present); proliferative fasciitis/myositis (similar features to nodular fasciitis but also large ganglion-like cells which are absent in fibromatosis); myofibroma/myofibromatosis (distinct myoid nodules, diffusely positive for SMA; it may have prominent hemangiopericytic vasculature, beta-catenin negative); calcifying fibrous pseudotumor (densely collagenized and hypocellular lesion with psammomatous calcifications and variable lymphoplasmacytic infiltrate; beta-catenin negative); sclerosing mesenteritis/idiopathic retroperitoneal fibrosis (nonneoplastic disease with variable histology based on the age of the lesion, from fasciitis-like to densely sclerotic; beta-catenin negative); solitary fibrous tumor (classic hemangiopericytic vasculature with a ropey collagenous background; it may be beta-catenin positive but is typically diffusely positive for CD34 and STAT6); gastrointestinal stromal tumor (GIST has a broad number of morphologies, including epithelioid and mixed type; positive for CD34, CD117, and DOG1; usually bears mutations in KIT or PDGFRA); leiomyoma (composed of smooth muscle cells positive for SMA, desmin, calponin, and h-caldesmon); nerve sheath tumors (more prominently fibrillary background, variable positivity for S100 and SOX10, with less staining in high-grade malignant peripheral nerve sheath tumors); fibrosarcoma (diagnosis of exclusion; typically more cellular with monotonous, hyperchromatic cells, mitotic activity and herringbone pattern; beta-catenin negative); inflammatory myofibroblastic tumor (usually background of inflammation composed of plasma cells and lymphocytes; 50% have ALK1 gene rearrangements; beta-catenin is not expressed); low-grade myofibroblastic sarcoma (very infiltrative lesion with at least focal atypia; predilection for head and neck; SMA positive and beta-catenin usually negative); and low-grade fibromyxoid sarcoma (alternating zones of hypocellular collagenous and more cellular myxoid tissue; prominent arcades of vessels in the myxoid areas; MUC4 positive and characteristic FUS-CREB3L2 fusion gene; beta-catenin negative).

Biomarkers

Cells stain positive for vimentin, variably positive for MSA[1] and SMA,[2] and typically negative for desmin, h-caldesmon, S100, CD34, cytokeratins, DOG1,[3] CD117 (KIT), and MUC4. Estrogen receptors are expressed in up to 80% of the lesions, especially in abdominal wall DTF.

---

[1] MSA: muscle-specific actin.
[2] SMA: smooth muscle actin.
[3] DOG1: discovered on GIST 1 (also known as ANO1, anoctamin 1).

Most tumors (approximately 80%) show nuclear positivity for beta-catenin. DTF arising within the frame of FAP harbor germline inactivating mutations of the APC (adenomatous polyposis coli) gene, whereas up to 90% of sporadic lesions harbor somatic mutations in the CTNNB1 gene (encoding beta-catenin), both mutations leading to nuclear accumulation of beta-catenin; of note, APC and CTNNB1 mutations are mutually exclusive, which implies that finding somatic CTNNB1 mutations excludes FAP, whereas a DTF negative for somatic CTNNB1 mutations should prompt further investigation for FAP. Since an increasing number of tumors are being recognized to express nuclear beta-catenin, the routine use of CTNNB1 somatic mutations for diagnostic purposes not only in difficult cases but also in the routine setting is being advocated by many experts. The most frequent CTNNB1 somatic mutations are T41A (50% of cases), S45F (25%), and S45P (10%). Of note, S45F has been associated with increased risk of disease relapse after surgery as well as better response to medical therapy with imatinib.

Prognosis

DTF is a locally aggressive tumor neoplasm without metastatic potential.

The natural course is highly variable and basically unpredictable, with 20–30% of cases undergoing spontaneous regression (observed at any site, but more frequently in case of abdominal wall DTF). Local recurrence is common, but is currently acknowledged to be inconsistently related to the microscopic completeness of surgical excision, while attempts to achieve tumor-free resection margins may lead to significant morbidity. Due to the lack of evidence that surgical margins have a prognostic role (fewer than half patients with positive margins will experience disease relapse), intraoperative frozen section evaluation of resection margins is not advised.

Despite the lack of metastatic potential, DTF can be fatal due to local effects of tumor growth, especially in the head and neck region and in the mesentery.

The rate of abdominal wall DTF local recurrence is reported to be 15–30%, which is less frequent than extra-abdominal fibromatosis (35–65%). As regards intra-abdominal fibromatosis, while surgical resection may be curative in sporadic cases, local recurrence is frequently encountered in patients with FAP: the overall relapse rate is 23%, but the rate is 90% within the frame of FAP and 12% in sporadic cases.

According to a recent meta-analysis, the role of CTNNB1 mutational status is uncertain: in particular, primary sporadic DTF harboring the CTNNB1 S45F mutation has a higher risk of disease recurrence after surgery as compared to both wild-type DTF and DTF with other CTNNB1 mutations (i.e., T41A and S45P), but this association appears to be mediated by tumor size.

Therapy

Due to the rarity of the disease, evidence is not high level for any indication; each case should be discussed within the frame of a multidisciplinary tumor board and the strategy shared with the patient.

Watchful waiting is currently considered the upfront treatment, as spontaneous regressions are observed in 20–30% of cases and 5-year progression-free survival rates of 50% are reported with simple follow-up; this strategy is advised in all cases (including those associated with pain and pregnancy or who will become pregnant) with the obvious exception of those presenting with a complication (e.g., small bowel occlusion). Magnetic resonance imaging is considered the best method to follow up these patients: in particular, lesions with muscle/tumor T2 signal ratio lower than 1 tend to be stable or regress over time; moreover, given the interobserver measurement variability and the technique in-plane spatial resolution, a variation higher than 40% in tumor volume is suggested to confirm disease progression.

In case of disease progression, medical therapy, radiotherapy, and surgery should be considered.

Systemic therapy consists of three drug classes: (a) hormonal therapy, usually tamoxifen, is still largely employed, alone or in combination with nonsteroidal anti-inflammatory drugs (NSAIDs) such as sulindac. However, tumor response rates are low at best and disease stabilization is variable: accordingly, many investigators suggest there is no evidence for the use of endocrine therapy; (b) chemotherapy (e.g., low-dose methotrexate or conventional-dose doxorubicin) is associated with the best volumetric responses; (c) target therapy (e.g., imatinib,[4] nilotinib,[5] sorafenib[6]) is associated with low response rates and high disease stabilization rates, although the evidence is based on small data sets; in the DESMOPAZ trial, pazopanib[7] has been recently associated with a high progression-free rate (almost twice higher than chemotherapy).

Surgery should theoretically aim to obtain microscopically negative margins, although the prognostic role of resection margins has been widely questioned (patients with R0 resection may experience disease recurrence, and patients with R1 resection may never experience disease relapse). In any case, surgery should be function sparing: if the planned exeresis implies loss of function, alternative treatments should be considered. Although **radiotherapy** has been proposed as an adjuvant treatment after incomplete surgical resection, there is no consensus on this strategy. Primary radiotherapy has been associated with adequate disease control and can be proposed as an alternative to surgery or in case of medical therapy failure.

In order to avoid amputation (e.g., DTF involving neurovascular bundles, multiple/recurrent lesions), **isolated limb perfusion** (ILP) with melphalan and tumor necrosis factor (TNF) has been advocated (without the need of post-ILP surgery in case of residual disease, as usually performed for soft tissue sarcomas of the extremities).

---

[4] Imatinib: tyrosine kinase inhibitor targeting the following—KIT, RET, BCR, PDGFRA.

[5] Nilotinib: tyrosine kinase inhibitor targeting the following—ABL1, KIT.

[6] Sorafenib: tyrosine kinase inhibitor targeting the following—BRAF, KIT, RET, FGFR1, FLT3, VEGFR1, VEGFR2, VEGFR3, PDGFRB.

[7] Pazopanib: tyrosine kinase inhibitor targeting the following—VEGFR, PDGFR, KIT.

Finally, **cryoablation** and **radiofrequency** have also been reported as alternative approaches to small- to medium-sized lesions which do not involve critical structures (e.g., neurovascular bundles) and can be reached with the specific devices.

Suggested Readings

Bhat (2015) Infantile fibromatosis: a rare cause of anterior mediastinal mass in a child. J Clin Imaging Sci 5:34

Cobianchi (2014) The challenge of extraabdominal desmoid tumour management in patients with Gardner's syndrome: radiofrequency ablation, a promising option. World J Surg Oncol 12:361

Fletcher (2020) WHO classification of tumours of soft tissue and bone, 5th edn. IARC Press, Lyon

Gondim Teixeira (2020) Evidence-based MR imaging follow-up strategy for desmoid-type fibromatosis. Eur Radiol 30(2):895–902

Kasper (2017) An update on the management of sporadic desmoid-type fibromatosis: a European Consensus Initiative between Sarcoma PAtients EuroNet (SPAEN) and European Organization for Research and Treatment of Cancer (EORTC)/Soft Tissue and Bone Sarcoma Group (STBSG). Ann Oncol 28(10):2399–2408

Martínez Trufero (2017) Desmoid-type fibromatosis: who, when, and how to treat. Curr Treat Options Oncol 18(5):29

Mullen (2012) Desmoid tumor: analysis of prognostic factors and outcomes in a surgical series. Ann Surg Oncol 19(13):4028–4035

Pannier (2019) Hormonal therapies in uterine sarcomas, aggressive angiomyxoma, and desmoid-type fibromatosis. Crit Rev Oncol Hematol 143:62–66

Penel (2017) Surgical versus non-surgical approach in primary desmoid-type fibromatosis patients: a nationwide prospective cohort from the French Sarcoma Group. Eur J Cancer 83:125–131

Timbergen (2019) The prognostic role of β-catenin mutations in desmoid-type fibromatosis undergoing resection only: a meta-analysis of individual patient data. Ann Surg [Epub ahead of print]. https://doi.org/10.1097/SLA.0000000000003698

Toulmonde (2019) Pazopanib or methotrexate-vinblastine combination chemotherapy in adult patients with progressive desmoid tumours (DESMOPAZ): a non-comparative, randomised, open-label, multicentre, phase 2 study. Lancet Oncol 20(9):1263–1272

Walker (2012) Imaging features of superficial and deep fibromatoses in the adult population. Sarcoma 2012:215810

Definition

Desmoplastic fibroblastoma is a benign lesion classified among fibroblastic-myofibroblastic tumors. It is also known as collagenous fibroma.

Epidemiology and Presentation

This is a relatively uncommon tumor with a male predominance (M:F = 2:1) generally diagnosed in adults and elderly people. The disease presents as an asymptomatic, slow-growing subcutaneous mass (but fascial and skeletal muscle involvement is quite common) most frequently affecting the upper arm, shoulder, lower limb, back, forearm, hands, and feet. The lesion is well circumscribed, displays a cartilage-like consistency, and generally reaches 1–4 cm in diameter (but much larger lesions have been described).

Pathology

The lesion is paucicellular (with bland, stellate-shaped, and spindled fibroblastic cells) with abundant collagenous or myxocollagenous matrix and low vascularity. Centered in the subcutis, the lesion extends into the skeletal muscle in approximately 25% of cases. Purely intramuscular cases have been rarely reported. Atypia is absent and mitotic figures are rare.

Differential diagnosis may be needed with fibromatosis (not circumscribed, more cellular, fascicular pattern, prominent vasculature).

S. Mocellin, *Soft Tissue Tumors*, https://doi.org/10.1007/978-3-030-58710-9_70

Biomarkers

Tumor cells stain positive for vimentin and may be focally positive for SMA;[1] they are negative for desmin, EMA,[2] S100, and CD34.

Desmoplastic fibroblastoma is characterized by the **chromosomal translocation** t(2;11)(q31;q12), which leads to increased expression of FOSL1.[3]

Prognosis

Desmoplastic fibroblastoma is a benign lesion.

Therapy

Surgical excision is the treatment of choice.

Suggested Readings

Fletcher (2020) WHO classification of tumours of soft tissue and bone, 5th edn. IARC Press, Lyon
Grewal (2018) Desmoplastic fibroblastoma of the left upper arm. BMJ Case Rep 2018. pii: bcr-2017-221738
Kato (2016) FOSL1 immunohistochemistry clarifies the distinction between desmoplastic fibroblastoma and fibroma of tendon sheath. Histopathology 69(6):1012–1020
Macchia (2012) FOSL1 as a candidate target gene for 11q12 rearrangements in desmoplastic fibroblastoma. Lab Investig 92(5):735–743

---

[1] SMA: smooth muscle actin.

[2] EMA: epithelial membrane antigen.

[3] FOSL1: the Fos gene family consists of four members: FOS, FOSB, FOSL1, and FOSL2. These genes encode leucine zipper proteins that can dimerize with proteins of the JUN family, thereby forming the transcription factor complex AP-1. As such, the FOS proteins have been implicated as regulators of cell proliferation, differentiation, and transformation.

Definition

Desmoplastic small round cell tumor (DSRCT) is a high-grade malignancy of uncertain differentiation. It is also known as intra-abdominal desmoplastic round cell tumor and polyphenotypic small round cell tumor.

Epidemiology and Presentation

DSRCT typically occurs in children and young adults (peak incidence: third decade of life), with a remarkable male prevalence. The great majority of these tumors occur in the abdominal cavity, frequently affecting the retroperitoneum, pelvis, omentum, and mesentery. At the time of first diagnosis, multiple peritoneum implants are already present. Other sites of involvement (mainly thoracic cavity and paratesticular location) are rare. Clinically, the disease presents with abdominal pain and distention, palpable mass, ascites, and bowel obstruction.

Pathology

Macroscopically, areas of hemorrhage and necrosis are frequent. Microscopically, the tumor is composed of small round neoplastic cells associated with prominent stromal desmoplasia and polyphenotypic differentiation. DSRCT belongs to the family of small blue round cell tumors → see also Chap. 93. Some tumors have larger cells with greater pleomorphism. Mitoses are frequent and cell necrosis is common. The desmoplastic stroma is composed of fibroblasts or myofibroblasts embedded in a loose extracellular matrix with prominent vascularization.

Biomarkers

DSRCT typically shows a polyphenotypic differentiation by expressing proteins associated with epithelial, muscular, and neural cells. Most cases stain positive for cytokeratins, EMA,[1] vimentin, desmin, and NSE.[2] WT1[3] nuclear expression is also generally detected, whereas myogenin and MyoD1 are consistently negative.

Cytogenetically, its hallmark is the chromosomal translocation t(11;22)(p13;q12) which leads to the generation of the **EWSR1-WT1 fusion gene**.

Prognosis

DSRCT is associated with a dismal prognosis, almost independently of the treatment. Cure in DSRCT is estimated to be possible in about 5% of patients.

Therapy

Given its rarity, optimal treatment has not been defined. A multimodality therapy including cytoreductive surgery, Ewing sarcoma-based systemic chemotherapy, whole abdomen radiotherapy (WART), and hyperthermic intraperitoneal intraoperative chemotherapy (HIPEC) is usually proposed, although the results are poor. In particular, the role of WART and HIPEC is unclear. As regards target therapy, pazopanib[4] has shown some activity against heavily pretreated DSRCT.

Suggested Readings

Bétrian (2017) Antiangiogenic effects in patients with progressive desmoplastic small round cell tumor: data from the French national registry dedicated to the use of off-labeled targeted therapy in sarcoma (OUTC's). Clin Sarcoma Res 7:10

Gani (2019) A national analysis of patterns of care and outcomes for adults diagnosed with desmoplastic small round cell tumors in the United States. J Surg Oncol 119(7):880–886

Hayes-Jordan (2018) Desmoplastic small round cell tumor treated with cytoreductive surgery and hyperthermic intraperitoneal chemotherapy: results of a phase 2 trial. Ann Surg Oncol 25(4):872–877

Honoré (2017) Abdominal desmoplastic small round cell tumor without extraperitoneal metastases: is there a benefit for HIPEC after macroscopically complete cytoreductive surgery? PLoS One 12(2):e0171639

Honoré (2019) Can we cure patients with abdominal desmoplastic small round cell tumor? Results of a retrospective multicentric study on 100 patients. Surg Oncol 29:107–112

---

[1] EMA: epithelial membrane antigen.

[2] NSE: neuron-specific enolase.

[3] WT1: Wilms tumor 1.

[4] Pazopanib: tyrosine kinase inhibitor targeting the following: VEGFR, PDGFR, KIT.

Menegaz (2018) Clinical activity of pazopanib in patients with advanced desmoplastic small round cell tumor. Oncologist 23(3):360–366

Stiles (2018) Desmoplastic small round cell tumor: a nationwide study of a rare sarcoma. J Surg Oncol 117(8):1759–1767

Subbiah (2018) Multimodality treatment of desmoplastic small round cell tumor: chemotherapy and complete cytoreductive surgery improve patient survival. Clin Cancer Res 24(19):4865–4873

Thway (2016) Desmoplastic small round cell tumor: pathology, genetics, and potential therapeutic strategies. Int J Surg Pathol 24(8):672–684

Definition

Diffuse pulmonary lymphangiomatosis (DPL) is a histologically benign mesenchymal tumor of the lungs. If the proliferation is focal, it corresponds to a lymphangioma.

Epidemiology and Presentation

DPL is a very rare condition that typically presents in children and young adults, without gender prevalence.

Although primarily localized to the lungs, it can also involve other organs such as the bone, spleen, soft tissue, and liver. The disease is progressive with recurrent pleural effusions and can lead to respiratory failure following infections and chylous accumulation. As it presents with dyspnea, wheezing, and cough, it may be confused with asthma. Although radiological imaging may be suggestive, in most cases the diagnosis is reached only after lung biopsy. Thoracentesis often shows chylous effusion (high levels of triglycerides).

Pathology

DPL is composed of a diffuse proliferation of abnormal lymphatic channels (lymphangiomas) lined by benign-appearing endothelial cells. It may contain a hemorrhagic "Kaposiform" component.

Biomarkers

DPL stains positive for CD31 and factor VIII in endothelial cells and for vimentin and desmin in spindle cells. It stains negative for HMB45, cytokeratins, and HHV8.

Differential diagnosis may be needed with the following: Kaposiform hemangioendothelioma, Kaposi sarcoma (HHV8 positive), and lymphangioleiomyomatosis (HMB45 positive).

Prognosis

Prognosis depends upon the severity of lung involvement (which can lead to respiratory failure). Children have a worse prognosis than adults.

Therapy

Treatment is mainly supportive. Surgical resection has been advocated for localized disease; pleurocentesis, pleurodesis, and ligation of thoracic duct have also been proposed. Lung transplantation has been reported as a therapeutic option.

As regards targeted therapy, anecdotal positive experiences have been reported with mTOR and VEGF inhibitors such as sirolimus and bevacizumab, respectively.

Suggested Readings

Averyanov (2019) Severe pulmonary lymphedema in a patient with diffuse pulmonary lymphangiomatosis. Am J Respir Crit Care Med 200(9):e91–e92

Gurskytė (2020) Successful treatment of diffuse pulmonary lymphangiomatosis with sirolimus. Respir Med Case Rep 101014:29

Kadakia (2013) Diffuse pulmonary lymphangiomatosis. Can Respir J 20(1):52–54

Onyeforo (2018) Diffuse pulmonary lymphangiomatosis treated with bevacizumab. Respirol Case Rep 7(1):e00384

Yu (2019) Diffuse pulmonary lymphangiomatosis: a rare case report in an adult. Medicine (Baltimore) 98(43):e17349

Definition

Diffuse tenosynovial giant cell tumor (DTGCT) is a locally aggressive tumor arising from the synovium of joints, bursae, and tendon sheaths. Along with the localized form, it is one of the two subtypes of tenosynovial giant cell tumor ($\rightarrow$ see Chap. 157).

It is also known as pigmented villonodular synovitis (PVNS), pigmented villonodular tenosynovitis, diffuse-type giant cell tumor, diffuse-type tenosynovial giant cell tumor, and giant cell tumor of tendon sheath.

Epidemiology and Presentation

DTGCT tends to affect younger patients (most lesions affect young adults aged <40 years) and larger joints as compared to the localized subtype. Intra-articular lesions (more frequent, as compared to the localized type which is more often extra-articular) affect predominantly the knee (75% of cases), followed by the hip (15%). Extra-articular tumors (less frequent) most commonly involve the knee region, thigh, and foot. Uncommon locations include the fingers, wrist, groin, elbow, and toe.

Patients complain of pain, tenderness, swelling, or limitation of motion. Hemorrhagic joint effusions are frequent. The symptoms are usually of relatively long duration (often several years). Usually the size is larger than the localized counterpart (often >5 cm).

Radiologically, most lesions present as ill-defined articular masses, frequently associated with degenerative joint disease.

S. Mocellin, *Soft Tissue Tumors*, https://doi.org/10.1007/978-3-030-58710-9_73

Etiology and Predisposition

Patients with **Noonan syndrome** are at higher than expected risk of developing DTGCT. The Noonan syndrome is a disease characterized by short stature, facial dysmorphic features such as hypertelorism, a downward eye slant and low-set posteriorly rotated ears, and a high incidence of congenital heart defects and hypertrophic cardiomyopathy. Other features can include a short neck with webbing or redundancy of skin, deafness, motor delay, variable intellectual deficits, multiple skeletal defects, cryptorchidism, and bleeding diathesis. Individuals with Noonan syndrome are also at risk of rhabdomyosarcoma ($\rightarrow$ see dedicated section) as well as juvenile myelomonocytic leukemia.

Noonan syndrome is inherited in an autosomal dominant pattern and is caused by germline mutations (usually activating mutations) in multiple genes. Mutations in the PTPN11 gene cause about 50% of all cases. SOS1 gene mutations cause an additional 10–15%, and RAF1 and RIT1 genes each account for about 5% of cases. The cause of Noonan syndrome in 15–20% of people with this disorder is unknown. The PTPN11, SOS1, RAF1, and RIT1 genes encode proteins involved in the RAS/ MAPK cell signaling pathway, which is why Noonan syndrome is classified as a RASopathy.

Pathology

DTGCT is composed of synovial-like mononuclear cells, admixed with multinucleate giant cells, foam cells, siderophages, and inflammatory cells, which may be intra-articular (more often) or extra-articular (less frequently). Most tumors are infiltrative and grow as diffuse sheets.

Biomarkers

The biomarkers are identical to those of the localized counterpart ($\rightarrow$ see Chap. 157). Histiocyte-like cells are positive for CD68, CD163, and CD45; multinucleate giant cells display an osteoclastic phenotype (they express CD68 and CD45).

A small percentage of cells (10%) of most cases of DTGCT harbor a **chromosomal translocation** leading to the formation of the COL6A3-CSF1 fusion gene.[1] This chromosomal translocation leads to CSF1 protein overexpression, which is believed to contribute to tumor growth.

---

[1] COL6A3-CSF1 fusion gene: COL6A3 (collagen type VI alpha 3 chain) encodes the alpha-3 chain, one of the three alpha chains of type VI collagen, a beaded filament collagen found in most connective tissues. CSF1 (colony-stimulating factor 1) encodes a cytokine that controls the production, differentiation, and function of macrophages; the active form of the protein is found extracellularly as a disulfide-linked homodimer and is thought to be produced by proteolytic cleavage of membrane-bound precursors.

Prognosis

Recurrences are common (20–40% for intra-articular lesions, 30–50% for extra-articular lesions), are often multiple, and may severely compromise joint function. The risk of recurrence does not correlate with any histological parameter, while it is associated with positive excision margins.

DTGCT should be considered as a locally aggressive but non-metastasizing neoplasm, although some rare cases of malignant tenosynovial giant cell tumor showing obvious sarcomatous areas and giving rise to pulmonary metastasis have been reported.

Therapy

The mainstay of treatment is wide surgical excision (for intra-articular lesions: synovectomy).

As regards target therapy, given the relatively high frequency of CSF1 overexpression, drugs (e.g., imatinib,[2] nilotinib,[3] emactuzumab,[4] cabiralizumab,[5] and pexidartinib[6]) blocking the CSFR pathway have been investigated with encouraging results. In particular, pexidartinib[6] has been recently approved for the treatment of adult patients with symptomatic DTGCT associated with severe morbidity or functional limitations and not amenable to surgery based on the findings of a randomized controlled trial.

Suggested Readings

Cassier (2012) Efficacy of imatinib mesylate for the treatment of locally advanced and/or metastatic tenosynovial giant cell tumor/pigmented villonodular synovitis. Cancer 118(6):1649–1655

Fletcher (2020) WHO classification of tumours of soft tissue and bone, 5th edn. IARC Press, Lyon

Gelderblom (2018) Nilotinib in locally advanced pigmented villonodular synovitis: a multicentre, open-label, single-arm, phase 2 trial. Lancet Oncol 19(5):639–648

Gouin (2017) Localized and diffuse forms of tenosynovial giant cell tumor (formerly giant cell tumor of the tendon sheath and pigmented villonodular synovitis). Orthop Traumatol Surg Res 103(1S):S91–S97

Lamb (2019) Pexidartinib: first approval. Drugs 79:1805–1812 [Epub ahead of print]

Mastboom (2019) Surgical outcomes of patients with diffuse-type tenosynovial giant-cell tumours: an international, retrospective, cohort study. Lancet Oncol 20(6):877–886

Miri A (2018) Multifocal pigmented villonodular synovitis in the noonan syndrome. Case Rep Orthop 2018:7698052

---

[2] Imatinib: tyrosine kinase inhibitor targeting the following: KIT, RET, BCR, PDGFRA.

[3] Nilotinib: tyrosine kinase inhibitor targeting the following: ABL1, KIT.

[4] Emactuzumab: humanized monoclonal antibody blocking CSF1R.

[5] Cabiralizumab: humanized monoclonal antibody blocking CSF1R.

[6] Pexidartinib: tyrosine kinase inhibitor targeting the following: CSF1R, KIT, FLT3.

Noailles (2017) Giant cell tumor of tendon sheath: open surgery or arthroscopic synovectomy? A systematic review of the literature. Orthop Traumatol Surg Res 103(5):809–814

Tap (2019) Pexidartinib versus placebo for advanced tenosynovial giant cell tumour (ENLIVEN): a randomised phase 3 trial. Lancet 394(10197):478–487

Verspoor (2019) Long-term efficacy of imatinib mesylate in patients with advanced Tenosynovial Giant Cell Tumor. Sci Rep 9(1):14551

The following is the list of soft tissue tumors that can affect the digestive system (including the esophagus, stomach, small intestine, colon and rectum, liver, biliary tract, and pancreas) according to the 2019 World Health Organization classification of digestive system tumors.

For details → see sections dedicated to each tumor.

Tumor	Notes
Angiosarcoma	→ See Chaps. 25 and 119
Calcifying nested stromal epithelial tumor of the liver	Specific to the digestive system
Desmoid-type fibromatosis	–
Hepatic embryonal sarcoma	Specific to the digestive system
Epithelioid hemangioendothelioma	–
Gastrointestinal clear cell sarcoma (GCCS)	Specific to the digestive system. Also known as gastrointestinal neuroectodermal tumor (GNET)
Gastrointestinal stromal tumor (GIST)	Specific to the digestive system
Glomus tumor	–
Granular cell tumor	–
Hemangioma	→ See Chaps. 117 and 123
Inflammatory fibroid polyp	Specific to the digestive system
Inflammatory myofibroblastic tumor	–
Kaposi sarcoma	–
Leiomyoma	Mainly esophageal location (→ see dedicated section)
Leiomyosarcoma	The diagnosis of leiomyosarcoma of the gastrointestinal tract can be made only after excluding GIST (most lesions once defined as gastrointestinal leiomyosarcomas are now classified as GIST)

S. Mocellin, *Soft Tissue Tumors*, https://doi.org/10.1007/978-3-030-58710-9_74

Tumor	Notes
Lipoma	Mainly found in the gastrointestinal tract with special regard to the stomach and colon
Lymphangioma	–
Mesenchymal hamartoma of the liver	Specific to the digestive system
PEComa (including angiomyolipoma)	–
Perineurioma	–
Plexiform fibromyxoma	Specific to the digestive system
Rhabdomyosarcoma	–
Schwannoma	–
Solitary fibrous tumor	–
Synovial sarcoma	–

Definition

EBV-associated smooth muscle tumor (ESMT) is a benign smooth muscle tumor developing only in immunocompromised patients.

Epidemiology and Presentation

ESMT is a rare entity occurring in immunocompromised patients (e.g., AIDS patients or transplanted patients). It occurs mainly (but not exclusively) in adults, with a slight male prevalence.

Of note, multifocal tumors are due to multiple infection events, not to metastatic disease; multifocal tumors can affect one or multiple organs (e.g., the liver, brain, spinal cord, and adrenal gland).

Etiology and Predisposition

ESMT is believed to be caused by Epstein-Barr virus (EBV) infection in immuno-compromised patients.

Of note, EBV is also associated with leiomyosarcoma in this type of patients.

Pathology

ESMT appears as a well-differentiated smooth muscle tumor with primitive round cell areas and prominent intratumoral T-cells. Atypia is mild or absent. Mitotic figures are rare or absent. No pleomorphism is present.

© The Editor(s) (if applicable) and The Author(s), under exclusive license to
Springer Nature Switzerland AG 2021
S. Mocellin, *Soft Tissue Tumors*, https://doi.org/10.1007/978-3-030-58710-9_75

ESMT is histologically distinct from classic soft tissue smooth muscle tumors and is not readily evaluated by conventional histologic criteria (as it can show incomplete smooth muscle differentiation).

Biomarkers

Epstein-Barr virus-encoded small RNAs (EBER) are small noncoding RNAs localized in the nucleus of human cells infected with EBV. EBER is the most important diagnostic feature of ESMT and can be revealed by FISH.

Prognosis

ESMT is a benign appearing tumor that usually shows a slow disease progression but can lead patients to death (less than 10% of cases).

Therapy

Surgery can be utilized for symptomatic lesions. Recently, mTOR inhibitors (e.g., sirolimus) have been associated with tumor response.

Suggested Readings

Hirama (2019) Epstein-Barr virus-associated smooth muscle tumors after lung transplantation. Transpl Infect Dis 21(3):e13068
Penney (2019) Treatment response with sirolimus for a pediatric patient with an EBV-associated smooth-muscle tumor after bone marrow transplantation. Pediatr Blood Cancer 66(5):e27585
Stubbins (2019) Epstein-Barr virus associated smooth muscle tumors in solid organ transplant recipients: incidence over 31 years at a single institution and review of the literature. Transpl Infect Dis 21(1):e13010
Willeke (2020) Epstein Barr virus associated smooth muscle tumors in the central nervous system: a case report and systematic review of the literature. J Neuro-Oncol 147(2):247–260

Definition

Disseminated peritoneal leiomyomatosis (DPL) is a benign entity due to the proliferation of smooth muscle cells throughout the peritoneal surface. It is also known as leiomyomatosis peritonealis disseminate. The term parasitic leiomyoma relates to a similar condition in which the lesion is single (nondisseminated disease).

Epidemiology and Presentation

DPL is an exceedingly rare condition usually occurring in females of reproductive age. Clinically, DPL must be differentiated from other peritoneal tumors (e.g., peritoneal carcinomatosis from colorectal or ovarian carcinoma).

Etiology and Predisposition

The etiology is unknown. The origin of this condition is unclear: some believe that DPL might derive from a histologically "bland" low-grade leiomyosarcoma that has been overlooked; others believe that DPL might develop from the implantation and proliferation of benign smooth muscle cells from a uterine leiomyoma. The latter theory has been recently supported by the observation of DPL occurring after laparoscopic morcellation of uterine leiomyomas.

Pathology

Histopathology usually reveals highly cellular interlacing bundles of smooth muscle cells, mimicking a leiomyoma; no nuclear atypia, mitotic figures, or signs of necrosis are present.

S. Mocellin, *Soft Tissue Tumors*, https://doi.org/10.1007/978-3-030-58710-9_76

Biomarkers

Immunochemical analysis shows that DPL expresses desmin, caldesmon, estrogen receptor and progesterone receptor.

Prognosis

DPL is a benign condition, although anecdotal cases have been reported to undergo progression and malignant transformation.

Therapy

Due to the rarity of the disease, there is no consensus on the treatment strategy. Surveillance or medical therapy (e.g., aromatase inhibitors or GnRH agonists) are two options. Surgery (i.e., DPL debulking) may be considered for symptomatic cases. In women who do not wish to bear a child, hysterectomy with salpingo-oophorectomy plus DPL debulking has also been proposed.

Suggested Readings

Anand (2016) Disseminated peritoneal leiomyomatosis status post laparoscopic hysterectomy with morcellation. J Radiol Case Rep 10(12):12–18

Glaser (2018) Laparoscopic myomectomy and morcellation: a review of techniques, outcomes, and practice guidelines. Best Pract Res Clin Obstet Gynaecol 46:99–112

Hiremath (2016) Disseminated peritoneal leiomyomatosis: a rare cause of enigmatic peritoneal masses. BJR Case Rep 2(3):20150252

Khan (2018) Parasitic leiomyoma of the greater omentum presenting as small bowel obstruction. J Surg Case Rep 2018(7):rjy164

Ma (2020) A clinicopathological and molecular analysis in uterine leiomyomas and concurrent/metachronous peritoneal nodules: new insights into disseminated peritoneal leiomyomatosis. Pathol Res Pract 216(5):152938

Ramos (2015) Surgical cytoreduction for disseminated benign disease after open power uterine morcellation. Obstet Gynecol 125(1):99–102

Soni (2020) Disseminated peritoneal leiomyomatosis: an unusual presentation of intra-abdominal lesion mimicking disseminated malignancy. Med Pharm Rep 93(1):113–116

Wu (2016) Leiomyomatosis peritonealis disseminata: a case report and review of the literature. Mol Clin Oncol 4(6):957–958

Definition

Ectomesenchymoma (EM) is a malignant tumor composed of both neuroectodermal elements and one or more mesenchymal elements (e.g., rhabdomyosarcoma); it is currently classified by the World Health Organization among skeletal muscle tumors. It is also known as gangliorhabdomyosarcoma.

Epidemiology and Presentation

This tumor is exceedingly rare and usually affects children under 15 years of age (only 20% of cases have been described in adults), with a slight male predominance (M:F = 3:2). The most frequent locations are the head and neck (orbit and nasopharynx), central nervous system, abdomen and retroperitoneum, pelvis, perineum, scrotum, and prostate. Clinically it presents as a mass of variable size (mean diameter: 5 cm) without specific signs/symptoms (mainly compression and infiltration by primary tumor and/or metastasis).

Pathology

EM is characterized by the coexistence of ectodermal derivatives (neuroblasts and ganglion cells, often with immature and atypical appearance, resembling those of ganglioneuroma, ganglioneuroblastoma, neuroblastoma, peripheral primitive neuroectodermal tumor), and mesenchymal components (mostly represented by plump elongated cells with rhabdomyoblastic differentiation, including strap-like and racket-shaped cells). Of note, the ectodermal component may be sometimes scarcely represented and thus can be overlooked. Differential diagnosis should consider rhabdomyosarcoma (NSE negative), triton tumor (loss of H3K27me3 expression in the MPNST component), teratoma, Wilms tumor (WT1 positive), and benign ectomesenchymoma (also known as ectomesenchymal hamartoma).

© The Editor(s) (if applicable) and The Author(s), under exclusive license to
Springer Nature Switzerland AG 2021
S. Mocellin, *Soft Tissue Tumors*, https://doi.org/10.1007/978-3-030-58710-9_77

Biomarkers

Skeletal muscle component is positive for myogenin, MyoD1, desmin, and MSA;[1] ganglioneuroma component is positive for S100 protein, and ganglion cells stain positive for NSE.[2] EM does not express cytokeratins.

EM is characterized by HRAS mutations in most cases and trimethylation at lysine 27 of histone H3 (H3K27me3) expression (typically lost in malignant peripheral nerve sheath tumor) retained in all cases analyzed.

Prognosis

EM is a rapidly growing malignancy which can metastasize.

Therapy

Surgery is the mainstay of primary tumor treatment. Metastatic disease is usually treated with chemotherapy protocols suitable for rhabdomyosarcoma or neuroblastoma.

Suggested Readings

Fletcher (2020) WHO classification of tumours of soft tissue and bone, 5th edn. IARC Press, Lyon
Griffin (2018) Malignant ectomesenchymoma: series analysis of a histologically and genetically heterogeneous tumor. Int J Surg Pathol 26(3):200–212
Huang (2016) Frequent HRAS mutations in malignant ectomesenchymoma: overlapping genetic abnormalities with embryonal rhabdomyosarcoma. Am J Surg Pathol 40(7):876–885
Mahajan (2019) Primary intracranial malignant ectomesenchymoma in an adult: report of a rare case and review of the literature. Neuropathology 39(3):200–206
Nael (2014) Metastatic malignant ectomesenchymoma initially presenting as a pelvic mass: report of a case and review of literature. Case Rep Pediatr 2014:792925

---

[1] MSA: muscle-specific actin.

[2] NSE: neuron-specific enolase.

Definition

Ectopic hamartomatous thymoma (EHT) is a benign soft tissue tumor of undefined differentiation. It is also known as branchial anlage mixed tumor and biphenotypic branchioma. Despite the term "thymoma," there is no evidence of thymic origin or differentiation.

Epidemiology and Presentation

EHT exclusively arises in the superficial or deep soft tissues of the lower neck (supraclavicular, suprasternal, or presternal areas). It occurs in adults (median age: 45 years), almost always in men (M:F = 10:1).

Pathology

The tumor is composed of spindle cells, epithelial islands, and adipose cells.

Biomarkers

Immunohistochemically, the spindle cells coexpress cytokeratins, CD34, and SMA (but do not express desmin), whereas the epithelial cells stain positive for cytokeratins only.

Prognosis

EHT is a benign lesion which rarely recurs after complete surgical excision.

© The Editor(s) (if applicable) and The Author(s), under exclusive license to
Springer Nature Switzerland AG 2021
S. Mocellin, *Soft Tissue Tumors*, https://doi.org/10.1007/978-3-030-58710-9_78

Therapy

Surgical excision is the treatment of choice.

Suggested Readings

Fetsch (2004) Ectopic hamartomatous thymoma: a clinicopathologic and immunohistochemical analysis of 21 cases with data supporting reclassification as a branchial anlage mixed tumor. Am J Surg Pathol 28(10):1360–1370

Fletcher (2013) WHO classification of tumours of soft tissue and bone, 4th edn. IARC Press, Lyon

Sato (2018) Ectopic hamartomatous thymoma: a review of the literature with report of new cases and proposal of a new name: biphenotypic branchioma. Head Neck Pathol 12(2):202–209

Weissferdt (2016) Ectopic hamartomatous thymoma—new insights into a challenging entity: a clinicopathologic and immunohistochemical study of 9 cases. Am J Surg Pathol 40(11):1571–1576

Definition

Like "conventional" meningioma,[1] ectopic meningioma is a tumor originating from meningothelial cells (i.e., cells forming the arachnoidal cap): however, it develops outside the intracranial and intraspinal compartments (which normally contain meningothelial cells and are the sites of "conventional" meningioma). It is currently classified by the World Health Organization (WHO) among benign nerve sheath tumors, although it can behave as a malignant tumor ($\rightarrow$ see below paragraph in Section "Prognosis").

It is also known as extracranial/extraspinal meningioma, extraneuraxial meningioma, heterotopic meningioma, cutaneous meningioma, calvarial meningioma, intraosseous meningioma, and meningothelial choristoma.

It should be distinguished from meningothelial hamartoma ($\rightarrow$ see Table 79.1).

Epidemiology and Presentation

"Conventional" meningioma is the most common extra-axial neoplasm and accounts for 15% of all intracranial tumors. Ectopic meningioma is a rare neoplasm (approximately 1.6% of all resected meningiomas) occurring at all ages (but most frequently in adults) without remarkable gender differences. It generally arises in the head and neck region (>90% of cases), with special regard to the orbit, bone (skull), sinonasal space, oropharynx, middle ear, scalp, parotid gland, and neck. Lesions originating in the orbit with a connection to the optic nerve dural sleeve should not be

---

[1] Meningioma arises from arachnoidal cap cells known as meningothelial cells: these cells derive from precursor cells characteristically positive for prostaglandin D2 synthase (PGDS). These precursor cells are of mesoderm origin at the skull base (PGDS+ meningeal cell) and neural crest derived at the cerebral convexity (telencephalic region).

Table 79.1 Comparison between ectopic meningioma and meningothelial hamartoma

	Ectopic meningioma	Meningothelial hamartoma
Age	Mainly adults	Mainly neonates or infants
Gender	M ≈ F	M ≈ F
Biology	Neoplasm	Developmental rest
Cells of origin	Meningothelial cells	Meningothelial cells
Prognosis	Usually benign, rarely malignant	Benign
Intracranial connection	Absent	Absent
Site	Mainly the head and neck	Mainly scalp
Pathology	Like "conventional" meningioma (grade I to III, with a range of variants)	Cutaneous slit-like spaces that resemble lymphatics or angiosarcoma but lined by meningothelial rather than endothelial cells

considered as ectopic but rather "conventional" meningiomas. By definition, no intracranial/spinal component must be present.

The lesion typically presents as a painless, slow-growing mass which can cause compression signs/symptoms over time.

Pathology

Macroscopically, the lesion is similar to "conventional" meningioma, except for the fact that invasion of adjacent tissues is much more frequent. Microscopically, ectopic meningioma presents the variety of histological appearances encountered in "conventional" meningioma (→ see Table 79.2).

Biomarkers

No specific biomarker exists. The tumor usually stains positive for EMA,[2] vimentin, and progesterone receptor and negative for chromogranin, synaptophysin CD31, and SMA.[3]

Prognosis

For meningiomas in general, three WHO grades are recognized:

– Grade I: by far the most frequent, benign.

---

[2] EMA: epithelial membrane antigen.
[3] SMA: smooth muscle actin.

Table 79.2 Meningioma variants

Grade I	Angiomatous	Rare, vascular component exceeds 50% of total tumor area, meningothelial cells are wrapped around small blood vessels, differential diagnosis with hemangioblastoma which stains positive for inhibin and NSE
	Fibroblastic	Composed of spindle cells, sheet-like architecture, resembles schwannoma or solitary fibrous tumor but is focally EMA positive and often has thick bundles of collagen
	Lymphocyte rich	May be associated with Castleman disease or other hematopoietic neoplasm
	Meningothelial	The most common variant, syncytial and epithelial cells, indistinct cell borders and classic whorls; may have sparse psammoma bodies
	Metaplastic	May contain foci of the bone, cartilage, or fat
	Microcystic	Overall resembles microcysts, variable pleomorphism
	Psammomatous	Numerous psammoma bodies
	Secretory	Eosinophilic secretions, may secrete CEA, may have cytologic atypia
	Transitional	Meningothelial and fibroblastic features; usually prominent whorls, psammoma bodies, and clusters of syncytial cells
Grade II	Atypical	
	Chordoid	
	Clear cell	
Grade III	Anaplastic	
	Papillary	
	Rhabdoid	

- Grade II: about 6% of cases, characterized by an increased probability of recurrence.
- Grade III: the rarest subgroup, malignant behavior.

As with "conventional" meningioma, tumor grade and completeness of resection are the most important prognostic factors for disease recurrence. Distant metastases have been reported in approximately 6% of cases, mostly in anaplastic (malignant) lesions.

Therapy

Like "conventional" meningiomas, asymptomatic stable ectopic lesions might be followed up. Otherwise, surgical excision is the treatment of choice.

Suggested Readings

Fletcher (2020) WHO classification of tumours of soft tissue and bone, 5th edn. IARC Press, Lyon
Fox (2013) Cutaneous meningioma: a potential diagnostic pitfall in p63 positive cutaneous neoplasms. J Cutan Pathol 40(10):891–895

Kalamarides (2011) Identification of a progenitor cell of origin capable of generating diverse meningioma histological subtypes. Oncogene 30:2333–2344

Ohashi-Nakatani (2019) Primary pulmonary meningioma: a rare case report of aspiration cytological features and immunohistochemical assessment. Diagn Cytopathol 47(4):330–333

Tan (2017) Ectopic orbital meningioma: fact or fiction? Orbit 36(3):144–146

Thompson (2016) Update on select benign mesenchymal and meningothelial sinonasal tract lesions. Head Neck Pathol 10(1):95–108

Elastofibroma

80

Definition

Elastofibroma is a benign lesion classified among fibroblastic-myofibroblastic tumors. It is also known as elastofibroma dorsi (due to its typical location).

Epidemiology and Presentation

Elastofibroma is a frequent soft tissue neoplasm occurring mainly in the elderly (peak incidence between 70 and 80 years), with a significant prevalence in females. Genetic evidence supports its neoplastic nature.

Elastofibroma typically develops in the deep soft tissue of the back, between the scapula and the thoracic wall. However, extracapsular locations have been rarely reported (e.g., other parts of the thoracic wall, extremities, limb girdles, gastrointestinal tract, and other viscera).

Elastofibroma presents as a slow-growing poorly circumscribed mass which is often oligo-symptomatic (it is often an incidental finding of radiological imaging performed with other indications) and can reach several centimeters in diameter.

Pathology

Elastofibroma presents as an ill-defined rubbery mass that microscopically shows a proliferation of elastofibrous tissue featuring an excessive number of abnormal elastic fibers, dispersed spindled fibroblasts, and a variable amount of mature adipose tissue.

Differential diagnosis may be needed with the following: desmoid fibromatosis (more cellular, infiltration of skeletal muscle, no elastic fibers); fibrolipoma (no elastic fibers); and nuchal fibroma (younger age, between scapula and vertebrae, no elastic fibers).

© The Editor(s) (if applicable) and The Author(s), under exclusive license to 265
Springer Nature Switzerland AG 2021
S. Mocellin, *Soft Tissue Tumors*, https://doi.org/10.1007/978-3-030-58710-9_80

Biomarkers

The lesion typically stains positive for elastin. Spindle cells are usually positive for CD34 and vimentin, but negative for SMA and desmin.

Prognosis

Elastofibroma is a benign tumor and post-surgery local recurrence is very rare.

Therapy

Surgical excision is the treatment of choice.

Suggested Readings

Andrés-Ramos (2019) Cutaneous elastic tissue anomalies. Am J Dermatopathol 41(2):85–117
Beenen (2016) Elastofibroma of the pylorus presenting as gastric outlet obstruction: a case report and review of literature. ANZ J Surg 86(11):946–947
Findikcioglu (2013) A thoracic surgeon's perspective on the elastofibroma dorsi: a benign tumor of the deep infrascapular region. Thorac Cancer 4(1):35–40
Fletcher (2020) WHO classification of tumours of soft tissue and bone, 5th edn

Embryonal Rhabdomyosarcoma

81

Definition

Embryonal rhabdomyosarcoma (ERMS) is a malignant tumor deriving from embryonic skeletal muscle cells. It is also known as myosarcoma, malignant rhabdomyoma, rhabdopoietic sarcoma, rhabdosarcoma, embryonal sarcoma, botryoid rhabdomyosarcoma, and sarcoma botryoides.

Along with alveolar (ARMS), pleomorphic (PRMS), and spindle cell/sclerosing (SRMS) rhabdomyosarcoma ($\rightarrow$ see dedicated sections), it belongs to the rhabdomyosarcoma family of tumors (for general details on these tumors $\rightarrow$ see section entitled "Rhabdomyosarcoma").

Epidemiology and Presentation

ERMS is the most common type of rhabdomyosarcoma and typically affects children aged less than 10 years (36% of all cases occur in children aged less than 5 years), with a slight male predominance. ERMS represents about 70% of childhood rhabdomyosarcoma cases and 20% of adulthood rhabdomyosarcoma cases.

Despite the name, fewer than 10% of ERMS cases develop within the skeletal muscles of the extremities. About 40% arise within the head and neck and 40% within the genitourinary system. Common sites include the urinary bladder, prostate, paratesticular soft tissues, periorbital soft tissues, oropharynx, parotid, auditory canal and middle ear, pterygoid fossa, nasopharynx, nasal passages and paranasal sinuses, tongue, and cheek. ERMS may also occur in the biliary tract, retroperitoneum, pelvis, perineum, as well as abdomen and viscera (e.g., the kidney and heart). The ERMS subtype called botryoid rhabdomyosarcoma is always confined to epithelial-lined viscera such as the urinary bladder, biliary tract, pharynx, conjunctiva, or auditory canal.

Clinically, ERMS causes symptoms related to the compression/infiltration of adjacent structures and organs, but it may simply present as a painless mass. Head and neck lesions may lead to proptosis, diplopia, sinusitis, or unilateral deafness; genitourinary lesions may cause a scrotal mass or urinary retention; biliary lesions may be associated with jaundice.

Etiology and Predisposition

Most ERMS cases are sporadic, but patients with some cancer predisposition syndromes are at higher risk of ERMS. For more details → see section entitled "Rhabdomyosarcoma" (paragraph "Predisposition").

Pathology

Macroscopically, ERMS presents as a poorly circumscribed, fleshy mass that impinges on adjacent structures; the botryoid subtype has a characteristic polypoid appearance (grape bunch appearance, hence the name) and abuts an epithelial surface.

Microscopically, ERMS (which resembles embryonic skeletal muscle) is composed of primitive mesenchymal cells in various stages of myogenesis, with a variable content of rhabdomyoblasts. Cell differentiation often becomes more evident after chemotherapy. Some tumors contain abundant, myxoid stroma (mimicking myxoma), while others comprise compact, patternless sheets of spindle and round cells. Especially in the case of a small biopsy, ERMS may only contain densely cellular sheets of round cells (rhabdomyosarcomas belong to the family of small blue round cell tumors → see also section entitled "Extraskeletal Ewing Sarcoma").

The botryoid variant (also known as sarcoma botryoides and botryoid embryonal rhabdomyosarcoma) contains linear aggregates of tumor cells (also known as the "cambium layer") that abut an epithelial surface.

Differential diagnosis may be needed with the following: alveolar rhabdomyosarcoma (strong nuclear staining for myogenin and MyoD1; molecular studies including FISH show PAX-FOXO1 fusion gene in approximately 80% of cases); desmoplastic small round cell tumor (tumor nodules on serosal surfaces, strongly positive for cytokeratin and EMA, it may be desmin positive but is MSA negative; it is associated with desmoplasia, and histologically it more closely mimics alveolar rather than embryonal rhabdomyosarcoma; it is negative for myogenin and MyoD1); Ewing/PNET (another small blue round cell tumor; it often displays Homer Wright rosettes, nuclei are far more uniform and pale, not dense and hyperchromatic; CD99 positive; desmin, MyoD1, and myogenin negative; it displays characteristic chromosomal rearrangements); lymphoma (positive for CD45, B-cell, or T-cell biomarkers; desmin, myogenin, MyoD1, and MSA negative); monophasic synovial sarcoma (negative for muscle biomarkers, usually far more spindled and organized in long fascicles; cytokeratin and EMA positive; it displays a typical chromosomal translocation); myxoid liposarcoma (typically is easy to distinguish from ERMS, but it may have a very similar background matrix; signet ring lipoblasts; more bland histology and more uniformity when compared to ERMS; immunostaining and molecular features are also useful); neuroblastoma (undifferentiated neuroblastoma may be very difficult to distinguish histologically; elevated urinary catecholamines, rosettes, granular chromatin; S100, chromogranin, synaptophysin, and GFAP positive; lack of myogenic biomarkers); pleomorphic rhabdomyosarcoma (exclusively adults, usually deep soft tissue of the extremity and remarkable for its diffuse cytologic atypia; uniformly pleomorphic; it does not contain elements of embryonal rhabdomyosarcoma); and Wilms tumor (it may have rhabdomyoblastic differentiation, especially in the setting of chemotherapy; epithelial and blastemal components can be very focal following chemotherapy; WT1 and cytokeratin positive, muscle biomarkers negative).

Biomarkers

ERMS is typically positive for biomarkers of skeletal muscle differentiation, which correlate with the degree of tumor cell differentiation: in fact, only vimentin is present in the cytoplasm of the most primitive cells, while desmin and actin are acquired by developing rhabdomyoblasts, and only differentiated cells show biomarkers of terminal differentiation (e.g., creatine kinase M). MyoD and myogenin are highly specific and sensitive for rhabdomyosarcoma and are routinely used for diagnostic purposes (of note, only nuclear staining is specific, since nonspecific staining is common in paraffin-embedded tissues). Without myogenic differentiation (MyoD1 or myogenin) it is very difficult to diagnose ERMS; however, ERMS typically stains weakly/focally positive for myogenin, which is instead strongly positive for most cases of alveolar rhabdomyosarcoma.

Sporadic ERMS is cytogenetically aneuploid, with multiple numerical chromosome changes. Most cases share a loss of heterozygosity (LOH) localized to chromosomal region 11p15.5, which suggests the presence of a tumor suppressor gene inactivated during ERMS tumorigenesis by allelic loss of the active allele.

Syndromic ERMS implies different genes in the pathogenesis of this malignancy ($\rightarrow$ see "Predisposition" paragraph of the section entitled "Rhabdomyosarcoma").

Prognosis

In general, ERMS has a better prognosis than the other types of rhabdomyosarcomas. Younger age is a favorable factor, while the outcome of parameningeal and extremity lesions is poorer than that of orbital and paratesticular lesions. Finally, botryoid rhabdomyosarcoma has a better prognosis as compared to standard ERMS.

For more details on staging and prognosis $\rightarrow$ see the section entitled "Rhabdomyosarcoma."

Therapy

Currently, risk-adapted multimodality treatment (personalized therapy) is the standard of care.

For details → see the section entitled "Rhabdomyosarcoma."

Suggested Readings

Fletcher (2020) WHO classification of tumours of soft tissue and bone, 5th edn

Garren (2020) NRAS associated RASopathy and embryonal rhabdomyosarcoma. Am J Med Genet A 182(1):195–200

McCluggage (2020) Embryonal rhabdomyosarcoma of the ovary and fallopian tube: rare neoplasms associated with germline and somatic DICER1 mutations. Am J Surg Pathol 44(6):738–747

Pappo (2018) Rhabdomyosarcoma, Ewing sarcoma, and other round cell sarcomas. J Clin Oncol 36(2):168–179

Skapek (2019) Rhabdomyosarcoma. Nat Rev Dis Primers 5(1):1

Tang (2018) The prognosis and effects of local treatment strategies for orbital embryonal rhabdomyosarcoma: a population-based study. Cancer Manag Res 10:1727–1734

Definition

The term endometrial stromal sarcoma (ESS) applies to malignant neoplasms typically composed of cells that resemble endometrial stromal cells of the proliferative endometrium. ESS are predominantly intramural neoplasms exhibiting myometrial invasion.

There are two ESS subtypes:

- Low-grade endometrial stromal sarcoma (LGESS)
- High-grade endometrial stromal sarcoma (HGESS)

Epidemiology and Presentation

LGESS occurs in women between 40 and 55 years old of whom >50% is premenopausal. Patients can present with vaginal bleeding, dysmenorrhea, or pelvic pain, but as many as 25% is asymptomatic.

HGESS present with abdominal bleeding, an enlarged uterus, or pelvic mass at a mean age of 50 years (range 28–67). The tumor may appear as intracavitary polypoid or mural masses.

For further details → see section entitled "Uterine Sarcomas."

Pathology

In LGESS, neoplastic cells resemble those of proliferative endometrial stroma and lack significant cytological atypia.

HGESS shows the "tongue-like" permeative pattern into the myometrium and angiolymphatic invasion typical of LGESS; however, the cytomorphology is distinctive as it does not exactly resemble proliferative endometrial stromal cells and is

S. Mocellin, *Soft Tissue Tumors*, https://doi.org/10.1007/978-3-030-58710-9_82

instead characterized by a monomorphic proliferation of round cells in a vaguely nested or pseudoglandular pattern; moreover, necrosis is common and mitotic rate is higher than in LGESS (usually >10/10 HPF).

For LGESS, **differential diagnosis** may be needed with the following: endometrial stromal nodule (not infiltrative, no angiolymphatic invasion); cellular leiomyoma (no infiltration, no angiolymphatic invasion); and metastatic lobular carcinoma (clinical history of primary tumor; strongly positive for cytokeratins).

For HGESS, **differential diagnosis** may be needed with the following: LGESS (pathology, chromosomal rearrangements → see below section on biomarkers); epithelioid leiomyosarcoma (positivity for smooth muscle immunomarkers, presence of at least focal marked atypia; lack of YWHAE-NUTM2 fusion gene); perivascular epithelioid cell tumor (PEComa may show "fingerlike" projections analogous to those of ESS but typically shows epithelioid and spindled cells, nested growth pattern, prominent vascular network, and coexpression of melanocytic and muscle markers); and epithelioid gastrointestinal stromal tumor (particularly in intraperitoneal/pelvic locations in view of the frequent extrauterine spread at presentation; CD117 and DOG1 positivity; lack of YWHAE-NUTM2 fusion gene).

Biomarkers

In LGESS, CD10 and hormone receptors (estrogen, progesterone) are typically positive on tumor cells. Most cases of LGESS harbor **chromosomal translocations**, the most common being translocation t(7;17)(p15;q21), which results in the JAZF1-SUZ12 fusion gene.[1]

In HGESS, CD10 is usually positive, whereas estrogen and progesterone receptors are negative. Recently, the **chromosomal translocation** t(10;17)(q22;p13) has been identified in a large proportion of HGESS. This rearrangement results in a fusion between YWHAE and one of the two highly homologous genes FAM22A and FAM22B: this fusion gene, formerly designated as YWHAE-FAM22, is now called YWHAE-NUTM2.[2] The presence of YWHAE-NUTM2 helps discriminate HGESS from the more common LGESS with JAZF1 rearrangement and from undifferentiated uterine sarcoma (UUS) which has no identifiable molecular aberrations. Cyclin D1 expression can be used as an immunohistochemical diagnostic

---

[1] JAZF1-SUZ12 fusion gene: JAZF1 (juxtaposed with another zinc finger protein 1) encodes a nuclear protein with three C2H2-type zinc fingers and functions as a transcriptional repressor. SUZ12 (suppressor of zeste 12) encodes a polycomb group (PcG) protein which acts as a component of the PRC2/EED-EZH2 complex, which methylates "Lys-9" (H3K9me) and "Lys-27" (H3K27me) of histone H3, leading to transcriptional repression of the affected target gene.

[2] YWHAE-NUTM2 fusion gene: YWHAE encodes tyrosine 3-monooxygenase/tryptophan 5-monooxygenase activation protein epsilon, a member of the 14-3-3 family of proteins which mediate signal transduction by binding to phosphoserine-containing proteins. NUTM2 (NUT family member 2B) is a protein-coding gene whose alterations have been linked to endometrial stromal sarcoma and kidney clear cell sarcoma.

Table 82.1 FIGO staging for endometrial stromal sarcoma (ESS)

Stage	Definition
I	Tumor limited to the uterus
IA	Tumor limited to the endometrium
IB	Up to half of the myometrium invaded
IC	More than half of the myometrium invaded
II	Tumor extends beyond the uterus, within the pelvis
IIA	Adnexal involvement
IIB	Involvement of other pelvic tissues
III	Tumor infiltrates abdominal tissues
IIIA	1 site
IIIB	>1 site
IIIC	Involves pelvic and/or para-aortic lymph nodes
IV	Tumor invades pelvic organs and/or distant metastasis
IVA	Invasion of bladder or rectum
IVB	Distant metastasis

indicator for HGESS with YWHAE-NUTM2 rearrangement. In a subset of HGESS with a more aggressive clinical course, the ZC3H7B-BCOR fusion gene[3] has been detected.

Prognosis

ESS is a malignant tumor. Prognosis of LGESS is favorable. Recurrences occur in up to one third of the patients and may occur after many years. Five-year survival for stages I–II is 90%, compared to 50% for stages III–IV.

Compared to LGESS, patients with HGESS more frequently experience disease relapse, which occurs earlier after primary diagnosis (HGESS prognosis is intermediate between that of LGESS and undifferentiated uterine sarcoma → see dedicated section).

ESS is usually staged according to the to the International Federation of Gynecology and Obstetrics (FIGO) staging system (→ see the below Table 82.1).

---

[3] ZC3H7B-BCOR fusion gene: ZC3H7B (zinc finger CCCH-type containing 7B) encodes a protein that contains a tetratricopeptide repeat domain. BCOR (BCL6 corepressor) encodes a transcriptional corepressor which specifically inhibits gene expression when recruited to promoter regions by sequence-specific DNA-binding proteins such as BCL6 and MLLT3; BCOR rearrangements have been described in clear cell sarcoma of the kidney, primitive myxoid mesenchymal tumor of infancy, central nervous system high-grade neuroepithelial tumor, undifferentiated round cell sarcoma, high-grade endometrial stromal sarcoma, and ossifying fibromyxoid tumor.

Therapy

- ***Early disease.*** Hysterectomy and bilateral salpingo-oophorectomy are the standard treatment. The risk of lymph node metastases from an ESS is <10%, which suggests to avoid lymphadenectomy (unless suspicious lymphadenopathy is observed on preoperative imaging or intraoperatively); moreover, evidence form retrospective series suggests that addition of lymphadenectomy does not lead to any survival advantage, either for LGESS or for HGESS.
- Altogether, there is no sufficient evidence to support the use of radiotherapy or chemotherapy in the adjuvant setting as standard of care in ESS.
- Since about 80% of ESS cases express estrogen receptor (ER) and progesterone receptor (PgR), some oncologists suggest the use of adjuvant hormonal therapy, although no definitive evidence exists to support this approach; in particular, for LGESS—which has a good prognosis—the therapeutic advantage must be balanced with side effects.
- ***Advanced/metastatic disease.*** LGESS usually has a very indolent behavior and relapses are often late: patients with a low volume of metastatic disease may be offered the option of radiologic surveillance or local therapies such as surgery, radiotherapy, or radiofrequency ablation; hormone receptor positivity may be exploited, with clinical benefit rates up to 90%; upon failure of hormonal therapy, systemic chemotherapy may be considered, although response rates are low.
- As regards HGESS, this tumor is associated with universally poor outcomes and low response rates to conventional chemotherapy (which is based on anthracyclines); these patients should be considered for clinical trials of novel agents.

Suggested Readings

Aldera (2020) Gene of the month: BCOR. J Clin Pathol [Epub ahead of print]

Ali (2015) Endometrial stromal tumours revisited: an update based on the 2014 WHO classification. J Clin Pathol 68(5):325–332

Desar (2018) Systemic treatment in adult uterine sarcomas. Crit Rev Oncol Hematol 122:10–20

Douglas (2020) Genomic profiling of BCOR-rearranged uterine sarcomas reveals novel gene fusion partners, frequent CDK4 amplification and CDKN2A loss. Gynecol Oncol 157(2):357–366

Makise (2019) Low-grade endometrial stromal sarcoma with a novel MEAF6-SUZ12 fusion. Virchows Arch 475(4):527–531

Pannier (2019) Hormonal therapies in uterine sarcomas, aggressive angiomyxoma, and desmoid-type fibromatosis. Crit Rev Oncol Hematol 143:62–66

Rauh-Hain (2013) Endometrial stromal sarcoma: a systematic review. Obstet Gynecol 122(3):676–683

Thiel (2018) Low-grade endometrial stromal sarcoma—a review. Oncol Res Treat 41(11):687–692

Definition

Epithelioid fibrous histiocytoma (EFH) is a variant of benign fibrous histiocytoma (→ see dedicated section). EFH is believed to originate from dermal fibroblasts and dendritic histiocytes.

It is also known as epithelioid cell histiocytoma, histiocytoid hemangioendothelioma, epithelioid benign fibrous histiocytoma, and cutaneous epithelioid cell histiocytoma.

Epidemiology and Presentation

EFH is a rare tumor representing approximately 1% all benign fibrous histiocytomas of the skin. It most commonly presents in the fifth decade of life with a slight male predominance. EFH affects the skin, the lower extremity being the most frequent site (up to 60% of cases). The solitary elevated nodule (mostly 0.5–2 cm in diameter) is usually skin-colored, although in some cases it presents with a pronounced vascular appearance mimicking pyogenic granuloma.

Pathology

Microscopically, EFH is characterized by rounded or angulated epithelioid cells with eosinophilic cytoplasm accounting for more than 50% of the tumor cell population, with low or no mitotic activity. A population of secondary elements including multinucleated giant cells and hemosiderin-laden macrophages is typically present (which can help distinguish EFH from other histiocytic neoplasms).

Differential diagnosis may be needed with the following: melanocytic proliferation with epithelioid morphology such as Spitz nevus (nested growth pattern, S100 and HMB-45 positive) or even melanoma (nuclear pleomorphism, brisk mitotic

S. Mocellin, *Soft Tissue Tumors*, https://doi.org/10.1007/978-3-030-58710-9_83

activity, S100 and HMB-45 positive); epithelioid sarcoma (tendency to occur in deep soft tissues or subcutis, cell atypia, grow in a multinodular or "pseudogranulomatous" pattern with geographic necrosis, cytokeratin positive, loss of INI1/SMARCB1 expression, CD163 negative); histiocytic sarcoma (macrophage malignancy with marked atypia and high mitotic activity); and Rosai-Dorfman disease (multiple skin lesions and adenopathy, histiocytes are S100 positive and pleomorphic with emperipolesis, also prominent B-cells and plasma cells).

Biomarkers

EFH may stain positive for EMA[1] and CD163, but stains negative for CD34, melanocytic markers, desmin, and cytokeratins.

Most EFH cases (>90%) harbor ALK[2] rearrangement due to **chromosomal translocations** leading to the formation of an ALK-based fusion gene. The most common fusion partners are SQSTM1 and VCL (more than 70% of cases), other fusion partners being DCTN1, ETV6, PPFIBP1, SPECC1K, TMP3, PRKAR2A, MLPH, and EML4. ALK rearrangement leads to ALK overexpression detectable on immunohistochemistry. This biomarker can be useful for differential diagnosis purposes.

Prognosis

EFH is a benign tumor.

Therapy

Surgical excision is the treatment of choice.

---

[1] EMA: epithelial membrane antigen.

[2] ALK: Anaplastic lymphoma receptor tyrosine kinase encodes a receptor tyrosine kinase belonging to the insulin receptor superfamily. It plays an important role in the development of the brain and exerts its effects on specific neurons in the nervous system. This gene has been found to be rearranged, mutated, or amplified in a series of tumors including anaplastic large cell lymphomas, neuroblastoma, non-small cell lung cancer, and inflammatory myofibroblastic tumor. The chromosomal rearrangements are the most common genetic alterations in this gene, which result in creation of multiple fusion genes including ALK (chromosome 2)/EML4 (chromosome 2), ALK/RANBP2 (chromosome 2), ALK/ATIC (chromosome 2), ALK/TFG (chromosome 3), ALK/NPM1 (chromosome 5), ALK/SQSTM1 (chromosome 5), ALK/KIF5B (chromosome 10), ALK/CLTC (chromosome 17), ALK/TPM4 (chromosome 19), and ALK/MSN (chromosome X).

Suggested Readings

Dickson (2018) Epithelioid fibrous histiocytoma: molecular characterization of ALK fusion partners in 23 cases. Mod Pathol 31(5):753–762

Felty (2019) Epithelioid fibrous histiocytoma: a concise review. Am J Dermatopathol 41(12):879–883

Definition

Epithelioid hemangioendothelioma (EHE) is a malignant vascular neoplasm. The outdated term intravascular bronchioloalveolar tumor (IVBAT) refers to a lung localization of EHE.

Epidemiology and Presentation

EHE is an uncommon neoplasm affecting most frequently (but not exclusively) patients in the second decade of life, with a slight female predominance. This malignancy typically develops as a solitary moderately painful tan-tinged mass in the soft tissues of the extremities, but it has been described in virtually any body site; among the viscera, liver, and lung are the most frequent locations (for hepatic EHE → see dedicated section). As an angiocentric tumor, EHE arising in a large vessel can cause vessel occlusion. Calcifications may be visible at X-rays.

Pathology

This angiocentric tumor expands the vessel wall, obliterates the lumen, and spreads centrifugally into the surrounding tissues. Microscopically, EHE displays chains and cords of epithelioid endothelial cells distributed in a myxohyaline stroma. The cells present with vacuoles that distinctively deform the cytoplasm (blister cells). In most cases the cells are of low nuclear grade, although a subset of cases has higher-grade morphology.

Differential diagnosis may be needed with the following: epithelioid angiosarcoma (irregular sinusoidal vascular channels, solid sheets of cells with marked atypia and prominent mitotic activity, necrosis); epithelioid sarcoma (distal extremities of young adults, tumor cells merge with collagenous stroma, cytokeratin strongly positive, CD31 negative); melanoma (S100 and HMB45 positive, CD31 negative); and metastatic carcinoma (marked atypia, mitotic activity, usually not angiocentric, cytokeratin strongly positive, CD31 negative).

Biomarkers

EHE stains positive for vascular biomarkers (e.g., CD34, CD31, FLI1, and ERG). Cytokeratins and EMA[1] are expressed in a minority of cases.

EHE is characterized (in virtually all cases) by the **chromosomal translocation** t(1;3)(p36;q23-25), which leads to the formation of the WWTR1-CAMTA1 fusion gene.[2] As this fusion gene is unique to EHE and is not detected in its mimics, this gene rearrangement can be used as a diagnostic tool. More recently, a histologically distinctive subset of EHE has been shown to harbor the YAP1-TFE3 fusion gene.[3]

Prognosis

EHE is a low-grade malignant tumor. Unlike angiosarcoma, most cases of EHE show an indolent course; nevertheless, up to 30% of patients experience metastatic disease and about 15% of patients die of the disease. EHE with more malignant features are usually also clinically more aggressive. In particular, patients with EHE larger than 3 cm in diameter and with more than 3 mitoses per 50 HPF have a 60% 5-year disease-specific survival rate as compared to the 100% rate of patients affected with tumors lacking these features.

---

[1] EMA: epithelial membrane antigen.

[2] WWTR1-CAMTA1 fusion gene: WWTR1 (WW domain-containing transcription regulator 1) encodes a transcriptional coactivator which acts as a downstream regulatory target in the Hippo signaling pathway that plays a pivotal role in organ size control and tumor suppression by restricting proliferation and promoting apoptosis. CAMTA1 (calmodulin-binding transcription activator 1) encodes a protein that contains a CG1 DNA-binding domain, a transcription factor immunoglobulin domain, ankyrin repeats, and calmodulin-binding IQ motifs. The encoded protein is thought to be a transcription factor.

[3] YAP1-TFE3 fusion gene: YAP1 encodes Yes-associated protein 1, a downstream nuclear effector of the Hippo signaling pathway (which is involved in development, growth, repair, and homeostasis); YAP1 is known to play a role in the development and progression of multiple cancers as a transcriptional regulator of this signaling pathway. TFE3 belongs to the microphthalmia family of bHLH-LZ transcription factors (MiT/TFE) which is composed of four members: MITF, TFEB, TFE3, and TFEC; neoplasms with alterations in these genes are also called MiT family tumors.

Therapy

Surgery is the treatment of choice, whenever feasible. Liver transplantation has been advocated for unresectable hepatic EHE. Treatment for metastatic disease is experimental and includes chemotherapy, immunotherapy, and targeted therapy (including antiangiogenic drugs and mTOR inhibitors).

In asymptomatic patients with disease not amenable to surgery, watchful waiting has been proposed as an option if the histology is favorable.

Suggested Readings

Antonescu (2013) Novel YAP1-TFE3 fusion defines a distinct subset of epithelioid hemangioendothelioma. Genes Chromosomes Cancer 52(8):775–784

Cao (2019) Selection of treatment for hepatic epithelioid hemangioendothelioma: a single-center experience. World J Surg Oncol 17(1):183

Cournoyer (2020) Clinical characterization and long-term outcomes in pediatric epithelioid hemangioendothelioma. Pediatr Blood Cancer 67(2):e28045

Engel (2019) A retrospective review of the use of sirolimus for pediatric patients with epithelioid hemangioendothelioma (EHE). J Pediatr Hematol Oncol [Epub ahead of print]

Errani (2011) A novel WWTR1-CAMTA1 gene fusion is a consistent abnormality in epithelioid hemangioendothelioma of different anatomic sites. Genes Chromosomes Cancer 50(8):644–653

Fletcher (2020). WHO classification of tumours of soft tissue and bone. 5th edition

Noh (2020) Treatment and prognosis of hepatic epithelioid hemangioendothelioma based on SEER data analysis from 1973 to 2014. Hepatobiliary Pancreat Dis Int 19(1):29–35

Papke (2020) What is new in endothelial neoplasia? Virchows Arch 476(1):17–28

Rosenberg (2018) Epithelioid hemangioendothelioma: update on diagnosis and treatment. Curr Treat Options in Oncol 19(4):19

Shon (2019) Epithelioid vascular tumors: a review. Adv Anat Pathol 26(3):186–197

Suurmeijer (2020) Variant WWTR1 gene fusions in epithelioid hemangioendothelioma—a genetic subset associated with cardiac involvement. Genes Chromosomes Cancer 59(7):389–395

Epithelioid Hemangioma

85

Definition

Epithelioid hemangioma (EHA) is a benign tumor of vascular differentiation. It is also known as angiolymphoid hyperplasia with eosinophilia, nodular angioblastic hyperplasia with eosinophilia and lymphofolliculosis, subcutaneous angioblastic lymphoid hyperplasia with eosinophilia, atypical pyogenic granuloma, inflammatory angiomatous nodule, and histiocytoid hemangioma.

Epidemiology and Presentation

EHA can arise at virtually any age, with an incidence peak in the third through fifth decade of life. Most lesions are subcutaneous, with dermal cases being less frequent. The most common sites are the head and distal extremities, where the disease presents as an indolent mass of 1–2 cm that the patient is aware of since up to 1 year before. Rare cases of EHA of the deep soft tissue, bone, lymph nodes, lung, eye, colon, heart, spleen, and penis have been reported.

Pathology

The tumor is composed by well-formed small, capillary-sized vessels lined by epithelioid endothelial cells (hence the name), most cases being rich in lymphocytes and eosinophils.

The morphologic spectrum of EHA includes a wide range of appearances, including intravascular growth, a heavy inflammatory infiltrate, a cellular/solid proliferation, or atypical histologic features with increased mitotic activity and necrosis.

Differential diagnosis may be needed with the following: epithelioid angiosarcoma (marked atypia); epithelioid hemangioendothelioma (usually not cutaneous lesion); and pyogenic granuloma (no epithelioid endothelial cells).

S. Mocellin, *Soft Tissue Tumors*, https://doi.org/10.1007/978-3-030-58710-9_85

Biomarkers

The epithelioid endothelial cells stain positive for ERG and CD31 and—though to a lesser degree—for CD34.

The ZFP36-FOSB fusion gene[1] has been found in a small subset with atypical features, which can be useful to distinguish EHA from malignant epithelioid vascular tumors such as angiosarcoma and epithelioid hemangioendothelioma.

Prognosis

Although it is a benign tumor, EHA can locally recur in up to one third of cases. Nevertheless, disease relapses are indolent and can be cured by redo surgery.

Therapy

Surgical excision.

Suggested Readings

Fletcher (2013) WHO classification of tumours of soft tissue and bone, 4th edn
Huang (2015) Frequent FOS gene rearrangements in epithelioid hemangioma: a molecular study of 58 cases with morphologic reappraisal. Am J Surg Pathol 39(10):1313–1321
Liu (2019) Characterization of long-term outcomes for pediatric patients with epithelioid hemangioma. Pediatr Blood Cancer 66(1):e27451
Papke What is new in endothelial neoplasia? Virchows Arch 2020, 476(1):17–28
Shon (2019) Epithelioid vascular tumors: a review. Adv Anat Pathol 26(3):186–197

---

[1] ZFP36-FOSB fusion gene: ZFP36 encodes a zinc finger RNA-binding protein that destabilizes several cytoplasmic AU-rich element (ARE)-containing mRNA transcripts by promoting their poly(A) tail removal or deadenylation and hence provides a mechanism for attenuating protein synthesis. FOSB: FosB proto-oncogene (AP-1 transcription factor subunit) encodes a member of the Fos gene family, which consists of four members: FOS, FOSB, FOSL1, and FOSL2; these genes encode leucine zipper proteins that can dimerize with proteins of the JUN family, thereby forming the transcription factor complex AP-1 (which is involved in the regulation of cell proliferation, differentiation, and transformation).

Definition

Epithelioid sarcoma (EpS) is a malignant tumor of uncertain differentiation. As described below, two variants are recognized:

- Distal-type epithelioid sarcoma (also known as classic epithelioid sarcoma or conventional epithelioid sarcoma)
- Proximal-type epithelioid sarcoma (also known as large cell epithelioid sarcoma)

Epidemiology and Presentation

EpS accounts for about 0.5–1% of soft tissue sarcomas (4–8% of non-rhabdomyosarcomas in children). The distal variant is twice more frequent than the proximal subtype. EpS can occur in a wide age range (generally affects young adults, but patients with distal variant are averagely younger), with a male prevalence (1.5- to 2-fold more frequent in males).

The classic variant mainly affects superficial or deep tissues of distal upper extremity (more than 60% of cases are located in the hand, where EpS is the most frequent type of soft tissue sarcoma), followed by the distal lower extremity, proximal extremities, trunk, and head and neck. The foot and hand are affected mostly in their volar surface. The proximal-type variant mainly develops in the deep soft tissues of the trunk (the pelvis and perineum, genital, and inguinal) and buttock/hip, followed by the thigh, head and neck, distal extremity, and axilla. Very rarely, EpS arises from other sites, including the viscera.

Superficial EpS presents as solitary or multiple, firm, slow-growing, usually painless, ill-defined, dermal, or subcutaneous nodule(s) (from few millimetres to 5 cm), which may appear as nonhealing skin ulcer(s). In contrast, deeply located EpS is usually a larger in size and more infiltrative multinodular mass that can reach up to 20 cm in diameter and involve tendons or fascia.

© The Editor(s) (if applicable) and The Author(s), under exclusive license to
Springer Nature Switzerland AG 2021
S. Mocellin, *Soft Tissue Tumors*, https://doi.org/10.1007/978-3-030-58710-9_86

EpS is one of the few soft tissue sarcomas that often metastasize to lymph nodes (about 30% of cases).

Calcifications may be present at radiological imaging studies.

Pathology

EpS is a mesenchymal tumor characterized by epithelioid cytomorphology.

Distal-type EpS predominately arises in subcutaneous tissue of extremities and consists of cellular nodules of epithelioid and spindled tumor cells with central degeneration and/or necrosis (so-called pseudogranulomatous growth pattern: bland histiocytoid cells with frequent central palisaded necrosis). Mitotic activity is usually low. Calcification and metaplastic bone formation are detected in 20% of cases, and chronic inflammatory cells are usually present at the periphery of the tumor nodules.

Proximal-type EpS is characterized by a multinodular and sheetlike growth of large and sometimes pleomorphic epithelioid (carcinoma-like) cells (large undifferentiated anaplastic cells with high-grade nuclear features and prominent nucleoli). Foci of necrosis are frequently found, without formation of a pseudogranulomatous pattern. Significant morphologic overlap exists with pediatric malignant rhabdoid tumor.

Cells with rhabdoid features occur in both forms, which can make difficult the differential diagnosis from extrarenal rhabdoid tumors. Rare cases of EpS show mixed histological features of both classic and proximal types.

Differential diagnosis may be needed with the following: squamous cell carcinoma (p63 positive, look for an epithelial component); epithelioid angiosarcoma (CD31 and factor VIII positivity); epithelioid MPNST (shows INI1 loss but also diffuse S100 positivity); and malignant rhabdoid tumor (pediatric).

Biomarkers

Both variants show positivity for epithelial biomarkers such as cytokeratins and EMA.[1] As opposed to carcinomas, vimentin and CD34 are often positive.

Loss of nuclear expression of SMARCB1 (also known as INI1) protein[2] is detected in both variants (in about 80–90% of cases). Cytogenetic studies have

---

[1] EMA: epithelial membrane antigen.

[2] SMARCB1: SWI/SNF-related matrix-associated actin-dependent regulator of chromatin, subfamily B, member 1 (also known as INI1) encodes a protein which is part of the BAF (hSWI/SNF) complex that relieves repressive chromatin structures, allowing the transcriptional machinery to access its targets more effectively. This ATP-dependent chromatin-remodeling complex plays an important role in different cell activities including cell differentiation; in particular, regulation of the stem cell-associated programme, which is maintained by the repressive effect of the EZH2-dependent PRC2 (polycomb repressive complex 2), is disrupted by SMARCB1. Overall, SMARCB1 has been found to act as a tumor suppressor, and its mutations have been associated with malignancies including sarcomas.

identified in chromosomal 22q11 abnormalities (e.g., mutation, deletions) the cause of SMARCB1 loss of expression, which is found also in pediatric rhabdoid tumors of the kidney and central nervous system as well as other sarcomas ($\rightarrow$ see section entitled "SMARC-Deficient Sarcomas").

Prognosis

EpS is generally considered a high-grade sarcoma. The 5-year and 10-year overall survival rates are 60–80% and 40–60%, respectively. Local recurrence rates range between 30 and 80%, while metastases develop in 40–50% of patients (involving mainly lungs and and regional lymph nodes). Adverse prognostic factors (for both variants) are male gender, older age, proximal extremity/axial location, deep location, primary tumor size >5 cm and multifocality, high mitotic rate, regional (lymph node) or distant metastasis, proximal-type histology (versus distal type), proximal-type histology with presence of rhabdoid cells (versus conventional proximal type), and extensive necrosis. The prognostic role of FNCLCC[3] histological grading system is debated.

Therapy

Surgery Surgical wide excision is the mainstay of treatment. The use of sentinel node biopsy is generally discouraged. Isolated limb perfusion can be utilized in case of limb-threatening EpS.

Radiotherapy Adjuvant/neoadjuvant radiotherapy is often used to increase local disease control, especially in high-risk lesions.

Chemotherapy Anthracycline-based and gemcitabine-based regimens have a moderate activity in EpS, with similar tumor response rate (about 20%) and survival rates; the efficacy of pazopanib is considered low. The role of adjuvant/neoadjuvant chemotherapy for high-risk lesions is debated. For metastatic disease, systemic chemotherapy yields generally poor results.

Target therapy Drugs of this category have been tested, with generally poor results. Attempts to therapeutically exploit the SMARCB1 deficiency are underway: in fact, aberrations of the switch/sucrose nonfermentable (SWI/SNF) complex (such as those deriving from SMARCB1 or SMARCA4 deficiency) can lead to aberrant histone methylation, oncogenic transformation, and proliferative depen-

---

[3] FNCLCC: Fédération Nationale des Centres de Lutte Contre Le Cancer.

dency on EZH2[4] activity. On the basis of a trial showing a 15% response rate, the FDA[5] has recently approved tazemetostat (an EZH2 inhibitor) for patients with locally advanced or metastatic EpS not eligible for complete resection.

Suggested Readings

Ahmad (2019) Primary pleural epithelioid sarcoma of the proximal type: a diagnostic and therapeutic challenge. Transl Lung Cancer Res 8(5):700–705

Andreou (2013) Sentinel node biopsy in soft tissue sarcoma subtypes with a high propensity for regional lymphatic spread—results of a large prospective trial. Ann Oncol 24(5):1400–1405

Elsamna (2020) Epithelioid sarcoma: half a century later. Acta Oncol 59(1):48–54

Emori (2017) A typical presentation of primary pulmonary epithelioid sarcoma misdiagnosed as non-small cell lung cancer. Pathol Int 67(4):222–224

Fletcher (2020) WHO classification of tumours of soft tissue and bone, 5th edn

Frezza (2018) Anthracycline, gemcitabine, and pazopanib in epithelioid sarcoma: a multi-institutional case series. JAMA Oncol 4(9):e180219

Gasparini (2011) Prognostic determinants in epithelioid sarcoma. Eur J Cancer 47(2):287–295

Hoy (2020) Tazemetostat: first approval. Drugs 80(5):513–521

Italiano (2018) Tazemetostat, an EZH2 inhibitor, in relapsed or refractory B-cell non-Hodgkin lymphoma and advanced solid tumours: a first-in-human, open-label, phase 1 study. Lancet Oncol 19(5):649–659

Jones (2012) Role of palliative chemotherapy in advanced epithelioid sarcoma. Am J Clin Oncol 35(4):351–357

Le Loarer (2014) Consistent SMARCB1 homozygous deletions in epithelioid sarcoma and in a subset of myoepithelial carcinomas can be reliably detected by FISH in archival material. Genes Chromosomes Cancer 53(6):475–486

Maduekwe (2009) Role of sentinel lymph node biopsy in the staging of synovial, epithelioid, and clear cell sarcomas. Ann Surg Oncol 16(5):1356–1363

Noujaim (2015) Epithelioid sarcoma: opportunities for biology-driven targeted therapy. Front Oncol 5:186

Schuetze (2017) Phase 2 study of dasatinib in patients with alveolar soft part sarcoma, chondrosarcoma, chordoma, epithelioid sarcoma, or solitary fibrous tumor. Cancer 123(1):90–97

Sparber-Sauer (2019) Epithelioid sarcoma in children, adolescents, and young adults: localized, primary metastatic and relapsed disease. Treatment results of five Cooperative Weichteilsarkom Studiengruppe (CWS) trials and one registry. Pediatr Blood Cancer 66(9):e27879

Spunt (2019) Clinical features and outcomes of young patients with epithelioid sarcoma: an analysis from the Children's Oncology Group and the European paediatric soft tissue Sarcoma Study Group prospective clinical trials. Eur J Cancer 112:98–106

Stacchiotti (2019) Safety and efficacy of tazemetostat, a first-in-class EZH2 inhibitor, in patients (pts) with epithelioid sarcoma (ES) (NCT02601950). J Clin Oncol 37(15) Suppl: Abstract 11003

Sullivan (2013) Epithelioid sarcoma is associated with a high percentage of SMARCB1 deletions. Mod Pathol 26(3):385–392

---

[4]EZH2: Enhancer of zeste 2 polycomb repressive complex 2 subunit encodes a member of the Polycomb group (PcG) family. In particular, it encodes the catalytic subunit of the PRC2/EED-EZH2 complex, which methylates Lys-9 (H3K9me) and Lys-27 (H3K27me) of histone H3, leading to transcriptional repression of the affected target gene. The dysregulation of this methylation is believed to be critical in the development of cancer.

[5]FDA: Food and Drug Administration.

Definition

This is a benign tumor originating from smooth muscle cells of the esophagus. It belongs to the leiomyoma family (see section entitled "Leiomyoma").

Epidemiology and Presentation

Esophageal leiomyoma is a rare tumor but is the most frequent type of benign neoplasm of the esophagus. It most frequently occurs between the ages of 20–50 years, with a higher incidence in males (M:F = 2:1). The most common location is in the lower two thirds of the esophagus (only 10% of cases occur in the upper one third of the esophagus). Most cases are detected when they are less than 5 cm in size; rarely, this neoplasm grows larger than 10 cm (in this case it is called giant leiomyoma of the esophagus). Multiple tumors may be observed. The most common symptoms are dysphagia, chest pain, vague retrosternal discomfort, heartburn, and occasionally regurgitation; gastrointestinal bleeding is rarely observed. In the rare case of a giant leiomyoma of the esophagus, patients report persistent cough. Large esophageal leiomyomas usually grow outward, so dysphagia need not be present and does not reflect the size of such tumor. Many of these tumors are discovered incidentally during endoscopic procedures or radiological tests. With the increasing use of endoscopy and radiological investigation, the number of cases diagnosed is growing.

The typical appearance is a smooth concave space-occupying lesion underlying a normal mucosa. It is easy to recognize a sharp angle at the junction of the tumor and healthy tissue. When an endoscopy is performed, these tumors can be identified as relatively mobile submucosal swellings. An upper GI endoscopy will confirm the presence of a submucosal tumor by clearly visualizing a mass protruding into the lumen of the esophagus, with normal-looking mucosa covering the swelling. A computed tomography scan is a valuable investigation in confirming the diagnosis.

© The Editor(s) (if applicable) and The Author(s), under exclusive license to
Springer Nature Switzerland AG 2021
S. Mocellin, *Soft Tissue Tumors*, https://doi.org/10.1007/978-3-030-58710-9_87

Currently, endoscopic ultrasonography (EUS) plays a critical role to diagnose esophageal leiomyoma.

Pathology

The tumor presents as a circumscribed lesions composed of intersecting fascicles of bland spindle cells with abundant cytoplasm. These well-differentiated smooth muscle cells which are of the spindle type are arranged as braids. These bundles are demarcated by adjacent tissue or a definite connective tissue capsule. The spindle cells intersect with each other at varying angles. The tumor cells have blunt elongated nuclei and display minimal atypia and very few mitotic figures.

Biomarkers

Tumor cells stain positive for desmin and alpha-smooth muscle actin, while they stain negative for CD34, CD117 (KIT), and S100.

Prognosis

Esophageal leiomyoma is a benign neoplasm.

Therapy

All patients with symptomatic tumors are advised to undergo excision or enucleation of the tumor. The conventional surgical approach is an open thoracotomy; after this, an enucleation of the tumor with an esophageal myotomy or a resection of the tumor with the esophagus is performed. Surgical esophageal resection may be indicated in giant leiomyoma of the esophagus or tumors involving long segments of the esophagus. Tumors of the middle third can be approached using a right thoracic route, and tumors of the distal one third can be accessed through a left-sided approach. Video-assisted thoracoscopic surgery (VATS) has progressively gained acceptance in the last few years. For extra-mucosal excision or enucleation, the outer esophageal muscle is incised longitudinally, and then careful dissection is performed to separate and remove the leiomyoma from the underlying mucosa. Recently, endoscopic submucosal dissection and enucleation of esophageal leiomyomas are increasingly being performed. The standard surgical practice is to approximate the muscle layer following a myotomy and enucleation, although some investigators believe that even large myotomies or extra-mucosal defects can be left open without the development of a subsequent complication. Esophageal resection as a treatment is reserved for those with very large tumors. Asymptomatic tumors which are less than 1 cm are managed by regular follow-up strategies.

Suggested Readings

Chen (2017) Minimally invasive surgery for giant esophageal leiomyoma: a case report & review of the literatures. J Thorac Dis 9(1):E26–E31

Chen (2019) A novel hybrid approach for enucleation of esophageal leiomyoma. J Thorac Dis 11(6):2576–2580

Donatelli (2017) Submucosal tunneling endoscopic resection (STER) with full-thickness muscle excision for a recurrent para-aortic esophageal leiomyoma after surgery. Endoscopy 49(S 01):E86–E87

Zhu (2019) Successful en bloc endoscopic full-thickness resection of a giant cervical esophageal leiomyoma originating from muscularis propria. J Cardiothorac Surg 14(1):16

Definition

Ewing-like sarcomas are also known as Ewing-like sarcoma family, Ewing-like tumor family, atypical Ewing sarcomas, and Ewing-like tumors. The terms Ewing sarcoma family of tumors and Ewing family of tumors include both Ewing sarcoma (osseous and extraosseous) and Ewing-like sarcomas.

These are highly aggressive sarcomas sharing some histological features (small round cell neoplasms, though some variability exists; see below) as well as chromosomal translocations (involving the EWSR1 gene, though not in all cases) with classical Ewing sarcoma (which includes bone and extraosseous Ewing sarcomas → see section entitled "Extraskeletal Ewing Sarcoma").

In the past, most Ewing-like sarcomas were classified among undifferentiated round cell sarcomas,[1] which belong to the sarcoma family known as undifferentiated pleomorphic sarcoma (→ see dedicated section).

The Ewing-like sarcoma family encompasses the following nosological entities:

(a) Non-EST-rearranged Ewing-like sarcoma
(b) CIC-rearranged Ewing-like sarcoma
(c) BCOR-rearranged Ewing-like sarcoma
(d) Adamantinoma-like Ewing sarcoma
(e) Askin tumor
(f) Peripheral primitive neuroectodermal tumor (pPNET)

---

[1] Round cell sarcomas are a heterogeneous group of mesenchymal neoplasms with overlapping morphology and immunohistochemical profile. Ewing sarcoma is the most well-known tumor in this group characterized by EWSR1/FUS rearrangements with members of the ETS family of transcription factors: undifferentiated round cell sarcomas lacking these rearrangements are known as Ewing-like sarcomas, described in this section.

A certain degree of overlapping exists in this terminology: for instance, the term pPNET is often utilized interchangeably with the term Ewing family of tumors (which Ewing and Ewing-like sarcomas).

Non-ETS-Rearranged Ewing-Like Sarcoma

This neoplasm is very rare and more commonly affects young and middle-aged adults (i.e., older people as compared to classical Ewing sarcoma). It is characterized by **chromosomal translocations** leading to the generation of fusion transcripts between EWSR1 and non-ETS genes: EWSR1-NFATC2 fusion gene from t(20;22) (q13;q12); EWSR1-POU5F1 from t(6;22)(p21;q12); EWSR1-SMARCA5 from t(4;22)(q31;q12); EWSR1-PATZ1 from t(1;22)(q36.1;q12); and EWSR1-SP3 from t(2;22)(q31;q12). NFATC2-rearranged sarcomas have been more frequently found in the bone, whereas other rearrangements are more often observed in sarcomas of the soft tissues.

The tumor is composed of round or epithelioid cells with nuclear polymorphism; CD99 expression is present in half cases.

Recently, EWSR1-NFATC2-rearranged sarcoma has been found to express NKX3-1, an immunohistochemical biomarker also positive in prostate carcinoma and mesenchymal chondrosarcoma ($\rightarrow$ see dedicated section) but not in Ewing sarcoma or other soft tissue sarcomas.

CIC-Rearranged Ewing-Like Sarcoma

This is the most frequent and best characterized of Ewing-like sarcomas. It is characterized by recurrent CIC gene rearrangements. The most common **chromosomal translocations** are t(4;19)(q35;q13) and t(10;19)(q26;q13), which both lead to the formation of the CIC-DUX4 fusion gene.[2] In a minority of cases, (5%) other chimeric products are CIC-FOXO4 (t(x;19)(q13;q13.3)), CIC-NUTM1 (t(15;19) (q14;q13.2)), and CIC-NUTM2B (t(10;19)(q23.3;q13)).

This sarcoma occurs most frequently in children and young adults, although it may develop at any age. Most lesions arise in the deep soft tissue of the trunk, limbs, or head and neck; superficial soft tissues are involved in about 10% of cases, whereas bone involvement is very rare; viscera are involved in approximately 10% of cases. Microscopically, the tumor is less monotonous than conventional Ewing sarcoma,

---

[2]CIC-DUX4 fusion gene: the CIC gene is the human homolog of the *Drosophila* gene capicua transcriptional repressor; CIC encodes a high-mobility group box transcription factor and is involved in the development of the central nervous system. DUX4 is a double homeodomain gene whose normal function is unclear. The transcription activity of the CIC-DUX4 fusion product (which is linked to the CIC component) leads to the upregulation of the PEA3 subclass of ETS family of genes, which includes ETV1, ETV4, and ETV-5.

with mild-to-moderate pleomorphism; neoplastic cells may organize in a lobular growth pattern, and confluent geographic areas of necrosis may be detected; mitotic count is generally high (frequently >40 mitoses/10 HPF). CD99 staining is positive in >80% of cases, but it is weaker than in Ewing sarcoma; nuclear expression of DUX4 is consistently observed. ETV4 is diffusely expressed as a consequence of the upregulation of ETV4 gene expression, which in turn is the result of the transcriptional activity of the CIC-DUX4 chimeric protein.

CIC-rearranged Ewing-like sarcoma generally has a poor prognosis, frequently presenting with lung metastasis at primary diagnosis, the 5-year overall survival rate being approximately 40%. Biological aggressiveness is also supported by a worse response to chemotherapy as compared to conventional Ewing sarcoma.

BCOR-Rearranged Ewing-Like Sarcoma

This rare Ewing-like tumor is characterized by recurrent BCOR gene rearrangements; the most frequent **chromosomal rearrangements** are inv(x)(p11;p11), t(4;x)(p11;q31), and t(x;22;)(p11;q13.2), which lead to the formation of BCOR-CCNB3 fusion gene[3] (60% of cases), BCOR-MAML3, and ZC3H7B-BCOR, respectively.

This sarcoma accounts for approximately 4% of all round cell sarcomas and occurs more often in the bone than in soft tissues, with a peak incidence in the second decade of life and a remarkable male predominance. The tumor affects more frequently the pelvis, lower limbs, and paraspinal region, the visceral location being very rare. The morphologic spectrum is quite broad, with tumors composed of a mixed proliferation of round and spindle cells arranged in sheets or fascicles. Mitotic activity is usually very high. Of note, recurrent and metastatic lesions show increased cellularity and higher pleomorphism as compared to the primary tumor, which calls for differential diagnosis with undifferentiated pleomorphic sarcoma.

Immunohistochemically, virtually all cases exhibit strong and diffuse cyclin B3 (CCNB3) nuclear positivity; BCOR expression may also be detected, but it is less specific than CCNB3. CD99 staining is usually weaker or absent.

Of note, BCOR-rearranged Ewing-like sarcoma is associated with a more indolent behavior as compared to classic Ewing sarcoma (5-year overall survival rate, 75%).

---

[3] BCOR-CCNB3 fusion gene: this fusion originates from a paracentric inversion on the X-chromosome and splicing of the end of the BCOR coding sequence to the CCNB3 exon 5 splice acceptor site. The resultant fusion protein is composed of full-length BCOR, a transcriptional repressor encoding the Bcl-6 co-repressor, and the C-terminus of cyclin CCNB3. The BCOR-CCNB3 fusion protein is oncogenic and is believed to drive cell proliferation in this sarcoma.

Adamantinoma-Like Ewing Sarcoma

Adamantinoma-like Ewing sarcoma (ALES) is a very rare and somewhat controversial variant of Ewing sarcoma. Although this neoplasm harbors the **chromosomal translocation** t(11;22) leading to the generation of the EWSR1-FLI1 fusion gene (typical of classic Ewing sarcoma), it also shows epithelial differentiation, including immunohistochemical expression of high molecular weight cytokeratins and p40 and often overt keratin pearl formation (which calls for differential diagnosis with carcinoma). Although it has been originally described in the extremities and thorax, ALES has been predominantly recognized in the head and neck (approximately 75% of all cases); in this location, ALES may pose a particularly challenging differential diagnosis with other small round blue cell tumors as well as basaloid carcinoma.

Askin Tumor

Askin tumor is a peripheral primitive neuroectodermal tumor (pPNET → see below paragraph) arising in the thoracic wall (where it represents 10–15% of all primary tumors): therefore, it should not be considered a separate entity. It affects children and adolescents. Askin tumor presents with respiratory problems such as pain, dyspnea, and mass and weight loss. Histologically, it shows small round blue cells; the chromosomal translocation t(11;22)(q24;q12) leads to the formation of the EWSR1-FLI1 fusion gene. It is highly malignant with poor prognosis (5-year overall survival rate, 60%). Because of rarity of condition, there is no defined treatment guideline for this condition. Most centers follow multimodality treatment of chemotherapy, surgery, and radiotherapy.

Peripheral Primary Neuroectodermal Tumor (pPNET)

For details → see dedicated section. It is also known as peripheral neuroepithelioma.

Suggested Readings

Aldera (2020) Gene of the month: BCOR. J Clin Pathol 73(6):314–317
Brčić (2020) Undifferentiated round cell sarcomas with CIC-DUX4 gene fusion: expanding the clinical spectrum. Pathology 52(2):236–242
Fletcher (2013) WHO classification of tumours of soft tissue and bone, 4th edn
Pappo (2018) Rhabdomyosarcoma, Ewing sarcoma, and other round cell sarcomas. J Clin Oncol 36(2):168–179
Renzi (2019) Ewing-like sarcoma: an emerging family of round cell sarcomas. J Cell Physiol 234(6):7999–8007

Rooper (2020) Soft tissue special issue: adamantinoma-like Ewing sarcoma of the head and neck: a practical review of a challenging emerging entity. Head Neck Pathol 14(1):59–69

Sbaraglia (2020) Ewing sarcoma and Ewing-like tumors. Virchows Arch 476(1):109–119

Yoshida (2020) NKX3-1 is a useful immunohistochemical marker of EWSR1-NFATC2 sarcoma and mesenchymal chondrosarcoma. Am J Surg Pathol 44(6):719–728

88

Extrarenal Rhabdoid Tumor

89

Definition

Extrarenal rhabdoid tumor (ERT) is a malignancy of uncertain differentiation. It is the extrarenal counterpart of rhabdoid tumor ($\rightarrow$ see dedicated section) which affects mainly the kidney and brain. It is also known as rhabdoid tumor of soft tissue and malignant rhabdoid tumor. It belongs to the family of SMARC-deficient sarcomas ($\rightarrow$ see dedicated section).

Epidemiology and Presentation

ERT is a very rare disease occurring mainly in infants and children (median age: 2 years). Considering fetal and neonatal rhabdoid tumors, ERT is more frequent than rhabdoid tumor of the kidney and brain.

This neoplasm mainly arises in deep axial sites, such as the neck, paraspinal region, perineal region, abdominal cavity, retroperitoneum, and pelvis; moreover, it may also affect the viscera (e.g., the liver, thymus, genitourinary tracts, and gastrointestinal system) and other sites (e.g., extremities).

Clinically, the lesion usually presents as a rapidly growing mass greater than 5 cm in diameter.

Etiology and Predisposition

ERT can be sporadic or familial. Familial ERT is associated with germline mutations of the SMARCB1 gene (also known as INI1) which is located in chromosome 22q11.2. As this genetic alteration can be found in one third of ERT cases, all patients newly diagnosed with rhabdoid tumors should be tested for germline SMARCB1 mutation or deletion. According to the classic "two-hit" hypothesis, the germline mutation inactivates the first allele, and then a somatic alteration of the

S. Mocellin, *Soft Tissue Tumors*, https://doi.org/10.1007/978-3-030-58710-9_89

second allele leads to the complete loss of function of the tumor suppressor gene. The SMARCB1 protein product contributes to the SWItch Sucrose NonFermentable (SWI/SNF) complex, a highly conserved multi-subunit complex regulating the process of chromatin remodeling (and thus involved in the epigenetic regulation of gene expression, cell proliferation, and differentiation).

Of note, people with germline SMARC mutations are at risk also for rhabdoid tumor of the kidney (RTK), atypical teratoid/rhabdoid tumor (ATRT) (linked to SMARCB1, rarely SMARCA4), familial schwannomatosis (linked to SMARCB1, → see section entitled "Schwannoma"), small cell carcinoma of the ovary hypercalcemic type (SCCOHT, linked to SMARCA4), and multiple meningiomas (linked to SMARCE1). Interestingly, also epithelioid sarcoma (→ see dedicated section) and other sarcomas are recognized as SWI/SNF-driven neoplasms (see section entitled "SMARC-Deficient Sarcomas").

Pathology

Macroscopically, the tumor is unencapsulated, infiltrates surrounding tissues, and frequently shows hemorrhagic necrosis. Microscopically, ERT consists of characteristic "rhabdoid cells" (rounded or polygonal, with large nuclei, prominent nucleoli, and abundant cytoplasm containing hyaline-like PAS-positive/diastase-resistant inclusion bodies) arranged in sheets or in a solid trabecular pattern. Nuclear pleomorphism is not evident, whereas mitotic figures are frequent.

In some cases, the predominant proliferation is of undifferentiated small round cells with only a few typical rhabdoid cells. Of note, rhabdoid cells are also focally or diffusely observed in other tumors such as carcinomas, sarcomas, meningiomas, melanomas, and mesotheliomas; among sarcomas, proximal-type epithelioid sarcoma is of special relevance because of similar morphology, immunohistochemical features, and SMARCB1 gene alterations (→ see section entitled "Rhabdoid Tumor").

Biomarkers

Most ERT coexpress vimentin and epithelial biomarkers (e.g., cytokeratins and EMA). The expression of neural cell biomarkers (e.g., CD99 and synaptophysin) is also frequently encountered. SMARCB1[1] expression is typically lost.

---

[1] SMARCB1: SWI/SNF-related matrix-associated actin-dependent regulator of chromatin, subfamily B, member 1 (also known as INI1) encodes a protein which is part of the BAF (hSWI/SNF) complex that relieves repressive chromatin structures, allowing the transcriptional machinery to access its targets more effectively. This ATP-dependent chromatin-remodeling complex plays an important role in different cell activities including cell differentiation; in particular, regulation of the stem cell-associated program, which is maintained by the repressive effect of the EZH2-dependent PRC2 (polycomb repressive complex 2), is disrupted by SMARCB1. Overall, SMARCB1 has been found to act as a tumor suppressor, and its mutations have been associated with a variety of malignancies including sarcomas.

From the genetic viewpoint, ERT is likely caused by homozygous inactivation of the SMARCB1 tumor suppressor gene. Of note, about 98% of ERT, rhabdoid tumor of kidney (→ see dedicated section), and atypical teratoid/rhabdoid tumor (ATRT) show different types of alterations of both gene alleles.

In the rare cases with retained SMARCB1 expression, loss of function alterations of the SMARCA4[2] gene have been described.

Prognosis

ERT is a highly malignant neoplasm characterized by a dismal prognosis, with many patients showing metastatic disease at presentation and a 5-year survival rate lower than 15%.

Therapy

Because of the rarity of ERT, no standard treatment is available. For more details → see section entitled "Rhabdoid Tumor".

Suggested Readings

Agaimy (2018) Hereditary SWI/SNF complex deficiency syndromes. Semin Diagn Pathol 35(3):193–198

Cheng (2019) Clinical and prognostic characteristics of 53 cases of extracranial malignant rhabdoid tumor in children. A single-institute experience from 2007 to 2017. Oncologist 24(7):e551–e558

Fletcher (2020) WHO classification of tumours of soft tissue and bone, 5th edn

Le Loarer (2014) Consistent SMARCB1 homozygous deletions in epithelioid sarcoma and in a subset of myoepithelial carcinomas can be reliably detected by FISH in archival material. Genes Chromosomes Cancer 53(6):475–486

Lu (2019) An in-depth look at small cell carcinoma of the ovary, hypercalcemic type (SCCOHT): clinical implications from recent molecular findings. J Cancer 10(1):223–237

---

[2] SMARCA4, located at 19p13, encodes the protein BRG1 and is part of the switch/sucrose-non-fermenting (SWI/SNF) chromatin remodeling complex that is also known as the BAF (BRG1-associated factor) complex. This complex is ATP-dependent and plays an important role in transcription, differentiation, and DNA repair and has been shown to behave as a tumor-suppressing complex. Each complex contains multiple subunits, each of which contains a mutually exclusive ATPase subunit, SMARCA4 (BRG1) or SMARCA2 (BRM).

Definition

Extraskeletal aneurysmal bone cyst (EABC) is a benign tumor also known as aneurysmal bone cyst of soft tissues.

Epidemiology and Presentation

EABC is the soft tissue counterpart of intraosseous aneurysmal bone cyst. Clinically it presents as a rapidly growing mass (median size, 5 cm; range, 2.5–10 cm) of deep soft tissues typically located in the upper extremities, thigh, or groin, without involvement of adjacent bones; it may be painful. The mean age of occurrence is 30 years (range: 10–40 years).

Pathology

The features are identical to those or intraosseous aneurysmal bone cyst. Macroscopically it presents as a mass made of hemorrhagic cystic spaces with fibrous septa and surrounded by a thin rim of bone.

Microscopically, EABC is composed of cystic spaces filled with blood, fibrous septa composed of fibroblasts, osteoclast-type giant cells, and woven bone.

Differential diagnosis may be needed with extraskeletal osteosarcoma.

Biomarkers

The **chromosomal translocation** t(17;22)(p13;q12) leading to the formation of the MYH9-USP6 fusion gene[1] is a frequent event in EABC (establishing its clonal neoplastic nature). Also nodular fasciitis and myositis ossificans often carry this chromosomal rearrangement, providing evidence that these three entities are genetically related.

Prognosis

EABC is a benign neoplasm that may recur locally if incompletely excised.

Therapy

Surgery is the treatment of choice.

Suggested Readings

Bekers (2018) Myositis ossificans—another condition with USP6 rearrangement, providing evidence of a relationship with nodular fasciitis and aneurysmal bone cyst. Ann Diagn Pathol 34:56–59
Song (2019) Soft tissue aneurysmal bone cyst: six new cases with imaging details, molecular pathology, and review of the literature. Skelet Radiol 48(7):1059–1067
Zhang (2020) Myositis ossificans-like soft tissue aneurysmal bone cyst: a clinical, radiological, and pathological study of seven cases with COL1A1-USP6 fusion and a novel ANGPTL2-USP6 fusion. Mod Pathol 33(8):1492–1504

---

[1] MYH9-USP6 fusion gene: MYH9 (myosin heavy chain 9) encodes a non-muscle myosin which is involved in cytokinesis, cell motility, and maintenance of cell shape. USP6 (ubiquitin-specific peptidase 6) encodes a deubiquitinase with an ATP-independent isopeptidase activity, cleaving at the C-terminus of the ubiquitin moiety.

Definition

Extraskeletal chondroma (ESC) is a benign mesenchymal tumor classified among the chondro-osseous neoplasms. It is also known as soft tissue chondroma and chondroma of soft parts. For pulmonary chondroma → see Chap. 161.

Epidemiology and Presentation

ESC occurs over a wide age range (mean age: 35 years), with males being affected more frequently (M:F = 3:2). Two thirds of lesions arise in the fingers, the other cases affecting the hands, toes, and feet (the head and neck and trunk are uncommon sites). Clinically, the lesion usually presents as a slow-growing solitary painless mass (mainly 1–2 cm in size) in the soft tissues adjacent to tendons and joints. Radiologically, the tumor is well demarcated and lobulated and shows central and peripheral calcifications. By definition, this neoplasm develops in the soft tissues without any connection to the bone cortex, intra-articular synovium, or periosteum.

Pathology

ESC is composed of hypercellular lobules of mature, hyaline cartilage containing cells with chondrocyte phenotype. Cartilage may undergo calcification or endochondral ossification. A chondroblastoma-like variant has been described (presence of cells with cleaved nuclei and scattered osteoclast-like giant cells). Mitotic activity is scarce and atypical mitoses are absent.

Differential diagnosis may be needed with chondrosarcoma, which is rare in the hands and feet, infiltrative and destructive, and typically high-grade.

S. Mocellin, *Soft Tissue Tumors*, https://doi.org/10.1007/978-3-030-58710-9_91

Prognosis

ESC is a benign neoplasm, with a recurrence rate of 15–20%.

Therapy

Surgery is the treatment of choice.

Suggested Readings

Cardia (2019) A large extraskeletal chondroma: an unusual location in the lower extremity, huge extraskeletal chondroma: an unusual localization in the leg. J Orthop Case Rep 9(1):74–77
Fletcher (2020) WHO classification of tumours of soft tissue and bone, 5th edn
Salvatori (2020) Extraskeletal chondroma: a rare cause of trigger finger in children. Case Rep Orthop 2020:8259089

Definition

Chordoma is a slow-growing bone tumor arising from cellular remnants of the notochord. It is also known as chordocarcinoma, chordoepithelioma, notochordal sarcoma, and notochordoma. When arising outside the skeleton, it is known as extraskeletal chordoma, soft tissue chordoma, and extraosseous chordoma.

Epidemiology and Presentation

The annual incidence of chordoma is about 1 case per million people, with a 2:1 male to female ratio. Although it can occur at any age, chordoma most often affects people between 50 and 70 years of age. It is typically located in the base skull and spine, with approximately 30–50% in the sacrococcygeal bones (in this site, it represents the most frequent tumor), 30% in the skull (with special regard to the clivus), and 20–30% in the remaining spine vertebral bones. Very rare cases have been described in extra-axial bones and in extraskeletal sites (soft tissue chordoma). Chordomas account for 1% of intracranial tumors and 1–5% of all primary bone tumors.

Skull chordomas most commonly present with headache, neck pain, and cranial nerve palsy (e.g., diplopia or facial nerve palsy). Chordoma of the mobile spine and sacrum/coccyx present with chronic back pain (or coccydynia, also known as tailbone pain). Sacrococcygeal chordoma can be palpable at physical examination. Spinal cord involvement can lead to changes in bowel and/or bladder function as well as limb paresthesia/paresis. The time lapse between onset of symptoms and diagnosis is generally long (>1 year) due to misdiagnosis with other causes of the same symptoms (mainly pain). Extraskeletal chordoma presents with signs and symptoms related to a mass effect.

Preoperative CT-guided core needle biopsy is recommended (the site of biopsy should be chosen so to be removed with definitive surgery: for instance, biopsy of sacral chordoma should be performed using a posterior route, not the transrectal route), although in some cases (e.g., clivus chordoma), it can be impossible or hazardous.

Magnetic resonance imaging (MRI) is the recommended modality for primary chordoma diagnosis because it allows for delineation of the different soft tissue components of the tumor and adjacent structures. Typically, the tumor exhibits a very high signal in the T2-weighted sequence.

Etiology and Predisposition

Most chordomas develop as sporadic disease. There is no conclusive proof that chordoma can arise from a benign notochordal cell tumor.

Chordoma rarely occurs in a familial setting, when the inheritance pattern is compatible with an autosomal dominant trait. In some of these families, the inherited disease is associated with duplication of the TBX1 gene, whose protein product called brachyury acts as a transcription factor required for notochordal development. Only 7% of sporadic chordomas show amplification of this gene.

People with tuberous sclerosis complex have a higher than expected risk of chordoma.

Pathology

Classic chordoma (or chordoma not otherwise specified, chordoma NOS) is composed of large cells (with vacuolated "bubbly" cytoplasm, also known as "physaliphorous cells") separated into lobules by fibrous septa. The cells are arranged as small ribbons and cords embedded in abundant extracellular myxoid matrix, or as more densely arranged epithelioid packets.

Chondroid chordoma refers to chordoma in which the matrix mimics hyaline cartilaginous neoplasms.

Dedifferentiated chordoma is a biphasic tumor comprising the features of a chordoma NOS as well as those of a high-grade undifferentiated spindle cell sarcoma; it occurs in about 1–5% of patients.

Differential diagnosis may be necessary with the following: chondrosarcoma (negative for cytokeratin, EMA, and brachyury); metastatic carcinoma (negative for S100 protein and brachyury; usually positive for "origin specific markers" such as PAX8 in renal cell carcinoma or TTF1 in metastatic pulmonary adenocarcinoma); schwannoma; osteosarcoma; Ewing sarcoma (including extraskeletal type); benign notochordal cell tumor (also known as notochordal hamartoma); giant cell tumor of the bone (or of the soft tissues); myxopapillary ependymoma (negative for epithelial markers); lymphoma; and multiple myeloma.

Biomarkers

Brachyury (protein product of TBX1 gene) is a highly specific marker for chordoma and helps distinguish chordoma from morphologically similar neoplasms including carcinoma, chondrosarcoma, and chordoid meningioma.

Chordoma NOS and chondroid chordoma express cytokeratins, EMA,[1] and S100. Brachyury, cytokeratins, EMA, and S100 are not expressed in the dedifferentiated component of a dedifferentiated chordoma.

Prognosis

Median overall survival is about 7 years (10-year survival rate $\approx$ 50%). Up to 30–40% chordomas metastasize. Chondroid chordoma has the same prognosis as conventional (or not otherwise specified, NOS) chordoma. Dedifferentiated chordoma is associated with a worse prognosis. The tumor can metastasize to the lung, bone, lymph nodes, and subcutaneous tissue. Data on extraskeletal chordoma are very scarce.

Therapy

Due to the rarity of extraskeletal chordoma, no standard therapy exists. The following is actually a summary of the therapeutic approach to osseous chordoma.

Surgery Surgical excision is the mainstay of treatment. For clivus tumors, endoscopic transnasal trans-sphenoidal approach can be an alternative to open surgery. Surgery should include the biopsy track and be aimed at achieving complete en bloc resection because this is the most important determinant of long-term outcome. Intralesional surgery followed by radiotherapy should not be regarded as an alternative to en bloc resection, if en bloc resection is feasible. Tumor rupture should be avoided because it inevitably results in locoregional seeding and subsequently in locoregional recurrences, which are difficult to treat successfully.

Due to the tumor proximity to neurological structures, surgery can result in significant morbidity. For instance, sacrum resection can lead to bowel, bladder, and motor impairment, depending on the level of sacral amputation, which must be balanced against the need for negative margins. For tumors arising from S4 and below, surgery should be offered as the treatment of choice. For lesions originating from S3, surgery remains the standard approach if preservation of S2 roots is possible, because some neurological recovery is possible in 40% of cases. For chordomas originating above S3, surgery is always associated with significant neurological deficits, and the chance of obtaining an R0 resection is lower as compared to chordoma arising below S3: accordingly, pros and cons of surgery versus radiotherapy alone should be

---

[1] EMA: epithelial membrane antigen.

discussed with the patient, taking into consideration that local disease control rates with radiotherapy alone are slightly lower than those achieved with surgery plus radiotherapy. For tumors arising from S1, surgery leads to high morbidity, which suggests that definitive radiotherapy should be regarded as a valid alternative to surgery. Rectal resection may be necessary to perform surgery with radical intent.

Radiotherapy Since radical surgery is not always possible (due to the tumor location close to vital/important nervous structures), adjuvant radiotherapy is usually recommended (though no RCT-based evidence is available). Also radiotherapy is burdened by significant morbidity due to the tumor proximity to neurological structures.

In this regard, particle radiotherapy (i.e., carbon ion radiotherapy or proton beam radiotherapy; also known as hadron therapy) might be preferred to conventional radiotherapy (i.e., photon therapy) due to lower toxicity rates, especially when radiation is used as definitive treatment (since chordoma is radioresistant, high radiation doses must be applied especially in the definitive treatment setting).

Chemotherapy Currently no drug is formally approved for the treatment of advanced/metastatic chordoma. Cytotoxic chemotherapy is generally inactive, and not enough evidence is available to recommend chemotherapy for chordoma.

Target therapy Based on the activation of PRGFR, EGFR, and VEGR pathways shown in chordoma cells, targeted therapy with drugs such as imatinib,[2] lapatinib,[3] sorafenib,[4] and dasatinib[5] has been tested in patients with advanced/metastatic disease with some evidence of anticancer activity (mainly disease stabilization). Patients unsuitable for surgery/radiotherapy should be offered targeted therapy or experimental trials.

Suggested Readings

Boronat (2018) Less common manifestations in TSC. Am J Med Genet C Semin Med Genet 178(3):348–354

Fletcher (2020) WHO classification of tumours of soft tissue and bone, 5th edn

Meng (2019) Molecular targeted therapy in the treatment of chordoma: a systematic review. Front Oncol 9:30

Schuetze (2017) Phase 2 study of dasatinib in patients with alveolar soft part sarcoma, chondrosarcoma, chordoma, epithelioid sarcoma, or solitary fibrous tumor. Cancer 123(1):90–97

Stacchiotti (2015) Building a global consensus approach to chordoma: a position paper from the medical and patient community. Lancet Oncol 16(2):e71–e83

---

[2] Imatinib: tyrosine kinase inhibitor targeting the following: KIT, RET, BCR, PDGFRA.

[3] Lapatinib: tyrosine kinase inhibitor targeting the following: EGFR/ERBB1, HER2/ERBB2.

[4] Sorafenib: tyrosine kinase inhibitor targeting the following: BRAF, KIT, RET, FGFR1, FLT3, VEGFR1, VEGFR2, VEGFR3, PDGFRB.

[5] Dasatinib: tyrosine kinase inhibitor targeting the following: ABL, SRC, KIT, EPHA2, PDGFRB.

Definition

Extraskeletal Ewing sarcoma (ESES) (also known as extraosseous Ewing sarcoma) is the soft tissue counterpart of Ewing sarcoma of the bone. This malignant tumor displays varying degrees of neuroectodermal differentiation, but the cell of origin is unknown. Lesions arising in the chest wall are also known as Askin tumor. For information on the Ewing-like sarcoma family → see dedicated section.

Epidemiology and Presentation

Although rare (approximately 1 case per million people per year), Ewing sarcoma is the second most frequent type of primary bone malignancy (after osteosarcoma) in children and adolescents, accounting for 6–8% of primary malignant bone neoplasms. Overall, Ewing sarcoma occurs mainly in people younger than 20 years (median age, 15 years), with a slight male predominance. ESES represents about 10–20% of all Ewing sarcoma cases (and less than 1% of all soft tissue sarcomas) and is usually found in older children and adolescents compared to Ewing sarcoma from bone origin. The clinical presentation of ESES is nonspecific and is that of a usually rapidly growing mass with its possible compression effects. ESES can affect the head and neck, retroperitoneum, omentum, paravertebral space, orbits, skin, chest wall, pelvis, lower extremities, and viscera.

Pathology

Macroscopically, the tumor shows invasive margins and both necrotic and hemorrhagic areas. Microscopically, the neoplasm belongs to the family of small round cell tumors (→ see Table 93.1). In fact, most cases (also called classical

© The Editor(s) (if applicable) and The Author(s), under exclusive license to
Springer Nature Switzerland AG 2021
S. Mocellin, *Soft Tissue Tumors*, https://doi.org/10.1007/978-3-030-58710-9_93

Table 93.1 List of small round cell tumors (SRCT, also known as small blue round cell tumors), highly aggressive malignant tumors composed of relatively small and monotonous poorly differentiated or undifferentiated cells with increased nuclear-cytoplasmic ratio

Ewing sarcoma	Leukemic infiltrate
Primitive neuroectodermal tumor (PNET)	Alveolar rhabdomyosarcoma (ARMS)
Merkel cell carcinoma	Neuroblastoma
Embryonal rhabdomyosarcoma (ERMS)	Poorly differentiated synovial sarcoma
Small cell carcinoma (e.g., SCLC)	Mesenchymal chondrosarcoma
Small cell lymphoma	Retinoblastoma
Neuroendocrine carcinoma	Small cell osteosarcoma
Medulloblastoma	Desmoplastic small round cell tumor (DSRCT)
Round cell liposarcoma	Nephroblastoma (Wilms tumor)
Hepatoblastoma	Melanoma

Ewing sarcoma) are composed of uniform small round cells with round nuclei and scanty clear or eosinophilic cytoplasm, without extracellular matrix. In others, tumor cells are larger with prominent nucleoli and irregular contours (atypical Ewing sarcoma). Sometimes, a more evident degree of neuroectodermal differentiation (i.e., presence of rosettes: ill-defined groups of up to ten cells oriented toward a central space, with/without consistent immunophenotype) is observed and is referred to as peripheral primitive neuroectodermal tumor (pPNET → see dedicated section). Upon electronic microscopy, no intermediate filaments or neurofilaments can be observed; PNET may show neurosecretory granules and neurite-like processes.

Differential diagnosis may be needed especially with other round cell tumors (→ see Table 93.1): differentiation-specific biomarkers and detection of specific fusion genes are of great help.

Biomarkers

Classic Ewing sarcoma lacks frank neural differentiation and usually shows only diffuse membranous CD99 (also known as MIC2) positivity (highly sensitive but not specific). Importantly, lymphoblastic leukemia, lymphoma, and myeloid sarcoma may show identical CD99 positivity, which calls for differential diagnosis with leukemic soft tissue infiltration and extra-nodal lymphoma. CD99 staining may be patchy or negative in Ewing-like sarcomas. FLI1 and ERG staining is often positive in tumors carrying the EWSR1-FLI1 and EWSR1-ERG fusion genes (see below). Vimentin is always expressed, whereas up to 30% of cases demonstrate positivity for cytokeratins. CD45 (leukocyte common antigen), myogenin, MyoD1, and chromogranin are not expressed.

Ewing sarcoma is characterized by the presence of recurrent balanced **chromosomal translocations** involving, in almost all cases, the EWSR1 gene[1] on chromosome 22 and a member of the ETS family of transcription factors,[2] which leads to the formation of fusion oncogenes believed to play a key role in the disease pathogenesis. About 85% of Ewing sarcomas harbor the somatic chromosomal translocation t(11;22)(q24;q12), which leads to the formation of the EWSR1-FLI1 fusion gene.[3] In other cases, alternate translocations are the following: t(21;22)(q22;q12), t(7;22)(p22;q12), t(17;22)(q21;q12), and t(2;22)(q35;q12), resulting in EWSR1-ERG fusion gene (about 10% of cases), EWSR1-ETV1 fusion gene, EWSR1-ETV4 fusion gene, and EWSR1-FEV fusion gene, respectively. In rarer cases, FUS-ERG fusion gene (FUS is also known as TLS) or FUS-FEV fusion gene derives from translocations t(16;21)(p11;q22) and t(2;16)(q35;p11), where the FUS protein (TLS)—which is similar to EWSR1 in amino acid sequence—belongs to the TET family of proteins (including TLS, EWSR1, and TAF15). The diagnosis of Ewing sarcoma can be confirmed by the presence of these translocations by RT-PCR or FISH, although one must still consider the diagnoses of other EWSR1-rearranged sarcomas (e.g., desmoplastic round cell tumor, extraskeletal myxoid chondrosarcoma, myxoid liposarcoma, or clear cell sarcoma). Detection of such fusion genes in the peripheral blood is being explored as a tool for the identification of minimal residual disease.

Mutations in TP53 and CDKN2A tumor suppressor genes have also been identified and appear to have prognostic significance.

---

[1] EWSR1 is a "promiscuous" gene because it can fuse with different partner genes in phenotypically similar neoplasms or with the same genes in morphologically and behaviorly different tumors. In fact, EWSR1-based chimeric genes can be found not only in Ewing and Ewing-like sarcomas but also in other tumors such as angiomatoid fibrous histiocytoma, clear cell sarcoma, low-grade fibromyxoid sarcoma, sclerosing epithelioid fibrosarcoma, hemangioma of the bone, desmoplastic small round cell tumor, extraskeletal myxoid chondrosarcoma, myoepithelial tumor of soft tissue, and myxoid liposarcoma.

It must be underscored that fluorescence in situ hybridization (FISH) analysis has a significant risk of false-negative results, making next-generation sequencing (NGS)-based diagnostic tools more sensitive for detecting EWSR1 rearrangements.

[2] ETS gene family: the erythroblastosis *t*ransforming *s*equence (ETS) family includes (among others) the following genes (encoding transcription factors): FLI1, ERG, ETV1, ETV4, FEV.

[3] EWSR1-FLI1 fusion gene: EWSR1 (Ewing sarcoma breakpoint region 1) encodes a multifunctional protein that is involved in various cellular processes, including gene expression, cell signaling, and RNA processing and transport. FLI1 (Friend leukemia integration 1) encodes a transcription factor containing an ETS DNA-binding domain. EWSR1-FLI1 chimeric protein is believed to act as an oncoprotein playing a key role in Ewing sarcoma pathogenesis; for instance, its activity leads to upregulation of c-Myc and GLI expression and inhibition of the transcriptional activity of p53, as well as blockage of the ability of Runx2 to induce osteoblast differentiation.

Prognosis

The most common form of ESES spread is hematogenous, primarily to the lungs; the incidence of distant metastatic disease at the time of diagnosis is reported at 10%, of which over 80% are located in the lungs.

ESES staging should probably consist of the same workup recommended for bone Ewing sarcoma: bone marrow biopsy, whole-body bone scan (skeletal scintigraphy), total body computed tomography scan (including the brain), lumbar puncture for cerebrospinal fluid evaluation, and LDH plasma levels; likely, the use of positron emission tomography combined with computed tomography (PET-CT) might reduce the need for bone marrow biopsy (and perhaps bone scintigraphy) due to the high diagnostic accuracy of this technique.

The prognosis for patients affected by localized Ewing sarcoma has been considerably improved by current therapeutic strategy (5-year survival rate: 75%). Nevertheless, the outcome of patients with metastatic disease remains poor (5-year survival rate: 30%).

Younger age, extremity location, smaller size (cutoff: 8 cm), stage (nonmetastatic), and tumor response to induction chemotherapy (i.e., histopathological assessment of tumor necrosis, or—as more recently proposed—imaging response at positron emission tomography) are associated with better outcome. Genetic alterations such as TP53 status and CDKN2A loss have been associated with prognosis, but the clinical implications are to be defined. Of note, EWSR1-ETS fusion type is not of prognostic value. ESES appears to have a worse prognosis as compared to bone Ewing sarcoma.

Therapy

Ewing sarcoma is considered both chemosensitive and radiosensitive. For localized primary Ewing sarcoma, neoadjuvant **chemotherapy** followed by local control therapy (**surgery** and/or **radiotherapy**) and then adjuvant chemotherapy is the standard approach. In patients who undergo surgery, surgical margins and histologic response are considered in planning postoperative radiotherapy. For metastatic disease, systemic chemotherapy is administered. Chemotherapy regimens most frequently utilized are the following: VDCA/IE (vincristine, doxorubicin, cyclophosphamide, and D-actinomycin alternating with ifosfamide and etoposide); VIDE (vincristine, ifosfamide, doxorubicin, and etoposide); VDC (vincristine, doxorubicin, and cyclophosphamide); and VAI (vincristine, doxorubicin [Adriamycin], and ifosfamide). In North America, standard chemotherapy for bone Ewing sarcoma consists of VDCA/IE based on the results of the randomized controlled trial Intergroup-0091, which demonstrated significantly better disease-free and overall survival with the addition of ifosfamide and etoposide to the standard VDCA regimen in patients with localized disease; of note, no such benefits were observed in the metastatic setting. Analogously, in the EuroEwing99 trial, consolidation high-dose chemotherapy with high-dose chemotherapy (busulfan and melphalan) and blood autologous stem-cell rescue (after induction chemotherapy with VIDE) improved both disease-free and overall survival in patients with localized high-risk Ewing sarcoma, but not with metastatic disease.

As regards **target therapy**, different compounds are under investigation; in a recent phase II trial, cabozantinib[4] has shown clinically meaningful activity against advanced Ewing sarcoma of the bone; following the role of EWSR1 rearrangements in Ewing sarcoma pathogenesis, efforts are underway to modulate the activity of disease-specific chimeric proteins, such as the use of inhibitors of the bromodomain and extra-terminal (BET) domain family proteins (based on the dependency of EWS/ETS transcription factors on BET epigenetic reader proteins). Knowledge on the role of **immunotherapy** is still in its infancy.

Suggested Readings

Bailey (2019) Emerging novel agents for patients with advanced Ewing sarcoma: a report from the Children's Oncology Group (COG) New Agents for Ewing Sarcoma Task Force. F1000Res 8. pii: F1000 Faculty Rev-493

Bosma (2019) Individual risk evaluation for local recurrence and distant metastasis in Ewing sarcoma: a multistate model: a multistate model for Ewing sarcoma. Pediatr Blood Cancer 66(11):e27943

Casey (2019) Exploiting signaling pathways and immune targets beyond the standard of care for Ewing sarcoma. Front Oncol 9:537

Cochran (2019) Bromodomains: a new target class for drug development. Nat Rev Drug Discov 18(8):609–628

Dirksen (2019) High-dose chemotherapy compared with standard chemotherapy and lung radiation in Ewing sarcoma with pulmonary metastases: results of the European Ewing Tumour Working Initiative of National Groups, 99 Trial and EWING 2008. J Clin Oncol 37(34):3192–3202

Fletcher (2020) WHO classification of tumours of soft tissue and bone, 5th edn

Gollavilli (2018) EWS/ETS-driven Ewing sarcoma requires BET bromodomain proteins. Cancer Res 78(16):4760–4773

Huang (2018) Effectiveness of 18F-FDG PET/CT in the diagnosis, staging and recurrence monitoring of Ewing sarcoma family of tumors: a meta-analysis of 23 studies. Medicine (Baltimore) 97(48):e13457

Inagaki (2019) Bone marrow examination in patients with Ewing sarcoma/peripheral primitive neuroectodermal tumor without metastasis based on 18F-fluorodeoxyglucose positron emission tomography/computed tomography. Med Oncol 36(7):58

Italiano (2020) Cabozantinib in patients with advanced Ewing sarcoma or osteosarcoma (CABONE): a multicentre, single-arm, phase 2 trial. Lancet Oncol 21(3):446–455

Jahanseir (2020) Ewing sarcoma in older adults: a clinicopathologic study of 50 cases occurring in patients aged ≥40 years, with emphasis on histologic mimics. Int J Surg Pathol 28(4):352–360

Krystel-Whittemore (2019) Novel and established EWSR1 gene fusions and associations identified by next-generation sequencing and fluorescence in-situ hybridization. Hum Pathol 93:65–73

Loganathan (2019) Targeting the IGF1R/PI3K/AKT pathway sensitizes Ewing sarcoma to BET bromodomain inhibitors. Mol Cancer Ther 18(5):929–936

McCaughan (2016) Programmed cell death-1 blockade in recurrent disseminated Ewing sarcoma. J Hematol Oncol 9(1):48

---

[4] Cabozantinib: small molecule tyrosine kinase inhibitor targeting the following: VEGFR2, RET, KIT, MET.

Pappo (2018) Rhabdomyosarcoma, Ewing sarcoma, and other round cell sarcomas. J Clin Oncol 36(2):168–179

Sbaraglia (2020) Ewing sarcoma and Ewing-like tumors. Virchows Arch 476(1):109–119

Schmidkonz (2020) Assessment of treatment responses in children and adolescents with Ewing sarcoma with metabolic tumor parameters derived from 18F-FDG-PET/CT and circulating tumor DNA. Eur J Nucl Med Mol Imaging 47(6):1613

Shukla (2017) Plasma DNA-based molecular diagnosis, prognostication, and monitoring of patients with EWSR1 fusion-positive sarcomas. JCO Precis Oncol 2017. https://doi.org/10.1200/PO.16.00028

Takigami (2019) Pazopanib confers a progression-free survival in a patient with Ewing's sarcoma/primitive neuroectodermal tumor of the lung. Intern Med 58(9):1335–1339

Whelan (2018) High-dose chemotherapy and blood autologous stem-cell rescue compared with standard chemotherapy in localized high-risk Ewing sarcoma: results of Euro-E.W.I.N.G.99 and Ewing-2008. J Clin Oncol 36(31):JCO2018782516

Xu (2019) Management of recurrent or refractory Ewing sarcoma: a systematic review of phase II clinical trials in the last 15 years. Oncol Lett 18(1):348–358

Definition

Extraskeletal myxoid chondrosarcoma (EMC) is a malignant tumor of uncertain differentiation. It is also known as chordoid sarcoma, extraskeletal chondrosarcoma, and extraosseous chondrosarcoma.

Epidemiology and Presentation

EMC is a rare mesenchymal neoplasm accounting for less than 3% of all soft tissue sarcomas. It typically (but not exclusively) arises in adults (median age: 50 years), with a male prevalence (ratio: 2:1). EMC usually develops in the deep soft tissues of proximal extremities and limb girdles (the thigh being the most frequent localization); other sites include the trunk, head and neck, paraspinal soft tissue, abdomen, pelvis, and feet. The bone location as primary location is extremely rare and few cases are reported.

Clinically, the lesion presents as a deep mass (median size, 7 cm; maximum size, 30 cm), which may be painful and may resemble a hematoma.

Pathology

Macroscopically, gelatinous areas separated by fibrous septa, intratumoral hemorrhage, cystic cavities, and areas of necrosis are frequently observed. Microscopically, the tumor is characterized by abundant myxoid matrix, multilobular hypocellular architecture, and uniform cells arranged in cords and clusters. The stroma is remarkably hypovascular. Despite the name, there is no clear evidence of cartilaginous differentiation. Mitotic activity is usually low. Rhabdoid features may be present. Only rare cases are hypercellular and have higher grade, often epithelioid cytomorphology.

S. Mocellin, *Soft Tissue Tumors*, https://doi.org/10.1007/978-3-030-58710-9_94

Biomarkers

No specific immunohistochemical pattern is observed (vimentin is positive in 90% of cases). A minority of cases show positivity for S100, CD117 (c-Kit), synaptophysin, and NSE.[1] EMC stains negative for cytokeratins and EMA. Cases with rhabdoid features are frequently negative for SMARCB1 (INI1).

The genetic hallmark of EMC is the **chromosomal translocation** t(9;22) (q22;q12) translocation which leads to the formation of the EWSR1-NR4A3 fusion gene.[2] Less frequently, the chromosomal translocation t(9;17)(q22;q11) leading to the generation of the TAF15-NR4A3 fusion gene is present. Overall, NR4A3-fusions (which act as strong transcriptional activators) are present in more than 90% of EMCs.

Prognosis

EMC is an aggressive malignancy: although it can be associated with prolonged survival, it is characterized by high rates of both local recurrence (50%) and distant metastasis (40%, generally to the lungs). The 5-year, 10-year, and 15-year overall survival rates have been reported to be 80–90%, 60–70%, and 50–60%, respectively. Negative prognostic factors are older age, large tumor size (>10 cm), and proximal location. Some investigators report that hypercellularity and atypia are also negative prognostic factors.

TAF15-translocated EMCs appear to feature a more aggressive behavior as compared to EWSR1-positive EMC.

Therapy

Surgery is the mainstay of treatment. **Radiotherapy** appears to play a positive role in the locoregional therapeutic management of this disease.

For advanced/metastatic disease, anthracycline-based **chemotherapy** is the standard treatment, to which EMC appears moderately sensitive. Trabectedin and **target therapy** with pazopanib[3] or sunitinib[4] are considered valuable options after failure of first-line chemotherapy.

---

[1] NSE: neuron-specific enolase.

[2] EWSR1-NR4A3 fusion gene: EWSR1 (Ewing sarcoma breakpoint region 1) encodes a multifunctional protein that is involved in various cellular processes, including gene expression, cell signaling, and RNA processing and transport. NR4A3 (also known as TEC and NOR1) encodes an orphan nuclear receptor belonging to the steroid/thyroid receptor gene family, whereas EWSR1 and TAF15 belong to the TET family of RNA- and DNA-binding proteins.

[3] Pazopanib: tyrosine kinase inhibitor targeting the following: VEGFR, PDGFR, KIT.

[4] Sunitinib: tyrosine kinase inhibitor targeting the following: PDGFR, VEGFR, KIT, FLT3, CSF1R, RET.

Suggested Readings

Agaimy (2019) SWI/SNF complex-deficient soft tissue neoplasms: a pattern-based approach to diagnosis and differential diagnosis. Surg Pathol Clin 12(1):149–163

Brenca (2019) NR4A3 fusion proteins trigger an axon guidance switch that marks the difference between EWSR1 and TAF15 translocated extraskeletal myxoid chondrosarcomas. J Pathol 249(1):90–101

Finos (2017) Primary extraskeletal myxoid chondrosarcoma of bone: report of three cases and review of the literature. Pathol Res Pract 213(5):461–466

Fletcher (2020) WHO classification of tumours of soft tissue and bone, 5th edn

Kemmerer (2018) Benefit of radiotherapy in extraskeletal myxoid chondrosarcoma: a propensity score weighted population-based analysis of the SEER database. Am J Clin Oncol 41(7):674–680

Morioka (2016) Results of sub-analysis of a phase 2 study on trabectedin treatment for extraskeletal myxoid chondrosarcoma and mesenchymal chondrosarcoma. BMC Cancer 16:479

Stacchiotti (2014) Activity of sunitinib in extraskeletal myxoid chondrosarcoma. Eur J Cancer 50(9):1657–1664

Stacchiotti (2019) Pazopanib for treatment of advanced extraskeletal myxoid chondrosarcoma: a multicentre, single-arm, phase 2 trial. Lancet Oncol 20(9):1252–1262

Urbini (2017) HSPA8 as a novel fusion partner of NR4A3 in extraskeletal myxoid chondrosarcoma. Genes Chromosomes Cancer 56(7):582–586

Definition

Extraskeletal osteosarcoma (ESO) is a malignant neoplasm that represents the soft tissue counterpart of bone osteosarcoma (it is also known as soft tissue osteosarcoma and extraosseous osteosarcoma).

Epidemiology and Presentation

ESO is rare as it accounts for 1–2% of all soft tissue sarcomas and 2–5% of all osteosarcomas (osteosarcoma is the most frequent type of bone primary malignancy, with an annual incidence of 3–4 cases per million). Unlike the bone counterpart, ESO typically occurs in mid-late adulthood (mainly during the fifth to seventh decades of life), with a male predominance (M:F = 2:1). Most ESO arise in the deep soft tissues, fewer than 10% being superficial (dermis or subcutis). The most common site is the thigh (50%), other locations being the buttock, shoulder girdle, trunk, and retroperitoneum (very rare cases have been also described in the breast and viscera). Clinically, the lesion presents as a deep enlarging mass (median size, 8 cm) that may be painful. Radiologically, calcifications are often detected. Positron emission tomography can be useful to exclude primary osteosarcoma of the bone, detect metastatic disease, and determine tumor response to medical treatments. For bone osteosarcoma, radionuclide bone scanning with technetium-99 (99mTc)-methylene diphosphonate (MDP/MDI) is routinely performed to evaluate the presence of metastatic disease to the skeleton: the utility in ESO is unknown.

Etiology and Predisposition

Although for most cases the etiology is unknown, 5–10% of cases are associated with radiation exposure, with a latency time of at least 2 years. Bone osteosarcoma is associated with cancer predisposition syndromes such as Li-Fraumeni and hereditary retinoblastoma (due to its rarity, virtually no data are available on the genetic predisposition to ESO).

Pathology

Macroscopically, ESO presents as a circumscribed tumor with possible hemorrhagic and necrotic areas; bone areas are usually located in the center of the lesion. Microscopically, ESO is composed of tumor cells that secrete bone matrix that can mineralize (the characteristic feature of osteosarcoma is the presence of osteoid in the lesion). All osteosarcoma subtypes observed in bone can be found in ESO: osteoblastic (the most frequent), fibroblastic, chondroblastic, telangiectatic, small cell, and well-differentiated variant. Tumor cells are spindle or polyhedral in shape, variably pleomorphic, cytologically atypical, and mitotically active (frequently with atypical mitotic figures). A common denominator across all variants is the presence of neoplastic bone intimately associated with tumor cells. The bone is typically most prominent in the center of the lesion, with more densely cellular areas located in the periphery (an opposite pattern as compared to myositis ossificans).

Differential diagnosis may be needed with the following: myositis ossificans (no atypia, reverse ossification) and other sarcomas that may produce metaplastic bone (e.g., undifferentiated pleomorphic sarcoma, synovial sarcoma, fibrosarcoma).

Biomarkers

The immunophenotypic pattern of ESO is nonspecific and rarely helpful for diagnosis.

Prognosis

ESO is associated with a very poor prognosis (5-year survival rate: 25%). Larger size and higher grade correlate with worse prognosis. ESO prognosis is reported to be poorer than that of skeletal osteosarcoma. In bone osteosarcoma, tumor necrosis after neoadjuvant chemotherapy is a strong predictor of survival.

Therapy

Surgery is the treatment of choice for localized primary ESO. **Radiotherapy** appears to increase the local disease control; in contrast, the role of perioperative **chemotherapy** is undefined (in patients with bone osteosarcoma, neoadjuvant and adjuvant chemotherapy is routinely used for high-grade tumors). For advanced/metastatic disease, chemotherapy regimens utilized for bone osteosarcoma (i.e., cisplatin plus doxorubicin; high-dose methotrexate plus cisplatin plus doxorubicin; doxorubicin plus cisplatin plus ifosfamide plus high-dose methotrexate; ifosfamide plus cisplatin plus epirubicin) are generally administered, although the results are not satisfactory.

As regards **target therapy**, regorafenib[1] appears to benefit patients with metastatic osteosarcoma.

Suggested Readings

Bernthal (2012) Long-term results (>25 years) of a randomized, prospective clinical trial evaluating chemotherapy in patients with high-grade, operable osteosarcoma. Cancer 118(23):5888–5893

Burk (2019) Diagnostic evaluation and treatment of primary breast osteosarcoma: a case report. Breast J 25(4):709–711

Duffaud (2019) Efficacy and safety of regorafenib in adult patients with metastatic osteosarcoma: a non-comparative, randomised, double-blind, placebo-controlled, phase 2 study. Lancet Oncol 20(1):120–133

Heng (2020) The role of chemotherapy and radiotherapy in localized extraskeletal osteosarcoma. Eur J Cancer 125:130–141

Longhi (2017) Extraskeletal osteosarcoma: a European musculoskeletal oncology society study on 266 patients. Eur J Cancer 74:9–16

McClelland (2020) Role of radiation therapy for pediatric upper extremity extraskeletal osteosarcoma: a case series. Pediatr Blood Cancer 67(2):e28018

Roller (2018) Clinical, radiological, and pathological features of extraskeletal osteosarcoma. Skelet Radiol 47(9):1213–1220

Shimizu (2019) Surgery and proton beam therapy for mediastinal extraskeletal osteosarcoma. Ann Thorac Surg 108(5):e289–e291

Yu (2018) Primary osteosarcoma of the liver: case report and literature review. Pathol Oncol Res 26(1):115–120

Zhang (2018) PET/CT in the diagnosis and prognosis of osteosarcoma. Front Biosci 23:2157–2165

---

[1] Regorafenib: tyrosine kinase inhibitor targeting the following: RET, VEGFR1, VEGFR2, VEGFR3, KIT, PDGFRA, PDGFRB, FGFR1, FGFR2.

Definition

Fetal rhabdomyoma is a benign neoplasm with rhabdomyoblastic differentiation. Along with adult rhabdomyoma and genital rhabdomyoma (→ see dedicated sections), it belongs to the extra-cardiac subgroup of rhabdomyomas (→ see Chap. 223).

Epidemiology and Presentation

Fetal rhabdomyoma is a rare tumor affecting more frequently males (M:F = 5:3) with mean age being 5 years (range: 2–58 years). Approximately 25% of cases are congenital. Most cases (70–90%) develop in the head and neck (especially the posterior auricular region), with a median size of 3 cm. Very rarely it localizes in the chest, abdomen, pelvis, and extremities.

Like all extra-cardiac rhabdomyomas, fetal rhabdomyoma is not associated with tuberous sclerosis complex.

Etiology and Predisposition

Fetal rhabdomyoma often occurs in association with **basal cell nevus syndrome** (also known as **Gorlin syndrome** and **nevoid basal cell carcinoma syndrome**), a cancer predisposition disease inherited in an autosomal dominant manner and caused by germline loss-of-function mutations in PTCH1 (9q22.1-q31), a tumor suppressor gene encoding an inhibitory receptor in the sonic hedgehog signaling pathway. This syndrome has a birth incidence of 1/19,000, equally affects both genders, and is characterized by the early onset of mandibular odontogenic keratocysts (second decade of life) and multiple basal cell carcinomas (most commonly on the face, back, and chest; third decade of life). Approximately 60% of individuals have a typical appearance with macrocephaly, frontal bossing, coarse facial features, and

S. Mocellin, *Soft Tissue Tumors*, https://doi.org/10.1007/978-3-030-58710-9_96

facial milia. Ectopic calcification of the falx is present in about 90% of patients by the age of 20 years. Palmar or plantar pits (asymmetrical, 2–3 mm in diameter, 1–3 mm in depth, second decade of life) and skeletal anomalies (fusion of vertebrae, wedge-shaped vertebrae, bifid or fused ribs, hemivertebra, kyphoscoliosis, pectus deformity, syndactyly, polydactyly) are also reported.

The Gorlin syndrome is associated also with other neoplasms such as medulloblastoma, meningioma, cardiac fibroma, ovarian fibroma (commonly bilateral and calcified), and nephroblastoma.

Pathology

The tumor is composed of irregular bundles of immature skeletal muscle fibers in a myxoid background. Cells have features of fetal myotubes. The cellular variant shows a more uniform population of differentiating myoblasts. The myxoid variant contains a more predominant stroma. Mitoses can be relatively frequent (up to 15 per 50 HPF), but cells lack significant nuclear atypia, infiltrative margins, atypical mitoses, or necrosis.

Differential diagnosis may be needed with the following: botryoid variant of embryonal rhabdomyosarcoma (resembles myxoid variant of fetal rhabdomyoma but has deep location, true cambium layer, atypia, numerous mitotic figures, tumor cell necrosis, infiltrative margins, no maturation of cells at periphery); infantile fibromatosis (deep location, fascicles of spindle cells, no cross striations, no undifferentiated cells); neuromuscular hamartoma (S100 positive; nerve fibers and skeletal muscle in same perimysial sheath); and spindle cell variant of embryonal rhabdomyosarcoma (mimics cellular variant of fetal rhabdomyoma but has cellular pleomorphism and tumor cell necrosis).

Biomarkers

Fetal rhabdomyoma stains positive for desmin, myogenin, and MSA,[1] whereas it stains negative for EMA[2] and CD68.

Prognosis

Fetal rhabdomyoma is a benign tumor.

---

[1] MSA: muscle-specific actin.
[2] EMA: epithelial membrane antigen.

Therapy

Complete excision is usually curative.

Suggested Readings

Diociaiuti (2015) Naevoid basal cell carcinoma syndrome in a 22-month-old child presenting with multiple basal cell carcinomas and a fetal rhabdomyoma. Acta Derm Venereol 95(2):243–244

Fletcher (2020) WHO classification of tumours of soft tissue and bone, 5th edn

Walsh (2008) Cutaneous fetal rhabdomyoma: a case report and historical review of the literature. Am J Surg Pathol 32(3):485–491

Calcifying aponeurotic *fibroma* (→ see dedicated section)
Cardiac *fibroma* (→ see cardiac soft tissue tumors)
Cellular digital *fibroma* (→ see acral fibromyxoma)
Collagenous *fibroma* (→ see desmoplastic fibroblastoma)
Fibroma of tendon sheath (→ see dedicated section)
Gardner *fibroma* (→ see dedicated section)
Infantile digital *fibroma* (→ see inclusion body fibromatosis)
Nuchal-type *fibroma* (→ see dedicated section)
Ovarian *fibroma* (→ see dedicated section)
Pleomorphic *fibroma* (→ see dedicated section)
Sclerotic *fibroma* (→ see dedicated section)
Skin *fibroma* (→ see cutaneous fibroepithelial polyp)
Uterine *fibroma* (→ see uterine leiomyoma)

Definition

Fibroma of tendon sheath (FTS) is a benign tumor classified among the fibroblastic-myofibroblastic neoplasms. It is also known as tenosynovial fibroma.

Epidemiology and Presentation

FTS is an uncommon lesion typically occurring in patients between 20 and 50 years of age. It develops in the finger tendons, where it presents as a well-circumscribed small (typically <3 cm) and slow-growing nodule.

Pathology

FTS is a fibroblastic nodular neoplasm attached to a tendon, with a lobular fibrous appearance resembling a localized-type tenosynovial giant cell tumor (but it lacks pigmentation). The lesion is composed of spindle cells in a collagenous background. There is generally no atypia and cellularity is typically low, although sometimes is higher resembling nodular fasciitis.

Biomarkers

Spindle cells are usually positive for smooth muscle actin (SMA).

Prognosis

Although benign, FTS can recur in up to 20% of cases.

© The Editor(s) (if applicable) and The Author(s), under exclusive license to
Springer Nature Switzerland AG 2021
S. Mocellin, *Soft Tissue Tumors*, https://doi.org/10.1007/978-3-030-58710-9_98

Therapy

Surgical excision is the treatment of choice.

Suggested Reading

Fletcher (2020) WHO classification of tumours of soft tissue and bone, 5th edn

Fibromatosis

There are two main types of fibromatosis (mainly in adults):

(a) **Superficial fibromatosis** is a family of fibromatoses of superficial tissues and includes palmar/plantar fibromatosis, penile fibromatosis, knuckle pads, pachydermodactyly, and infantile digital fibromatosis. For more details → see Chap. 240.
(b) **Deep fibromatosis** (fibromatosis of the deep tissues): for details → see Chap. 69.

Other types of fibromatosis are typical of pediatric age:

– Fibromatosis colli (→ see dedicated section)
– Juvenile hyaline fibromatosis (→ see dedicated section)
– Inclusion body fibromatosis (→ see dedicated section)
– Infantile fibromatosis (→ see lipofibromatosis)

© The Editor(s) (if applicable) and The Author(s), under exclusive license to   333
Springer Nature Switzerland AG 2021
S. Mocellin, *Soft Tissue Tumors*, https://doi.org/10.1007/978-3-030-58710-9_99

Definition

Fibromatosis colli is a benign soft tissue lesion classified among the fibroblastic-myofibroblastic tumors. It is also known as congenital muscular torticollis, sterno-cleidomastoid tumor of infancy, or pseudotumor of infancy.

Epidemiology and Presentation

Fibromatosis colli occurs in approximately 0.4% of live births, with a slight male prevalence. In most infants, the diagnosis is made by the age of 6 months. The disease is site-specific as the lesion develops exclusively in the distal sternocleidomastoid muscle: the nodule presents as a fusiform thickening of the muscle and leads to cervicofacial asymmetry due to muscle shortening (torticollis). There is a significant association with some musculoskeletal developmental abnormalities including forefoot anomalies and congenital hip dislocation.

Both ultrasound and magnetic resonance imaging usually provide useful information to make a correct diagnosis.

Pathology

When a doubt exists on the diagnosis, fine needle aspiration cytology can be useful. Microscopic findings vary depending on the time of examination: in the early phase, cellular specimens show aggregates of uniform plump spindle cells embedded in myxoid to collagenous matrix; later examination (e.g., at the time of surgery for persistent torticollis) usually demonstrates less cellular collagen-rich tissue mimicking a scar.

© The Editor(s) (if applicable) and The Author(s), under exclusive license to
Springer Nature Switzerland AG 2021
S. Mocellin, *Soft Tissue Tumors*, https://doi.org/10.1007/978-3-030-58710-9_100

Biomarkers

Fibromatosis colli stains positive for vimentin and MSA (muscle specific actin), while stains negative for nuclear beta-catenin.

Prognosis

Fibromatosis colli is a benign condition.

Therapy

The mainstay of treatment is passive stretching and physiotherapy, which lead to cure in the majority of infants. Surgery (tenotomy) is required in <10% of patients. Residual deformity is more frequently observed in patients diagnosed and treated beyond 1 year of age.

Suggested Readings

Fletcher (2020) WHO classification of tumours of soft tissue and bone, 5th edn
Kumar (2019) Fibromatosis colli: a rare cause of neck mass with cytological soft pointers. Cytopathology 30(5):549–551
Oliveira (2018) Sternocleidomastoid tumour in neonate: fibromatosis colli. BMJ Case Rep 2018. pii: bcr-2017-223543

Fibro-osseous pseudotumor of digits (FOPD) is a benign lesion classified among the fibroblastic and myofibroblastic soft tissue tumors and is usually considered together with myositis ossificans.

For details → see Chap. 180.

Fibrosarcoma is a malignant neoplasm arising from fibroblasts and can develop in the soft tissues as well as in the bones (bone fibrosarcoma and ameloblastic fibrosarcoma are not covered in this book).

There are five soft tissue fibrosarcoma subtypes ($\rightarrow$ see dedicated sections):

1. Infantile fibrosarcoma (IFS)
2. Adult fibrosarcoma (AFS)
3. Dermatofibrosarcoma protuberans (DFSP)
4. Myxofibrosarcoma (MFS)
5. Sclerosing epithelioid fibrosarcoma (SEF)

Many cases previously designated as soft tissue fibrosarcomas are now classified otherwise, such as dedifferentiated liposarcoma, fibromatosis, fibrosarcomatous DFSP, low-grade fibromyxoid sarcoma, malignant peripheral nerve sheath tumor (MPNST), synovial sarcoma, or undifferentiated pleomorphic sarcoma (UPS) ($\rightarrow$ see sections dedicated to each tumor).

Definition

Fibrous hamartoma of infancy (FHI) is a benign soft tissue lesion classified among fibroblastic-myofibroblastic tumors. It is also known as subdermal fibromatous tumor of infancy.

Epidemiology and Presentation

FHI is a very rare lesion which can be congenital (about 20% of cases) or develops by the first 2 years of life, males being more frequently affected than females.

FHI mainly affects the axillary and inguinal regions, upper arms, and trunk, although other body sites may be affected. The lesion usually grows as a solitary painless dermal and subcutaneous nodule.

Pathology

FHI presents as a poorly circumscribed superficial soft tissue nodule (sometimes reaching several centimeters in diameter) featuring an organoid pattern of three histological components: fibrocollagenous tissue, immature mesenchymal cells, and mature adipose tissue. Mitotic figures are infrequent.

Biomarkers

The fibroblastic areas express smooth muscle actin (SMA), while the mature adipose tissue is reactive for S100.

© The Editor(s) (if applicable) and The Author(s), under exclusive license to
Springer Nature Switzerland AG 2021
S. Mocellin, *Soft Tissue Tumors*, https://doi.org/10.1007/978-3-030-58710-9_103

Prognosis

FHI is a benign lesion (local recurrence is rare and probably follows incomplete resection).

Therapy

Surgical excision is the treatment of choice.

Suggested Readings

Fletcher (2020) WHO classification of tumours of soft tissue and bone, 5th edn

Ji (2019) Fibrous hamartoma of infancy: radiologic features and literature review. BMC Musculoskelet Disord 20(1):356

Scott (1999) Fibrous hamartoma of infancy. J Am Acad Dermatol 41(5 Pt 2):857–859

The term fibrous histiocytoma is included in several tumor types with very different biological behavior (clinical aggressiveness), as schematized in Table 104.1.

For more details on each neoplasm → see dedicated sections.

Table 104.1 List of fibrous histiocytoma types

Tumor	Behavior[a]	Comment
Malignant fibrous histiocytoma	Malignant	This term should no longer be used, as recommended by the World Health Organization
Benign fibrous histiocytoma	Benign	The superficial subtype is also called dermatofibroma (note that a malignant counterpart exists, i.e., the dermatofibrosarcoma protuberans)
Aneurismal fibrous histiocytoma	Intermediate	It is generally considered a variant of benign fibrous histiocytoma
Cellular fibrous histiocytoma	Intermediate	It is generally considered a variant of benign fibrous histiocytoma
Epithelioid fibrous histiocytoma	Benign	It is generally considered a variant of benign fibrous histiocytoma
Angiomatoid fibrous histiocytoma	Intermediate	Despite the name, the World Health Organization does not classify it along with previous tumors (which are included among fibrohistiocytic tumors) but separately (among tumors of uncertain differentiation)

[a]According to the World Health Organization classification

S. Mocellin, *Soft Tissue Tumors*, https://doi.org/10.1007/978-3-030-58710-9_104

Definition

Gardner fibroma is a benign lesion classified among the fibroblastic-myofibroblastic tumors. It is also known as Gardner-type fibroma, soft fibroma, and—when localized in the mesentery—desmoid precursor lesion.

Epidemiology and Presentation

Gardner fibroma usually occurs in the first decade of life, without gender differences. Most cases (approximately 80–90%) are associated with Gardner-type familial adenomatous polyposis (FAP): in particular, Gardner fibroma is considered a sentinel event for FAP.

This fibroma usually locates in superficial and deep soft tissues of the paraspinal region, back, chest wall, abdomen, head and neck, limbs, and mesentery (desmoid precursor lesion).

The lesion, which can range from 1 to 10 cm in diameter, is an ill-defined mass and is generally asymptomatic.

Etiology and Predisposition

Classic FAP is inherited in an autosomal dominant manner and is due to inactivating germline mutations of the APC tumor suppressor gene, whose protein product promotes rapid degradation of CTNNB1 (encoding beta-catenin) and thus negatively regulates the Wnt signaling pathway. FAP has a birth incidence of about 1/8300 and manifests equally in both sexes. The disease causes the formation of hundreds of colorectal adenomatous polyps, with a lifetime risk of developing colorectal carcinoma greater than 90% (FAP accounts for about 1% of all colorectal cancer cases).

FAP may present some extraintestinal manifestations such as osteoma, dental abnormalities, congenital hypertrophy of the retinal pigment epithelium (CHRPE), desmoid-type fibromatosis ($\rightarrow$ see dedicated section), and extracolonic cancers (thyroid, liver, bile ducts, and central nervous system).

Some lesions (skull and mandible osteoma, dental abnormalities, and fibroma) are indicative of the Gardner syndrome, whereas the association of FAP and medulloblastoma is referred to as the Turcot syndrome.

Pathology

Gardner fibroma is a plaque-like hypocellular proliferation of thick, haphazardly arranged collagen fibers with interspersed fibroblasts. In young patients with suspected nuchal-type fibroma (which usually develops later in life), Gardner fibroma should be taken into consideration.

Biomarkers

Gardner fibroma stains positive for CD34 and vimentin, whereas it is negative for SMA,[1] MSA,[2] desmin, estrogen receptor, and progesterone receptor. Focal nuclear positivity for beta-catenin is frequent.

Prognosis

Gardner fibroma is a benign tumor. However, approximately 50% of these patients develop a desmoid-type fibromatosis ($\rightarrow$ see dedicated section) at the site of the fibroma, either spontaneously or after surgery.

Diagnosis of Gardner fibroma (especially in young patients) should prompt investigation for FAP.

Therapy

Surgical excision is the treatment of choice.

---

[1] SMA: smooth muscle actin.
[2] MSA: muscle specific actin.

Suggested Readings

Fletcher (2020) WHO classification of tumours of soft tissue and bone, 5th edn
Santoro (2017) From Gardner fibroma diagnosis to constitutional APC mutation detection: a one-
    way street. Clin Case Rep 5(10):1557–1560

Definition

Gastrointestinal clear cell sarcoma (GCCS) is a malignancy that resembles clear cell sarcoma of soft tissues (see Chap. 52) without evidence of melanocytic differentiation. It is also known as clear cell sarcoma-like tumor of the gastrointestinal tract.

Although it is generally considered a mesenchymal tumor, there is evidence that it might arise from primitive cells of the neural crest, which is why some have proposed the name gastrointestinal neuroectodermal tumor (GNET).

Epidemiology and Presentation

This very rare tumor occurs in adults (median age: 35 years) without gender predilection. It most commonly localizes in the small intestine (about 60% of cases), followed by the stomach (15%), colon (10%), ileocecal junction (5%), esophagus (5%), and anal canal (5%). Clinically, GCCS presents as a mass ranging in size from 2 to 15 cm and often shows transmural involvement of the bowel wall (typically extends into the serosa and is accompanied occasionally by mucosal ulceration); most common symptoms are abdominal pain and intestinal obstruction.

Pathology

Microscopically, the tumor is composed of epithelioid cells with eosinophilic or clear cytoplasm arranged in nest, sheetlike, papillary, or pseudoalveolar patterns and/or spindle tumor cells with eosinophilic cytoplasm arranged in a fascicular pattern; osteoclast-like giant cells may be present.

Differential diagnosis may be needed with the following: gastrointestinal stromal tumor (positive for CD117 and DOG1), clear cell sarcoma (positive for HMB45 and Melan-A; it may metastasize to the gastrointestinal tract or possibly arise there), malignant peripheral nerve sheath tumor, alveolar rhabdomyosarcoma (positive for myogenin and myoD1, harbors characteristic translocation), and synovial sarcoma (positive for cytokeratins; characteristic chromosomal translocation).

Biomarkers

Immunohistochemically, tumor cells stain positively for S100, SOX10, and vimentin and negatively for CD117 (with very rare exceptions), HMB45, Melan-A, DOG1, CD34, cytokeratins, SMA, and desmin.

Almost all cases (>90%) carry a **chromosomal translocation** leading to the formation of the EWSR1-CREB1 fusion gene or the EWSR1-ATF1 fusion gene.

Prognosis

GCCS is a malignant neoplasm that can metastasize to lymph nodes, liver, lungs, and bone.

Therapy

Surgery is the mainstay of treatment. GCCS is poorly responsive to conventional chemotherapy.

A few advanced/metastatic cases responding to target therapy drugs such as apatinib,[1] anlotinib,[2] and a combination of crizotinib[3] with pazopanib[4] have been described.

Suggested Readings

Chang (2019) Malignant gastrointestinal neuroectodermal tumor: clinicopathologic, immunohistochemical, and molecular analysis of 19 cases. Am J Surg Pathol [Epub ahead of print]
Green (2018) Clear cell sarcoma of the gastrointestinal tract and malignant gastrointestinal neuroectodermal tumour: distinct or related entities? A review. Pathology 50(5):490–498
Libertini (2018) Clear cell sarcoma-like tumor of the gastrointestinal tract: clinical outcome and pathologic features of a molecularly characterized tertiary center case series. Anticancer Res 38(3):1479–1483

---

[1] Apatinib: tyrosin.

[2] Anlotinib: VEGFR, FGFR, PDGFR, KIT.

[3] Crizotinib: small molecule tyrosine kinase inhibitor targeting the following—ALK, MET.

[4] Pazopanib: tyrosine kinase inhibitor targeting the following—VEGFR, PDGFR, KIT.

Stockman (2012) Malignant gastrointestinal neuroectodermal tumor: clinicopathologic, immuno-histochemical, ultrastructural, and molecular analysis of 16 cases with a reappraisal of clear cell sarcoma-like tumors of the gastrointestinal tract. Am J Surg Pathol 36(6):857–868

Subbiah (2016) Activity of c-Met/ALK inhibitor crizotinib and multi-kinase VEGF inhibitor pazopanib in metastatic gastrointestinal neuroectodermal tumor harboring EWSR1-CREB1 fusion. Oncology 91(6):348–353

Wolak (2018) Malignant gastrointestinal neuroectodermal tumor (clear cell sarcoma-like tumor of the gastrointestinal tract) of the small intestine in a 12-year-old boy. Dev Period Med 22(4):358–363

For details → see Chap. 74.

Definition

Gastrointestinal stromal tumor (GIST) is a mesenchymal neoplasm believed to originate from myenteric interstitial cells of Cajal (ICC, which are involved in the pacemaker activity of the digestive tract). Of note, most smooth muscle (e.g., leiomyoma and leiomyosarcoma) and nerve sheath tumors (e.g., schwannoma) diagnosed in the gastrointestinal tract before the current definition of GIST as well as neoplasms formerly designated as leiomyoblastoma and gastrointestinal autonomic nerve tumor (GANT) are actually GISTs.

Epidemiology and Presentation

GIST is the most frequent type of primary mesenchymal tumor in the gastrointestinal tract (about 80% of cases) and one of the most frequent sarcomas (15% of all cases, including bone neoplasms), its annual incidence being estimated to be 1 per 100,000 (however, autopsy studies reveal much higher rates, especially for micro-GIST, e.g., lesions <10 mm) and its prevalence being estimated to be 10–15 per 100,000. The tumor typically occurs in older adults (median age: 60 years) without remarkable gender differences, children being very rarely affected (nearly always in the stomach). Approximately 55% of all GISTs occur in the stomach (where the tumor represents 2–3% of all malignant gastric tumors), 30% in the small intestine (including duodenum), 5% in the colon-rectum, and 1% in the esophagus, and the remaining 9% are primarily disseminated with an unknown site of origin. So-called extragastrointestinal GISTs arising in the omentum or mesentery are usually metastatic disease originating somewhere in the gastrointestinal tract.

Clinically, the tumor presents with vague abdominal complaints or complications such as bowel obstruction, bleeding (acute or chronic), and bowel perforation (rare). A significant proportion of (smaller) GISTs are detected incidentally during

S. Mocellin, *Soft Tissue Tumors*, https://doi.org/10.1007/978-3-030-58710-9_108

endoscopy (e.g., gastroscopy, often coupled with ultrasound scan), surgery, or radiological imaging studies (incidentaloma).

Computed tomography scan appears to yield the highest diagnostic accuracy; endoscopic ultrasound is often utilized in the workup of gastric GIST; positron emission tomography scan may be useful as GIST typically exhibits strong fluoro-deoxyglucose uptake. Histological diagnosis is needed to make differential diagnosis with other gastrointestinal/abdominal tumors/masses (e.g., carcinoma, lymphoma, mesenteric fibromatosis, and retroperitoneal germ cell tumors or soft tissue sarcoma) and to personalize treatment (e.g., neoadjuvant/primary medical therapy in locally advanced/metastatic disease). A diagnostic biopsy may be obtained endoscopically (e.g., gastric GIST); if this is not possible, percutaneous core needle biopsy (under radiological guidance) is the standard approach; surgical biopsy is the last option. For (small) localized primary lesions suspected for GIST which cannot be biopsied preoperatively, definitive surgery can be both diagnostic and therapeutic.

Etiology and Predisposition

Although most GISTs are sporadic, about 5–10% are associated with the following tumor predisposition syndromes:

(a) **Familiar GIST**: this is an autosomal dominant condition due to germline mutations in KIT[1] or PDGFRA[2] oncogenes. It is characterized by multifocal GISTs (usually occurring in middle-aged adults), ICC hyperplasia (possibly leading to dysphagia), hyperpigmentation, and mast cell tumors.

---

[1] KIT: this gene encodes the human homolog of the proto-oncogene c-Kit (which was first identified as the cellular homolog of the feline sarcoma viral oncogene v-Kit). The encoded protein is a type 3 transmembrane receptor for mast cell growth factor (MGF, also known as stem cell factor or SCF); it is a receptor tyrosine kinase and is recognized by the monoclonal antibody CD117. KIT mutations are associated with gastrointestinal stromal tumors, mast cell disease, acute myelogenous leukemia, and piebaldism. In particular, activating mutations lead to upregulation of downstream signaling pathways, including RAS/RAF/MAPK and PI3K/AKT/mTOR.

[2] PDGFRA: platelet-derived growth factor receptor alpha encodes a cell surface tyrosine kinase receptor for members of the platelet-derived growth factor family, which are mitogens for cells of mesenchymal origin. The type of ligand bound to a receptor monomer determines whether the functional receptor is a homodimer or a heterodimer, composed of both PDGFRA and platelet-derived growth factor receptor beta (PDGFRB) polypeptides. This gene plays a role in organ development, wound healing, and tumor progression. Mutations in this gene have been associated with idiopathic hypereosinophilic syndrome, gastrointestinal stromal tumors, as well as a variety of other neoplasms. In particular, activating mutations lead to upregulation of downstream signaling pathways, including RAS/RAF/MAPK and PI3K/AKT/mTOR.

(b) **Neurofibromatosis type 1**: this is an inheritable disease caused by biallelic loss of the NF1 tumor suppressor gene.[3] These patients are at high risk of developing GIST, as well as other tumors: for more details → see Chap. 187. GISTs are characterized by younger age at onset, location in the duodenum and small intestine, small size, tumor multiplicity, and an indolent clinical course. Most GISTs are CD117 positive, have a spindle cell morphology, and generally show low mitotic rates. NF1-associated GISTs do not harbor KIT/PDGFRA mutations; instead, loss of NF1 leads to MAPK signal activation.
(c) **Carney-Stratakis syndrome**: this autosomal dominant inheritable disease is due to germline mutations in the succinate dehydrogenase (SDH) mitochondrial tumor suppressor gene pathway.[4] Patients are typically at risk to develop both GIST and paraganglioma (Carney-Stratakis dyad).
(d) **Carney triad**: this non-hereditary condition is characterized by the development of GIST, pulmonary chondroma (→ see dedicated section), and extra-adrenal paraganglioma. It is due to epigenetic hypermethylation in the SDH complex genes. It predominantly affects young females.

Pathology

Macroscopically, GISTs vary from small mural nodules to large masses (up to 30 cm), with variable intraluminal and extra-luminal components. Hemorrhage and cystic change are typical of larger lesions.

Microscopically, GISTs show a relatively broad morphological spectrum. Most lesions are spindle cell GISTs (easier diagnosis, also due to CD117 consistent positivity), but epithelioid GISTs are observed in 20–30% of cases (more difficult diagnosis, also due to inconsistent/negative staining for CD117), and some cases display mixed histology. Nuclear pleomorphism is not common and is observed more often in epithelioid lesions. Other subtypes have been described such as sclerosing GIST (especially observed in small lesions), palisaded-vacuolated GIST (one of the most common), cellular GIST (with diffuse hypercellularity), sarcomatoid GIST (with significant nuclear atypia and mitotic activity), and dedifferentiated GIST (which can occur either de novo or after prolonged treatment with imatinib). Epithelioid

---

[3] NF1: neurofibromin 1 contains a GAP-related domain that is responsible for converting active Ras-GTP to inactive Ras-GDP and ultimately negatively regulates RAS signaling. Mutations in this gene have been associated with neurofibromatosis type 1, juvenile myelomonocytic leukemia, and Watson syndrome.

[4] SDH: the SDH enzyme is composed of the subunits A (SDHA), B (SDHB), C (SDHC), and D (SDHD). These genes encode the catalytic subunits of succinate-ubiquinone oxidoreductase, a complex of the mitochondrial respiratory chain. SDH deficiency results in the accumulation of succinate, which is a competitive inhibitor of alpha-ketoglutarate-dependent dioxygenases, including the TET family of 5-methylcytosine hydroxylases. Members of the TET family are active DNA demethylases, and inhibition of TET activities can lead to aberrant DNA methylation in GISTs. Accumulation of succinate is also involved in the stabilization of HIF1-alpha, which controls oncogene transcription.

GIST may show sclerosing, hypercellular, or sarcomatous morphology with significant atypia and mitotic activity. SDH-deficient GIST characteristically shows epithelioid morphology and is multinodular (with plexiform mural involvement): it frequently features lymphovascular invasion and occasionally lymph node metastasis, which is not observed in conventional GIST.

Differential diagnosis may be needed with the following: smooth muscle tumors (desmin positive, CD117 negative); schwannoma (S100 positive, CD117 negative); desmoid-type fibromatosis; solitary fibrous tumor (spindle to epithelioid cells arranged in a "patternless pattern" with characteristic staghorn vessels; CD34 and STAT6 positive, CD117 negative); inflammatory myofibroblastic tumor; perivascular epithelioid cell tumor (PEComa); and inflammatory fibroid polyp.

Biomarkers

GIST is characterized by strong immunopositivity upon staining with CD117.[5] However, 5% of GISTs (especially gastric GIST with mutant PDGFRA) may result weakly positive or negative upon CD117 staining. Staining with DOG1[6] is equally sensitive and specific and often reacts also with CD117-negative GISTs. Most spindle cell GISTs (especially the gastric ones) are positive for CD34 (epithelioid GIST is less consistently positive). Immunohistochemical loss of SDHB (succinate dehydrogenase subunit B) is a practical biomarker to identify SDH-deficient GIST. Most GISTs do not stain with smooth muscle biomarkers (e.g., desmin, SMA, myosin).

Most GISTs contain KIT or PDGFRA **activating mutations**, which play a key role in the disease pathogenesis.

KIT oncogenic mutations (leading to constitutive activation of the KIT signaling pathway) are found in about 80% of sporadic GISTs; these mutations most often occur in KIT exon 11 (70%). KIT exon 9 mutations occur in approximately 10% of cases and are almost invariably associated with intestinal tumor location. KIT exons 13 and 17 are rarely involved (1–2%). A subset of GISTs carry PDGFRA mutations (10–15%): they are characterized by gastric location, epithelioid morphology, and an indolent clinical course. The most common PDGFRA mutation is D842V in exon 18, which accounts for 60–65% of PDGFRA mutations in GISTs (approximately 5% of all GISTs) and is associated with extremely favorable disease-free survival as compared to other mutation types. GISTs that are deficient in SDH or associated with neurofibromatosis type 1 do not contain KIT or PDGFRA mutations.

The most frequent molecular alteration in GISTs with wild-type KIT/PDGFRA is SDH deficiency. SDH consists of four subunits (SDHA, SDHB, SDHC, and SDHD) and is a component of the citric acid cycle and respiratory electron transfer chain. SDH deficiency underlies Leigh syndrome (a neurodegenerative disorder

---

[5]CD117: it is a monoclonal antibody specific for c-Kit, the protein product of the KIT oncogene, which is also expressed on ICC, hematopoietic stem cells, mast cells, melanocytes, and germ cells.

[6]DOG1: discovered on GIST 1 is an alias for ANO1 a gene encoding anoctamin-1 (a chloride-channel protein), which has been associated with GIST and frontal sinus squamous cell carcinoma.

caused by mitochondrial dysfunction) or different types of neoplasms (e.g., paraganglioma, GIST, renal cell carcinoma, and pituitary adenoma). **SDH-deficient GISTs** are immunohistochemically negative for SDHB: this is helpful in the diagnostic workup as presence of mutated SDH suggests Carney-Stratakis syndrome, whereas wild-type SDH suggests Carney triad. SDH-deficient GISTs occur almost exclusively in the stomach, exhibit a unique growth pattern of nests of tumor cells separated by septa of smooth muscle cells, and usually follow an indolent course. The Carney triad, Carney-Stratakis syndrome, and some sporadic GISTs (wild type for KIT/PDGFRA) are included among the SDH-deficient GISTs.

In very rare cases, the GIST does not carry mutations in KIT/PDGFRA and is SDH-proficient: after excluding a NF1-related syndromic GIST, the case can be named **wild-type GIST**; this type of GIST is often characterized by overexpression of CALCRL/COL22A1, NTRK2 (for which specific inhibitors for clinical use already exist), CDK6 (for which specific inhibitors for clinical use already exist), or ERG or mutations *in KRAS, BRAF (e.g., activating mutation V600E, for which specific inhibitors for clinical use already exist), TP53, MEN1, or MAX.*

Mutational analysis for known mutations involving KIT and PDGFRA can confirm a doubtful diagnosis of GIST (especially in rare CD117-/DOG1-negative lesions). Mutational analysis has a predictive value for sensitivity to molecular-targeted therapy and to prognostic value ($\rightarrow$ see below paragraphs): therefore, its inclusion in the diagnostic workup of all GISTs should be considered a standard practice (with the possible exclusion of low-risk lesions such as gastric <2 cm nodules).

Prognosis

Approximately 25% of GISTs are malignant (this figure mainly refers to gastric GIST, as for non-gastric lesions, the rate increases up to 40%). Malignant GISTs can infiltrate surrounding structures (e.g., spleen, pancreas, and bowel), spread into the peritoneal cavity (and retroperitoneal space), and often metastasize to the liver (lymph node, bone, skin, and soft tissue metastases occur infrequently). Distinctively, pulmonary metastasis is rare, in contrast with leiomyosarcoma. GIST may metastasize after a long delay, which calls for long-term follow-up. Of note, some (rare) patients with metastatic GIST may survive for long time even without treatment. While many metastatic GISTs resulted formerly fatal within 1–2 years, patients often now survive 5 years or more with tyrosine kinase inhibitor therapy. Spontaneous or iatrogenic tumor rupture is associated with high risk for peritoneal metastasis (which is why laparoscopic surgery is discouraged).

The most reliable prognostic factors are tumor size, mitotic activity, and anatomical site (gastric GISTs fare better than non-gastric lesions). There is no formal grading system for GIST (grading for soft tissue sarcoma is not applicable). For details on the TNM staging system $\rightarrow$ see Tables 108.1, 108.2 and 108.3; of note, the system differs for tumors arising in the stomach or in other sites; moreover,

Table 108.1 AJCC pathologic TNM staging system for GIST (eighth edition): definition of TNM categories

Category	Definition
pT	
pTX	Primary tumor cannot be assessed
pT0	No evidence of primary tumor
pT1	Tumor ≤2 cm in greatest dimension
pT2	Tumor >2 cm and ≤ 5 cm
pT3	Tumor >5 cm and ≤ 10 cm
pT4	Tumor >10 cm in greatest dimension
pN	
pN0	No regional lymph node metastasis
pN1	Regional lymph node metastasis
pM	
pM0	No distant metastasis
pM1	Distant metastasis
Grading[a]	
Low mitotic rate	≤ 5 mitoses per 5 mm^2
High mitotic rate	> 5 mitoses per 5 mm^2

[a]Mitotic rate per 5 mm^2 roughly corresponds to 50 high-power fields (HPF) in older microscopes and 20–25 HPF in newer microscopes

pediatric GIST, familial GIST (germline mutant KIT or PDGFRA), or syndromic GIST is not staged according to the AJCC system.

About 60–80% of patients with SDH-deficient GIST develop distant metastasis, but their prognosis is less predictable (lesions with low mitotic counts in this group can develop liver metastases, while lesions with high mitotic counts may never metastasize).

Gastric GIST with exon 11 deletions has a worse prognosis than those with missense mutations.

High expression of ROR2 (receptor tyrosine kinase-like orphan receptor 2) has been identified in a subset of GISTs; this is associated with a poor clinical outcome.

Most KIT mutations are heterozygous, but homozygous mutations can occur (via hemizygosity), and these tumors are often more aggressive than corresponding heterozygous mutants.

Therapy

Surgery is the treatment of choice for primary localized GIST and is curative in about 60% of patients. Due to the very rare occurrence of lymph node metastasis, lymphadenectomy is not recommended. Since tumor rupture worsens the prognosis, the laparotomic approach is preferred over the laparoscopic route (especially for

Table 108.2 AJCC TNM staging system (eighth edition): definition of TNM stages for gastric and omental GIST

Stage I		
IA	T1–T2	
	N0	
	M0	
	Low mitotic rate	
IB	T3	
	N0	
	M0	
	Low mitotic rate	
Stage II		
	T1–T2	
	N0	
	M0	
	High mitotic rate	
	T4	
	N0	
	M0	
	Low mitotic rate	
Stage III		
IIIA	T3	
	N0	
	M0	
	High mitotic rate	
IIIB	T4	
	N0	
	M0	
	High mitotic rate	
Stage IV		
	Any T	
	N1	
	M0	
	Any mitotic rate	
	Any T	
	Any N	
	M1	
	Any mitotic rate	

lesions >5 cm). Risk of postoperative disease recurrence correlates with the above described prognostic factors.

Due to their low risk of malignancy, for suspected GISTs <2 cm arising in the esophagus, stomach, and duodenum, a valid option (alternative to surgery) is endoscopic ultrasound assessment and then follow-up, reserving excision for patients willing to do it or those whose tumor increases in size or becomes symptomatic. For histologically proven esophago-gastro-duodenal GIST <2 cm, the choice of surgery depends upon the risk. Patients with duodenal GIST should not undergo mutilating surgery (i.e., Whipple pancreatico-duodenectomy) if the tumor can be removed with conservative surgery.

Table 108.3 AJCC TNM staging system (eighth edition): definition of TNM stages for small intestinal, esophageal, colorectal, mesenteric, and peritoneal GIST

Stage I		
	T1–T2	
	N0	
	M0	
	Low mitotic rate	
Stage II		
	T3	
	N0	
	M0	
	Low mitotic rate	
Stage III		
IIIA	T1	
	N0	
	M0	
	High mitotic rate	
	T4	
	N0	
	M0	
	Low mitotic rate	
IIIB	T2–T3–T4	
	N0	
	M0	
	High mitotic rate	
Stage IV		
	Any T	
	N1	
	M0	
	Any mitotic rate	
	Any T	
	Any N	
	M1	
	Any mitotic rate	

Target therapy has revolutionized the management of patients with GIST: the key randomized controlled trials in this field are reported in Table 108.4. In particular, imatinib[7] is the first choice in the metastatic, neoadjuvant, and adjuvant setting. Most KIT exon 11 (90%) and exon 13 (1%) mutant GISTs are extremely sensitive to imatinib; in contrast, KIT exon 9 (8%) and PDGFR exon 12, exon 14, and exon 18 mutant GISTs respond less well to imatinib, prompting dose escalation (800 mg daily instead of 400 mg daily) or use of alternative inhibitors (e.g., sunitinib or nilotinib). GISTs with PDGFR exon 18 D842V mutation (8%) and those lacking KIT

---

[7] Imatinib: tyrosine kinase inhibitor targeting the following—KIT, RET, BCR, PDGFRA.

Table 108.4 Pivotal randomized controlled trials of target therapy in patients with GIST

Author (year)	Comparison	Setting	Line	Main findings
Verweij (2004)	Imatinib 800 mg vs 400 mg	Metastatic/ advanced	First-line	Imatinib 800 mg improved PFS (HR = 0.82).[a] No difference in tumor response rates
Blanke (2008)	Imatinib 800 mg vs 400 mg	Metastatic/ advanced	First-line	No difference in tumor response rates, PFS or OS
Le Cesne (2010)	Imatinib continuous vs 3 years	Metastatic/ advanced	First-line	Imatinib continuous improved PFS (HR not reported)[a]
Blay (2015)	Nilotinib vs imatinib	Metastatic/ advanced	First-line	PFS was worse with nilotinib (HR = 1.47)[a]
Demetri (2006)	Sunitinib vs placebo	Metastatic/ advanced	Second-line (after failure of imatinib)	Sunitinib improved PFS (HR = 0.33)[a]
Demetri (2013)	Regorafenib vs placebo	Metastatic/ advanced	Third-line (after failure of imatinib and sunitinib)	Regorafenib improved PFS (HR = 0.27)[a]
Mir (2016)	Pazopanib vs BSC	Metastatic/ advanced	Third-line (after failure of imatinib and sunitinib)	Pazopanib improved (HR = 0.59)[a]
Dematteo (2009)	Imatinib vs placebo	Adjuvant (high-risk GIST)	–	Imatinib improved DFS (HR = 0.35)[a]
Casali (2015)	Imatinib vs placebo	Adjuvant (high-risk GIST)	–	Imatinib improved DFS (HR = 0.35)[a]
Joensuu (2016)	Imatinib 3 years vs 1 year	Adjuvant (high-risk GIST)	–	Imatinib 3-y improved DFS (HR = 0.60)[a]

BSC best supportive care, *DFS* disease-free survival, *HR* hazard ratio, *PFS* progression-free survival, *OS* overall survival
[a]Statistically significant result

and PDGFR mutations are notoriously resistant to imatinib. The NCCN and ESMO guidelines recommend mutational testing for optimal management of GIST.

Neoadjuvant imatinib is indicated for locally advanced tumors (likely not amenable to radical surgery) to shrink large tumors and limit surgical resections; the optimal duration of preoperative treatment is unknown, but considering that the aim is to achieve maximum response, imatinib is usually given for 6–12 months.

For localized GIST, a 3-year **adjuvant** treatment with imatinib is recommended for high-risk tumors (→ see Tables 108.5 and 108.6), the 5-year disease-free survival being about 70%. Since tumor rupture at the time of surgery is a well-known

Table 108.5 Risk classification for primary GIST as described in Miettinen (2006a, b)

Tumor parameters		Risk of progressive disease			
Mitotic index[a]	Size	Stomach	Duodenum	Jejunum-ileum	Rectum
≤5 per 50 HPF	≤2 cm	Very low (≈ 0%)	Very low (≈ 0%)	Very low (≈ 0%)	Very low (≈ 0%)
	>2 ≤ 5 cm	Very low (1.9%)	Low (8.3%)	Low (4.3%)	Low (8.5%)
	>5 ≤ 10 cm	Low (3.6%)	No data	Moderate (24%)	No data
	>10 cm	Moderate (10%)	High (34%)	High (52%)	High (57%)
>5 per 50 HPF	≤2 cm	Very low (≈ 0%)	No data	High	High (54%)
	>2 ≤ 5 cm	Moderate (16%)	High (50%)	High (73%)	High (52%)
	>5 ≤ 10 cm	High (55%)	No data	High (85%)	No data
	>10 cm	High (86%)	High (86%)	High (90%)	High (71%)

This classification has been adopted by the National Comprehensive Cancer Network. The recurrence risk is evaluated as high (>30%), moderate (10–30%), low (<10%), or very low (0–2%)

[a]Mitotic count is determined by Miettinen on a 5 mm² surface, not on 50 HPF (5 mm² correspond to 20–25 HPF on modern microscopes)

<table>
<tr><td rowspan="9">Table 108.6 Risk classification for primary GIST as described in Fletcher (2002)</td><td>Risk category</td><td>Tumor size</td><td>Mitotic count</td></tr>
<tr><td>Very low risk</td><td><2 cm</td><td><5 per 50 HPF</td></tr>
<tr><td>Low risk</td><td>2–5 cm</td><td><5 per 50 HPF</td></tr>
<tr><td>Intermediate risk</td><td><5 cm</td><td>6–10 per 50 HPF</td></tr>
<tr><td>5–10 cm</td><td><5 per 50 HPF</td></tr>
<tr><td>High risk</td><td>>5 cm</td><td>>5 per 50 HPF</td></tr>
<tr><td>>10 cm</td><td>Any mitotic rate</td></tr>
<tr><td>Any size</td><td>>10 per 50 HPF</td></tr>
</table>

This classification has been endorsed by the National Institutes of Health. The recurrence risk is evaluated as high (>30%), moderate (10–30%), low (< 10%), or very low (0–2%)

risk factor for peritoneal recurrence, these patients should be considered for adjuvant therapy as well.

In the **metastatic** setting, some GISTs can be controlled for many years with imatinib although many develop resistance due to secondary KIT mutations. Imatinib is associated with a tumor response >50% (which increases to 80% when stable disease is considered) and has extended the median overall survival for patients with metastatic GIST from 1.5 to 5 years. In the metastatic setting, treatment with imatinib should be continued indefinitely, since treatment interruption is generally followed by relatively rapid tumor progression. When feasible, surgical excision of residual metastatic disease (in responding patients) has been shown to be associated with a good prognosis, although it has not been demonstrated prospectively whether this is due to surgery or to patient selection. In the case of tumor progression on 400 mg, an option may be to increase the imatinib dose to 800 mg daily.

In the case of confirmed progression or rare intolerance to imatinib, the approved second-line treatment is sunitinib.[8] Regorafenib[9] is currently approved as the third-line medication after failure to imatinib and sunitinib.

In 2020, the FDA has approved avapritinib[10] for the treatment of unresectable or metastatic GIST carrying mutations in exon 18 of PDGFRA that render tumors insensitive to all previously approved therapies.

Suggested Readings

Anon (2020) Avapritinib approved for GIST subgroup. Cancer Discov Epub ahead of print]

---

[8] Sunitinib: tyrosine kinase inhibitor targeting the following—PDGFR, VEGFR, KIT, FLT3, CSF1R, RET.

[9] Regorafenib: tyrosine kinase inhibitor targeting the following—RET, VEGFR1, VEGFR2, VEGFR3, KIT, PDGFRA, PDGFRB, FGFR1, FGFR2.

[10] Avapritinib: tyrosine kinase inhibitor targeting the following—PDGFRA, KIT.

Blanke (2008) Phase III randomized, intergroup trial assessing imatinib mesylate at two dose levels in patients with unresectable or metastatic gastrointestinal stromal tumors expressing the kit receptor tyrosine kinase: S0033. J Clin Oncol 26(4):626–632

Casali (2015) Time to definitive failure to the first tyrosine kinase inhibitor in localized GI stromal tumors treated with Imatinib as an adjuvant: A European Organisation for Research and Treatment of Cancer Soft Tissue and Bone Sarcoma Group Intergroup Randomized Trial in Collaboration With the Australasian Gastro-Intestinal Trials Group, UNICANCER, French Sarcoma Group, Italian Sarcoma Group, and Spanish Group for Research on Sarcomas. J Clin Oncol 33(36):4276–4283

Casali (2018) Gastrointestinal stromal tumours: ESMO-EURACAN Clinical Practice Guidelines for diagnosis, treatment and follow-up. Ann Oncol 29(Suppl 4):iv68–iv78

Dematteo (2009) Adjuvant imatinib mesylate after resection of localised, primary gastrointestinal stromal tumour: a randomised, double-blind, placebo-controlled trial. Lancet 373(9669):1097–1104

Demetri (2006) Efficacy and safety of sunitinib in patients with advanced gastrointestinal stromal tumour after failure of imatinib: a randomised controlled trial. Lancet 368(9544):1329–1338

Demetri (2013) Efficacy and safety of regorafenib for advanced gastrointestinal stromal tumours after failure of imatinib and sunitinib (GRID): an international, multicentre, randomised, placebo-controlled, phase 3 trial. Lancet 381(9863):295–302

Duffaud (2014) Conservative surgery vs. duodeneopancreatectomy in primary duodenal gastrointestinal stromal tumors (GIST): a retrospective review of 114 patients from the French sarcoma group (FSG). Eur J Surg Oncol 40(10):1369–1375

Falkenhorst (2019) New therapeutic agents in gastrointestinal stromal tumours. Curr Opin Oncol 31(4):322–328

Fletcher (2002) Diagnosis of gastrointestinal stromal tumors: a consensus approach. Hum Pathol 33(5):459–465

Fletcher (2020) WHO classification of tumours of soft tissue and bone, 5th ed.

Gold (2009) Development and validation of a prognostic nomogram for recurrence-free survival after complete surgical resection of localised primary gastrointestinal stromal tumour: a retrospective analysis. Lancet Oncol 10(11):1045–1052

Hemming (2018) Translational insights into gastrointestinal stromal tumor and current clinical advances. Ann Oncol 29(10):2037–2045

Hirota (2018) Differential diagnosis of gastrointestinal stromal tumor by histopathology and immunohistochemistry. Transl Gastroenterol Hepatol 3:27

Jones (2014) Practical aspects of risk assessment in gastrointestinal stromal tumors. J Gastrointest Cancer 45(3):262–267

Joensuu (2016) Adjuvant Imatinib for high-risk GI stromal tumor: analysis of a randomized trial. J Clin Oncol 34(3):244–250

Judson (2017) UK clinical practice guidelines for the management of gastrointestinal stromal tumours (GIST). Clin Sarcoma Res 7:6

Karakas (2019) Dedifferentiated gastrointestinal stromal tumor: recent advances. Ann Diagn Pathol 39:118–124

Landi (2019) Gastrointestinal stromal tumours (GISTs): French Intergroup Clinical Practice Guidelines for diagnosis, treatments and follow-up (SNFGE, FFCD, GERCOR, UNICANCER, SFCD, SFED, SFRO). Dig Liver Dis 51(9):1223–1231

Laurent (2019) Adjuvant therapy with imatinib in gastrointestinal stromal tumors (GISTs)-review and perspectives. Transl Gastroenterol Hepatol 4:24

Le Cesne (2010) Discontinuation of imatinib in patients with advanced gastrointestinal stromal tumours after 3 years of treatment: an open-label multicentre randomised phase 3 trial. Lancet Oncol 11(10):942–949

Liu (2017) Randomized clinical trials in gastrointestinal stromal tumors. Surg Oncol Clin N Am 26(4):545–557

Mantese (2019) Gastrointestinal stromal tumor: epidemiology, diagnosis, and treatment. Curr Opin Gastroenterol 35(6):555–559

Mason (2016) Conventional risk stratification fails to predict progression of succinate dehydrogenase-deficient gastrointestinal stromal tumors: a clinicopathologic study of 76 cases. Am J Surg Pathol 40(12):1616–1621

Miettinen (2006a) Gastrointestinal stromal tumors of the jejunum and ileum: a clinicopathologic, immunohistochemical, and molecular genetic study of 906 cases before imatinib with long-term follow-up. Am J Surg Pathol 30(4):477–489

Miettinen (2006b) Gastrointestinal stromal tumors: pathology and prognosis at different sites. Semin Diagn Pathol 23(2):70–83

Mir (2016) Pazopanib plus best supportive care versus best supportive care alone in advanced gastrointestinal stromal tumours resistant to imatinib and sunitinib (PAZOGIST): a randomised, multicentre, open-label phase 2 trial. Lancet Oncol 17(5):632–641

Niinuma (2018) Molecular characterization and pathogenesis of gastrointestinal stromal tumor. Transl Gastroenterol Hepatol 3:2

Osoegawa (2019) Mucosal incision-assisted biopsy versus endoscopic ultrasound-guided fine-needle aspiration with a rapid on-site evaluation for gastric subepithelial lesions: a randomized cross-over study. Dig Endosc 31(4):413–421

Pantaleo (2017) Genome-wide analysis identifies MEN1 and MAX mutations and a neuroendocrine-like molecular heterogeneity in quadruple WT GIST. Mol Cancer Res 15(5):553–562

Prior (2009) Early prediction of response to sunitinib after imatinib failure by ^{18}F-fluorodeoxyglucose positron emission tomography in patients with gastrointestinal stromal tumor. J Clin Oncol 27(3):439–445

Verweij (2004) Progression-free survival in gastrointestinal stromal tumours with high-dose imatinib: randomised trial. Lancet 364(9440):1127–1134

Mehren v (2018) Gastrointestinal stromal tumors. J Clin Oncol 36(2):136–143

Wang (2019) Mutational testing in gastrointestinal stromal tumor. Curr Cancer Drug Targets 19(9):688–697

Definition

Genital rhabdomyoma is a benign rhabdomyoblastic neoplasm showing mature skeletal (striated) muscle differentiation. Along with fetal rhabdomyoma and adult rhabdomyoma ($\rightarrow$ see dedicated sections), it belongs to the extra-cardiac subgroup of rhabdomyomas ($\rightarrow$ see also Chap. 223).

Epidemiology and Presentation

Genital rhabdomyoma is the rarest of rhabdomyomas and affects the female or male genital tract. Most cases occur in women (usually adults), but males may also be affected. Most cases arise from the vagina, although the vulva and cervix can also be affected. In males, this tumor arises from the spermatic cord, tunica vaginalis, or paratesticular soft tissues. In females, the lesion presents as a painless mass (discovered upon clinical examination) which can cause bleeding. In males, the tumor presents as a scrotal swelling or as a painful mass.

Like all extra-cardiac rhabdomyomas, genital rhabdomyoma is not associated with tuberous sclerosis complex.

Pathology

The lesion is composed of loose fibrous connective tissue with differentiated spindled, polygonal, or elongate rhabdomyoblasts. The microscopic assessment shows neither mitotic figures, cambium layer, spider cells, necrosis, nor nuclear pleomorphism.

Differential diagnosis may be needed with botryoid variant of embryonal rhabdomyosarcoma (usually <25 years old with rapidly growing mass, cambium layer, atypia, and mitotic activity).

© The Editor(s) (if applicable) and The Author(s), under exclusive license to
Springer Nature Switzerland AG 2021
S. Mocellin, *Soft Tissue Tumors*, https://doi.org/10.1007/978-3-030-58710-9_109

Biomarkers

The tumor stains positive for desmin, myogenin, actin, and myosin, whereas it stains negative for cytokeratins, EMA, and CD68.

Prognosis

Genital rhabdomyoma is a benign tumor with excellent prognosis.

Therapy

Surgical excision is the treatment of choice.

Suggested Readings

Fletcher (2013) WHO classification of tumours of soft tissue and bone, 4th edn
Schoolmeester (2018) Genital rhabdomyoma of the lower female genital tract: a study of 12 cases with molecular cytogenetic findings. Int J Gynecol Pathol 37(4):349–355

Definition

Giant cell fibroblastoma (GCF) is a neoplasm with intermediate biological aggressiveness classified among the fibroblastic-myofibroblastic tumors. It is considered a variant of dermatofibrosarcoma protuberans (DFSP → see dedicated section for more details).

Epidemiology and Presentation

GCF is a rare tumor which develops mainly in childhood (mean age: 6 years) with a male predominance (M/F = 2:1). Most lesions arise in the trunk wall, groin, and axillary area, but some cases have been described in extremities and the head and neck. As for DFSP, GCF affects superficial soft tissues, with special regard to dermis and subcutaneous fat. The lesion presents usually as a slow-growing painless cutaneous mass that can be protuberant and even polypoid (mean diameter: 3–4 cm).

Pathology

GCF consists of an ill-defined hypocellular proliferation of spindle cells and scattered giant cells (with a myxoid or collagenous stroma) infiltrating the deep dermis, the subcutaneous fat (with honeycomb or parallel growth patterns and adnexal sparing), and only rarely the superficial skeletal muscle. Giant cells are characteristic of the lesion (hence the name); pseudovascular tissue spaces lined by multinucleated giant cells are often observed. Mitotic activity is low and there is no necrosis. The lesion contains areas of conventional DFSP in about 15% of cases. Rare cases may contain pigmented cells (Bednar tumor), myoid whorls, or fibrosarcomatous areas.

© The Editor(s) (if applicable) and The Author(s), under exclusive license to
Springer Nature Switzerland AG 2021
S. Mocellin, *Soft Tissue Tumors*, https://doi.org/10.1007/978-3-030-58710-9_110

Biomarkers

Both spindle and giant cells are positive for CD34 but negative for SMA, desmin, and S100.

Like DFSP, GCF is characterized by the **chromosomal translocation** t(17,22) (q22;q13), leading to the formation of the COL1A1-PDGFB fusion gene.

Prognosis

GCF is a locally aggressive tumor (local disease recurrence occurs in about half cases) with no metastatic potential.

Therapy

Surgical excision is the treatment of choice.

Suggested Readings

Fletcher (2020) WHO classification of tumours of soft tissue and bone, 5th ed.
Iwasaki (2019) Current update on the molecular biology of cutaneous sarcoma: dermatofibrosarcoma protuberans. Curr Treat Options in Oncol 20(4):29
Karagianni (2016) Recurrent giant cell fibroblastoma: malignancy predisposition in Kabuki syndrome revisited. Am J Med Genet A 170A(5):1333–1338

Definition

Giant cell tumor (GCT) is a soft tissue tumor with intermediate malignant potential and is classified among fibrohistiocytic tumors. It might represent the counterpart of GCT of bone. It is also known as giant cell tumor of soft tissue (to differentiate it from the giant cell tumor of bone), osteoclastoma of soft tissue, and giant cell tumor of low malignant potential.

Epidemiology and Presentation

GCT may occur at any age but is more frequent in the fifth decade of life, without gender differences. The lesion typically develops in the superficial soft tissues of the upper and lower extremities (70% of cases); less frequently it can be found in the trunk and head and neck. About one fourth of cases are situated deep to muscle fascia.

Clinically, GCT presents as well-circumscribed painless mass ranging in size from 1 to 10 cm (mean: 3 cm). In analogy with giant cell tumor of the bone, calcifications can be observed at radiology imaging.

Pathology

GCT is histologically similar to giant cell tumor of the bone. It characteristically displays a multinodular architecture (nodules ranging in size up to 15 mm); cellular nodules (composed of round to oval mononuclear cells and osteoclast-like giant cells immersed in a richly vascularized stroma) are separated by fibrous septa containing hemosiderin-laden macrophages. Mitotic activity generally ranges from 1 to

S. Mocellin, *Soft Tissue Tumors*, https://doi.org/10.1007/978-3-030-58710-9_111

30 figures per 10 HPF.[1] Atypia, nuclear pleomorphism, and bizarre giant cells are absent, and necrosis is rarely found. Metaplastic bone formation can be found in about half cases. Cystic change with formation of blood-filled lakes (similar to aneurysmal bone cyst) and vascular invasion are observed in about 30% of cases.

Although GCT soft tissue shows a striking histological resemblance to GCT of bone, the two entities appear to be genetically distinct.

Differential diagnosis might be needed with the following: GCT of tendon sheaths, cellular dermatofibroma with osteoclast-like giant cells, ossifying dermato-fibroma with osteoclast-like giant cells, reparative giant cell granuloma, nodular fasciitis, leiomyosarcoma with osteoclast-like giant cells, epithelioid sarcoma with giant cells, extraskeletal osteosarcoma, atypical fibroxanthoma with osteoclast-like giant cells, and plexiform fibrohistiocytic tumor.

Biomarkers

GCT stains positive for CD68 (multinucleated giant cells) and SMA[2] (mononuclear cells). Mononuclear cells express RANKL[3] (an activator of osteoclast activity).

Prognosis

GCT is associated with a local recurrence rate of 12% (incomplete surgical excision is associated with an increased risk) and very rare cases of distant metastasis. No clinicopathological prognostic factors have been thus far identified.

Giant cell tumor of the soft tissues is associated with a lower local recurrence rate compared to GCT of bone but with a higher metastatic and death rate: thus, close clinical follow-up is recommended.

Therapy

Surgical excision is the treatment of choice. While denosumab (a monoclonal anti-body against RANKL) has been approved for the treatment of GCT of bone, no data exist on the use of this target therapy for GCT of soft tissue.

---

[1] HPF: high-power field.

[2] SMA: smooth muscle actin.

[3] RANKL: receptor activator of nuclear factor kappa-B Ligand, which is currently better named TNF superfamily member 11 (TNFSF11), encodes a member of the tumor necrosis factor (TNF) cytokine family that acts as a ligand for osteoprotegerin and promotes osteoclast differentiation and activation.

Suggested Readings

Aramin (2019) Skin and superficial soft tissue neoplasms with multinucleated giant cells: clinical, histologic, phenotypic, and molecular differentiating features. Ann Diagn Pathol 42:18–32
Fletcher (2020) WHO classification of tumours of soft tissue and bone, 5th edn
López-Pousa (2015) Giant cell tumour of bone: new treatments in development. Clin Transl Oncol 17(6):419–430
Mavrogenis (2019) Giant Cell Tumor of Soft Tissue: A Rare Entity. Orthopedics 42(4):e364–e369

Definition

Glomeruloid hemangioma (GHA) is a benign tumor of vascular origin.

Epidemiology and Presentation

GHA is an extremely rare skin tumor: it presents as small, red-to-violaceous cutaneous papules, usually on the trunk and proximal extremities.

Etiology and Predisposition

GHA is observed exclusively in patients with the so-called POEMS syndrome (polyneuropathy, organomegaly, endocrinopathy, monoclonal protein, skin lesions). Such lesions are observed in up to 45% of patients with this syndrome. Although patients with POEMS syndrome may develop other benign vascular tumors (e.g., cherry hemangioma), GHA is specific for this syndrome.

The lesion may appear well before the full POEMS syndrome develops: therefore, a follow-up of patients with diagnosis of GHA is recommended for early identification of other POEMS manifestations.

Pathology

GHA is located in the dermis and consists of collections of ectatic small vessels containing intraluminal nests of proliferating capillaries, which mimics kidney glomeruli. A distinctive feature is the presence of large, vacuolated endothelial cells that contain eosinophilic protein-derived material (polytypic immunoglobulin).

© The Editor(s) (if applicable) and The Author(s), under exclusive license to
Springer Nature Switzerland AG 2021
S. Mocellin, *Soft Tissue Tumors*, https://doi.org/10.1007/978-3-030-58710-9_112

Biomarkers

GHA stains positive for biomarkers of normal endothelium, such as CD31 and CD34.

Prognosis

GHA per se is an innocuous lesion. However, patients with POEMS syndrome have a poor prognosis (5-year survival rate: approximately 60%).

Therapy

Surgical excision is requested for diagnostic purposes more than for cure.

Suggested Reading

Lee (2017) Glomeruloid hemangioma as a marker for the early diagnosis of POEMS syndrome. Ann Dermatol 2017;29(2):249-251

Definition

Glomus tumor is a neoplasm with variable clinical behavior and is classified pericytic (perivascular) tumors. Other names: glomangioma, glomic tumor, glomangiopericytoma, glomangiomyoma, glomuvenous malformation, malignant glomus tumor, and glomangiosarcoma.

Epidemiology and Presentation

Glomus tumor is a rare mesenchymal neoplasm accounting for <2% of soft tissue tumors. Multiple lesions may be observed in 10% of patients. Most lesions are diagnosed in young adults, although it may occur at any age, without gender prevalence (except for subungual lesions, which are much more common in females with a 3:1 ratio). Most lesions occur in the distal extremities (skin or superficial soft tissues), with special regard to the subungual region, the hand, the wrist, and the foot. Rare cases have been reported in almost every body site, including viscera (e.g., kidney, stomach) and bones. The rare malignant variant is usually deeply situated, but may be cutaneous. Clinically, skin glomus tumors are usually small (<1 cm), red-blue nodules often associated with a long history of pain (especially upon cold exposure or minor pressure). Deeply seated or visceral glomus tumors present as a nonspecific mass.

Etiology and Predisposition

(a) The vascular tumors in blue rubber bleb nevus syndrome (BRBNS) are commonly known as glomovenous malformations. This rare sporadically occurring disorder is a condition in which the blood vessels do not develop properly in an area of the skin or other body organ, particularly the bowel. The vascular lesion

379

S. Mocellin, *Soft Tissue Tumors*, https://doi.org/10.1007/978-3-030-58710-9_113

is called "nevus" (hence the name). The lesions are congenital even though they may not be visible until later in life; skin lesions can be painful, while intestinal nevi can bleed spontaneously and cause anemia or other complications. Glomovenous malformations are caused by autosomal dominant mutations in glomulin (GLMN) gene (the penetrance varying from 80% at the age of 20 years to 100% at 30 years) which is predominantly expressed in vascular smooth muscle cells).

(b) An association between digital glomus tumor and neurofibromatosis type I (NF1) has been reported, with frequent involvement of multiple digits.

Pathology

The tumor is composed of cells resembling the modified smooth muscle cells of the normal glomus body (small, uniform, and rounded with a centrally placed, round nucleus), a specialized arteriovenous anastomosis that regulates heat in the skin and is surrounded by layers of epithelioid, SMA-positive glomus cells.

Solid glomus tumor comprises approximately 75% of cases: it is composed of nests of glomus cells surrounding capillary-sized vessels. Glomovenous malformation, also known as glomangioma, is commonest in patients with multiple or familial lesions, comprises approximately 20% of cases, and is characterized by cavernous hemangioma-like vascular structures surrounded by small clusters of glomus cells. Glomangiomyoma shows transition from typical glomus cells to elongated cells resembling mature smooth muscle. In glomangiopericytoma, a branching, hemangiopericytoma-like vasculature is present. Symplastic glomus tumor shows striking nuclear atypia in the absence of any other features indicative of negative outcome (e.g., large size, deep location, mitotic activity, necrosis).

The diagnosis of "malignant glomus tumor" (also known as glomangiosarcoma) should be reserved for lesions showing (a) marked nuclear atypia and any level of mitotic activity or (b) atypical mitotic figures. There are two types of malignant glomus tumor: in the first, the malignant component resembles a leiomyosarcoma or fibrosarcoma; in the second, the malignant component consists of sheets of highly malignant-appearing round cells. Immunohistochemical demonstration of SMA expression and pericellular type IV collagen is required for this diagnosis, in the absence of a clear-cut benign precursor. A glomus tumor not fulfilling the criteria for malignancy but showing at least one atypical feature other than nuclear pleomorphism should be defined as "glomus tumor of uncertain malignant potential."

Finally, although in the past glomus tumors greater than 2 cm in size and deep location were considered "malignant," subsequent experience suggests that these have "uncertain malignant potential."

Differential diagnosis may be needed with the following: myopericytoma and other pericytic tumors (→ see dedicated sections; histologic and immunohistochemical overlap in areas with more prominent spindled differentiation); benign adnexal tumors like nodular hidradenoma/eccrine spiradenoma (variable epithelial or sebaceous differentiation, positivity for cytokeratins and negativity for SMA);

paraganglioma (prominent Zellballen growth pattern, positivity for synaptophysin, chromogranin, and S100); neuroendocrine tumor (salt and pepper chromatin; negative for SMA and positive for cytokeratin, synaptophysin, and chromogranin); dermal nevus (nests of melanocytes, with or without pigmentation, lacking association with blood vessels; positive for S100 and melanocytic biomarkers; negative for SMA and h-caldesmon); and angioleiomyoma (bundles of smooth muscle cells that lack a prominent round cell component; desmin typically positive).

Biomarkers

Glomus tumors of all types typically express SMA and show abundant pericellular production of type IV collagen. Staining for h-caldesmon, vimentin, and SMA is also positive.

It negatively stains for the following: cytokeratin, CD31, S100, HMB45, CD117, desmin, chromogranin, synaptophysin, CD20, CD45, and WT1.

NOTCH-base fusion genes have been described in many (but not all) glomus tumors examined.

Prognosis

Most glomus tumors are benign neoplasms; nevertheless, glomovenous malformations of the bowel can be lethal due to severe bleeding. Malignant glomus tumors are exceedingly rare; they are particularly aggressive, with metastases and death from disease in up to 40% of patients. Glomus tumors of uncertain malignant potential may behave aggressively.

Therapy

Surgery is the mainstay of treatment (the reported recurrence rate of 10% is likely due to incomplete resection).

As regards target therapy, mTOR inhibitors (e.g., sirolimus) have been reported to be effective for the treatment of glomovenous malformations in patients with blue rubber bleb nevus syndrome.

Suggested Readings

Amyere (2013) Somatic uniparental isodisomy explains multifocality of glomuvenous malformations. Am J Hum Genet 92(2):188–196

Borroni (2014) Incomplete penetrance of GLMN gene c.395-1G>C mutation in a family with glomuvenous malformations. Int J Dermatol 53(11):1362–1364

Chang (2019) Pericytes in sarcomas and other mesenchymal tumors. Adv Exp Med Biol 1147:109–124

Chen (2020) Glomus tumor of the colon: a rare case report and review of literature. Int J Surg Pathol [Epub ahead of print]

Fletcher (2020) WHO classification of tumours of soft tissue and bone, 5th ed.

Isoldi (2019) Diagnosis and management of children with Blue Rubber Bleb Nevus Syndrome: a multi-center case series. Dig Liver Dis 51(11):1537–1546

Mosquera (2013) Novel MIR143-NOTCH fusions in benign and malignant glomus tumors. Genes Chromosomes Cancer 52(11):1075–1087

Nakajima (2018) Blue Rubber Bleb Nevus Syndrome with long-term follow-up: a case report and review of the literature. Case Rep Gastrointest Med 2018:8087659

Nambi (2019) Excision of subungual glomus tumor by subungual approach: a useful yet underutilized technique. J Cutan Aesthet Surg 12(3):187–190

Santoshi (2019) Glomus tumor of the fingertips: a frequently missed diagnosis. J Family Med Prim Care 8(3):904–908

Definition

Granular cell tumor (GCT) is a benign neoplasm classified among nerve sheath tumors. It is also known as granular cell schwannoma, granular cell nerve sheath tumor, granular cell myoblastoma, and Abrikossoff tumor. For details on malignant granular cell tumor → see dedicated section.

Epidemiology and Presentation

GCT is a rare neoplasm typically occurring in adults in the fourth to sixth decade of life (although it can develop at any age), with a male prevalence (M/F = 2.5:1); it is also more common in African-Americans.

The most frequent site of involvement is the head and neck (including the tongue); other locations are the breast and proximal extremities. GCT usually arises in the cutis/subcutis or submucosa, but visceral involvement (especially gastrointestinal and respiratory tracts) is also common. While most lesions are solitary, up to 10% are multiple. Clinically, it presents as an asymptomatic slow-growing nodule (size: 0.5–3 cm), but GCT can be painful in the skin and tongue. Cutaneous lesions are firm, flesh-colored to reddish-brown.

Etiology and Predisposition

Multiple GCTs may be part of the **Noonan syndrome**, a condition characterized by mildly unusual facial features, short stature, heart defects, bleeding problems, skeletal malformations, predisposition to some tumors (e.g., leukemia and granular cell tumor), and many other signs and symptoms.

S. Mocellin, *Soft Tissue Tumors*, https://doi.org/10.1007/978-3-030-58710-9_114

Along with cardiofaciocutaneous syndrome, Costello syndrome, neurofibromatosis type 1, and Legius syndrome, Noonan syndrome is a RASopathy (syndromes due to the alteration of the RAS signaling pathway).

Noonan syndrome occurs in approximately 1 out of 1000–2500 people and is inherited in an autosomal dominant pattern.

Mutations in multiple genes can cause Noonan syndrome. Mutations in the PTPN11 gene cause about 50% of all cases.[1] Other causal mutations are located in the SOS1 gene (10–15% of cases), RAF1 gene (5%), and RIT1 gene (5%) (see footnote 1). For the other cases, the responsible gene has not yet been identified. Many of the mutations in the genes associated with Noonan syndrome cause the activation of the corresponding protein which in turn leads to cell proliferation.

Pathology

GCT is a neoplasm showing neuroectodermal differentiation (likely Schwann cell type) and composed of large, oval to round cells with abundant eosinophilic and distinctively granular cytoplasm, organized in nests and trabeculae. Mitoses are variable in number but not numerous. The granular appearance of the cytoplasm (hence the name) is due to massive accumulation of lysosomes. Perineural infiltration is common. For lesions arising below the squamous epithelium (e.g., GCT of the skin, tongue, and esophagus), pseudoepitheliomatous hyperplasia is sometimes present and may need to be differentiated from squamous cell carcinoma.

Differential diagnosis may be needed with the following: reactive histiocytic lesions such as mycobacterial pseudotumor/histoid leprosy (presence of acid-fast bacilli, often in immunocompromised patients; S100 negative); malakoplakia (histiocytic proliferation with small calcospherocytes called Michaelis-Gutmann bodies; S100 negative); Rosai-Dorfman disease (syncytial proliferation with lymphoid background and emperipolesis; positive for S100 and CD68); granular cell reaction (cells surround nodules of granular, amorphous debris and are filled with an acid-fast and autofluorescent ceroid lipofuscin substance); crystal storing histiocytosis (cells filled with refractile crystalline material such as immunoglobulin, Charcot-Leyden, or clofazimine crystals; S100 negative); cellular spindled histiocytic pseudotumor complicating fat necrosis (arises in the setting of fat necrosis around the breast; S100 negative); alveolar soft part sarcoma (alveolar pattern, prominent nucleoli, cytoplasm filled with more crystalline material and glycogen; usually variable/focal S100 positivity; TFE3 is positive as in GCT); rhabdomyoma (cytoplasmic vacuolization, rare spider cells, cross striations, or inclusions can be observed; positive for desmin, MyoD1, and myogenin, negative for S100); hibernoma (multivacuolated cells and admixed mature fat can be observed; S100 is more variable; negative for CD68); congenital granular cell tumor (also known as congenital epulis; exclusively in newborns, typically in the alveolar ridge; prominent stromal

---

[1] The PTPN11, SOS1, RAF1, and RIT1 genes encode proteins involved in the RAS/MAPK cell signaling pathway, which is involved in many cell activities including cell proliferation.

capillaries, overlying epithelium ulcerated; negative for S100 and CD68); and tumors that can (though) rarely have granular cell morphology (melanoma, ameloblastoma, benign fibrous histiocytoma, leiomyoma, leiomyosarcoma, angiosarcoma, undifferentiated pleomorphic sarcoma, atypical fibroxanthoma).

Biomarkers

GCT stains usually positive for S100, SOX10, CD68, CD63, inhibin-A, EMA,[2] and NSE.[3] MITF and TFE3 are expressed in most cases, but HMB45 and Melan-A are not expressed. Staining for CD31, CD34, SMA,[4] desmin, NFP,[5] GFAP,[6] synaptophysin, chromogranin, and cytokeratins is also negative. Cytoplasmatic granules are PAS positive and diastase resistant.

Sporadic GCT does not carry (somatic) mutations in PTPN11 (like those associated with Noonan syndrome), but carry (somatic) inactivating mutations in endosomal pH regulators ATP6AP1 or ATP6AP2 in 72% of cases (providing a link between the cardinal feature of lysosome accumulation and tumorigenesis).

Prognosis

GCT is a benign neoplasm, although local recurrence is possible, especially after incomplete excision. For details on malignant granular cell tumor → see dedicated section.

Therapy

Surgery is the treatment of choice.

Suggested Readings

Barakat (2018) Gastrointestinal and biliary granular cell tumor: diagnosis and management. Ann Gastroenterol 31(4):439–447
Fletcher (2020) WHO classification of tumours of soft tissue and bone, 5th ed.
França (2018) Sporadic granular cell tumours lack recurrent mutations in PTPN11, PTEN and other cancer-related genes. J Clin Pathol 71(1):93–94
Meani (2019) Granular cell tumor of the breast: a multidisciplinary challenge. Crit Rev. Oncol Hematol 144:102828

---

[2] EMA: epithelial membrane antigen.

[3] NSE: neuron-specific enolase.

[4] SMA: smooth muscle actin.

[5] NFP: neurofilament protein.

[6] GFAP: glial fibrillary acidic protein.

Mobarki (2020) Granular cell tumor a study of 42 cases and systemic review of the literature. Pathol Res Pract [Epub ahead of print]

Moten (2018) Granular cell tumor experience at a comprehensive cancer center. J Surg Res 226:1–7

Pareja (2018) Loss-of-function mutations in ATP6AP1 and ATP6AP2 in granular cell tumors. Nat Commun 9(1):3533

Definition

Hemangioblastoma is a benign tumor of vascular origin (tumor of grade I according to the World Health Organization).

Epidemiology and Presentation

This is a rare neoplasm of the central nervous system (most often arising in the cerebellum or spinal cord) where it represents about 2% of all tumors. It presents in adults with dizziness, headache, bladder or bowel dysfunction, numbness, weakness, and pain in the upper or lower extremities.

Polycythemia due to the ectopic production of erythropoietin by tumor cells can be present as a paraneoplastic syndrome.

Exceptional cases located outside of the central nervous system (e.g., kidney, retroperitoneum) have been reported.

Etiology and Predisposition

Hemangioblastoma can be sporadic (about 70% of cases) or associated with the **von Hippel-Lindau** (VHL) **disease**, a cancer predisposition syndrome inherited as an autosomal dominant trait and due to the loss of function of the VHL gene that leads to increased activity of hypoxia-inducible factor (HIF), which in turn increases the levels of angiogenic factors such as VEGF. Besides hemangioblastoma of the cerebellum and retina, the VHL syndrome also includes the development cysts of the liver and pancreas, pheochromocytoma, and kidney cancer.

© The Editor(s) (if applicable) and The Author(s), under exclusive license to
Springer Nature Switzerland AG 2021
S. Mocellin, *Soft Tissue Tumors*, https://doi.org/10.1007/978-3-030-58710-9_115

Pathology

Macroscopically, it presents as a well-circumscribed mural nodule (which contains the tumor cells) associated with a large fluid-filled cyst (hence, it is important to obtain a frozen section of the mural nodule, and not of the cyst wall).

Differential diagnosis may be needed with renal cell carcinoma (nuclear atypia, mitotic figures, cytokeratin positive, EMA positive, NSE negative).

Biomarkers

Hemangioblastoma stains positive for NSE,[1] reticulin, and CD34. It stains negative for EMA,[2] cytokeratins, and CD10.

Prognosis

The prognosis is good as long as the tumor is amenable to complete surgical excision, which is the case in most patients.

Therapy

Surgical excision is the treatment of choice (microsurgical resection or stereotactic radiosurgery).

Suggested Readings

Aronow (2019) Von Hippel-Lindau disease: update on pathogenesis and systemic aspects. Retina [Epub ahead of print]

Bisceglia (2018) Extraneuraxial hemangioblastoma: clinicopathologic features and review of the literature. Adv Anat Pathol 25(3):197–215

Pan (2018) Stereotactic radiosurgery for central nervous system hemangioblastoma: systematic review and meta-analysis. J Neurooncol 137(1):11–22

---

[1] NSE: neuron-specific enolase.

[2] EMA: epithelial membrane antigen.

Hemangioendotheliomas are a group of tumors of vascular differentiation. For details on single hemangioendothelioma types, → see the sections dedicated to each of the following tumors:

- Composite hemangioendothelioma
- Epithelioid hemangioendothelioma
- Histiocytoid hemangioendothelioma (→ see Chap. 83)
- Hobnail hemangioendothelioma (→ see Chap. 197)
- Kaposiform hemangioendothelioma
- Pseudomyogenic hemangioendothelioma
- Malignant hemangioendothelioma (→ see Chap. 25)
- Retiform hemangioendothelioma
- Spindle cell hemangioendothelioma (→ see Chap. 235)

Definition

Hemangioma is a benign blood-containing vascular tumor, as opposed to lymphangioma which is a lymph-containing lesion. Since lymphangioma is by far much less frequent, hemangioma is often simply called angioma.

The nomenclature regarding vascular anomalies (tumors and malformations) is not always consistent in the literature: a dedicated classification of anomalies is provided by the International Society for the Study of Vascular Anomalies (ISSVA, *www.issva.org*).

According to the diameter of the vascular channels forming the lesion, it is classified as capillary hemangioma (small vascular channels) and cavernous hemangioma (large vascular channels).

For details on the following types of hemangioma, → see dedicated sections:

- Anastomosing hemangioma
- Arteriovenous malformation hemangioma
- Cherry hemangioma
- Congenital hemangioma
- Glomeruloid hemangioma
- Hepatic hemangioma
- Hobnail hemangioma
- Infantile hemangioma
- Intramuscular hemangioma
- Lobular capillary hemangioma (→ see Chap. 220)
- Microvenular hemangioma
- Spindle cell hemangioma
- Synovial hemangioma
- Tufted hemangioma

- Venous hemangioma
- Epithelioid hemangioma
- Tufted hemangioma

Epidemiology and Presentation

Hemangioma (which can be congenital or acquired) is overall a frequently occurring lesion and can arise in virtually any site of the body, the most frequent locations being the skin and liver. In the skin, liver, and spleen, hemangioma represents the most common primary tumor. Depending on the location (and the size), symptoms can vary from completely absent to life-threatening. For instance, gastrointestinal hemangioma (which can affect more frequently the small bowel, where it represents about 10% of all benign tumors of this site) can lead to bleeding (most frequent), occlusion, and perforation. Yet, hemangioma of the kidney or bladder is a very rare cause of bleeding in the urinary tract. For more details on hemangioma complications, → see specific hemangioma types.

Pathology

Hemangioma is characterized by endothelial cell proliferation and should be distinguished from vascular malformations (e.g., port-wine stain, telangiectasia, angiokeratoma, arteriovenous malformation), which are always congenital and are caused by defects of vascular morphogenesis.

For details on single hemangioma types, → see the following dedicated sections:

Biomarkers

Hemangioma typically stains positive for endothelial cell biomarkers.

For details on single hemangioma types, → see the following dedicated sections:

Prognosis

Hemangioma is a benign lesion and the prognosis in most cases is definitely favorable. However, in rare cases specific types of hemangiomas can lead to even lethal complications (such as Kasabach-Merritt syndrome in tufted hemangioma of the liver).

Therapy

In most cases, no therapy is needed. The treatment of specific hemangiomas is described in the dedicated sections.

Definition

Hemosiderotic fibrolipomatous tumor (HFT) is a neoplasm of uncertain differentiation and intermediate malignant potential. It is also referred to as hemosiderotic fibrohistiocytic lipomatous lesion.

Epidemiology and Presentation

HFT develops most frequently in females during the fifth to and sixth decade of life. It affects mainly the foot (dorsum), followed by ankle, hand (dorsum), calf, thigh, and cheek. The lesion typically presents as a slowly growing, sometimes painful, subcutaneous mass of variable size (mean diameter, 8 cm; maximum, 20 cm).

Pathology

HFT is an unencapsulated tumor composed of fascicles of fibroblastic spindle cells containing hemosiderin, admixed with adipocytes, hemosiderin-laden macrophages, osteoclast-like giant cells, and scattered chronic inflammatory cells. Mitoses and necrosis are generally absent, and atypia is rare.

HFT may display hybrid features with myxoinflammatory fibroblastic sarcoma (→ see dedicated section).

Biomarkers

The spindled cells are positive for CD34 and calponin and negative for S100, h-caldesmon, desmin, and cytokeratins.

© The Editor(s) (if applicable) and The Author(s), under exclusive license to Springer Nature Switzerland AG 2021
S. Mocellin, *Soft Tissue Tumors*, https://doi.org/10.1007/978-3-030-58710-9_118

In a subset of cases, the **chromosomal translocation** t(1;10)(p22;q24) leads to the formation of the TGFBR3-MGEA5 fusion gene (whose functional effect appears to be the transcriptional upregulation of the FGF8 gene, located close to MGEA5 on chromosome 10), which has been described also in pleomorphic hyalinizing angiectatic tumor (→ see dedicated section) and myxoinflammatory fibroblastic sarcoma (→ see dedicated section). VGLL3 amplification has also been reported. Unlike myxoinflammatory fibroblastic sarcoma, HFT does not carry BRAF rearrangements.

Prognosis

HFT is a locally aggressive tumor with a rate of local recurrence of 30–50% (especially in case of incomplete resection).

Therapy

Wide surgical excision is the standard treatment.

Suggested Readings

Boland (2017) Hemosiderotic fibrolipomatous tumor, pleomorphic hyalinizing angiectatic tumor, and myxoinflammatory fibroblastic sarcoma: related or not? Adv Anat Pathol 24(5):268–277
Fletcher (2020) WHO classification of tumours of soft tissue and bone, 5th ed.
Kao (2017) Recurrent BRAF gene rearrangements in myxoinflammatory fibroblastic sarcomas, but not hemosiderotic fibrolipomatous tumors. Am J Surg Pathol 41(11):1456–1465
Liu (2019) The t(1;10)(p22;q24) TGFBR3/MGEA5 Translocation in pleomorphic hyalinizing angiectatic tumor, myxoinflammatory fibroblastic sarcoma, and hemosiderotic fibrolipomatous tumor. Arch Pathol Lab Med 143(2):212–221

Definition

Hepatic angiosarcoma (HAS) is the liver localization of angiosarcoma ($\rightarrow$ see dedicated section). It is also known as liver angiosarcoma.

Epidemiology and Presentation

HAS accounts for approximately 5% of all angiosarcomas and 2% of primary liver malignancies (it ranks third after hepatocellular carcinoma and cholangiocarcinoma and represents the most frequent type of liver sarcoma). Unlike other hepatic cancers, it develops in otherwise healthy liver. The initial presentation of HA is nonspecific (including abdominal pain, weight loss, and fatigue), and no plasma biomarkers are associated with it. As the disease progresses, hepatomegaly, ascites, and jaundice become clinically apparent; spontaneous hemoperitoneum is a potentially fatal complication. In general, liver function is maintained until later stages of the disease, often leading to diagnosis once the disease is already advanced or metastatic.

HAS incidence has a male predominance (M:F = 3:1), with the majority of patients diagnosed in their sixth decade of life.

The tumor may present as a single mass, but the multifocal bilateral growth pattern is the most common type of presentation. Metastases are common at the time of diagnosis, with the lungs, spleen, and bone being the most frequent metastatic sites. Plain computed tomography images of these masses are observed to be hypodense when compared to normal hepatic parenchyma, while lesions observed with contrast-enhanced computed tomography may be either hypodense or hyperdense, depending on the presence of hemorrhage within the tumor. Magnetic resonance imaging may be required to rule out both benign and malignant mimickers.

© The Editor(s) (if applicable) and The Author(s), under exclusive license to
Springer Nature Switzerland AG 2021
S. Mocellin, *Soft Tissue Tumors*, https://doi.org/10.1007/978-3-030-58710-9_119

Etiology and Predisposition

Although HAS has been historically linked to the exposure to chemical carcinogens (e.g., thorotrast, arsenic, vinyl chloride, anabolic steroids, and exogenous estrogens) or ionizing radiation, most cases of HAS are not associated with a causative factor.

Pathology

Pathological examination is needed for diagnosis (and differential diagnosis with other liver neoplasms). For pathological details → see Chap. 25.

Prognosis

HAS is a high-grade, aggressive tumor carrying a dismal prognosis independently of therapy (average life expectancy: 10–12 months). The majority of patients have metastatic disease at the time of presentation. Liver failure, intra-abdominal bleeding (due to liver rupture), and metastatic disease are the usual causes of death.

Therapy

Any treatment has yielded so far poor results. Better prognosis is observed in patients with a single tumor mass, small tumor size, lack of metastases, and negative surgical resection margins. Liver transplant is contraindicated due to the biological aggressiveness of HAS. The tumor is quite chemoresistant and radioresistant. Transarterial embolization might be useful in case of hemoperitoneum by tumor rupture.

Suggested Readings

Li (2018) A pooled analysis of treatment and prognosis of hepatic angiosarcoma in adults. Hepatobiliary Pancreat Dis Int 17(3):198–203

Tripke (2019) Surgical therapy of primary hepatic angiosarcoma. BMC Surg 19(1):5

Wilson (2019) Hepatic angiosarcoma: a multi-institutional, international experience with 44 cases. Ann Surg Oncol 26(2):576–582

Zeng (2020) A pooled analysis of primary hepatic angiosarcoma. Jpn J Clin Oncol Epub ahead of print]

Definition

Hepatic calcifying nested stromal epithelial tumor (CNSET) is a low-grade primary malignancy of the liver and is believed to be of mesenchymal origin (non-hepatocytic and non-biliary origin), although the true histogenesis remains uncertain.

It is also known as calcifying nested stromal epithelial tumor of the liver, ossifying malignant mixed epithelial and stromal tumor, ossifying stromal epithelial tumor, and desmoplastic nested spindle cell tumor of the liver.

Epidemiology and Presentation

This rare primary tumor of the liver occurs in children of all ages (range 2–34 years) with a female predominance (M:F = 1:2.5). It usually presents as a solitary well-demarcated and lobulated mass with variable calcifications.

CNSET has been associated with Beckwith-Wiedemann syndrome, Cushing-type syndrome, and Klinefelter syndrome.

Clinically, no specific features are present: it may present with abdominal pain/distention, normal liver function tests, and normal serum tumor markers such as alpha-fetoprotein (AFP) and carcinoembryonic antigen (CEA). At computed tomography scan, CNSET presents as a well-circumscribed, macrolobulated mass, with enhancement and calcifications; at magnetic resonance imaging, the lesion shows T1 hypointensity and T2 hyperintensity; main differential diagnosis on radiology includes hepatoblastoma, fibrolamellar hepatocellular carcinoma, and calcified hemangioma.

Pathology

Macroscopically it presents as a solitary or multiple, well-demarcated and lobulated mass of 3–30 cm in diameter (mean: 12 cm) with variable calcifications.

Microscopically, CNSET is composed of nests of epithelioid and spindle cells with an associated desmoplastic myofibroblastic stroma and variable calcification or ossification. In most cases, mitotic activity is < 1 per 10 HPF but may be higher. Vascular invasion is rare.

Differential diagnosis may be needed with the following: synovial sarcoma (positive for SYT-SSX1 or SYT-SSX2 fusion genes); hepatoblastoma (presence of fetal or embryonal hepatocytes and the positivity for AFP or HepPar1; extramedullary hematopoiesis is common in fetal and embryonal subtypes); desmoplastic small round cell tumor (typically positive for WT1 and bears characteristic chromosomal translocation); and metastatic gastrointestinal stromal tumor (no desmoplastic stroma; positive for CD34, CD117, and DOG1).

Biomarkers

CNSET stains usually positive for cytokeratins, vimentin, cytoplasmic, and nuclear beta-catenin; it may stain positive for nuclear WT1. It stains negative for synaptophysin, chromogranin A, desmin, CD34, HepPar1, CEA, alpha-fetoprotein (AFP), HMB45, and inhibin-A.

Prognosis

CNSET has an indolent behavior but may recur if not completely excised. Large size, infiltrative growth, vascular invasion, necrosis, and increased mitotic activity are risk factors associated with disease recurrence.

Therapy

Liver resection is the mainstay of treatment. Liver transplantation has been proposed for unresectable lesions. The role of medical treatments is basically unknown.

Suggested Readings

Lefkowitch (2010) Advances in hepatobiliary pathology: update for 2010. Clin Liver Dis 14(4):747–762

Makhlouf (2009) Calcifying nested stromal-epithelial tumors of the liver: a clinicopathologic, immunohistochemical, and molecular genetic study of 9 cases with a long-term follow-up. Am J Surg Pathol 33(7):976–983

Olin (2020) Surgical resection of calcifying nested stromal-epithelial tumor in an adolescent female: a case report. Int J Surg Case Rep 66:1–3

Schaffer (2016) Calcifying nested stromal-epithelial tumor (CNSET) of the liver: a newly recognized entity to be considered in the radiologist's differential diagnosis. Clin Imaging 40(1):137–139

Tsuruta (2018) Calcifying nested stromal epithelial tumor of the liver in a patient with Klinefelter syndrome: a case report and review of the literature. World J Surg Oncol 16(1):227

Definition

Hepatic embryonal sarcoma (HES) is a malignancy classified among soft tissue tumors of uncertain differentiation. It is also known as liver embryonal sarcoma, embryonal sarcoma of the liver, undifferentiated embryonal sarcoma, malignant mesenchymoma of the liver, and mesenchymal sarcoma of the liver.

Epidemiology and Presentation

HES occurs mainly in children (usually between ages of 6 and 10 years, without gender preference), representing 10–15% of pediatric hepatic tumors (in this population it is the third malignancy after hepatoblastoma and hepatocellular carcinoma). Rare cases have been described in adults.

In children, HES has been associated with mesenchymal hamartoma of the liver (→ see dedicated section); some investigators believe that HES might be an evolution of mesenchymal hamartoma (mainly based on cytogenetics similarities).

It typically presents with pain, fever, abdominal mass, and normal serum levels of alpha-fetoprotein (AFP).

Magnetic resonance imaging is helpful in the surgical planning because it may detect vascular invasion, biliary obstruction, and hilar lymphadenopathy.

Pathology

Macroscopically it presents as a solitary, well-demarcated mass (usually 10–30 cm in diameter) with cystic, gelatinous, hemorrhagic, and necrotic foci.

Microscopically the tumor shows a pseudocapsule and is variably cellular with anaplastic, spindled-to-oval cells with prominent PAS-positive diastase-resistant hyaline globules and frequent mitotic activity. Multinucleated cells and bizarre cells with hyperchromatic nuclei can often be observed between the sarcomatoid cells. The stroma is variably myxoid, with numerous thin-walled veins. Extramedullary hematopoiesis is common. Areas of myogenic, lipoblastic, or endothelial differentiation can be found (hence the name "mesenchymoma").

Biomarkers

HES cells are characterized by PAS-positive diastase-resistant hyaline globules and often stain positive for vimentin and desmin.

Glypican 3 (GPC3), known to be a diagnostic marker for hepatoblastoma and hepatocellular carcinoma, can be positive in a subset of HES and thus is not a reliable biomarker to differentiate HES from these neoplasms. HES is usually negative for AFP, hepatocyte paraffin 1 (HepPar1), myogenin, CD34, c-Kit (CD117), anaplastic lymphoma kinase 1 (ALK1), cytokeratins, and S100.

Differential diagnosis may be needed with the following: embryonal rhabdomyosarcoma (usually 2–6 years old, myxoid mass extending into bile duct, rhabdomyoblastic differentiation with cytoplasmic cross striations, cambium layer present, no diffuse anaplasia or hyaline globules, myogenin and MyoD1 positive); gastrointestinal stromal tumor (adults, CD117, DOG1, and CD34 positive); hepatoblastoma (cytokeratin and AFP positive); mesenchymal hamartoma (the second most common benign hepatic tumor in the pediatric population after infantile hemangioma, usually <1 year old, cystic, bland tumor cells and no giant cells); sarcomatoid hepatocellular carcinoma (variably positive to cytokeratin); and sclerosing variant of hepatocellular carcinoma (rare in children, has intracellular bile, Mallory-Denk bodies, HepPar1 positive).

Prognosis

HES is an aggressive malignancy. Before the introduction of multimodality approach, the prognosis was dismal, whereas the current 5-year overall survival rate is approximately 80%. Large tumors can undergo rupture and cause (even fatal) hemoperitoneum.

Therapy

Surgery remains the treatment of choice, if feasible. Neoadjuvant chemotherapy is often helpful in initially unresectable cases. In addition, postoperative (adjuvant) chemotherapy and radiation therapy are often reasonable options, particularly in surgical cases with positive margins.

For unresectable, refractory, or recurrent HES, liver transplantation is an option.

Suggested Readings

Chavhan (2019) Rare malignant liver tumors in children. Pediatr Radiol 49(11):1404–1421

Pandit (2019) Undifferentiated embryonal sarcoma of liver in an adult with spontaneous rupture and tumour thrombus in the right atrium. ANZ J Surg 89(9):E396–E397

Perl (2020) Paraneoplastic syndrome in undifferentiated embryonic sarcoma of the liver. EJNMMI Res 10(1):11

Putra (2015) Undifferentiated embryonal sarcoma of the liver: a concise review. Arch Pathol Lab Med 139(2):269–273

Saeed (2017) Primary mesenchymal liver tumors of childhood. Semin Diagn Pathol 34(2):201–207

Shi (2017) Characteristics and outcomes in children with undifferentiated embryonal sarcoma of the liver: a report from the National Cancer Database. Pediatr Blood Cancer 64:4. https://doi.org/10.1002/pbc.26272

Techavichit (2016) Undifferentiated Embryonal Sarcoma of the Liver (UESL): a single-center experience and review of the literature. J Pediatr Hematol Oncol 38(4):261–268

Definition

Hepatic epithelioid hemangioendothelioma (HEHE) is the liver localization of epithelioid hemangioendothelioma ($\rightarrow$ see dedicated section), a malignant tumor of vascular differentiation.

Epidemiology and Presentation

HEHE typically occurs in middle-aged adults with a slight female predominance (M:F = 2:3). The most frequent symptoms are right upper quadrant abdominal pain, hepatomegaly, and weight loss, but it can remain asymptomatic for long time.

Generally, it presents as multiple nodules involving both hepatic lobes and can be misdiagnosed as metastatic carcinoma on the basis of its radiologic appearance. Most HEHE are hypoechoic on ultrasonography, hypodense on computed tomography, and hypointense on T1-weighted magnetic resonance imaging (MRI) and hyperintense on T2-weighted MRI.

Pathology

Macroscopically, HEHE lesions are usually multifocal with ill-defined nodules often scattered throughout the liver. Microscopically, HEHE is composed of neoplastic endothelial cells that mimic epithelial cells (hence the term "epithelioid"). It shows a characteristic zoning phenomenon: at the periphery, malignant cells with moderate nuclear atypia infiltrate preexisting sinusoids and terminal hepatic venules (these cells exhibit intracytoplasmic structures resembling those of signet ring cells, but mucin staining is always negative); the center of the lesion reveals a marked desmoplastic stromal reaction with dense sclerosis and scanty tumor cells (these

S. Mocellin, *Soft Tissue Tumors*, https://doi.org/10.1007/978-3-030-58710-9_122

findings may resemble those of cholangiocarcinoma). Immunohistochemistry for endothelial cell markers is needed to confirm the vascular origin of the neoplasm. Fine needle aspiration-based cytology can be misleading.

Differential diagnosis may be needed with the following: hemangioma (well circumscribed, no venous invasion, no atypia); angiosarcoma (similar biomarker profile, but it is much more destructive than HEHE and obliterates acinar landmarks with extensive hemorrhage; more atypia); cholangiocarcinoma (epithelial biomarkers positive, endothelial biomarkers negative), and metastasis from signet ring cell carcinoma (epithelial biomarkers positive, endothelial biomarkers negative).

Biomarkers

HEHE stains positive for endothelial biomarkers such as Factor VIII-related antigen, CD34, CD31, FLI1, and podoplanin. It stains negative for epithelial biomarkers such as cytokeratins; it also stains negative for alpha-fetoprotein and CEA.

While 90% of epithelioid hemangioendotheliomas are characterized by the **chromosomal translocation** t(1;3)(p36.3;q25) which leads to the formation of the WWTR1-CAMTA1 fusion gene,[1] a histologically distinctive subset of EHE has been more recently shown to harbor YAP1-TFE3 fusion gene[2] as a new gene rearrangement.

Prognosis

Epithelioid hemangioendothelioma represents the most aggressive member of the hemangioendothelioma family of tumors ($\rightarrow$ see Chap. 116). The prognosis is intermediate between hemangioma (benign tumor) and angiosarcoma (highly malignant tumor) in terms of recurrence and metastatic potential. In 50% of cases HEHE shows extrahepatic involvement at diagnosis (mainly abdominal lymph nodes, lung, omentum or peritoneum, spleen), which does not necessarily preclude long survival.

---

[1] WWTR1-CAMTA1 fusion gene: WWTR1 (WW domain-containing transcription regulator 1) encodes a transcriptional coactivator which acts as a downstream regulatory target in the Hippo signaling pathway that plays a pivotal role in organ size control and tumor suppression by restricting proliferation and promoting apoptosis. CAMTA1 (calmodulin-binding transcription activator 1) encodes a protein that contains a CG1 DNA-binding domain, a transcription factor immunoglobulin domain, ankyrin repeats, and calmodulin-binding IQ motifs. The encoded protein is thought to be a transcription factor.

[2] YAP1-TFE3 fusion gene: YAP1 encodes yes-associated protein 1, a downstream nuclear effector of the Hippo signaling pathway (which is involved in development, growth, repair, and homeostasis); YAP1 is known to play a role in the development and progression of multiple cancers as a transcriptional regulator of this signaling pathway. TFE3 belongs to the microphthalmia family of bHLH-LZ transcription factors (MiT/TFE) which is composed of four members – MITF, TFEB, TFE3, and TFEC; neoplasms with alterations in these genes are also called MiT family tumors.

Therapy

When feasible, surgical liver resection is the best therapeutic option (5-year survival rate: 75%). However, since bilateral disease is present in more than 80% of cases, most patients are not amenable to surgery. In these cases, liver transplantation is considered the best approach (5-year survival rate: 60–80%).

EHE is poorly sensitive to both chemotherapy and radiotherapy. The use of anti-angiogenic drugs is being explored.

Suggested Readings

Alves (2018) Vascular tumours of the liver: a particular story. Transl Gastroenterol Hepatol 3:62

Antonescu (2013) Novel YAP1-TFE3 fusion defines a distinct subset of epithelioid hemangioendothelioma. Genes Chromosomes Cancer 52(8):775–784

Errani (2011) A novel WWTR1-CAMTA1 gene fusion is a consistent abnormality in epithelioid hemangioendothelioma of different anatomic sites. Genes Chromosomes Cancer 50(8):644–653

Krasnodębski (2020) Hepatic epithelioid hemangioendothelioma: a rare disease with favorable outcomes after liver transplantation. Transplant Proc [Epub ahead of print]

Kobayashi (2016) Sorafenib monotherapy in a patient with unresectable hepatic epithelioid hemangioendothelioma. Case Rep Oncol 9(1):134–137

Lerut (2019) Malignant vascular tumors of the liver in adults. Semin Liver Dis 39(1):1–12

Studer (2018) Hepatic epithelioid hemangioendothelioma. Arch Pathol Lab Med 142(2):263–267

Definition

Hepatic hemangioma (HHA) is a benign tumor of vascular origin. It is often referred to as liver angioma. For general concepts on hemangioma, → see dedicated section.

Epidemiology and Presentation

HHA is the most common liver tumor: its prevalence is estimated to be as high as 20% (this observation is confirmed by the increasing recognition of HHA in asymptomatic patients undergoing radiologic imaging of the liver for other reasons). Hemangioma is often solitary (about 70–80%), but multiple lesions can be present. HHA ranges in size from a few millimeters to over 20 cm, but most cases are small (<5 cm); any HHA larger than 5 cm is defined as giant hemangioma of the liver.

Although HHA can be diagnosed at any age, up to 80% of cases are diagnosed in patients aged between 30 and 50 years. In adults, hemangiomas occur more frequently in women (M:F = 1:3). Most cases are asymptomatic and are discovered incidentally. Liver function tests are usually normal (unless there has been a complication such as thrombosis), as well as alpha-fetoprotein levels.

Giant HHA are more likely to be symptomatic. The most common symptoms are mild abdominal pain and right upper quadrant discomfort. Acute abdominal pain may derive from thrombosis or bleeding within the neoplasm, which can last up to 3 weeks and be associated with fever and abnormality of liver function tests.

In infancy, both congenital hemangioma (→ see dedicated section) and infantile hemangioma (→ see dedicated section) can localize in the liver, where they represent the most frequent benign neoplasm. More than five cutaneous hemangiomas in children may be predictive for the presence of HHA. Infantile hemangioma of the liver can have three distinct patterns of hepatic involvement: (1) focal, there is a single hepatic lesion that is typically asymptomatic and rarely associated with

© The Editor(s) (if applicable) and The Author(s), under exclusive license to
Springer Nature Switzerland AG 2021
S. Mocellin, *Soft Tissue Tumors*, https://doi.org/10.1007/978-3-030-58710-9_123

cutaneous hemangiomas; (2) multifocal, there are several distinct lesions in the liver, which are often but not always asymptomatic and can be associated with cutaneous hemangiomas; and (3) diffuse, this condition is also known as diffuse neonatal hemangiomatosis and is characterized by extensive liver involvement and multiple skin hemangiomas; these children are much more likely to develop complications.

Diagnosis is usually radiological, as HHA presents typical ultrasound, computed tomography, and magnetic resonance imaging features that allow a diagnosis in most cases (including the differential diagnosis with malignant primary and metastatic liver tumors): in particular, the use of contrast medium allows to recognize the characteristic centripetal enhancement of the signal ("filling in" phenomenon).

Pathology

Microscopically, most cases are cavernous hemangiomas composed of cavernous vascular spaces of varying sizes, lined by a single layer of flat endothelium and filled with blood. The vascular compartments are separated by thin fibrous septae and may contain thrombi. Rarely, there may be focal calcifications. Cavernous hemangiomas of the liver may be associated with hemangiomas in other organs, bile duct hamartomas, and focal nodular hyperplasia. Capillary hemangiomas are very rare in the liver.

Due to the risk of iatrogenic rupture following liver biopsy or fine needle aspiration, most clinicians are reluctant to perform such tests in these patients.

Biomarkers

For details on biomarkers, → see sections dedicated to specific subtypes of hemangiomas.

Prognosis

Most patients with hepatic hemangiomas are asymptomatic and have an excellent prognosis. Symptoms are more likely with large lesions and in women. Up to 10% enlarge during follow-up, especially but not exclusively during pregnancy or use of oral contraceptives.

Since there is no risk of malignant transformation, most cases can be simply followed up. Giant HHA located on the liver surface may rupture and cause hemoperitoneum (especially in case of liver blunt trauma) or compress adjacent structures (e.g., biliary tree, inferior vena cava). Giant HHA in children have been associated with high-output cardiac failure (due to an arterovenous shunt-like effect) and hypothyroidism (due to the presence of high levels of 3-iodothyronine deiodinase activity in the hemangioma tissue, which catalyzes the conversion of thyroxine and tri-iodothyronine into biologically inactive hormones). Diffuse infantile hemangioma of the liver may lead to liver failure due to extensive replacement of normal hepatic parenchyma.

The Kasabach-Merritt syndrome is characterized by severe thrombocytopenia and consumptive coagulopathy in children affected with giant HHA. However, the association with simple hemangiomas has been questioned, and currently this syndrome is associated only with tufted angioma (→ see dedicated section) and kaposiform hemangioendothelioma (→ see dedicated section).

Therapy

Most patients have small asymptomatic HHA and do not need either therapy or follow-up. In particular, the absence of symptoms the risk of bleeding is too low to justify prophylactic liver resection. Patients with giant HHA may be followed up. Patients with pain or symptoms suggestive of extrinsic compression of adjacent structures (e.g., biliary tree) should be considered for surgical resection. However, it is important that all other causes of pain have been evaluated and excluded prior to surgery. Emergency surgery is required in case of HHA rupture causing hemoperitoneum.

Arterial embolization has been used as an alternative to surgery, but it can be complicated by abscess formation, and there is no evidence on long-term efficacy.

Liver transplantation has been utilized to treat severely symptomatic patients with very large unresectable HHA.

In many cases of infantile hemangioma and congenital hemangioma of the liver, treatment is not needed because the tumors spontaneously regress (→ see dedicated sections); medical therapy (i.e., propranolol) has been reported to be effective in are cases of non-regressing symptomatic (complicated) infantile hemangioma of the liver.

Suggested Readings

Bajenaru (2015) Hepatic hemangioma review. J Med Life 8:4–11

Dong (2019) Invasive management of symptomatic hepatic hemangioma. Eur J Gastroenterol Hepatol 31(9):1079–1084

Gnarra (2016) History of the infantile hepatic hemangioma: from imaging to generating a differential diagnosis. World J Clin Pediatr 5(3):273–280

Jinhuan (2020) Is laparoscopic hepatectomy suitable for giant hepatic hemangioma larger than 10 cm in diameter? Surg Endosc 34(3):1224–1230

Leon (2020) Hepatic hemangioma: what internists need to know. World J Gastroenterol 26(1):11–20

Prodromidou (2019) Liver transplantation for giant hepatic hemangioma: a systematic review. Transplant Proc 51(2):440–442

Tuxun (2014) Surgery vs. observation for liver hemangioma: a systematic review and meta-analysis. Hepato-Gastroenterology 61(136):2377–2382

Wu (2020) Differentiation of atypical hepatic hemangioma from liver metastases: diagnostic performance of a novel type of color contrast enhanced ultrasound. World J Gastroenterol 26(9):960–972

Definition

Hepatic mesenchymal hamartoma (HMH) is a benign tumor of the liver with uncertain cell differentiation. It is also known as mesenchymal hamartoma of the liver, giant cell lymphangioma, bile cell fibroadenoma, cavernous lymphangiomatoid tumor, benign mesenchymoma, cystic hamartoma, and pseudocystic mesenchymal tumor.

Epidemiology and Presentation

With a reported incidence of 0.7 cases per million per year, HMH accounts for approximately 10% of liver tumors in persons younger than 21 years of age, is the second most common benign liver tumor in children (after hemangioma), and is the third most common tumor of liver in the pediatric age group (after hepatoblastoma and hemangioma). More than two thirds of the cases are observed in children younger than 2 years; HMH is extremely rare in older children and adults.

The clinical presentation is nonspecific (enlarging, often painless liver mass sometimes accompanied by fever; compression on surrounding structures can be the first sign of presentation; laboratory findings: nonspecific, with normal/slightly elevated alpha-fetoprotein plasma levels). Radiology is important to suspect the diagnosis, which can only be confirmed after pathology assessment (differential diagnosis with other liver tumors such as undifferentiated embryonal sarcoma is difficult/impossible based on imaging alone).

Etiology and Predisposition

Recently, HMH has been added to the phenotypes of the **DICER1 syndrome**, a genetic disease inherited in an autosomal dominant manner and due to germline mutations of the gene DICER1, whose protein product is involved in the metabolism of microRNA. People with this cancer predisposition syndrome most commonly develop pleuropulmonary blastoma ($\rightarrow$ see dedicated section).

Cystic nephroma, which involves multiple benign fluid-filled cysts in the kidneys, can also occur in people with DICER1 syndrome. DICER1 syndrome is also associated with tumors in the ovaries (known as Sertoli-Leydig cell tumors) as well as multinodular goiter of the thyroid.

Tumors occurring in this syndrome are characterized by biallelic pathogenic variants in DICER1: a germline variant (which typically results in loss of DICER1 function) accompanied by a characteristic somatic missense mutation that modifies one of five "hot spot" amino acids in the RNase IIIb domain.

Pathology

Macroscopically, the lesion presents as a multicystic, well-circumscribed, solitary, 5–25 cm in diameter, myxoid mass with fluid-filled cysts.

Microscopically, HMH shows both epithelial and mesenchymal components; the lesion is typically composed of loose mesenchyme (myxoid stroma) with variably sized cysts lined with biliary type epithelium (dilated bile ducts without atypia), accompanied by islands or cords of hepatocytes admixed with and blood vessels. No tumor giant cells are present. Extramedullary hematopoiesis is often found (90% of cases).

Differential diagnosis may be needed with the following: bile duct adenoma (no hepatocyte islands) or cystadenoma (adults); bile duct hamartoma (also known as von Meyenburg complex; usually multiple lesions with fibrous background); hepatic embryonal sarcoma (marked cellularity and atypical cells, hyaline globules; for more details $\rightarrow$ see dedicated section); infantile hemangioendothelioma (more vascular); infantile hemangioma (females more common, vascular channels of variable size); and mixed epithelial mesenchymal hepatoblastoma (epithelial component has embryonal and fetal hepatocytes; mesenchymal component has spindle cells, osteoid, cartilage).

Biomarkers

HMH may stain positive for CK7, vimentin, SMA, desmin, and glypican-3, but the biomarker profile is not specific.

Prognosis

HMH is a benign neoplasm. After surgical resection, the prognosis is excellent. However, it has been associated with a risk of malignant transformation (into hepatic mesenchymal sarcoma).

Therapy

The gold standard for the diagnosis and treatment of HMH is complete surgical excision. If the tumor is unresectable or recurs after partial hepatectomy, liver transplantation has been proposed.

Suggested Readings

Apellaniz-Ruiz (2019) Mesenchymal hamartoma of the liver and DICER1 syndrome. N Engl J Med 380(19):1834–1842

Khan (2019) Mesenchymal hamartoma in children: a diagnostic challenge. Case Rep Pediatr 2019:4132842

Thampy (2017) Imaging features of rare mesenchymal liver tumours: beyond haemangiomas. Br J Radiol 90(1079):20170373

Definition

Hibernoma is a benign adipocytic neoplasm.

Epidemiology and Presentation

Hibernoma is a rare neoplasm, including about 1% of all adipocytic tumors. It occurs predominantly in young adults, with a mean age of 40 years. The most common site is the thigh, followed by the trunk, upper extremity, and head and neck. The main location is the subcutis, but intramuscular cases can occur (20%); rare cases have been reported in other sites such as the mediastinum, breast, retroperitoneum, and spermatic cord.

Pathology

It presents as an encapsulated and richly vascularized tumor composed of variable proportions of brown fat cells (with multivacuolated cytoplasm) admixed with white adipose tissue. No or mild atypia is present.

Differential diagnosis may be needed with well-differentiated liposarcoma (deep location, atypia is present; specific genetic aberrations) and lipoma (lipocytes are not multivacuolated).

Biomarkers

Hibernoma cells are often positive for UCP1 and S100, while they are negative for CD34; nonetheless, CD34 positivity indicates the spindled fibroblastic component in the spindle cell hibernoma variant.

© The Editor(s) (if applicable) and The Author(s), under exclusive license to
Springer Nature Switzerland AG 2021
S. Mocellin, *Soft Tissue Tumors*, https://doi.org/10.1007/978-3-030-58710-9_125

From the cytogenetic viewpoint, almost all hibernomas show **chromosomal rearrangements** targeting chromosome 11q13-21 with special regard to deletions in a region covering the tumor suppressor genes MEN1 and AIP.

Prognosis

Hibernoma is a benign tumor with no significant potential for recurrence after surgical excision.

Therapy

Surgical excision is the treatment of choice.

Suggested Readings

Fletcher (2020) WHO classification of tumours of soft tissue and bone, 5th ed.
Kovitwanichkanont (2018) Hibernoma: a rare benign soft tissue tumour resembling liposarcoma. BJR Case Rep 4(3):20170067
Malzahn (2019) Immunophenotypic expression of UCP1 in hibernoma and other adipose/non adipose soft tissue tumours. Clin Sarcoma Res 9:8

High-grade endometrial stromal sarcoma is a uterine sarcoma arising from the endometrial stroma.

For details → see Chap. 82.

Definition

Hobnail hemangioma is a benign vascular tumor of the skin. It is also known as superficial hemosiderotic lymphovascular malformation and targetoid hemosiderotic hemangioma.

Epidemiology and Presentation

Hobnail hemangioma is an uncommon cutaneous lesion that clinically presents as a small solitary red to purple papule or macule, located on the limbs or trunk. Multiple lesions and atypical locations have also been described.

Pathology

It presents as a proliferation of irregular dissecting vascular channels lined by plump endothelial cells that protrude into vessel lumina (so-called hobnail appearance, hence the name). Usually it exhibits a biphasic pattern, with dilated vessels in the superficial dermis and angulated vessels in the deeper dermis. There is controversy about the histogenetic origin of hobnail hemangioma (some evidence supporting it is a lymphatic malformation rather than a tumor).

Differential diagnosis may be needed with other benign vascular tumors and Kaposi sarcoma (patch stage; HHVS8 positive).

Biomarkers

It positively stains for CD31 and CD34, while it results negative for HHV8 (human herpes virus 8).

Prognosis

Hobnail hemangioma is a benign neoplasm.

Therapy

Surgical excision is the treatment of choice.

Suggested Readings

AbuHilal (2016) Hobnail hemangioma (superficial hemosiderotic lymphovascular malformation) in children: a series of 6 pediatric cases and review of the literature. J Cutan Med Surg 20(3):216–220

Joyce (2014) Superficial hemosiderotic lymphovascular malformation (hobnail hemangioma): a report of six cases. Pediatr Dermatol 31(3):281–285

Porrino-Bustamante (2017) Hobnail hemangioma with an unusual clinical presentation. J Cutan Med Surg 21(2):164–166

Definition

Hybrid nerve sheath tumor (HNST) is a benign tumor which combines features of two or more conventional type peripheral nerve sheath tumors (neurofibroma, schwannoma, perineurioma; for details on these neoplasms, → see dedicated sections).

Epidemiology and Presentation

HNST is a very rare neoplasm, the most common type being schwannoma/perineurioma. It occurs in a wide age range, without gender differences. HNST may arise in many body sites, including viscera (mainly gastrointestinal tract), and usually presents as an asymptomatic nodule/mass.

Etiology and Predisposition

Hybrid schwannoma/perineurioma occurs sporadically, whereas hybrid neurofibroma/schwannoma may be syndromic within the frame of schwannomatosis or neurofibromatosis (→ see sections dedicated to neurofibroma and schwannoma).

Pathology

The microscopic appearance is that of the nerve sheath tumors composing the lesion. For details → see sections dedicated to neurofibroma and schwannoma.

Biomarkers

Schwann cells stain positive for S100; perineurial cells stain positive for EMA. Hybrid neurofibroma/schwannoma includes neurofilament-positive axons, and CD34 is often positive in a subset of cells in the neurofibromatous component. For more details → see sections dedicated to single tumors.

Prognosis

HNST is a benign neoplasm.

Therapy

Surgery is the treatment of choice.

Suggested Readings

Fletcher (2020) WHO classification of tumours of soft tissue and bone, 5th ed.

Hong (2019) Hybrid nerve sheath tumor in the orbit: a case report and review of literature. Surg Neurol Int 10:250

Ronellenfitsch (2020) Targetable ERBB2 mutations identified in neurofibroma/schwannoma hybrid nerve sheath tumors. J Clin Invest 130(5):2488–2495

Definition

Inclusion body fibromatosis (IBF) is a benign lesion classified among the fibroblastic—myofibroblastic tumors.

It is also known as infantile digital fibroma, infantile digital fibromatosis, and recurring digital fibrous tumor of childhood.

Epidemiology and Presentation

IBF accounts for 0.1% of soft tissue tumors and 2% of pediatric fibroblastic tumors. It generally develops within the first 2 years of life (30% of cases are congenital). This neoplasm, which equally affects males and females, rarely occurs in adults. IBF classically involves the digits (except the first digit) and (less frequently) the hand and foot. Extra-digital cases have been rarely reported.

Usually it presents as an asymptomatic dome-shaped or polypoid cutaneous nodule (generally <2 cm). Synchronous and metachronous lesions may occur.

Pathology

IBF is a predominantly myofibroblastic tumor characterized by eosinophilic paranuclear inclusions (hence the name). Spindle cells characteristically grow perpendicular to the epidermis within a variably collagenous dermis. The paranuclear inclusion is highlighted by trichrome (red), phosphotungstic acid-hematoxylin (dark purple), and Movat (pink) stains. Mitoses are rare, and atypia is absent.

Differential diagnosis may be needed with the following: infantile fibrosarcoma (not digits, usually >2 cm, more cellular, more mitotic figures, no inclusions) and infantile desmoid fibromatosis (rare on hand, usually >2 cm, more cellular, no inclusions).

© The Editor(s) (if applicable) and The Author(s), under exclusive license to
Springer Nature Switzerland AG 2021
S. Mocellin, *Soft Tissue Tumors*, https://doi.org/10.1007/978-3-030-58710-9_129

Biomarkers

Spindle cells express muscle-specific actin (MSA), calponin, and desmin, whereas they are negative for cytokeratin, estrogen receptor, progesterone receptor, and beta-catenin.

Prognosis

This is a benign tumor, although with a high potential for local recurrence (up to 60–70%). Spontaneous regressions have been reported.

Therapy

Surgical wide excision is the treatment of choice.

Suggested Readings

Fletcher (2020) WHO classification of tumours of soft tissue and bone, 5th ed.
Marks (2016) Infantile digital fibroma: a rare fibromatosis. Arch Pathol Lab Med 140(10):1153–1156

Definition

Infantile fibrosarcoma (IFS) is a malignant tumor originating from fibroblasts. Histologically it resembles adult fibrosarcoma (→ see dedicated section) but shows distinctive epidemiological, molecular, and prognostic characteristics.

It is also known as congenital fibrosarcoma, congenital infantile fibrosarcoma, juvenile fibrosarcoma, medullary fibromatosis of infancy, congenital fibrosarcoma-like fibromatosis, and desmoplastic fibrosarcoma of infancy.

The renal counterpart is congenital mesoblastic nephroma (→ see dedicated section).

Epidemiology and Presentation

Nearly all cases occur in the first year of life, up to 30–80% being congenital. Superficial and deep soft tissues of distal extremities are the origin in about 66% of cases. The trunk and head and neck are other major sites; rare cases arise from visceral sites. IFS presents as a solitary rapidly growing mass, sometimes of very large dimension.

Pathology

IFS is a densely cellular tumor composed of intersecting fascicles of primitive round, ovoid, and spindle cells. Focal necrosis and hemorrhage may be associated with calcifications. Cells show little pleomorphism, and mitotic activity may be prominent.

Differential diagnosis may be needed with the following: infantile fibromatosis (no pleomorphism, no mitotic figures, no NTRK3 rearrangement); myofibromatosis (myofibroblastic features, no NTRK3 rearrangement); and primitive myxoid mesenchymal tumor of infancy (BCOR internal tandem duplication and/or nuclear immunoreactivity for BCOR or BCL6).

Biomarkers

Vimentin is the most constant positive staining but is not specific.

Almost all cases of IFS are characterized by the **chromosomal translocation** t(12;15)(p13;q25), which generates the ETV6-NTRK3 fusion gene,[1] which in turn encodes the ETV6-NTRK3 chimeric tyrosine kinase. ETV6-NTRK3 is a potent oncogene that constitutively activates signal transduction cascades of the NTRK3 tyrosine kinase, namely, the Ras-Erk and PI3K-Akt pathways. ETV6-NTRK3 fusions are absent in infantile myofibromatosis and adult fibrosarcoma.

ETV6-NTRK3 fusions have also been reported in other malignancies including congenital mesoblastic nephroma ($\rightarrow$ see dedicated section), myeloid leukemia, secretory breast carcinoma, and mammary-type secretory carcinoma of the skin and salivary gland.

Prognosis

Unlike adult fibrosarcoma, IFS has a relatively favorable outcome, with a 10-year survival rate >90% and a recurrence rate of 10–50%. Metastasis is rare (mainly to lungs). No definitive prognostic factors are known. Spontaneous regression and non-recurrence of incompletely excised IFS have been reported.

Therapy

Conventional therapy. Traditional management consists of surgical resection, along with neoadjuvant and adjuvant chemotherapy (unlike its adult counterpart, IFS is typically chemosensitive). Initial surgery is suggested only if possible

---

[1] ETV6-NTRK3 fusion gene: ETV6 encodes an ETS family transcription factor associated with leukemia and congenital fibrosarcoma. NTRK3 encodes neurotrophic receptor tyrosine kinase 3 and belongs to the tropomyosin receptor kinases (TRK) family which also includes NTRK1 (encoding neurotrophic receptor tyrosine kinase 1) and NTRK2 (neurotrophic receptor tyrosine kinase 2). The encoded proteins elicit activities that regulate the natural growth, differentiation, and survival of neurons when they interact with endogenous neurotrophin ligands. Chromosomal rearrangements involving in-frame fusions of these genes with various partners, translocations in the TRK kinase domains, mutations in the TRK ligand-binding site, amplifications of NTRK, or the expression of TRK splice variants can result in constitutively activated chimeric TRK fusion proteins that can act as oncogenic drivers that promote cell proliferation and survival in tumor cell lines.

without mutilation. Patients with initial complete or microscopic incomplete resection usually have no further therapy.

Patients with an initially inoperable tumor receive first-line vincristine plus actinomycin-D chemotherapy, conservative surgery being planned after tumor shrinkage. Aggressive local therapy (mutilating surgery or external radiotherapy) is not usually needed.

Target therapy. NTRK inhibitors such as larotrectinib[2] and entrectinib[3] have shown high anticancer activity against IFS and are currently considered a valid therapeutic option.

Suggested Readings

Fletcher (2020) WHO classification of tumours of soft tissue and bone, 5th ed.

Hung (2018) Evaluation of pan-TRK immunohistochemistry in infantile fibrosarcoma, lipofibromatosis-like neural tumour and histological mimics. Histopathology 73(4):634–644

Kheder (2018) emerging targeted therapy for tumors with NTRK Fusion Proteins. Clin Cancer Res 24(23):5807–5814

Marchiò (2019) ESMO recommendations on the standard methods to detect NTRK fusions in daily practice and clinical research. Ann Oncol 2019 [Epub ahead of print]

Orbach (2016) Conservative strategy in infantile fibrosarcoma is possible: The European paediatric Soft tissue sarcoma Study Group experience. Eur J Cancer 57:1–9

---

[2] Larotrectinib: tyrosine kinase inhibitor targeting the following: NTRK1, NTRK2, NTRK3.

[3] Entrectinib: tyrosine kinase inhibitor targeting the following: NTRK1, NTRK2, NTRK3, ROS1, ALK.

Definition

Infantile hemangioma (IHA) is a benign tumor of vascular origin. It is also known as juvenile capillary hemangioma, juvenile hemangioma, strawberry hemangioma, strawberry mark, strawberry birthmark, and capillary hemangioma. For further details on the hemangioma family, → see the dedicated section entitled "Hemangioma."

Epidemiology and Presentation

IHA is the most common benign tumor of infancy and childhood, occurring in 5–10% of all children. As compared to congenital hemangioma (→ see dedicated section), IHA is significantly more frequent (in a retrospective review of 6459 children with vascular anomalies observed in a specialized Chinese center, IHA, congenital hemangioma, and vascular malformations were diagnosed in 43%, 14%, and 43% of patients, respectively).

IHA is found more frequently in females (M:F = 1:4), whites, premature infants, and twins. IHA occurs in the skin of the head and neck region (60%), followed by trunk (25%) and extremities (15%). Color can vary depending on the depth of the lesion: from bright red (superficial) to blue or normal skin color (deep). According to the extension of the disease, IHA is categorized into the localized (70%), segmental (25%), and multifocal (5%) type.

Unlike congenital hemangioma (which is fully developed at birth), IHA (which is absent at birth) arises during the first 8 weeks of life as an area of discoloration or telangiectasia. The lesion exhibits a rapid proliferative phase (when it raises above the normal skin level) during early childhood for 6–12 months. This is followed by gradual involution and a spontaneous regression by the age of 5–9 years; after regression, the skin may return to normal, but often there are residual changes (excessive fibrofatty tissue, telangiectasia, skin laxity).

S. Mocellin, *Soft Tissue Tumors*, https://doi.org/10.1007/978-3-030-58710-9_131

Most lesions are solitary, but multiple lesions occur in up to 20% of infants. IHA has a predilection for the head and neck region, but it can occur anywhere in the skin, mucous membranes, or viscera (mainly the liver, → see Chap. 123). IHA ranges from some millimeters to many centimeters in diameter. It can be superficial, deep, or combined (so-called compound hemangioma). Superficial IHA is the most common variant and appears as a bright red papule, nodule, or plaque raised above clinically normal skin (hence the name strawberry hemangioma). Deep IHA is a subcutaneous hemangioma that presents as a raised skin-colored nodule, which often has a bluish hue with or without central telangiectatic patch.

For details on differential diagnosis with other common cutaneous infantile vascular anomalies, → see Table 131.1.

Table 131.1 Differential diagnosis between common cutaneous infantile vascular anomalies

Infantile hemangioma	Congenital hemangioma	Port-wine stain	Nevus simplex
Not present at birth	Congenital	Congenital	Congenital
Benign tumor	Benign tumor	Malformation	Malformation
Mainly but not only head and neck	Mainly but not only head and neck	Unilateral (midline respected)	Crosses the midline
Associated with: PHACE syndrome and SACRAL/LUMBAR/PELVIS syndrome	–	Associated with: Sturge-Weber syndrome, Klippel-Trenaunay syndrome, Proteus syndrome, Bannayan-Riley-Ruvalcaba syndrome, Macrocephaly-capillary malformation syndrome, Microcephaly-capillary malformation syndrome, Beckwith-Wiedemann syndrome, Parkes-Weber syndrome	–
Rapidly becomes a raised lesion	Raised lesion	Starts as a flat lesion, may become thicker and nodular over years	Remains a flat lesion
Often regresses	Often regresses	No regression	Some (not nuchal) regress
Synonyms: strawberry hemangioma, capillary hemangioma	–	Synonyms: nevus flammeus, capillary malformation	Synonyms: salmon patch, angel kiss
Bright red color (superficial lesions) or skin-colored nodule, with a bluish hue with or without central telangiectatic patch (deep lesions)	Reddish mass with overlying telangiectasias and peripheral vasoconstriction	Pink-red, may become darker (violaceous) over years	Pale red color
5–10% of all children	Unknown (lower than IHA)	1% of all newborns	30% of all newborns

Etiology and Predisposition

IHA can be associated with the **PHACE syndrome** (*p*osterior fossa malformations, *h*emangioma, *a*rterial anomalies, *c*ardiovascular anomalies, *e*ye anomalies) and **LUMBAR syndrome** (*l*ower body hemangioma, *u*rogenital anomalies, *u*lceration, *m*yelopathy, *b*ony deformities, *a*norectal malformations, *a*rterial anomalies, and *r*enal anomalies and also known as SACRAL syndrome and PELVIS syndrome).

Pathology

Diagnosis is usually clinical. Microscopically, the lesion (usually multinodular) is composed of hyperplastic endothelial cells, pericytes with and without lumens, and prominent basement membranes. Fibrosis becomes dominant as the involution progresses.

Biomarkers

IHA always stains positive for GLUT1 (as opposed to congenital hemangioma and vascular malformations).

Like congenital hemangioma, tumor cells are positive for CD31, CD34, and WT1.

Prognosis

IHA is a benign tumor, and complete involution occurs in the majority of cases (90% by 9 years). Nonetheless, the following complications can occur: (1) ulceration (the most common, occurs in up to 10% of cases); (2) ophthalmologic complications (amblyopia, astigmatism, myopia, retrobulbar involvement, and tear duct obstruction); (3) airway obstruction (nasal lesions); (4) feeding difficulties (perioral or lip lesions); (5) visceral hemangiomatosis (patients with five or more skin lesions are recommended to undergo liver ultrasound due to the association with liver involvement); and (6) cosmetic disfigurement (lesions located in the face).

Therapy

Most cases of IHA do not require treatment because they regress spontaneously. However, complicated IHA may require treatment.

Beta-blockers (e.g., oral propranolol) have been shown to be effective as first-line therapy according to randomized controlled trial-based evidence. Oral prednisone is an alternative therapy for patients who do not tolerate that can be used.

Surgical excision may be considered to prevent complications or to treat lesions unresponsive to medical therapy. Surgery may be needed also when regression leaves cosmetic disfigurement (approximately 8% of cases).

Topical beta-blockers (i.e., timolol) and laser therapy can be used for small, superficial, and uncomplicated lesions.

Suggested Readings

Darrow (2015) Diagnosis and management of infantile hemangioma. Pediatrics 136(4):e1060–e1104

Johnson (2018) Vascular tumors in infants: case report and review of clinical, histopathologic, and immunohistochemical characteristics of infantile hemangioma, pyogenic granuloma, noninvoluting congenital hemangioma, tufted angioma, and kaposiform hemangioendothelioma. Am J Dermatopathol 40(4):231–239

Kim (2017) Comparison of efficacy and safety between propranolol and steroid for infantile hemangioma: a randomized clinical trial. JAMA Dermatol 153(6):529–536

Léauté-Labrèze (2008) Propranolol for severe hemangiomas of infancy. N Engl J Med 358(24):2649–2651

Léauté-Labrèze (2017) Infantile haemangioma. Lancet 390(10089):85–94

Mo (2004) GLUT1 endothelial reactivity distinguishes hepatic infantile hemangioma from congenital hepatic vascular malformation with associated capillary proliferation. Hum Pathol 35(2):200–209

PDQ Pediatric Treatment Editorial Board (2019). Childhood vascular tumors treatment (PDQ®): health professional version. PMID: 26844334

Smith (2017) Infantile hemangiomas: an updated review on risk factors, pathogenesis, and treatment. Birth Defects Res 109(11):809–815

Soukoulis (2015) Gastrointestinal infantile hemangioma: presentation and management. J Pediatr Gastroenterol Nutr 61(4):415–420

Wildgruber (2019) Vascular tumors in infants and adolescents. Insights Imaging 10(1):30

Yang (2015) Clinical characteristics and treatment options of infantile vascular anomalies. Medicine (Baltimore) 94(40):e1717

Definition

Inflammatory fibroid polyp (IFP) is a benign neoplasm of the gastrointestinal tract. It is also referred to as Vanek polyp and eosinophilic granuloma. Recently, telocytes (CD34 and PDGFRA-positive stromal cells) have been proposed as the physiological cell counterpart for IFP, and the term telocytoma has been suggested to replace the name IFP.

Epidemiology and Presentation

IFP is a mesenchymal polyp that may arise anywhere in the gastrointestinal tract but most frequently affects the stomach and the small bowel.

The tumor has a peak incidence in the sixth to seventh decade of life. It presents as a solitary, small, and sessile polyp (median size: 1.5 cm but can measure up to 9 cm).

Etiology and Predisposition

A recently described cancer predisposition syndrome called **familial PDGFRA-mutation syndrome** is associated with the development of mesenchymal tumors of the gastrointestinal tract, namely, gastrointestinal stromal tumor (GIST) and IFP. The syndrome is caused by germline-activating mutations of the platelet-derived growth factor receptor alpha (PDGFRA). The inheritance appears to be autosomal dominant but thus far has displayed incomplete penetrance and variable expressivity.

S. Mocellin, *Soft Tissue Tumors*, https://doi.org/10.1007/978-3-030-58710-9_132

Pathology

IFP is a submucosal lesion composed of spindle and stellate stromal cells. The loose edematous stroma contains thin-walled blood vessels with characteristic "onion skin" arrangement of spindled cells around vessels. An inflammatory infiltrate rich in eosinophils is present. The mitotic activity is minimal.

Differential diagnosis may be needed with the following: GIST (centered in muscularis propria, more hypercellular, CD117 and DOG1 positive); plexiform fibromyxoma (multinodular, centered on muscularis propria, lacks concentric vessels, CD34 negative); and schwannoma (usually arise from muscularis propria, peripheral lymphoid cuffing, S100 positive).

Biomarkers

IFP stains positively for CD34 (SMA is only variably expressed) and negatively for CD117 (although mast cells are CD117 positive), S100, and DOG1.

PDGFRA exon 12, 14, and 18 gain-of-function mutations have been reported in both sporadic and familial cases of IFP.

Prognosis

IFP is a benign tumor. No endoscopic surveillance is required after the histological diagnosis is confirmed.

Therapy

Local excision (during endoscopy) is the gold standard treatment.

Suggested Readings

Cunningham (2019) A large inflammatory fibroid polyp of the rectum removed by transanal excision. J Surg Case Rep 2019(6):rjz164

Hirota (2018) Differential diagnosis of gastrointestinal stromal tumor by histopathology and immunohistochemistry. Transl Gastroenterol Hepatol 3:27

Manley (2018) Familial PDGFRA-mutation syndrome: somatic and gastrointestinal phenotype. Hum Pathol 76:52–57

Nagao (2020) Inflammatory fibroid polyp mimicking an early gastric cancer. Gastrointest Endosc 92(1):217–218

Ricci (2018) Telocytes are the physiological counterpart of inflammatory fibroid polyps and PDGFRA-mutant GISTs. J Cell Mol Med 22(10):4856–4862

Definition

Inflammatory myofibroblastic tumor (IMT) is a neoplasm of intermediate biological aggressiveness and is classified among the fibroblastic—myofibroblastic tumors. It is also known as plasma cell granuloma, inflammatory myofibrohistiocytic proliferation, omental mesenteric myxoid hamartoma, inflammatory pseudotumor, inflammatory fibrosarcoma, and inflammatory myofibroblastic sarcoma.

Epidemiology and Presentation

IMT usually affects children and young adults (mean age at diagnosis: 10 years), without significant gender predominance. It can arise virtually in any body site but most frequently localizes in the mesentery, omentum, retroperitoneum, pelvis, and abdominal soft tissue (75% of cases), followed by the lung, mediastinum, and head and neck. Unusual locations include somatic soft tissue, gastrointestinal tract, uterus, bladder, pancreas, and central nervous system.

IMT presents as a nodular, circumscribed, or multinodular mass (with variable hemorrhage, necrosis, and calcification) ranging from 1 to more than 20 cm in diameter. Symptoms depend on the site of origin. About one third of patients show fever, malaise, weight loss, and laboratory abnormalities including anemia, thrombocytosis, polyclonal hyperglobulinemia, and elevated C-reactive protein serum levels: after tumor excision, these signs disappear, and their later occurrence can prelude disease recurrence.

Of note, IMT is to be considered a nosological entity different from IgG4-related sclerosing disease (a multi-organ, fibro-inflammatory condition with lesions which respond very well to steroids; virtually any organ can be involved, but the most common locations are the pancreas, kidneys, orbital adnexal structures, salivary glands, and retroperitoneum).

S. Mocellin, *Soft Tissue Tumors*, https://doi.org/10.1007/978-3-030-58710-9_133

Pathology

IMT is neoplasm composed of myofibroblastic and fibroblastic spindle cells accompanied by an inflammatory infiltrate of plasma cells, lymphocytes, eosinophils, and histiocytes. Necrosis is uncommon, and mitotic rate varies but is usually low. In case of disease recurrence, rare cases progress to frankly sarcomatous morphology.

An IMT variant with plump round epithelioid or histiocytoid tumor cells is associated with RANBP2-ALK gene rearrangement and appears to be associated with a more aggressive clinical behavior (so-called epithelioid inflammatory myofibroblastic sarcoma).

In a background of abundant blood vessels, IMT generally presents as a mixture of three patterns:

(a) One resembling nodular fasciitis with elongated myofibroblasts containing abundant eosinophilic cytoplasm and vesicular nuclei, loose myxoid stroma with neutrophils, lymphocytes, and eosinophils, but few plasma cells.
(b) A cellular pattern with spindled myofibroblasts and fibroblasts in more compact stroma, arranged as islands surrounded by fibromyxoid stroma with prominent plasma cells and mitotic figures.
(c) A densely hyalinized stroma with few spindle cells, few plasma cells, or lymphocytes.

All three patterns are characterized by lack of nuclear pleomorphism and lack of atypical mitotic figures.

In any case, ganglion cell-like myofibroblasts can be present. Malignant behavior is usually associated with highly atypical polygonal cells with oval nuclei, prominent nucleoli, Reed-Sternberg-like cells, and atypical mitotic figures.

Differential diagnosis may be needed with the following: calcifying fibrous tumor (calcification, no myofibroblastic proliferation, actin negative); IgG4-related sclerosing disease (IgG4-positive plasma cells; the ratio of IgG4+/IgG+ plasma cells is higher); low-grade myofibroblastic sarcoma (more uniform appearance with higher cellularity, more prominent hyperchromasia, more infiltrative, ALK negative); and nodular fasciitis (smaller size, older patients, less inflammation).

Biomarkers

IMT shows strong vimentin positivity and variable staining for SMA,[1] MSA,[2] desmin, and cytokeratins. Focal positivity for CD68 can be observed in histiocyte-like cells. It negatively stains for S100, c-Kit/CD117, HHV8,[3] CD34, and h-caldesmon.

---

[1] SMA: smooth muscle actin.

[2] MSA: muscle-specific actin.

[3] HHV8: human herpesvirus 8.

In about 50–60% of cases, a **chromosomal translocation** leads to the formation of an ALK-based fusion gene,[4] the most common partners being TPM3, TPM4, CLTC, RANBP2, ATIC, NUMA1, and SQSTM1. The chimeric proteins generated by these gene fusions function act as constitutively activated ALK, which is believed to play a key role in carcinogenesis. ALK staining (restricted to the neoplastic myofibroblastic component) strongly correlates with the presence of the fusion gene.

Prognosis

IMT is a neoplasm of intermediate aggressiveness: local disease relapse occurs in 25–35% of cases, and metastatic disease (usually involving the lungs, brain, liver, and bone) develops in about 2–4% of cases.

Overall, IMT has a good prognosis (especially in younger patients), even for initially unresectable disease and in ALK-negative cases (especially in pediatric cases).

Tumor size, cellularity, and histological features are not reliable prognostic indicators. ALK-negative IMT may have a higher likelihood of metastasis; on the other hand, metastasis may be associated with specific ALK fusion partners (such as RANBP2).

Therapy

Surgery is the mainstay of treatment. For locally advanced/metastatic disease, there is no standard of care, although traditional **chemotherapy** (e.g., doxorubicin or vinblastine-methotrexate) remains the most frequently adopted treatment.

Recently, **target therapy** with ALK inhibitors such as crizotinib,[5] alectinib,[6] and ceritinib[7] has been shown to be useful in cases harboring ALK rearrangements.

Suggested Readings

Brivio (2019) ALK inhibition in two emblematic cases of pediatric inflammatory myofibroblastic tumor: efficacy and side effects. Pediatr Blood Cancer 66(5):e27645

Butrynski (2010) Crizotinib in ALK-rearranged inflammatory myofibroblastic tumor. N Engl J Med 363(18):1727–1733

---

[4] ALK-based fusion gene: ALK (anaplastic lymphoma kinase) encodes a receptor tyrosine kinase, which belongs to the insulin receptor superfamily. It plays an important role in the development of the brain. ALK has been found to be rearranged, mutated, or amplified in a series of tumors including anaplastic large cell lymphomas, neuroblastoma, and non-small cell lung cancer.

[5] Crizotinib: small molecule tyrosine kinase inhibitor targeting the following: ALK, MET.

[6] Alectinib: small molecule tyrosine kinase inhibitor targeting the following: ALK.

[7] Ceritinib: small molecule tyrosine kinase inhibitor targeting the following: ALK.

Casanova (2020) Inflammatory myofibroblastic tumor: the experience of the European pediatric Soft Tissue Sarcoma Study Group (EpSSG). Eur J Cancer 127:123–129

Fletcher (2020) WHO classification of tumours of soft tissue and bone, 5th ed.

Fu (2019) Inflammatory myofibroblastic tumor: A demographic, clinical and therapeutic study of 92 cases. Math Biosci Eng 16(6):6794–6804

Honda (2019) Durable response to the ALK inhibitor alectinib in inflammatory myofibroblastic tumor of the head and neck with a novel SQSTM1-ALK fusion: a case report. Investig New Drugs 37(4):791–795

Lee (2017) ALK oncoproteins in atypical inflammatory myofibroblastic tumours: novel RRBP1-ALK fusions in epithelioid inflammatory myofibroblastic sarcoma. J Pathol 241(3):316–323

Michels (2017) ALK G1269A mutation as a potential mechanism of acquired resistance to crizotinib in an ALK-rearranged inflammatory myofibroblastic tumor. NPJ Precis Oncol 1(1):4

Mohammad (2018) ALK Is a specific diagnostic marker for inflammatory myofibroblastic tumor of the uterus. Am J Surg Pathol 42(10):1353–1359

Mossé (2017) Targeting ALK with crizotinib in pediatric anaplastic large cell lymphoma and inflammatory myofibroblastic tumor: a children's oncology group study. J Clin Oncol 35(28):3215–3221

Ogata (2019) Effectiveness of crizotinib for inflammatory myofibroblastic tumor with ALK mutation. Intern Med 58(7):1029–1032

Rao (2018) Inflammatory myofibroblastic tumor driven by novel NUMA1-ALK fusion responds to ALK inhibition. J Natl Compr Cancer Netw 16(2):115–121

Schöffski (2018) Crizotinib in patients with advanced, inoperable inflammatory myofibroblastic tumours with and without anaplastic lymphoma kinase gene alterations (European Organisation for Research and Treatment of Cancer 90,101 CREATE): a multicentre, single-drug, prospective, non-randomised phase 2 trial. Lancet Respir Med 6(6):431–441

Taylor (2019) Morphologic overlap between inflammatory myofibroblastic tumor and IgG4-related disease: lessons from next-generation sequencing. Am J Surg Pathol 43(3):314–324

Definition

Intimal sarcoma is a malignant high-grade sarcoma of unclear cell origin developing in large blood vessels.

Epidemiology and Presentation

Intimal sarcoma is a very rare tumor, the median age being 50 years for pulmonary lesions and 60 years for aortic lesions. Main sites are the pulmonary artery and aorta, but other arteries and veins can be involved. Cases originating from the heart have been also described (where it represents one of the most frequent primary sarcoma types). The main feature is the predominantly intraluminal growth, which has two main clinical consequences: vessel obstruction and embolization to peripheral vessels. Intimal sarcoma can be the cause of sudden death. Correct diagnosis is often possible only with pathology examination after death. It can be misdiagnosed with blood thrombosis and embolism.

Pathology

Intimal sarcoma is a poorly differentiated mesenchymal neoplasm of unclear cell origin consisting of atypical spindle cells with varying degrees of mitotic activity, necrosis, and nuclear polymorphism.

Differential diagnosis may be needed with the following: angiosarcoma (CD31 is positive), leiomyosarcoma (desmin and SMA positivity, MDM2 negative), and cardiac myxoma (low-grade neoplasm).

S. Mocellin, *Soft Tissue Tumors*, https://doi.org/10.1007/978-3-030-58710-9_134

Biomarkers

The tumor may stain positive for smooth muscle actin (SMA) and desmin; it stains negative for endothelial biomarkers.

MDM2 **gene amplification** and protein expression are found in the majority of cases.

Prognosis

The prognosis is poor, with metastases often being present at presentation. The mean survival of patients with aortic and pulmonary artery lesions is about 5–10 months and 12–18 months, respectively.

Therapy

Surgery should be performed, when feasible. The role of chemotherapy and target therapy appears limited: in a recent series including 72 patients, anthracycline-based regimens obtained a 38% overall response rate (with a median progression-free survival of 7–14 months, depending on the stage), whereas for gemcitabine and pazopanib (a tyrosine kinase inhibitor targeting VEGFR, PDGFR, and KIT), the same rate was 8% (median survival: 3 months). The role of radiotherapy is unclear.

Suggested Readings

Fletcher (2020) WHO classification of tumours of soft tissue and bone (5th edition)

Frezza (2020) Systemic treatments in MDM2 positive intimal sarcoma: a multicentre experience with anthracycline, gemcitabine, and pazopanib within the World Sarcoma Network. Cancer 126(1):98–104

Neuville (2014) Intimal sarcoma is the most frequent primary cardiac sarcoma: clinicopathologic and molecular retrospective analysis of 100 primary cardiac sarcomas. Am J Surg Pathol 38(4):461–469

Van Dievel (2017) Single-center experience with intimal sarcoma, an ultra-orphan, commonly fatal mesenchymal malignancy. Oncol Res Treat 40(6):353–359

Definition

Intramuscular hemangioma is a benign lesion of vascular origin. It is still debated whether to consider intramuscular hemangioma a tumor or a malformation. It is also known as intramuscular angioma and intramuscular infiltrating angiolipoma. It belongs to the family of hemangiomas ($\rightarrow$ see Chap. 117).

Epidemiology and Presentation

Intramuscular hemangioma is one of the most frequent deep-seated soft tissue tumors. Adolescents and young adults are most frequently affected (up to 90% of cases), with no difference between males and females. It arises most commonly in the lower limbs, followed by the head and neck, upper limbs, and trunk. Exceptional cases have been described in the cardiac muscle.

Typically, the lesion presents as a slow-growing mass that can be painful, especially after exercise and when the lesion is located in the lower limbs. X-ray-based imaging often shows the presence of calcification, but magnetic resonance imaging is the best radiological technique to establish the diagnosis.

Pathology

Intramuscular hemangioma is a proliferation of benign vascular channels within skeletal muscle, typically associated with variable amounts of mature adipose tissue. Like other hemangiomas, intramuscular hemangioma is traditionally classified into capillary and cavernous subtypes based on the vessel size (small and large, respectively), although mixed forms are frequent.

© The Editor(s) (if applicable) and The Author(s), under exclusive license to
Springer Nature Switzerland AG 2021
S. Mocellin, *Soft Tissue Tumors*, https://doi.org/10.1007/978-3-030-58710-9_135

Prognosis

Although classified as a benign lesion, intramuscular hemangioma tends to recur frequently (up to 50% of cases).

Therapy

Surgical (wide) excision is the treatment of choice.

Suggested Readings

Fletcher (2020) WHO classification of tumours of soft tissue and bone (5th edition)

Kandil (2009) Image of the month. Rectus abdominis intramuscular hemangioma. Arch Surg 144(2):191–192

Liu (2019) Intramuscular hemangioma within the biceps brachii causing the limitations of elbow extension and forearm pronation: A case report. Medicine (Baltimore) 98(5):e14343

Definition

Intramuscular myxoma is a benign neoplasm currently classified among soft tissue tumors of uncertain differentiation.

Epidemiology and Presentation

It occurs mainly in adult or elderly patients (more frequently females) as a painless intramuscular mass. The combination of intramuscular myxoma with bone fibrous dysplasia defines the Mazabraud's syndrome. Magnetic resonance imaging shows a poorly vascularized tumor (which can measure up to 20 cm in diameter) hyperintense on T2-weighted images.

Pathology

Macroscopically, the mass – which may show undefined margins – displays a gelatinous lobulated cut surface and may present fluid-filled cystic spaces.

Miscroscopically, intramuscular myxoma is composed of uniform spindled and stellated cells separated by abundant extracellular myxoid stroma composed of glycosaminoglycans (similar to low-grade myxofibrosarcoma, → see dedicated section). Mitoses, pleomorphism, and necrosis are not present even in the most cellular areas. Intramuscular myxoma with more cellularity is also called cellular myxoma. **Differential diagnosis** may be needed with the following: chondrosarcoma (bone or soft tissue tumor mimicking chordoma with rows of cuboidal cells separated by myxoid background; stains positive for S100 and vimentin, negative for cytokeratins); myxoid liposarcoma (mitotic figures, lipoblasts, positive for FUS-DDIT3 fusion gene); and myxoid leiomyosarcoma (invasive, highly myxomatous; see

© The Editor(s) (if applicable) and The Author(s), under exclusive license to   447
Springer Nature Switzerland AG 2021
S. Mocellin, *Soft Tissue Tumors*, https://doi.org/10.1007/978-3-030-58710-9_136

typical smooth muscle cells alternating with mesenchymal cells); intramuscular cellular myxoma may need to be differentiated from low-grade myxofibrosarcoma (no GNAS mutations).

Biomarkers

At immunohistochemistry, the cells stain variably positive for CD34 and desmin and negative for S100. From the genetics viewpoint, point mutations of the GNAS gene[1] are commonly observed (about 60% of all cases).

Prognosis

Intramuscular myxoma is a benign tumor, although cellular myxomas may recur.

Therapy

Surgical excision is the treatment of choice.

Suggested Readings

Allen (2000) Myxoma is not a single entity: a review of the concept of myxoma. Ann Diagn Pathol 4(2):99–123
Delaney (2009) GNAS1 mutations occur more commonly than previously thought in intramuscular myxoma. Mod Pathol 22(5):718–724
Fletcher (2020) WHO classification of tumours of soft tissue and bone (5th edition)
Vescini (2019) Mazabraud's syndrome: a case report and up-to-date literature review. Endocr Metab Immune Disord Drug Targets 19(6):885–893

---

[1] GNAS: alternative splicing of downstream exons of this gene (also named GNAS complex locus and guanine nucleotide-binding protein alpha-stimulating activity polypeptide 1) results in different forms of the stimulatory G-protein alpha subunit, a key element of the classical signal transduction pathway linking G protein-coupled receptors (GPCR) with the activation of adenylyl cyclase and ultimately a variety of cell activities.

Definition

Ischemic fasciitis is a benign fibroblastic-myofibroblastic proliferation also known as atypical decubital fibroplasia.

Epidemiology and Presentation

Ischemic fasciitis develops usually in elderly people (peak incidence between 70 and 90 years), with slight male prevalence. Often the disease is associated with physical immobility, where constant pressure can cause ischemia and initiate the pathological proliferation of fibroblastic – myofibroblastic cells.

Ischemic fasciitis typically locates around the limb girdles, sacral region, and greater trochanter; nevertheless, other locations have been described such as the chest wall and back.

Clinically, the lesion presents as a painless mass with an average diameter of 5 cm.

Pathology

Macroscopically, ischemic fasciitis develops as a white fibrous lesion with central necrosis in the deep subcutis, although infiltration of the dermis, tendons, and skeletal muscle may occur.

Histologically, the hallmark of this disease is a distinct zonal appearance: the central part is composed by a hypocellular area of necrosis surrounded by a granulation tissue-like vascular proliferation mixed with atypical fibroblasts and myofibroblasts (these cells can display ganglion cell-like appearance similar to proliferative fasciitis). Ischemic fasciitis is considered an example of pseudosarcoma as its appearance can mimic malignant soft tissue tumors.

Differential diagnosis may be needed with the following: epithelioid sarcoma (young adults on distal extremities, more cellular, atypical mitotic figures, cytokeratin positive); myxofibrosarcoma (marked atypia, lacks zonation and degenerative features); myxoid liposarcoma (prominent plexiform vasculature and lipoblasts, small monotonous cells rather than larger myofibroblasts); and proliferative fasciitis (younger patients, lesions not associated with pressure; myofibroblasts and fibroblasts with tissue culture type growth).

Biomarkers

Lesional cells express smooth muscle actin (SMA), vimentin, and (variably) desmin, confirming the fibroblastic-myofibroblastic nature of the lesion.

Prognosis

Ischemic fasciitis is a benign lesion with excellent prognosis.

Therapy

Surgical excision is usually curative, although disease recurrence may rarely occur in immobilized patients probably because of persistence of the underlying cause.

Suggested Readings

Fletcher (2020) WHO classification of tumours of soft tissue and bone (5th edition)
Lehmer (2016) Ischemic fasciitis: enhanced diagnostic resolution through clinical, histopathologic and radiologic correlation in 17 cases. J Cutan Pathol 43(9):740–748
Sachak (2018) Novel t(1;2)(p36.1;q23) and t(7;19)(q32;q13.3) chromosomal translocations in ischemic fasciitis: expanding the spectrum of pseudosarcomatous lesions with clonal pathogenetic link. Diagn Pathol 13(1):18
Sayeed (2014) Management of recurrent ischemic fasciitis, a rare soft tissue pseudosarcoma. Arch Plast Surg 41(1):89–90

Definition

Juvenile hyaline fibromatosis (JHF) is a hereditary disease characterized by the formation of tumor-like benign lesions (classified among fibroblastic-myofibroblastic tumors). The condition is also known as molluscum fibrosum, mesenchymal dysplasia, and hyaline fibromatosis syndrome.

Epidemiology and Presentation

This rare disorder typically presents in infancy and is characterized by the accumulation of extracellular hyaline material (produced by fibroblasts) which leads to the formation of tumor-like masses in the skin (generally as papules and nodules of face and neck), somatic soft tissues (especially periarticular soft tissues, leading to joint contractures), and skeleton (usually as lytic lesions of the skull, long bones, and phalanges).

Generally, the number and size of superficial and deep nodules progressively increase, leading to deformity and dysfunction, although survival into adulthood is possible.

Infantile systemic hyalinosis is a disorder clinically related to JHF but with earlier onset, visceral involvement (e.g., gastrointestinal tract, which results in severe diarrhea), and more severe prognosis (it is usually fatal by 2 years of life); it is caused by similar genetic alterations and is currently considered a variant of JHF.

Of note, patients affected with these two disorders are often the progeny of consanguineous parents.

S. Mocellin, *Soft Tissue Tumors*, https://doi.org/10.1007/978-3-030-58710-9_138

Etiology and Predisposition

JHF is inherited in an autosomal recessive fashion, and it is due to inactivating mutations of the ANTXR2 gene (which encodes capillary morphogenesis protein 2), located on chromosome 4.

Pathology

The nodules are composed of plump fibroblastic cells associated with extracellular uniform hyaline material. Nuclear atypia or necrosis is absent.

Biomarkers

PAS (periodic acid-Schiff) staining is strongly positive and diastase-resistant. The cells stain negative for MSA (muscle specific actin) and S100.

Prognosis

Although the nodules are benign, the prognosis is determined by their number, size, and location.

Therapy

Tumor-like nodules can be surgically removed, although local recurrence is frequent.

Suggested Readings

Fletcher (2020) WHO classification of tumours of soft tissue and bone (5th edition)
Härter (2020) Clinical aspects of hyaline fibromatosis syndrome and identification of a novel mutation. Mol Genet Genomic Med 8(6):e1203
Kalgaonkar (2017) Juvenile hyaline fibromatosis- A rare autosomal recessive disease. J Clin Diagn Res 11(7):SD04–SD06

Definition

Juxta-articular myxoma is a benign tumor with histological features mimicking a cellular myxoma (→ see Chap. 136). It is currently classified among soft tissue tumors of uncertain differentiation and is also known as parameniscal cyst or peri-articular myxoma.

Epidemiology and Presentation

This rare tumor usually arises close to a large joint (especially the knee, about 90% of cases). The median age of occurrence is 40 years. The swelling can be painful or tender. Radiologically the mass presents similar to intramuscular myxoma (→ see dedicated section).

Pathology

This tumor resembles the cellular variant of intramuscular myxoma (bland-appearing spindle cells embedded in a hypovascular myxoid stroma). Mitotic figures are absent or very rare. Cystic ganglion-like spaces are found in most cases. The periphery of the lesion is not well defined and tends to infiltrate adjacent tissues.

Biomarkers

Juxta-articular myxoma lacks the GNAS mutations detected in many intramuscular myxomas.

Prognosis

This is a benign tumor, but disease relapses occur in up to one third of cases.

Therapy

Surgical excision is the treatment of choice.

Suggested Readings

Fletcher (2020). WHO classification of tumours of soft tissue and bone (5th edition)
Raffaele (2019) Juxta-articular myxoma of the hip: a rare pediatric tumor. J Am Acad Orthop Surg Glob Res Rev 3(11):e070
Somford (2011) Juxta-articular myxoma of the knee. J Knee Surg 24(4):299–301

Juxtaglomerular Cell Tumor

Definition

Juxtaglomerular cell tumor (JGCT) is a benign neoplasm of the kidney. It originates from the smooth muscle cells of the glomerular afferent arteriole (juxtaglomerular apparatus). It is also known as reninoma.

Epidemiology and Presentation

JGCT is an exceedingly rare neoplasm typically presenting in young adults (mainly between 25 and 40 years), with a female prevalence. It is often associated with signs/symptoms of hyperreninism such as hypertension, hyperaldosteronism, and hypokalemia. Clinical differential diagnosis includes other renin-producing neoplasms (e.g., renal cell carcinoma, Wilms tumor, mesoblastic nephroma, hepatoblastoma, lung carcinoma, pancreatic adenocarcinoma).

Pathology

JGCT microscopic appearance is variable. The lesion is generally composed of sheets of homogenous round cells with granular eosinophilic or clear cytoplasm; capillaries with hemangiopericytoma-like growth pattern are usually numerous, and the stroma (composed of hyalinized or myxoid tissue) can be scarce or abundant. Mitoses, necrosis, or pleomorphism is rare.

Biomarkers

JGCT stain positive for PAS (cytoplasmic granules), vimentin, renin (strong and diffuse), SMA, and CD34; it stains negative for cytokeratins and HMB45.

S. Mocellin, *Soft Tissue Tumors*, https://doi.org/10.1007/978-3-030-58710-9_140

Prognosis

JGCT is a benign tumor.

Therapy

Nephron-sparing surgery is the treatment of choice.

Suggested Readings

Hagiya (2020) Juxtaglomerular cell tumor with atypical pathological features: report of a case and review of literature. Int J Surg Pathol 28(1):87–91

Inam (2019) Juxtaglomerular cell tumor: reviewing a cryptic cause of surgically correctable hypertension. Curr Urol 13(1):7–12

Jiang (2020) Increased FDG uptake on juxtaglomerular cell tumor in the left kidney mimicking malignancy. Clin Nucl Med 45(3):252–254

Krishnan (2020) Juxtaglomerular cell tumor in a young male presenting with new onset congestive heart failure. Urol Case Rep 31:101189

Definition

Kaposiform hemangioendothelioma (KHE) is a vascular tumor of intermediate malignant behavior. It is also known as Kaposi-like hemangioendothelioma. Although still often classified as separate nosological entities, KHE and tufted hemangioma ($\rightarrow$ see dedicated section) are becoming increasingly recognized as a spectrum of the same pathology.

Epidemiology and Presentation

KHE occurs almost exclusively in children, with more than 50% of cases presenting during the first year of life (with slight male prevalence). Exceptional cases in adults have been described. Unlike Kaposi sarcoma, this tumor is not associated with infection by human herpes virus 8 (HHV8).

KHE arises most frequently in the skin of the extremities, but it can also locate in other superficial and deep sites (including viscera). Superficial cases present as a tender violaceous mass that causes pain when the coagulation cascade is activated within the tumor. Unlike some types of hemangioma ($\rightarrow$ see dedicated section), KHE does not spontaneously regress.

Pathology

KHE is characterized by the presence of abundant vascular structures that infiltrate the surrounding soft tissues. Tumor nodules have irregular borders, and they are composed of fascicles of spindle endothelial cells organized as irregular vascular lobules that infiltrate soft tissue in a "cannonball" manner. Mitoses are rare, while nuclear atypia and necrosis are absent. It displays features recalling both capillary

© The Editor(s) (if applicable) and The Author(s), under exclusive license to
Springer Nature Switzerland AG 2021
S. Mocellin, *Soft Tissue Tumors*, https://doi.org/10.1007/978-3-030-58710-9_141

hemangioma and Kaposi sarcoma (hence the name; → see dedicated section). KHE appears morphologically identical to tufted hemangioma.

Biomarkers

Endothelial cells are positive for vascular markers such as CD31 and CD34 and negative for GLUT1 (as opposed to infantile hemangioma, → see dedicated section).

Prognosis

KHE is locally aggressive, but it may be life-threatening if associated with the Kasabach-Merritt syndrome (characterized by thrombocytopenia and coagulopathy) which occurs in about 50% of cases and is associated with 10% mortality rate.

Therapy

Surgery is the definitive treatment for KHE. However, it is often not possible given ill-defined tumor borders and the invasion of multiple tissue planes and local structures. Furthermore, once the Kasabach-Merritt syndrome develops, surgery is contraindicated given the hemodynamic risks. **Embolization** may be an alternative to surgery if a single feeding vessel is demonstrated (which is infrequent), although this strategy carries the risk of necrosis and superinfection. **Radiotherapy** can induce regression of the lesion but is associated with the risk of developmental delay, growth delay, and secondary malignancy. Multiple types of **medical therapy** are available. Historically, corticosteroids are the first-line treatment. In case of steroid failure (about 33% of cases), vincristine and **target therapy** with mTOR inhibitors (e.g., sirolimus) can be used. International guidelines currently recommend combination of steroid and vincristine as first-line therapy.

Suggested Readings

Fletcher (2020) WHO classification of tumours of soft tissue and bone (5th edition)
Ji (2020) Kaposiform hemangioendothelioma: current knowledge and future perspectives. Orphanet J Rare Dis 15(1):39
Papke (2019) What is new in endothelial neoplasia? Virchows Arch 476(1):17–28
Schmid (2018) Kaposiform hemangioendothelioma in children: a benign vascular tumor with multiple treatment options. World J Pediatr 14(4):322–329
Wang (2020) Sirolimus for Kaposiform Hemangioendothelioma With Kasabach-Merritt Phenomenon in Two Infants. J Craniofac Surg 31(4):1074–1077
Yao (2020) Retroperitoneal kaposiform hemangioendothelioma complicated by Kasabach-Merritt phenomenon and obstructive jaundice: a retrospective series of 3 patients treated with sirolimus. Pediatr Dermatol 37(4):677–680

Definition

Kaposi sarcoma (KS) is a vascular tumor of intermediate biological aggressiveness. It is also known as idiopathic multiple pigmented sarcoma of the skin, angiosarcoma multiplex, and granuloma multiplex hemorrhagicum.

Epidemiology and Presentation

Kaposi sarcoma presents in four different clinical forms:

1. **Sporadic Kaposi sarcoma** (also known as classic KS) occurs most commonly in elderly men of Mediterranean descent.
2. **Endemic Kaposi sarcoma** occurs in middle-aged adults and children in equatorial Africa who are not infected with human immunodeficiency virus (HIV, which causes AIDS, i.e., acquired immunodeficiency syndrome).
3. **Iatrogenic Kaposi sarcoma** develops in patients treated with immunosuppressive therapy such as those undergoing organ transplantation, corticosteroid therapy for autoimmune diseases, or chemotherapy.
4. **Epidemic Kaposi sarcoma** (also known as AIDS-associated KS) develops in people infected with HIV-1 (which is particularly frequent in homosexual and bisexual men); the risk of KS in this group has significantly decreased after the implementation of highly active antiretroviral therapy (HAART) and combined antiretroviral therapy (cART); of note, in this population, KS can be the first manifestation of HIV infection or a manifestation of cART failure. Although the widespread introduction of effective antiretrovirals to control HIV by restoring immunocompetence has reduced the prevalence of AIDS-related KS, KS does occur in individuals with well-controlled HIV infection.

© The Editor(s) (if applicable) and The Author(s), under exclusive license to
Springer Nature Switzerland AG 2021
S. Mocellin, *Soft Tissue Tumors*, https://doi.org/10.1007/978-3-030-58710-9_142

KS typically involves the skin. However, it can also spread to mucosal membranes (e.g., oral mucosa), lymph nodes, and viscera (virtually any body site can be affected), sometimes even without skin involvement. In general, the involvement of viscera may be silent or symptomatic, depending on the extent and specific site of the lesions.

In typical cases, cutaneous KS is characterized by the occurrence of purplish, reddish-blue, or dark brown macules, plaques, and nodules (from few millimeters to several centimeters) that localize preferably in distal extremities and can ulcerate. Lesions involving the mucosa, soft tissues, lymph nodes, and viscera present as hemorrhagic nodules of various sizes that may become coalescent.

According to a Surveillance, Epidemiology, and End Results (SEER) analysis, KS is the most frequent skin sarcoma in the USA, accounting for approximately 70% of all cases (followed by dermatofibrosarcoma protuberans, which accounts for about 18% of cases).

Etiology and Predisposition

KS is caused by a viral infection by human herpes virus 8 (HHV8), also known as KS-associated herpesvirus (KSHV), which is found in KS cells of all clinical forms of KS. Currently, most cases of KS occur in sub-Saharan Africa, where KSHV infection is prevalent due to virus transmission by saliva in childhood combined with the ongoing AIDS epidemic. Despite a decline in incidence since the introduction of combination anti-retroviral therapy, KS remains the most common malignancy in patients living with HIV in sub-Saharan Africa, where it causes significant morbidity and mortality.

Pathology

Histology is mandatory to make diagnosis. Microscopic appearance of KS does not vary across the four clinical types of disease. The tumor is composed of vascular proliferation where lining endothelial cells are typically spindled and show little or no atypia. Mitoses are common, but pleomorphism is usually minimal. Although the spindle-shaped cells in KS lesions are believed to be of endothelial lineage, they also have features of smooth muscles cells and pericytes. These spindle-shaped cells are present in all forms of KS, are the basis of diagnosis, and constitute the bulk of the proliferating cell fraction.

Recognized variants of KS include anaplastic KS (characterized by pleomorphism and atypia as well as an aggressive clinical course with increased metastatic potential), telangiectatic KS, lymphangioma-like KS, cavernous hemangioma-like KS, pyogenic granuloma-like KS, intravascular KS, bullous KS, ecchymotic KS, hyperkeratotic KS, keloidal KS, micronodular KS, glomeruloid KS, solid KS, keloidal KS, desmoplastic KS, KS with myoid nodules, KS with sarcoid-like granulomas, and pigmented KS.

Differential diagnosis may be needed with the following: angiosarcoma (usually arises in head and neck of sun-damaged skin of elderly or at site of irradiation; usually marked nuclear atypia; HHV8 negative); acroangiodermatitis (also known as pseudo-Kaposi sarcoma; it is due to severe vascular stasis and is a benign condition which clinically presents as violaceous macules and indurated plaques or nodules usually bilaterally on the extensor surfaces of lower extremities; fibroblastic spindle cell component rather than endothelial cells is present; negative for vascular biomarkers; HHV8 negative); hobnail hemangioma (also known as targetoid hemosiderotic hemangioma; lit-like vascular channels but no spindle cell proliferation, HHV8 negative); spindle cell hemangioma (spindled endothelial cells with slit-like channels but also has epithelioid cells, HHV8 negative); and Kaposiform hemangioendothelioma (unique whorled and nodular pattern of spindled endothelial cells, usually in young children or infants, HHV8 negative).

Biomarkers

The lining cells of vascular structures and the spindle tumor cells stain positive for endothelial biomarkers (e.g., CD31, CD34, and ERG), as well as lymphatic biomarkers (e.g., podoplanin).

However, since all KS cases are associated with HHV8 infection, the most specific biomarker is the viral antigen LANA (latency-associated nuclear antigen). Of note, LANA expression may also be present in other HHV8-associated conditions including multicentric Castleman disease and primary effusion lymphoma.

KS stains negative for SMA, desmin, cytokeratins, S100, Melan-A/MART1, and HMB45.

Prognosis

KS is classified by the World Health Organization as a malignant tumor of intermediate aggressiveness (as a rarely metastasizing tumor). Classic KS is the most indolent form of this disease, lymph node and visceral involvement being rare. Endemic KS localizes to the skin and displays a prolonged course; in children, this form can spread to the lymph nodes and behave aggressively (high mortality rates). Iatrogenic KS may regress after immunosuppressive drug withdrawal, although its course can be unpredictable and patients developing visceral involvement may succumb to the disease. Epidemic KS is the most aggressive form of KS: in the skin, lesions are most common on the face, genitals, and lower extremities; the oral mucosa, lymph nodes, gastrointestinal tract, and lungs are frequently involved, and lymph node or visceral disease may occur without mucocutaneous lesions. Unlike western countries (where the clinical outcome has substantially improved), in sub-Saharan Africa, KS continues to have a poor prognosis.

Therapy

Treatment for early AIDS-related KS in previously untreated patients should start with the control of HIV with antiretrovirals. About 50% of patients with epidemic KS respond to immune reconstitution and HIV suppression by cART. A fraction of AIDS-related KS experience tumor progression upon cART initiation: this phenomenon is called KS immune reconstitution syndrome (KS-IRIS) and is observed in approximately 10% of patients exposed to cART for the first time; in these patients (who cannot stop cART), concurrent chemotherapy is the most suitable choice. Of note, one third of AIDS-related KS develops in the context of successful cART (i.e., undetectable HIV viral load and near-normal CD4 counts).

Transplanted patients with iatrogenic KS respond to immune reconstitution, though lowering the immunosuppressive dose increases the risk of graft rejection. Switching the immune suppressive regimen from cyclosporine-A or FK506 (tacrolimus) to mTOR inhibitors (e.g., rapamycin, sirolimus, everolimus) often leads to KS regression.

Cytotoxic chemotherapy represents the standard of care for KS (including in children) that cannot be treated as above outlined: doxorubicin (and its liposomal formulation to minimize toxicity) is the first choice drug and is effective in 75% of patients; paclitaxel also shows clinical efficacy and is usually considered as second line therapy. Although in advanced-stage KS chemotherapy with pegylated liposomal doxorubicin or paclitaxel is the most commonly used treatment, these drugs are rarely curative.

Interferon-alpha has been used with some success in the past, but chemotherapy agents have largely replaced it. Other compounds such as anti-angiogenic agents (e.g., bevacizumab), imiquimod (a TLR7 agonist acting as an immunostimulating drug), and thalidomide (and its derivatives pomalidomide and lenalidomide) have been used with inconsistent results; among these medications, thalidomide and pomalidomide have been designated (but not approved) by the US Food and Drug Administration as orphan drugs for KS. Immunotherapy (with anti-PD1 monoclonal antibodies) is being explored with some encouraging results.

Suggested Readings

Cesarman (2019) Kaposi sarcoma. Nat Rev Dis Primers 5(1):9
Dupin (2020) Update on oncogenesis and therapy for Kaposi sarcoma. Curr Opin Oncol 32(2):122–128
Etemad (2019) Kaposi sarcoma updates. Dermatol Clin 37(4):505–517
Fletcher (2020) WHO classification of tumours of soft tissue and bone (5th edition)
Galanina (2018) Successful treatment of HIV-associated Kaposi sarcoma with immune checkpoint blockade. Cancer Immunol Res 6(10):1129–1135

Krown (2020) Treatment of advanced AIDS-associated Kaposi sarcoma in resource-limited settings: a three-arm, open-label, randomised, non-inferiority trial. Lancet 395(10231):1195–1207

Polizzotto (2016) Pomalidomide for symptomatic Kaposi's sarcoma in people with and without HIV infection: a phase I/II study. J Clin Oncol 34(34):4125–4131

Rouhani (2008) Cutaneous soft tissue sarcoma incidence patterns in the U.S.: an analysis of 12,114 cases. Cancer 113(3):616–627

Schneider (2017) Diagnosis and treatment of Kaposi sarcoma. Am J Clin Dermatol 18(4):529–539

Definition

Kidney clear cell sarcoma (KCCS) is a distinctive malignant neoplasm of the kidney. It is also known as clear cell sarcoma of the kidney.

Epidemiology and Presentation

KCCS is an uncommon neoplasm that typically presents in 2–3 years old children (with male prevalence 3:1); it represents 3–5% of all pediatric renal tumors and is the second most common primary renal malignancy in childhood (after Wilms tumor).

Pathology

Accurate diagnosis of KCCS can be challenging because this tumor can have diverse histologic features. Although many histological variants exist, the classic appearance is that of a tumor composed of uniform, small round cells with a clear appearance separated by a delicate vascular network into nests or cords. Despite its name, clear cells occur in only 20% of cases. Although the classic pattern is almost always at least focally present, other patterns may be present such as myxoid (50%), sclerosing (35%), cellular (25%), epithelioid (15%), palisading verocay body (10%), spindle cell (7%), storiform (4%), and anaplastic (2%).

Differential diagnosis may be needed with the following: clear cell carcinoma of kidney (extremely rare in children; cytokeratin positive); malignant rhabdoid tumor of the kidney (vimentin staining in a dot-like pattern); mesoblastic nephroma (WT1 and SMA positive); and Wilms tumor (nephrogenic rests rule out KCCS; WT1 positive; cytokeratin positivity in epithelioid areas; in a pure stromal-type Wilms tumor treated with preoperative chemotherapy, the tumor may show a

S. Mocellin, *Soft Tissue Tumors*, https://doi.org/10.1007/978-3-030-58710-9_143

KCCS-like appearance, and extensive sampling may be required to detect areas with other Wilms tumor components).

Biomarkers

KCCS is usually only positive for vimentin, although Cyclin D1 may also be expressed. Most importantly, BCOR[1] immunoreactivity is a sensitive and highly specific marker for KCCS. The tumor stains negative for WT1, CD56, EMA, S100, CD99, desmin, CEA, synaptophysin, and cytokeratins.

Internal tandem duplication in the BCOR gene (see footnote 1) is found in most cases of KCCS.

The **chromosomal translocation** t(10;17)(q22;p13) resulting in the YWHAE-NUTM2 fusion gene[2] has been reported in a subset of KCCS cases.

Prognosis

KCCS is characterized by aggressive behavior and late relapses. About 5% of patients have metastatic disease (including bone, brain, lung and liver) at presentation. It was initially named bone metastasizing renal tumor of childhood due to its propensity for skeletal metastasis (bone metastases occur in 20% to 40% of patients, as compared to less than 2% in Wilms tumor).

Therapy

Surgery (total nephrectomy) is the mainstay of treatment for localized disease; adjuvant chemoradiation is often utilized to consolidate the results of surgery. Of note, KCCS is highly responsive to doxorubicin (which makes extremely important to correctly diagnose this entity), which is usually combined with vincristine and D-actinomycin.

---

[1] BCOR (BCL6 corepressor) encodes a transcriptional corepressor which specifically inhibits gene expression when recruited to promoter regions by sequence-specific DNA-binding proteins such as BCL6 and MLLT3; BCOR rearrangements have been described in clear cell sarcoma of the kidney, primitive myxoid mesenchymal tumor of infancy, central nervous system high-grade neuroepithelial tumor, undifferentiated round cell sarcoma, high-grade endometrial stromal sarcoma, and ossifying fibromyxoid tumor.

[2] YWHAE-NUTM2 fusion gene: YWHAE encodes tyrosine 3-monooxygenase/tryptophan 5-monooxygenase activation protein epsilon, a member of the 14-3-3 family of proteins which mediate signal transduction by binding to phosphoserine-containing proteins. NUTM2 (NUT family member 2B) is a protein-coding gene whose alterations have been linked to endometrial stromal sarcoma and kidney clear cell sarcoma.

Suggested Readings

Aldera (2020) Clear cell sarcoma of the kidney. Arch Pathol Lab Med 144(1):119–123

Aw (2019) Clear cell sarcoma of the kidney. Arch Pathol Lab Med 143(8):1022–1026

Han (2020) BCOR-CCNB3 fusion-positive clear cell sarcoma of the kidney. Pediatr Blood Cancer 67(4):e28151

Khan (2019) Diagnostic utility of BCOR antibody in clear cell sarcomas of kidney. Int J Surg Pathol [Epub ahead of print]

Kusumakumary (1999) Clear cell sarcoma kidney: clinical features and outcome. Pediatr Hematol Oncol 16(2):169–174

Seibel (2019) Impact of cyclophosphamide and etoposide on outcome of clear cell sarcoma of the kidney treated on the National Wilms Tumor Study-5 (NWTS-5). Pediatr Blood Cancer 66(1):e27450

This neoplasm is also known as rhabdoid tumor of the kidney (RTK).
    For details → see Chap. 144.

The following is the list of soft tissue tumors of the kidney according the WHO Classification published in 2016.

For details on each single tumor, → see dedicated sections.

Tumor	Notes
Angiomyolipoma	–
Angiosarcoma	–
Congenital mesoblastic nephroma	Occurring mainly in children
Epithelioid angiomyolipoma	→ See Chap. 24
Ewing sarcoma	→ See Chap. 93
Hemangioblastoma	–
Hemangioma	–
Juxtaglomerular cell tumor	–
Kidney clear cell sarcoma	Occurring mainly in children; also known as clear cell sarcoma of the kidney
Kidney rhabdoid tumor	Occurring mainly in children; also known as rhabdoid tumor of the kidney
Leiomyoma	–
Leiomyosarcoma	–
Lymphangioma	–
Osteosarcoma	→ See Chap. 95
Rhabdomyosarcoma	–
Schwannoma	–
Solitary fibrous tumor	–
Synovial sarcoma	–

Leiomyoma is a benign tumor originating from smooth muscle cells.
For more details → see the sections dedicated to the following topics:

- Angioleiomyoma.
- Benign metastasizing leiomyoma.
- Cutaneous leiomyoma.
- Esophageal leiomyoma.
- Leiomyoma of deep tissue.
- Uterine leiomyoma.

Definition

Leiomyoma of deep tissue (LDT) is a benign tumor originating from smooth muscle cells. It is also known as leiomyoma of deep soft tissue. It belongs to the leiomyoma family of tumors (→ see Chap. 146).

Epidemiology and Presentation

LDT is a very rare mesenchymal tumor that mainly occurs in the retroperitoneum and other sites of the abdominal cavity (e.g., mesentery, omentum, and abdominal wall). LDT may also occur in the inguinal region (e.g., round ligament). Typically, LDT affects almost exclusively young to middle-aged women.

Occurrence in other sites (e.g., somatic soft tissues such as subcutis and muscles) is very rare and is characterized by equal frequency between males and females.

Clinically, LDT may become very large (>30 cm) and be multiple; calcifications may be present upon X-ray imaging.

Pathology

LDT is composed of intersecting fascicles of spindled cells that mimic normal smooth muscle cells with eosinophilic cytoplasm and uniform cigar-shaped nuclei. Neither nuclear atypia nor necrosis is present and mitotic activity is scarce to absent (generally <5 per 50 HPF).

Overall the lesion resembles uterine leiomyoma (→ see dedicated section). The presence of focal nuclear atypia and higher number of mitoses should raise the suspicion of leiomyosarcoma.

© The Editor(s) (if applicable) and The Author(s), under exclusive license to
Springer Nature Switzerland AG 2021
S. Mocellin, *Soft Tissue Tumors*, https://doi.org/10.1007/978-3-030-58710-9_147

Biomarkers

LDT stains positive for SMA, desmin, and h-caldesmon but negative for S100. Abdominal, retroperitoneal, and inguinal LDT in women stains consistently positive for estrogen receptor, progesterone receptor, and WT1.

Prognosis

LDT is a benign tumor.

Therapy

Surgical excision is usually curative, although local disease recurrence has been rarely reported especially with long-term follow-up.

Suggested Readings

Batihan (2018) Atypical deep somatic soft-tissue leiomyoma of extrathoracic chest wall: first case of the literature. BMJ Case Rep 11(1):e226668

Fletcher (2020) WHO classification of tumours of soft tissue and bone (5th edition)

Nakamura (2007) Intermuscular leiomyoma of deep soft tissue arising in the lower chest. Dermatol Surg 33(8):986–989

Panagopoulos (2017) Genetic heterogeneity in leiomyomas of deep soft tissue. Oncotarget 8(30):48769–48781

Definition

Leiomyosarcoma (LMS) is a malignant tumor originating from smooth muscle cells. In this section the so-called deep soft tissue LMS is considered; for superficial LMS (i.e., LMS of the skin), → see Chap. 62; for uterine leiomyosarcoma → see dedicated section.

Epidemiology and Presentation

LMS accounts for about 10–15% of all adult soft tissue sarcomas. LMS generally occurs in middle-aged or older adults, although cases in young adults and even in children have been reported.

LMS is one of the most frequent types of retroperitoneal/pelvic sarcomas and is the most frequent type of sarcoma of the large blood vessels (e.g., vena cava). It represents about 10–15% of extremity sarcomas. Females are overrepresented in patients with retroperitoneal or large vessel LMS, but this is not the case for LMS arising elsewhere. Gastrointestinal cases of LMS should be carefully reviewed in order to rule out the much more likely diagnosis of gastrointestinal stromal tumor (GIST).

Clinically, the tumor presents as a mass that can reach large diameters before diagnosis, especially when it is located in the retroperitoneum. The lesion may be painful and/or cause symptoms related to the compression/infiltration of adjacent structures.

Etiology and Predisposition

The cancer predisposition condition known as **Li-Fraumeni syndrome** is associated with a significant risk of developing LMS. This syndrome has an estimated prevalence of 1/20,000 people. The lifetime risk of cancer is about 70% for men and close to 100% for women. Typical cancers observed in this condition include breast carcinoma, soft tissue and bone sarcomas (including rhabdomyosarcoma, osteosarcoma, and LMS), and brain tumors (choroid plexus carcinoma, astrocytoma, medulloblastoma, and glioblastoma). However, other malignancies have been associated with the syndrome, which is caused by germline mutations in the tumor suppressor gene TP53 (located on chromosome 17p13.1) in about 80% of families. The syndrome is inherited in an autosomal dominant pattern. Most patients with Li-Fraumeni syndrome inherit an altered copy of the gene from an affected parent; however, in up to 20% of cases, the altered gene is the result of a new gene mutation in germ cells. The development of a malignancy in Li-Fraumeni syndrome requires a somatic mutation involving the other copy of the TP53 gene (during the patient lifetime), according to the classic two-hit hypothesis formulated by Knudson.

Finally, infection by **Epstein-Barr virus** (EBV) in immunocompromised patients has been associated with a higher than expected risk of developing LMS.

Pathology

Macroscopically, the lesion may show hemorrhage, necrosis, or cystic change. The tumor may be well circumscribed but can also frankly infiltrate surrounding structures. Microscopically, the common appearance is that of intersecting fascicles of spindle cells. The tumor is typically compactly cellular, but fibrosis or myxoid change as well as hypocellular zones and coagulative tumor necrosis may be present. Cell nuclei are characteristically elongated and blunt-ended.

Nuclear hyperchromasia and pleomorphism are generally evident although they may be mild or even absent. Mitotic figures are usually found readily, although they may be few; atypical mitoses are often found.

Rarely, areas with poorly differentiated, pleomorphic appearance (in addition to conventional areas) can be observed, which leads to the definition of so-called dedifferentiated leiomyosarcoma.

The tumor may show hemangiopericytoma-like vasculature, nuclear palisading, myxoid change, and osteoclast-like giant cells; some lesions have extensive pleomorphism mimicking undifferentiated pleomorphic sarcoma.

The following malignant criteria by site have been proposed:

- Deep soft tissues: 1–2 mitoses/10 high-power field (HPF).
- Cutis/subcutis: 1–2 mitoses/10 HPF.
- Retroperitoneum: 5 mitoses/10 HPF or 1–4 mitoses/10 HPF plus necrosis and size >7.5 cm.
- Vascular: 1–4 mitoses/10 HPF, plus large size and necrosis.

Cases with fewer mitoses should be probably better diagnosed as smooth muscle tumors of unknown malignant potential (STUMP → see dedicated section).

Differential diagnosis may be needed with dedifferentiated liposarcoma (better prognosis, well-differentiated component present, MDM2 and CDK4 amplification), leiomyoma (mitotic activity rare or absent, atypia minimal or absent, smaller size, neither hemorrhage nor necrosis, never infiltrating), and STUMP.

Biomarkers

LMS usually stains positive for smooth muscle actin (SMA), desmin, and h-caldesmon, although none of these biomarkers is completely specific for smooth muscle (positivity for at least two of these biomarkers confers more specificity). Of note, "dedifferentiated" areas are negative for SMA and desmin. CD117 (c-Kit) is typically negative (as opposed to GIST).

From the cytogenetics viewpoint, LMS is characterized by highly complex karyotypes. Tumor suppressor genes frequently altered in LMS are TP53, RB1, and PTEN. **Gene amplification** of myocardin (MYOCD, located on chromosome 17p and encoding a smooth muscle-specific transcriptional coactivator) is found in approximately 70% of cases.

Prognosis

LMS is a malignant neoplasm associated with both local recurrence and distant metastasis (mainly lungs; lymph node metastasis is rare). Of note, LMS is the sarcoma that most frequently metastasizes to the skin; soft tissue and bone metastases can also be observed.

The most significant prognostic factors are tumor location (superficial versus deep) and size (which are correlated). Retroperitoneal LMS is typically large (>10 cm), is often difficult or impossible to remove with clear margins, tends to recur locally recurrence and metastasize, and ultimately results fatal in most cases. LMS of large vessels is also associated with a poor prognosis, although generally better than that of retroperitoneal LMS. LMS arising from other sites are usually smaller and associated with a better prognosis. Superficial LMS (i.e., LMS developing above the muscular fascia) have a better prognosis as compared to deep tissue LMS.

Histological grading is another reliable prognostic factor; of note, the World Health Organization recognizes the classic three differentiation grades for LMS (G1, well differentiated; G2, moderately differentiated; and G3, poorly differentiated).

LMS arising in immunocompromised patients tends to involve parenchymal organs rather than soft tissues, occurs predominantly in children and young adults who are HIV positive or have been transplanted, and is associated with EBV infection; on average, these tumors have a better prognosis as compared to conventional LMS.

Therapy

Surgery is the mainstay of treatment for localized (resectable) LMS. For cases located in the somatic soft tissues (i.e., extremities and trunk wall), neoadjuvant or adjuvant **chemotherapy** and **radiotherapy** are generally considered for large and high-grade lesions. For retroperitoneal LMS, the only available randomized controlled trial (RCT) called STRASS failed to demonstrate any advantage for patients undergoing neoadjuvant radiotherapy.

For locally advanced (i.e., non resectable) and metastatic disease, anthracyclines remain the first choice agents. Although LMS is deemed to be somewhat more sensitive to gemcitabine plus dacarbazine, this drug combination resulted inferior to epirubicin plus ifosfamide in terms of disease-free survival in a RCT of neoadjuvant chemotherapy for soft tissue sarcomas including LMS (ISG-STS 1001). Doxorubicin plus dacarbazine appears to provide some tumor response and survival advantage (as compared to doxorubicin alone or combined with ifosfamide), but no RCT-based evidence is available. Based on the results of a RCT, trabectedin has been approved for the treatment of patients with unresectable or metastatic LMS (as well as liposarcoma) who received a prior anthracycline-containing regimen.

As regards **target therapy**, anti-angiogenic agent pazopanib (a tyrosine kinase inhibitor targeting VEGFR, PDGFR, and KIT) has been approved (based on the findings of the RCT PALETTE) for the treatment of advanced/metastatic soft tissue sarcomas (including LMS but excluding both adipocytic sarcomas and GIST) in patients who have received prior chemotherapy.

Suggested Readings

Bonvalot (2019) STRASS (EORTC 62092): a phase III randomized study of preoperative radiotherapy plus surgery versus surgery alone for patients with retroperitoneal sarcoma. J Clin Oncol 37(15_suppl):11001

D'Ambrosio (2020) Doxorubicin plus dacarbazine, doxorubicin plus ifosfamide, or doxorubicin alone as a first-line treatment for advanced leiomyosarcoma: a propensity score matching analysis from the European Organization for Research and Treatment of Cancer Soft Tissue and Bone Sarcoma Group. Cancer 126(11):2637–2647

Demetri (2016) Efficacy and safety of trabectedin or dacarbazine for metastatic liposarcoma or leiomyosarcoma after failure of conventional chemotherapy: results of a phase III randomized multicenter clinical trial. J Clin Oncol 34(8):786–793

Fletcher (2020) WHO classification of tumours of soft tissue and bone (5th edition)

Gronchi (2017) Histotype-tailored neoadjuvant chemotherapy versus standard chemotherapy in patients with high-risk soft-tissue sarcomas (ISG-STS 1001): an international, open-label, randomised, controlled, phase 3, multicentre trial. Lancet Oncol 18(6):812–822

Pantoja (2020) Caval reconstruction with undersized ringed graft after resection of inferior vena cava leiomyosarcoma. Ann Vasc Surg 65:25–32

Patel (2019) Overall survival and histology-specific subgroup analyses from a phase 3, randomized controlled study of trabectedin or dacarbazine in patients with advanced liposarcoma or leiomyosarcoma. Cancer 125(15):2610–2620

Shannon-Lowe (2019) The global landscape of EBV-associated tumors. Front Oncol 9:713

van der Graaf Winette (2012) Pazopanib for metastatic soft-tissue sarcoma (PALETTE): a randomised, double-blind, placebo-controlled phase 3 trial. Lancet 379:1879–1886

Vella (2020) Case of primary hepatic leiomyosarcoma successfully treated with laparoscopic right hepatectomy. BMJ Case Rep 13(2):e233567

Definition

Lipoblastoma is a benign neoplasm of embryonal white fat. It is also known as fetal lipoma, fetal fat tumor, embryonal lipoma, and lipoblastic tumor of childhood.

Epidemiology and Presentation

Lipoblastoma occurs almost exclusively in infancy and early childhood (90% of cases occur before age 3 years). Trunk and extremities are the most common sites; however, lipoblastoma cases have been rarely described in the retroperitoneum, pelvis, abdomen, mesentery, mediastinum, head and neck, and even viscera.

Pathology

Lipoblastoma shows a lobular architecture with sheets of adipocytes separated by fibrovascular septa. The fat cells display a spectrum of maturation, ranging from primitive stellate or spindled mesenchymal cells, to multivacuolated or small signet ring lipoblasts, to mature adipocytes. It is associated with plexiform vascular pattern and abundant myxoid stroma.

Differential diagnosis may be needed with the following: lipofibromatosis/infantile fibromatosis (fibrous tissue only which may entrap mature fat cells; no myxoid stroma, no plexiform vascular pattern); myxoid liposarcoma (rare in children, no distinct lobulation, usually more cellular with giant cells containing pleomorphic nuclei; different genetic aberrations); and well-differentiated liposarcoma (rare in children, mature fat but no lipoblasts; spindle cells with large nuclei and marked nuclear enlargement or pleomorphism; low cellularity; MDM2 and CDK4 immunostains are sensitive and specific).

Biomarkers

The adipocytes of lipoblastoma stain positive for S100 protein and CD34, and the primitive mesenchymal cells are often reactive for desmin.

Rearrangements of the PLAG1 gene (located in in 8q12.1 and coding for a transcription factor) are frequently present (>80%) and can be a diagnostic aid: besides **gene amplification, chromosomal translocations** lead to the formation of HAS2-PLAG1 fusion gene and COL1A2-PLAG1 fusion gene. These rearrangements generally lead to PLAG1 overexpression.

Prognosis

Lipoblastoma is a benign tumor, the recurrence rate of 15–45% being attributable to incomplete excision. Diffuse lipoblastoma (also known as lipoblastomatosis) is more infiltrative than circumscribed lipoblastoma, but this distinction has little clinical relevance since both types can recur.

There is no risk of metastasis or malignant transformation.

Therapy

Surgical excision is the treatment of choice.

Suggested Readings

Fletcher (2020) WHO classification of tumours of soft tissue and bone (5th edition)
Nitta (2019) Identification of a novel BOC-PLAG1 fusion gene in a case of lipoblastoma. Biochem Biophys Res Commun 512(1):49–52
Wang (2019) Three novel aberrations involving PLAG1 leading to lipoblastoma in three different patients: high amplification, partial deletion, and a unique complex rearrangement. Cytogenet Genome Res 159(2):81–87

Definition

Lipofibromatosis is a benign neoplasm classified among the fibroblastic-myofibroblastic tumors. It is also known as infantile fibromatosis (non-desmoid type), juvenile fibromatosis (non-desmoid type), and fibrous hamartoma of infancy.

Epidemiology and Presentation

Lipofibromatosis is a very rare tumor developing in childhood (about 20% of cases are congenital), with a male prevalence (M:F = 2:1). This neoplasm localizes mainly in the hand or foot and less frequently in the head and neck or trunk.

The lesion typically presents as an ill-defined, slow-growing, painless mass (usually 1–5 cm in diameter), with fatty appearance and located in the subcutis or deep soft tissue.

Pathology

The lesion is composed of abundant, usually mature adipose tissue (>50% of the tumor) mixed with a spindle cell (fibromatosis-like) component.

Fat cells are usually mature and lack atypia, while the fibroblastic component shows only mild atypia and a low mitotic rate; the fibroblastic component does not show the diffuse sheetlike and destructive growth pattern of desmoid-type fibromatosis (→ see dedicated section).

Differential diagnosis may be needed with the following: fibromatosis (solid sheetlike fibrous growth, minimal to no fat, beta-catenin positive) and fibrous hamartoma of infancy (primitive oval cell component with myxoid stroma).

© The Editor(s) (if applicable) and The Author(s), under exclusive license to
Springer Nature Switzerland AG 2021
S. Mocellin, *Soft Tissue Tumors*, https://doi.org/10.1007/978-3-030-58710-9_150

Biomarkers

Fibroblasts usually express CD34 and SMA.[1] Focal staining for S100, MSA,[2] and EMA[3] may occur. Staining for desmin, cytokeratins, and nuclear beta-catenin is negative.

Prognosis

Despite its benign nature (it has no metastatic potential), lipofibromatosis is burdened by a high rate of local recurrence.

Therapy

Surgical excision is the treatment of choice.

Suggested Readings

Al-Ibraheemi (2019) Aberrant receptor tyrosine kinase signaling in lipofibromatosis: a clinicopathological and molecular genetic study of 20 cases. Mod Pathol 32(3):423–434
Fletcher (2020) WHO classification of tumours of soft tissue and bone (5th edition)

---

[1] SMA: smooth muscle actin.

[2] MSA: muscle-specific actin.

[3] EMA: epithelial membrane antigen.

Definition

Lipofibromatosis-like neural tumor (LNT) is a soft tissue tumor closely resembling lipofibromatosis (→ see dedicated section) and characterized by intermediate biological aggressiveness.

Epidemiology and Presentation

LNT is a recently described nosological entity, and only a few cases have been described. It usually arises in childhood and young adulthood and locates in superficial soft tissues as a nodule of averagely 4 cm in diameter.

Pathology

LNT is a mesenchymal tumor that mimics lipofibromatosis (→ see dedicated section) but differs from it because it exhibits a mild degree of nuclear atypia, coexpresses S100 and CD34, and bears recurrent neurotrophic tyrosine kinase receptor 1 (NTRK1) gene rearrangements. The typical lesion is composed of streaming fascicles of spindle cells that infiltrate the subcutaneous adipose tissue in a fashion closely reminiscent of lipofibromatosis; the spindled tumor cells display a mild degree of nuclear atypia, the mitotic rate being low (lower than 1 per 10 HPF).

Differential diagnosis may be needed with spindle cell mesenchymal neoplasms arising in superficial soft tissues (in particular of young patients) such as the following: fibroma, infantile fibromatosis, congenital fibrosarcoma, solitary fibrous tumor, and DFSP. These fibroblastic neoplasms differ from LNT by consistent negativity for S100 protein; moreover, diffuse expression of CD34 is usually not a feature of fibroma, infantile fibromatosis, and congenital fibrosarcoma; besides the positive staining of S100, lack of STAT6 immunoreactivity also distinguishes LNT from solitary fibrous tumor. LNT can be confused with DFSP due to CD34 positivity and subcutaneous infiltration: however, the expression of S100, the presence of NTRK1 fusion genes, and the lack of PDGFB rearrangement favor the diagnosis of LNT. Finally, LNT should be differentiated from low-grade malignant peripheral nerve sheath tumor (MPNST), which usually occurs in the setting of neurofibromatosis type I: neoplastic cells in low-grade MPNST not only show positivity for S100 but also express SOX10; in addition, MPNST also exhibits loss of H3K27me3 protein expression, a feature that favors the diagnosis of MPNST over its mimics.

Biomarkers

LNT is characterized by coexpression of S100 and CD34. SOX10 and melanocytic markers are negative.

Characteristically, LNT bears **chromosomal translocations** leading to the formation of fusion genes involving NTRK1[1] such as TPR-NTRK1 gene fusion, TPM3-NTRK1 gene fusion, or LMNA-NTRK1 gene fusion.

Prognosis

LNT is a locally aggressive neoplasm (local recurrence has been described). No metastatic disease has been reported yet.

Therapy

Wide surgical excision is recommended. The presence of NTRK1 gene fusions in LNT is a potential therapeutic opportunity for the use of NTRK inhibitors already available in the clinical setting.

---

[1] NTRK1 encodes Neurotrophic Receptor Tyrosine Kinase 1 and belongs to the tropomyosin receptor kinases (TRK) family which also includes NTRK2 (encoding Neurotrophic Receptor Tyrosine Kinase 2) and NTRK3 (Neurotrophic Receptor Tyrosine Kinase 3). The encoded proteins elicit activities that regulate the natural growth, differentiation, and survival of neurons when they interact with endogenous neutrotrophin ligands. Chromosomal rearrangements involving in-frame fusions of these genes with various partners, translocations in the TRK kinase domains, mutations in the TRK ligand-binding site, amplifications of NTRK, or the expression of TRK splice variants can result in constitutively activated chimeric TRK fusion proteins that can act as oncogenic drivers that promote cell proliferation and survival in tumor cell lines.

Suggested Readings

Agaram (2016) Recurrent NTRK1 gene fusions define a novel subset of locally aggressive lipofibromatosis-like neural tumors. Am J Surg Pathol 40(10):1407–1416

Hung (2018) Evaluation of pan-TRK immunohistochemistry in infantile fibrosarcoma, lipofibromatosis-like neural tumour and histological mimics. Histopathology 73(4):634–644

Lao (2018) Lipofibromatosis-like neural tumour: a clinicopathological study of ten additional cases of an emerging novel entity. Pathology 50(5):519–523

Malik (2020) An addition to the evolving spectrum of lipofibromatosis and lipofibromatosis-like neural tumor: molecular findings in an unusual phenotype aid in accurate classification. Pathol Res Pract 216(6):152942

Definition

Lipoma is a benign tumor originating from adipocytes. It can develop in the subcutaneous tissue (superficial lipoma) or underneath the muscular fascia (deep lipoma, also known as intramuscular lipoma).

For details on specific subtypes (i.e., angiolipoma, myelolipoma, myolipoma, chondroid lipoma, spindle cell lipoma, pleomorphic lipoma) → see dedicated sections.

Epidemiology and Presentation

Lipoma is the most common soft tissue tumor in adults (it accounts for about 15% of all mesenchymal tumors and is at least 100-fold more common than liposarcoma) and is most frequent in people aged between 40 and 60 years. The prevalence of lipomas has been estimated to affect up to 1% of the population.

Most frequent sites of development are limbs, thoraco-abdominal wall and neck. Retroperitoneal, mediastinal, and visceral lipomas are rare (liposarcoma must be excluded, especially in the retroperitoneum). About 5% of patients have multiple lipomas; for details on a related condition possibly characterized by multiple lipomas → see Chap. 153.

The adipocytic tissue of lipomas is usually easily detected by ultrasound scan, magnetic resonance imaging, and computed tomography scan: any tissue heterogeneity, more than minimal vascularization or large size, should prompt differential diagnosis with liposarcoma.

Etiology and Predisposition

In rare cases, lipoma arises within the frame of syndromes such as the following:

- **Adiposis dolorosa** (→ see Chap. 153).
- **Encephalocraniocutaneous lipomatosis** (→ see Chap. 153).
- **Myoclonic epilepsy with ragged-red fibers** (MERRF) is a condition mainly affecting the muscles (e.g., weakness, spasticity) and nervous system (e.g., epilepsy, ataxia, peripheral neuropathy, dementia). Less frequently, patients with MERRF develop lipomas. MERRF is a rare disorder, its prevalence being unknown (MERRF belongs to a group of mitochondrial disorders with an estimated prevalence of 1 in 5000 people). Mutations in the MT-TK gene are the most frequent cause of MERRF (80% of all cases); less often, mutations in the MT-TL1, MT-TH, and MT-TS1 genes have been reported. These genes are located in mitochondrial DNA (mtDNA) and encode proteins in oxidative phosphorylation. MERRF is inherited in a mitochondrial pattern (also known as maternal inheritance), because egg cells (but not sperm cells) contribute mitochondria to the developing embryo, and thus the condition can only be inherited from the mother (who may or may not show symptoms of the disorder).
- **Bannayan-Riley-Ruvalcaba syndrome** is a genetic condition characterized by macrocephaly, intellectual disability or delayed development, multiple hamartomas (bowel hamartomatous polyps), and dark freckles on the penis in males. Other features often associated with the syndrome include lipomas and angiolipomas. The signs and symptoms are present from birth or become apparent in early childhood. The features of this disorder at least in part overlap with those of Cowden syndrome: both conditions can be caused by mutations in the PTEN gene (based on these commonalities, investigators believe the two syndromes represent a spectrum of overlapping features known as PTEN hamartoma tumor syndrome). Bannayan-Riley-Ruvalcaba syndrome is rare but is prevalence is unknown. About 60% percent of all cases result from mutations in the PTEN tumor suppressor gene which is a negative regulator of the Akt/mTOR pathway. This condition is inherited in an autosomal dominant pattern.
- **Giant congenital melanocytic nevus** is a congenital skin condition characterized by the presence of a nevus which may be small in infants but then grows (at the same rate the body grows) to be at least 40 cm in diameter. The nevus may arise anywhere on the skin but more frequently affects trunk and limbs (hypertrichosis can occur within the nevus). Patients have an increased risk of developing melanoma from the congenital nevus (5–10% lifetime risk). Other types of tumors associated with the condition are soft tissue sarcoma, lipoma, and schwannoma. Some patients develop neurocutaneous melanosis (growth of melanocytes in the leptomeninges which can cause intracranial hypertension leading to headache, vomiting, irritability, and seizures), and the risk of brain tumors is increased. Giant congenital melanocytic nevus occurs in approximately

1 out of 20,000 newborns. NRAS oncogene mutations cause most cases of this syndrome; rarely, mutations in the BRAF oncogene are responsible for this condition. These mutations are somatic (the condition is not inherited), and the alteration in one copy of the NRAS or BRAF gene is sufficient to cause the disorder.

Pathology

Lipoma is composed of mature white adipocytes with uniform nuclei resembling normal white fat. Lipomas may occasionally show areas of bone formation (osteolipoma), cartilage (chondrolipoma), or fibrous tissue (fibrolipoma). Lipoma with extensive myxoid change (also known as myxolipoma) is a variant of spindle cell lipoma. Intramuscular lipoma may be either well-demarcated from the adjacent skeletal muscle or, more frequently, displays an infiltrative growth pattern with mature adipocytes infiltrating skeletal muscle fibers. Lipoma arborescens (also known as synovial lipoma) shows infiltration of the subsynovial connective tissue.

The most important **differential diagnosis** is with well-differentiated liposarcoma (WDLS), which is positive for MDM2 and CDK4 amplification ($\rightarrow$ see WDLS for more details).

Biomarkers

Lipoma stains positive for S100 and HMGA2. Lipomas carry a range of **chromosomal translocations** leading to the formation of gene fusions involving HMGA2 [1] in up to 70% of cases. The most common chimeric product (about 20% of lipomas) derives from the HMGA2-LPP fusion gene, resulting from the translocation t(3;12); other partner genes are CXCR7 (chromosome 2q37.3), EBF1 (5q33.3), NFIB (9p22.3), and LHFP (13q13.3).

Of note, lipomas do not carry MDM2 or CDK4 gene amplification.

Prognosis

Lipomas rarely recur. Neither the classification into lipoma histological subtypes nor the presence of fusion genes has any prognostic significance; however, intramuscular lipoma has a higher rate of local recurrence. Neoplasms greater than 5 cm and deep are at higher risk of being liposarcoma and thus should be investigated (e.g., core needle biopsy to test for MDM2/CDK4 amplification).

Therapy

Surgical excision is the treatment of choice.

Suggested Readings

Donovan (2019) Life-threatening gastrointestinal bleeding from a giant ileal lipoma. ANZ J Surg [Epub ahead of print]

Fletcher (2020) WHO classification of tumours of soft tissue and bone (5th edition)

Karangelis (2019) Surgical resection of a cardiac lipoma of the right ventricle. Ann Card Anaesth 22(4):452–454

Krishnaraj (2018) Gastric lipoma: a rare cause of haematemesis. Ann R Coll Surg Engl 100(3):e41–e43

Ramírez-Montaño (2013) Giant lipoma of the breast. Arch Plast Surg 40(3):244–246

Definition

It is a benign overgrowth of mature adipose tissue which occurs in a variety of clinical settings, such as the following:

1. Diffuse lipomatosis (it usually occurs in individuals aged <2 years).
2. Pelvic lipomatosis (it most frequently affects black males ranging in age between 9 and 80 years).
3. Symmetric lipomatosis (also known as Madelung disease or Launois-Bensaude syndrome; it develops in middle-aged men of Mediterranean origin; many patients have a history of liver disease or excessive alcohol consumption).
4. Steroid lipomatosis (it manifests in patients on hormonal therapy or have increased endogenous production of adrenocortical steroids).
5. Lipodystrophy (it is frequently seen in HIV-positive patients treated with protease inhibitors but is also seen in patients receiving other forms of antiretroviral therapy).
6. Adiposis dolorosa (also known as Dercum's disease and lipomatosis dolorosa; multiple painful lipomas that arise in adult life, most often affecting obese women aged between 35 and 50 years).
7. Spinal epidural lipomatosis (a rare pathologic growth of histologically normal non-encapsulated adipose tissue in the epidural space).
8. Familial lipomatosis (also known as familial multiple lipomatosis and multiple hereditary lipomatosis, a rare hereditary syndrome with a proposed autosomal dominant inheritance; lipomas are typically painless).
9. Encephalocraniocutaneous lipomatosis (or Haberland syndrome, it is an uncommon sporadic neurocutaneous syndrome of unknown origin).
10. Lipomatosis of nerve: → see dedicated section.

Epidemiology and Presentation

In most cases of lipomatosis, patients present with abnormal accumulation of fat in the affected areas that may resemble a neoplasm.

Diffuse lipomatosis may involve the trunk, a larges portion of an extremity, the head and neck, abdomen, pelvis, or intestinal tract; it may be associated with macrodactyly or gigantism of a digit.

Symmetric lipomatosis manifests as symmetric deposition of fat in the upper part of the body, particularly the neck; these patients can experience neuropathy and involvement of the CNS; moreover, accumulation of fat in the lower neck areas can also cause laryngeal obstruction (potentially leading to death).

In pelvic lipomatosis there is diffuse overgrowth of fat in the perivesical and perirectal areas; these patients frequently complain of urinary frequency, perineal pain, constipation, and abdominal and back pain; bowel obstruction and hydronephrosis may eventually develop.

Steroid lipomatosis is characterized by the accumulation of fat in the face, sternal region, or the upper.

middle back (buffalo hump); the fat accumulation regresses after steroid levels have been lowered.

Lipodystrophy typically shows the accumulation of visceral fat, breast adiposity, cervical fat pads, hyperlipidemia, insulin resistance, and fat wasting in the face and limbs.

Adiposis dolorosa is characterized by pain, which can seriously affect quality of life.

Spinal epidural lipomatosis can compress the spinal cord or nerve roots causing myelopathy or radiculopathy (it is a cause of backache as well as neurogenic claudication); while it has been classically associated with long-term exposure to endogenous or exogenous steroids and obesity, idiopathic forms are much rarer.

Familial lipomatosis is characterized by multiple discrete; encapsulated lipomas are found on the trunk and extremities, with relative sparing of the head and shoulders.

Encephalocraniocutaneous lipomatosis is characterized by the hallmark triad of unilateral cutaneous lipomas, connective tissue nevi and alopecia, and ipsilateral ophthalmologic and neurological malformations.

Diagnosis

Pathology examination can only show normal fat tissue either encapsulated (lipoma-like) or diffuse.

Imaging studies in all forms of lipomatosis show accumulation of fat and are only helpful in determining the extent of its accumulation and excluding other processes.

Biomarkers

Encephalocraniocutaneous lipomatosis can result from mutations in the FGFR1 gene which arise randomly in one cell during the early stages of development before birth. As cells continue to grow and divide, some cells will have the mutation and others will not (mosaicism). In cells with an altered FGFR1 gene, the resulting FGFR1 protein is overactive, triggering abnormal signaling that affects cell growth and division.

Familial lipomatosis is associated with chromosomal translocations involving the HMGIC gene on chromosome 12.

Prognosis

Lipomatosis is a benign disease. All types of lipomatosis tend to recur locally after surgery. Lipomatosis in the neck can cause death due to laryngeal obstruction. In steroid lipomatosis the fat regresses upon steroid withdrawal or reduction.

Because multiple lipomas are often linked with mutations in tumor suppressor genes, familial multiple lipomatosis can be considered a marker for the presence of an underlying tumor predisposition syndrome.

For instance, multiple lipomas have been described in multiple endocrine neoplasia 1 (MEN-1, causative gene: MEN1, encoding for menin protein), hereditary retinoblastoma (causative gene: RB1), Cowden's disease (causative gene: PTEN). For this reason, people with multiple lipomas should be considered at increased risk for cancers, and a referral to a geneticist should be considered for appropriate screening.

Therapy

Surgical excision (or liposuction) is usually palliative because it results virtually impossible to completely remove the entire overgrowth of fat tissue.

Suggested Readings

Eliason (2019) Adiposis dolorosa pain management. Fed Pract 36(11):529–533
Fletcher (2020) WHO classification of tumours of soft tissue and bone (5th edition)
Ge (2019) Surgical treatment for pelvic lipomatosis using a bladder-sparing technique: a STROBE-compliant study. Medicine (Baltimore) 98(26):e16198
Genuardi (2001) Multiple lipomas linked to an RB1 gene mutation in a large pedigree with low penetrance retinoblastoma. Eur J Hum Genet 9(9):690–694
Li (2012) Multiple endocrine neoplasia type 1- presenting multiple lipomas and hypoglycemia onset. Am J Case Rep 13:224–229
Lotan (2020) Progressive myelopathy associated with spinal epidural lipomatosis in three non-obese patients with type 1 diabetes mellitus. J Neurol Sci 411:116688

Maximiano (2018) Madelung disease (multiple symmetric lipomatosis). Autops Case Rep 8(3):e2018030

Mrozek (1993) Chromosome 12 breakpoints are cytogenetically different in benign and malignant lipogenic tumors. Cancer Res 53:1670

Pathak (2020) Encephalocraniocutaneous lipomatosis: A rare congenital neurocutaneous syndrome. Radiol Case Rep 15(5):576–579

Schoenmakers (1995) Recurrent rearrangements in the high mobility group protein gene, HMGI-C, in benign mesenchymal tumours. Nat Genet 10:436

Ure (2016) CT and MR imaging features of diffuse lipomatosis of the abdomen. Diagn Interv Imaging 97(11):1189–1191

Definition

Lipomatosis of nerve is a benign expansion of the epineurium by adipose and fibrous tissue. It is also known as lipofibroma, fibrolipomatosis, intraneural lipoma of the median nerve, perineural lipoma, median nerve lipoma, macrodystrophia lipomatosa, and neural fibrolipoma.

Because it is made of normal components of the epineurium, some investigators have considered this lesion to be a hamartoma (fibrolipomatous hamartoma). For other related conditions → see the dedicated Chap. 153.

Epidemiology and Presentation

It most commonly affects the median nerve and its digital branches, followed by the ulnar nerve. In most patients age of diagnosis ranges between 10 and 40 years.

Pathology

Macroscopically the nerve is enlarged by yellow fibrofatty tissue. Microscopically, the fibrofatty tissue is composed by mature adipose tissue admixed with fibrous tissue.

Therapy

There is no fully effective therapy for this benign lesion (surgical excision can lead to severe damage of the involved nerve).

S. Mocellin, *Soft Tissue Tumors*, https://doi.org/10.1007/978-3-030-58710-9_154

Suggested Readings

Fletcher (2020) WHO classification of tumours of soft tissue and bone (5th edition)
Marek (2019) Surgical treatment of lipomatosis of nerve: a systematic review. World Neurosurg 128:587–592.e2

Definition

Liposarcoma is a malignant tumor with adipocytic differentiation.

There are four liposarcoma subtypes:

1. Well-differentiated liposarcoma (WDLS, also known as atypical lipomatous tumor).
2. Dedifferentiated liposarcoma (DDLS).
3. Myxoid/round cell liposarcoma (MRLS).
4. Pleomorphic liposarcoma (PLS).

For details on each subtype → see dedicated sections.

Epidemiology and Presentation

Liposarcoma is one of the most common types of soft tissue sarcomas (about 20% of all cases), representing approximately 50% of retroperitoneal and 25% of extremity soft tissue sarcomas.

Etiology and Predisposition

Liposarcoma is almost always a sporadic disease. However, it may (rarely) arise within the frame of the cancer predisposition disease known as **Li-Fraumeni syndrome**, a rare, autosomal dominant, hereditary cancer predisposition disease due to germline mutations of the TP53 tumor suppressor gene. The penetrance of these genetic alterations is high (close to 100%). It is also known as the sarcoma breast leukemia and adrenal gland syndrome (SBLA) due to the increased risk especially

© The Editor(s) (if applicable) and The Author(s), under exclusive license to
Springer Nature Switzerland AG 2021
S. Mocellin, *Soft Tissue Tumors*, https://doi.org/10.1007/978-3-030-58710-9_155

of these tumors. The most frequent types of sarcomas occurring in these patients are osteosarcoma and rhabdomyosarcoma. Li-Fraumeni syndrome is estimated to occur in 1 out of 5000 to 1 out of 20,000 people.

Most patients with Li-Fraumeni syndrome inherit an altered copy of the gene from an affected parent. However, in up to 20% of cases, the altered gene is the result of a new TP53 mutation occurring during the formation of reproductive cells or very early in development.

For a cancer to develop in Li-Fraumeni syndrome, a somatic mutation involving the other allele of the TP53 gene must occur during patient life, according to the classical two-hit hypothesis.

Classic diagnostic criteria for Li-Fraumeni syndrome are proband diagnosed with sarcoma before 45 years plus a first-degree relative with cancer before 45 years plus another first- or second-degree relative with any cancer diagnosed under the age of 45 years or with sarcoma at any age.

Pathology

For details → see sections dedicated to each liposarcoma subtype.

Biomarkers

For details → see sections dedicated to each liposarcoma subtype.

Prognosis

The four liposarcoma subtypes are characterized by a wide range of biological aggressiveness and response to medical treatments, as illustrated below:

Liposarcoma	Local recurrence[a]	Distant recurrence	Chemosensitivity	Radiosensitivity
Well-differentiated	Low	Null	Low	Low
Dedifferentiated	Moderate	Moderate	Low	Moderate
Myxoid	Low	Low	High	High
Round cell	Moderate	High	High	High
Pleomorphic	Moderate	High	Moderate	Moderate

[a]Liposarcomas arising in the retroperitoneum are characterized by high rates of local recurrence

For more details → see sections dedicated to each liposarcoma subtype.

Suggested Readings

Lee (2017) Clinical and molecular spectrum of liposarcoma. J Clin Oncol 36:151–159

Kast (2012) Late onset Li-Fraumeni Syndrome with bilateral breast cancer and other malignancies: case report and review of the literature. BMC Cancer 12:217

Tandon (2017) Association of Li-Fraumeni Syndrome with small cell carcinoma of the ovary, hypercalcemic type and concurrent pleomorphic liposarcoma of the cervix. Int J Gynecol Pathol 36(6):593–599

Yang (2020) Liposarcoma: advances in cellular and molecular genetics alterations and corresponding clinical treatment. J Cancer 11(1):100–107

Zare (2020) Recurrent pleomorphic myxoid liposarcoma in a patient with Li-Fraumeni Syndrome. Int J Surg Pathol 28(2):225–228

Definition

Littoral cell angioma (LCA) is a benign vascular tumor of the spleen. It is also known as littoral cell hemangioma. For general information on hemangiomas/angiomas → see the dedicated Chap. 117.

Epidemiology and Presentation

LCA is a rare splenic tumor occurring at any age (although most commonly presents in middle age) and without gender predilection.

It is typically identified incidentally in asymptomatic patients undergoing radiological imaging for other reasons or in subjects undergoing splenectomy for splenomegaly not otherwise specified (incidentaloma). LCA-associated splenomegaly can lead to thrombocytopenia or anemia.

An association with other neoplasms has been reported, which is why some investigators recommend careful investigation and close follow-up to rule out the coexistence or the development of a second tumor.

Pathology

Macroscopically, splenic involvement is characterized by multiple, spongy, cystic blood-filled, circumscribed nodules, ranging from 1 to 10 cm in diameter. Less commonly, the lesion is solitary or it completely replaces the splenic parenchyma.

Microscopically, LCA is composed by the lining cells of the splenic red pulp sinuses, which normally demonstrate both endothelial, and histiocyte/macrophage appearances and properties. A typical characteristic of LCA is represented by focal aggregates of eosinophilic globules 0.5–2 mm in size, which often entirely fill the cytoplasm of tumor cells: these globules most likely originate from the phagocytized red blood cells, lymphocytes, and plasma cells.

Differential diagnosis may be needed with the following: angiosarcoma (atypical sarcomatous cells with hyperchromatic nuclei and CD34 positivity; frequent tumor necrosis); hamartoma (disorganized blood vessels with entrapped adipocytes); hemangioendothelioma (typically mild to moderate cytological atypia, solid areas may be present; potentially metastasizing); Kaposi sarcoma (atypical spindle cells with HHV8 and CD34 positivity); hemangioma (usually asymptomatic, incidental finding, single layer of bland endothelial cells with CD34 positivity); hemangiopericytoma (oval to spindle cells surrounding staghorn blood vessels, CD34 positive; relatively high malignant potential); and lymphangioma (cystic, malformed lymphatic channels, often subcapsular; attenuated endothelial lining).

Biomarkers

LCA stains positive for both endothelial (factor VIII, CD31, ERG) and histiocytic (CD4, CD68, CD163, FLI1) biomarkers. It is negative for CD34, CD45, CD117, HHV8, and WT1.

Prognosis

LCA is a benign tumor. If present, associated malignancies determine the prognosis.

Therapy

Splenectomy is performed mainly to exclude a splenic malignancy or to treat hypersplenism linked to splenomegaly.

Suggested Readings

Anbardar (2017) Littoral cell angioma of the spleen: cytological findings and review of the literature. J Cytol 34(2):121–124

De Ridder (2015) Persistent thrombocytopaenia in a young man with splenomegaly, rebound thrombocytosis after splenectomy and subsequent pulmonary embolism: splenic littoral cell angioma and associated events. BMJ Case Rep 2015. pii: bcr2015212882

Karapolat (2020) A rare vascular tumor of the spleen: Littoral cell angioma. Acta Chir Belg 2020:1–3

Peckova (2016) Littoral cell angioma of the spleen: a study of 25 cases with confirmation of frequent association with visceral malignancies. Histopathology 69(5):762–774

Truong (2019) Littoral cell angioma of spleen. ANZ J Surg 89(4):E158–E159

Definition

Localized tenosynovial giant cell tumor (LTGCT) is a benign tumor arising from the synovium of joints, bursae, and tendon sheaths. Along with the diffuse form, it is one of the two types of tenosynovial giant cell tumor ($\rightarrow$ see Chap. 73).

It is also known as: giant cell tumor of tendon sheath and nodular tenosynovitis.

Epidemiology and Presentation

LTGCT is one of the most common tumors of the hand (after ganglion cyst). It is the most common subtype of giant cell tumors. It can occur at any age, most frequently between 30 and 50 years, with a female predominance. LTGCT most commonly occurs in the digits, especially of the hands (>80%). Intra-articular lesions are possible, especially in the knee.

On average, as compared to the diffuse counterpart, it is more often extra-articular, lower in size, painless, and affects smaller joints. Typically presents as a painless swelling. The tumor develops gradually over a long period (usually many years).

Radiological studies usually demonstrate a well-circumscribed soft tissue mass (generally 0.5–4 cm), with occasional erosion of the adjacent bone.

Pathology

It is composed of synovial-like mononuclear cells, accompanied by a variable number of multinucleate osteoclast-like cells, foam cells, siderophages, and inflammatory cells.

Differential diagnosis may be needed with the following: diffuse tenosynovial giant cell tumor (essentially identical microscopic appearance to localized type,

© The Editor(s) (if applicable) and The Author(s), under exclusive license to   507
Springer Nature Switzerland AG 2021
S. Mocellin, *Soft Tissue Tumors*, https://doi.org/10.1007/978-3-030-58710-9_157

distinguished only by large size, infiltrative growth, or anatomic site which is often intra-articular and in larger joints; in intra-articular cases the diffuse type shows a villonodular architecture); and giant cell tumor of soft tissue (more uniform background of mononuclear cells, typically shows sheets of osteoclastic giant cells similar to giant cell tumor of bone).

Biomarkers

The biomarkers are identical to those of the diffuse counterpart. Histiocyte-like cells are positive for CD68, CD163, and CD45; multinucleate giant cells display an osteoclastic phenotype (they express CD68 and CD45).

A small percentage of cells (10%) of most cases of LTGCT harbor a **chromosomal translocation** involving the CSF1 gene (located on chromosome 1), the fusion gene partner being most often COL6A3 (chromosome 2). This chromosomal translocation[1] leads to CSF1 protein overexpression, which is believed to contribute to tumor growth.

Prognosis

This tumor is considered benign, although it can relapse in 4–30% of cases. Recurrences are usually nondestructive and can be controlled by surgical re-excision.

Therapy

Surgical excision is the mainstay of treatment.

Suggested Readings

Fletcher (2020) WHO classification of tumours of soft tissue and bone (5th edition)
Gouin (2017) Localized and diffuse forms of tenosynovial giant cell tumor (formerly giant cell tumor of the tendon sheath and pigmented villonodular synovitis). Orthop Traumatol Surg Res 103(1S):S91–S97

---

[1] COL6A3-CSF1 fusion gene: COL6A3 (collagen type VI alpha 3 chain) encodes the alpha 3 chain, one of the three alpha chains of type VI collagen, a beaded filament collagen found in most connective tissues. CSF1 (colony stimulating factor 1) encodes a cytokine that controls the production, differentiation, and function of macrophages; the active form of the protein is found extracellularly as a disulfide-linked homodimer and is thought to be produced by proteolytic cleavage of membrane-bound precursors.

Low-grade endometrial stromal sarcoma is a uterine sarcoma arising from the endometrial stroma.

For details → see Chap. 82.

Definition

Low-grade fibromyxoid sarcoma (LGFMS) is a malignant soft tissue tumor classified among fibroblastic-myofibroblastic neoplasms. It is also known as Evans tumor.

Epidemiology and Presentation

LGFMS is a very rare tumor with a misleadingly bland histological appearance that typically arises in the deep soft tissues of the proximal extremities (thigh is the most common site) or trunk of young adults (median age, 34 years; range, 3–78 years) with a slight male predominance. It has been rarely described in the retroperitoneum, mediastinum, and superficial acral sites.

The lesion usually presents as a painless mass (2–20 cm in diameter) which can remain undiagnosed for years.

Pathology

The tumor is characterized by an admixture of heavily collagenized hypocellular zones and more cellular myxoid nodules. Short fascicular and characteristic whorling growth patterns are observed. Tumor vasculature is made of arcades of small vessels with perivascular sclerosis. Mitotic figures are rare.

Rarely the lesion is hardly distinguishable from sclerosing epithelioid fibrosarcoma (→ see dedicated section), a likely related neoplasm. Hybrid tumors displaying composite histologic features of LGFMS and sclerosing epithelioid fibrosarcoma have been recently described.

The hyalinizing spindle cell tumor with giant rosettes (HSCTGR), which is now accepted as a subtype of LGFMS, is much more rarely described: the immunohistochemical features and biological behavior of the two neoplasms are identical.

© The Editor(s) (if applicable) and The Author(s), under exclusive license to
Springer Nature Switzerland AG 2021
S. Mocellin, *Soft Tissue Tumors*, https://doi.org/10.1007/978-3-030-58710-9_159

Differential diagnosis may be needed with the following: fibromatosis (usually it lacks myxoid areas; fibrous cells are aligned in broad sweeping fascicles; cells appear more like reactive fibroblasts; distinct ectatic vessels are present; diffuse or occasionally focal nuclear beta-catenin staining); fibrosarcoma (no myxoid component; "herringbone" fascicular pattern, a diagnosis of exclusion); myxofibrosarcoma (more myxoid and less fibrous, more nuclear pleomorphism and hyperchromatism in contrast to LGFMS which is almost always bland and monomorphic with little to no pleomorphism; more developed vascular network, tumor cells aggregate around vessels); myxoid neurofibroma (wavy nuclei, background of thick collagen bundles, S100 positive); nodular fasciitis (tissue culture histology, extravasated erythrocytes, myxoid cystic degeneration); and sclerosing epithelioid fibrosarcoma (MUC4 positive like LGFMS but characterized by EWSR1 rearrangements and not by FUS rearrangements).

Biomarkers

MUC4, an epithelial glycoprotein, is constantly expressed by LGFMS. CD99 is frequently expressed (90% of cases). LGFMS stains negative for S100, desmin, cytokeratins, CD34, MDM2, SMA,[1] h-caldesmon, CD117, and nuclear beta-catenin.

The majority of LGFMS cases harbor the **chromosomal translocation** t(7;16) (q34;p11), which results in the formation of the FUS-CREB3L2 fusion gene.[2] A minority of cases have been shown to carry the FUS-CREB3L1 fusion gene resulting from chromosomal translocation t(11;16)(p11;p11).

Though less frequently, the FUS-CREB3L2 fusion gene has been reported also in sclerosing epithelioid fibrosarcoma (→ see dedicated section), which has led to the hypothesis that the two entities are related.

Prognosis

Despite the low-grade histological appearance, LGFMS is a malignant, often late-metastasizing tumor. Disease relapse and metastasis rates are low during the first years of follow-up, but they increase over time (up to >60% and >40%, respectively). No histological feature is known to correlate with prognosis.

---

[1] SMA: smooth muscle actin.

[2] FUS-CREB3L2 fusion gene: it derives from the fusion of FUS (fused in sarcoma, also known as TLS: translocated in liposarcoma) located on chromosome 16p11 and CREB3L2 (cAMP responsive element-binding protein 3-like 2) located on chromosome 17q33. FUS encodes a multifunctional protein component of the heterogeneous nuclear ribonucleoprotein (hnRNP) complex, which is involved in pre-mRNA splicing and the export of fully processed mRNA to the cytoplasm: this protein belongs to the FET family of RNA-binding proteins which are involved in regulation of gene expression, maintenance of genomic integrity, and mRNA/microRNA processing. CREB3L2 encodes a member of the oasis bZIP transcription factor family.

Therapy

Surgery is the mainstay of treatment.

Suggested Readings

Doyle (2011) MUC4 is a highly sensitive and specific marker for low-grade fibromyxoid sarcoma. Am J Surg Pathol 35(5):733–741

Fletcher (2020) WHO classification of tumours of soft tissue and bone (5th edition)

Lau (2013) EWSR1-CREB3L1 gene fusion: a novel alternative molecular aberration of low-grade fibromyxoid sarcoma. Am J Surg Pathol 37(5):734–738

Linos (2014) MUC 4-negative FUS-CREB3L2 rearranged low-grade fibromyxoid sarcoma. Histopathology 65(5):722–724

Maretty-Nielsen (2013) Low-Grade Fibromyxoid Sarcoma: Incidence, Treatment Strategy of Metastases, and Clinical Significance of the FUS Gene. Sarcoma 2013:256280

Mohamed (2017) Low-grade fibromyxoid sarcoma: clinical, morphologic and genetic features. Ann Diagn Pathol 28:60–67

Prieto-Granada (2015) A genetic dichotomy between pure sclerosing epithelioid fibrosarcoma (SEF) and hybrid SEF/low-grade fibromyxoid sarcoma: a pathologic and molecular study of 18 cases. Genes Chromosomes Cancer 54(1):28–38

Puls (2020) Recurrent fusions between YAP1 and KMT2A in morphologically distinct neoplasms within the spectrum of low-grade fibromyxoid sarcoma and sclerosing epithelioid fibrosarcoma. Am J Surg Pathol 44(5):594–606

Saab-Chalhoub (2019) Low-grade fibromyxoid sarcoma of acral sites: Case report and literature review. J Cutan Pathol 46(4):271–276

Scheer (2020) Low-grade fibromyxoid sarcoma: a report of the Cooperative Weichteilsarkom Studiengruppe (CWS). Pediatr Blood Cancer 67(2):e28009

Definition

Low-grade myofibroblastic sarcoma (LGMS) is a neoplasm with intermediate biological aggressiveness and is classified among fibroblastic-myofibroblastic tumors. It is also known as myofibrosarcoma.

Epidemiology and Presentation

LGMS usually occurs in adults (with a slight male preference). This tumor has been described in a variety of anatomical sites, most frequent locations being extremities and the head and neck region (especially tongue and oral cavity). It mainly develops in subcutaneous and deeper soft tissues (e.g., muscles). Usually it presents as a painless, enlarging mass with ill-defined margins.

Pathology

LGMS is characterized by an infiltrative growth pattern. Spindle cells are arranged in cellular fascicles or in a storiform growth pattern (often having fibromatosis-like features). Less frequently, the lesion is hypocellular with a more prominent collageneous (sometimes hyalinized) matrix. Mitotic rate ranges typically between 1 and 6 mitoses per 10 HPF. No histiocytic giant cells or prominent inflammation is found. Importantly, tumor cells show at least focally moderate nuclear atypia with enlarged, hyperchromatic, and irregular nuclei.

A corresponding high-grade variant is not recognized: a lesion with high-grade features should be classified as undifferentiated pleomorphic sarcoma ($\rightarrow$ see dedicated section).

Differential diagnosis may be needed with the following: fibromatosis (minimal nuclear atypia, usually negative for myogenic markers); fibrosarcoma (it may have

© The Editor(s) (if applicable) and The Author(s), under exclusive license to
Springer Nature Switzerland AG 2021
S. Mocellin, *Soft Tissue Tumors*, https://doi.org/10.1007/978-3-030-58710-9_160

focal but not diffuse myofibroblastic differentiation; herringbone fascicular pattern; often a diagnosis of exclusion); inflammatory myofibroblastic tumor (tumor of myofibroblasts with prominent lymphoplasmacytic infiltrate scattered amongst tumor cells, usually less atypia than myofibroblastic sarcoma; often ALK positive); leiomyosarcoma (alternating fascicular pattern, more eosinophilic cytoplasm, more evident and diffuse staining for multiple myogenic makers); myofibroma/myofibromatosis (often multiple and often in children, although solitary lesions and lesions in adults are also common; generally zonated with peripheral myoid nodules and central cellular spindle areas with dilated hemangiopericytic vessels; atypical forms of myofibroma may be challenging to differentiate from LGMS, zonation being an useful clue); nodular fasciitis (not infiltrative, not deep, <3 cm usually); and solitary fibrous tumor (diffusely positive for CD34, generally patternless arrangement of cells, usually no atypia except in malignant variant; STAT6 positive).

Biomarkers

Tumor cells are positive at least for one myogenic marker such as desmin, calponin, SMA,[1] and MSA.[2] Staining is instead negative for S100, cytokeratins, EMA,[3] ALK, nuclear beta-catenin, and h-caldesmon.

Prognosis

LGMS is classified as an intermediate aggressive neoplasm: local recurrences are common, but metastases are very rare (they may occur even many years after primary diagnosis).

Therapy

Surgical excision is the mainstay of treatment.

Suggested Readings

Bai (2019) Management of Low-Grade Myofibroblastic Sarcoma of the Larynx. Ear Nose Throat J 2019:145561319840140
Chan (2017) Low-grade myofibroblastic sarcoma: A population-based study. Laryngoscope 127(1):116–121
Fletcher (2013) WHO classification of tumours of soft tissue and bone (fourth edition)

---

[1] SMA: smooth muscle actin.

[2] MSA: muscle specific actin.

[3] EMA: epithelial membrane antigen.

Magro (2018) Differential Diagnosis of Benign Spindle Cell Lesions. Surg Pathol Clin 11(1):91–121

Wang (2019) Low-grade Myofibroblastic sarcoma: clinical and imaging findings. BMC Med Imaging 19(1):36

Wu (2020) Low-grade myofibroblastic sarcoma with abdominal pain, a stuffy nose, hearing loss, and multiple cavity effusion: a case report and literature review. J Int Med Res 48(1):300060519895661

Definition

Lung chondroma (LC) is a benign mesenchymal tumor of the lungs. It is also known as lung hamartoma and pulmonary chondromatous hamartoma.

Epidemiology and Presentation

LC is the most common benign tumor of lung, generally affecting adults between 40s and 60s. Usually is a solitary slow-growing lesion, measuring (generally) fewer than 4 cm. Calcification/ossification may be present and can be observed upon radiological imaging (so called "popcorn" calcifications).

Generally, it localizes peripherally (endobronchial cases occur in fewer than 10% of patients). In most cases the lesion is discovered incidentally upon radiological imaging performed for other reasons (incidentaloma); hemoptysis may occur in endobronchial cases.

Etiology and Predisposition

It is debated whether LC is the same entity occurring in the so-called Carney triad, a condition characterized by the occurrence of gastrointestinal stromal tumor (GIST), functional extra-adrenal paraganglioma, and pulmonary chondroma.

As a matter of fact, non-syndromic LC (as opposed to Carney triad) tends to be single rather than multiple, predominates in men rather than women, and displays entrapped respiratory epithelium, without a fibrous pseudocapsule.

Pathology

LC is typically composed of mature hyaline cartilage, fibrous tissue, smooth muscle, and fat, with a component of entrapped respiratory epithelium; calcification/ossification may be present.

If the lesion lacks the cartilagineous component, then it should be diagnosed as lipoma, myxoma, leiomyoma, or fibroadenoma (quite similar to breast fibroadenoma).

Other diagnosis must be considered if multinucleated cells, pleomorphism, mitoses, or necrosis is present.

Differential diagnosis may be needed with the following: benign metastasizing leiomyoma, leiomyosarcoma, lymphangioleiomyomatosis, primary or metastatic mesenchymal malignancy, and sarcomatoid carcinoma.

Biomarkers

LC fibromyxoid cells are vimentin positive and cytokeratin negative.

Prognosis

LC is a benign tumor.

Therapy

Surveillance for biopsy proven asymptomatic lesions is acceptable. Surgery (which is curative) is needed for symptomatic patients or when diagnosis is uncertain.

Suggest Readings

Kishore (2016) Pulmonary hamartoma mimicking malignancy: a cytopathological diagnosis. J Clin Diagn Res 10(11):ED06–ED07

Kitamura (2020) Peripheral pulmonary hamartoma with haemoptysis from the non-adjacent bronchus. Respirol Case Rep 8(4):e00553

Rodriguez (2007) Pulmonary chondroma: a tumor associated with Carney triad and different from pulmonary hamartoma. Am J Surg Pathol 31(12):1844–1853

Tian (2016) Pulmonary chondroma: a clinicopathological study of 29 cases and a review of the literature. Mol Clin Oncol 5(3):211–215

Wang (2018) Computed tomography imaging findings of pulmonary chondroma. Biomed Res Int 2018:4387689

The following is the list of primary soft tissue tumors of the lungs according to the World Health Organization classification published in 2015.

Since lungs are the most frequent site of soft tissue sarcoma metastases, sarcomas arising in the lungs are collectively known as primary pulmonary sarcomas.

For details on each single neoplasm → see dedicated sections.

Tumor	Notes
Diffuse pulmonary lymphangiomatosis	–
Epithelioid hemangioendothelioma	–
Intimal sarcoma	Referred to an intimal sarcoma arising in the pulmonary artery
Inflammatory myofibroblastic tumor	–
Lung chondroma	–
Myoepithelioma	–
PEComa	Including lymphangioleiomyomatosis, PEComa benign, PEComa malignant and clear cell sugar tumor of the lung
Pleuropulmonary blastoma	–
Pulmonary hamartoma	See section entitled "Lung Chondroma"
Pulmonary myxoid sarcoma	–
Synovial sarcoma	–

Other soft tissue tumors such as (extrapleural) solitary fibrous tumor and SMARC-deficient thoracic sarcoma can arise in the lungs and are described in this book (→ see dedicated sections).

Definition

Lymphangioleiomyomatosis (LAM) is a benign neoplasm belonging to the PEComa family (→ see Chap. 198). In the past LAM has been named also lymphangiomyomatosis, lymphangiomyoma, lymphangiopericytoma, leiomyomatosis, and intrathoracic angiomatous hyperplasia.

Epidemiology and Presentation

LAM is a rare progressive lung disease (often bilateral) typically occurring in women of reproductive age (only very few cases described in men or postmenopausal women on hormone replacement). The lesion can cause severe impairment of oxygen diffusion, dyspnea, pneumothorax, or emphysema (in the absence of a smoking history); fever, cough, chest pain, chylous pleural effusion, and hemoptysis may also be present. LAM is worsened by pregnancy, oral contraceptives, or menstruation, while it usually improves after menopause.

Angiomyolipoma (→ see dedicated section) can coexist. Extrapulmonary locations are infrequent (e.g., lymph nodes in the pelvis, mediastinum, retroperitoneum).

Serum VEGF-D >800 pg/ml in woman with typical cystic changes on computed tomography is considered to be highly accurate for diagnosis: otherwise, transbronchial or video-assisted thoracoscopic lung biopsy (and consequent histopathological evaluation) may be needed to confirm diagnosis. Positron emission tomography generally is not useful due to lack of fluorodeoxyglucose uptake by LAM.

Etiology and Predisposition

LAM is due to mutations in tuberous sclerosis complex (TSC) tumor suppressor genes TSC1 and TSC2, which leads to activation of the mTOR pathway (which in turn promotes cellular proliferation, migration, and invasion).

Besides sporadic cases, LAM can develop within the frame of tuberous sclerosis syndrome, an autosomal dominant hereditary condition due to germline inactivating mutations of TSC1 and TSC2. About 30% of females with TSC develop LAM, while 10–15% of males with TSC develop LAM.

For more details on tuberous sclerosis complex → see Chap. 198.

Pathology

Macroscopically, LAM shows diffuse emphysematous-like changes to cystic spaces (typically ranging from 0.5 to 2 cm) separated by thick, gray-white septa (honeycomb appearance).

Microscopically, LAM presents as a progressive cystic destruction of lung tissue due to proliferation of both perivascular epithelioid cells and bland spindled smooth muscle-like cells. Spindle cells are located centrally while epithelioid cells locate at the periphery. Cyst walls are lined by alveolar and bronchiolar epithelial cells. In the early stage, changes may mimic emphysema.

Differential diagnosis may be needed with the following: benign metastasizing leiomyoma (well-circumscribed single or multiple nodules of smooth muscle cells staining negative for HMB45); metastatic low-grade sarcoma; Langerhans cell histiocytosis (positivity for CD1a, S100, langerin); diffuse pulmonary lymphangiomatosis (less smooth muscle proliferation; HMB45 negative).

Biomarkers

LAM stains positive for HMB45, estrogen receptor, progesterone receptor, Melan-A/MART1, MITF, SMA, vimentin, desmin.

Prognosis

Although LAM is a benign tumor, respiratory insufficiency can lead to death.

Therapy

Symptomatic treatment consists of bronchodilators and pleurodesis (for pneumothorax). Hormone manipulation (e.g., oophorectomy, progesterone, or antiestrogens) have shown mixed results. More recently, mTOR inhibitor sirolimus has been approved for LAM treatment. Lung transplantation has been proposed for end stage respiratory failure, although LAM can recur in lung allografts.

Suggested Readings

Ando (2020) Lymphangioleiomyoma of the uterus and pelvic lymph nodes: a report of 3 cases, including the potentially earlicst manifestation of extrapulmonary lymphangioleiomyomatosis. Int J Gynecol Pathol 39(3):227–232

Bittmann (2003) Recurrence of lymphangioleiomyomatosis after single lung transplantation: new insights into pathogenesis. Hum Pathol 34(1):95–98

Hirose (2019) Serum vascular endothelial growth factor-D as a diagnostic and therapeutic biomarker for lymphangioleiomyomatosis. PLoS One 14(2):e0212776

Khawar (2019) Clinical outcomes and survival following lung transplantation in patients with lymphangioleiomyomatosis. J Heart Lung Transplant 38(9):949–955

McCormack (2011) Efficacy and safety of sirolimus in lymphangioleiomyomatosis. N Engl J Med 364(17):1595–1606

Miller (2020) Evolution of lung pathology in lymphangioleiomyomatosis: associations with disease course and treatment response. J Pathol Clin Res 2020 [Epub ahead of print]

Nijmeh (2018) Emerging biomarkers of lymphangioleiomyomatosis. Expert Rev. Respir Med 12(2):95–102

Xu (2020) Lymphangioleiomyomatosis. Semin Respir Crit Care Med 41(2):256–268

Yoshida (2020) Diagnostic usefulness of transbronchial lung cryobiopsy in two patients mildly affected with pulmonary lymphangioleiomyomatosis. Respir Investig 2020. pii: S2212-5345(20)30033-2

Young (2010) Serum vascular endothelial growth factor-D prospectively distinguishes lymphangioleiomyomatosis from other diseases. Chest 138(3):674–681

Definition

Lymphangioma is a benign lesion of vascular origin. Although included in the World Health Organization list of vascular tumors, it is unclear whether lymphangioma should be rather considered a malformation. It is also known as cystic hygroma and lymphatic malformation.

Epidemiology and Presentation

Lymphangioma represents 4% of all vascular tumors and approximately 25% of all benign pediatric vascular tumors. It is a pediatric lesion presenting most often at birth or during the first years of life. Rare cases have been described also in adults.

Head and neck, axilla, and groin represent the most frequent sites, although cases developing in upper trunk, limbs, and abdominal cavity have been described.

The mass presents as a circumscribed painless swelling fluctuant on palpation, which can displace adjacent structures (compression of trachea and esophagus or intestine for abdominal cases).

Pathology

Macroscopically, lymphangioma appears as a multicystic or spongy mass containing watery or milky fluid. Microscopically, lymphangioma presents as a cystic lesion composed of dilated lymphatic channels.

Biomarkers

Endothelial cells expresses podoplanin and PROX1 selectively, CD31 consistently, and CD34 variably.

Prognosis

Lymphangioma is a benign lesion without potential of malignant transformation. Disease relapse is due to incomplete surgical removal.

Therapy

Surgical excision is the mainstay of treatment. Sclerotherapy has been advocated as an alternative treatment.

Suggested Readings

Chen (2018) Experience in the diagnosis and treatment of mesenteric lymphangioma in adults: a case report and review of literature. World J Gastrointest Oncol 10(12):522–527

Chen (2020) Adult lymphangioma of the oropharynx: a case report. Anticancer Res 40(3):1631–1636

Dionísio (2019) Giant cystic mediastinal lymphangioma. Eur J Case Rep Intern Med 7(1):001323

Fletcher (2020) WHO classification of tumours of soft tissue and bone (5th edition)

Kumar (2020) Surgical management of giant retroperitoneal lymphangioma in a child. BMJ Case Rep 13(2):e234447

Parker (2020) Complete resection of a massive mesenteric lymphangioma in an adult. BMJ Case Rep 13(3):e233714

Sonmez (2020) Macrocystic lymphangioma in children treated by sclerotherapy with bleomycin. J Craniofac Surg 31(3):e250–e251

Tanaka (2020) Effective use of EUS for diagnosing a jejunal lymphangioma accompanied with hemorrhage. Gastrointest Endosc 91(1):199–200

Malignant fibrous histiocytoma (MFH) is currently considered an obsolete term used in the past for tumors now classified mainly as undifferentiated pleomorphic sarcoma ($\rightarrow$ see dedicated section).

Definition

Malignant granular cell tumor (MGCT) is a malignant neoplasm classified among the nerve sheath tumors due to its origin from Schwann cells. A benign counterpart exists ($\rightarrow$ see Chap. 114).

Epidemiology and Presentation

MGCT is an extremely rare neoplasm which accounts for less than 2% of all granular cell tumors. It occurs in a wide age range (mean of 40 years), with a female predominance. Despite a Schwann cell phenotype, the origin from a nerve cannot be usually identified.

The most frequent sites of involvement are the soft tissue of the thigh, proximal arm, trunk, and then distal extremities. Less commonly it affects the head and neck. The lesion is 1–20 cm in diameter (median: 4 cm) and usually locates in subcutaneous or intramuscular tissues.

Pathology

MGCT is a sarcoma composed of malignant granular cells characterized by abundant cytoplasmic lysosomes filled with amorphous granular material (hence the name). Most cases have high-grade spindle or polygonal cell morphology with eosinophilic granular cytoplasm, high mitotic rate (>2 mitoses per 10 HPF), geographic necrosis, marked pleomorphism, and high nucleus-to-cytoplasm ratio.

A minority of cases are morphologically bland and not overtly malignant in appearance, although they still behave aggressively (i.e., give rise to metastasis). Some investigators argue that metastasis remains the only definite criterion for malignancy.

Biomarkers

Like the benign counterpart, MGCT stain is strongly and diffusely positive for S100 and CD68.

Prognosis

MGCT is highly aggressive with metastatic disease in up to 50% of patients (about 12% to lymph nodes, the remaining to distant sites). Larger primary tumor size, local disease recurrence, metastasis, and older patient age are adverse prognostic factors.

Therapy

Surgery is the treatment of choice for localized primary tumor. Due to the rarity of the disease, no standard therapy exists for metastatic disease; besides conventional chemotherapy, target therapy (e.g., pazopanib) has been utilized in anecdotal cases.

Suggested Readings

Bradford Bell (2020) Benign and malignant granular cell tumor of the hypopharynx: two faces of a rare entity. Head Neck Pathol. [Epub ahead of print]

Cheng (2014) A rare case of pulmonary malignant granular cell tumor detected with 18F-FDG PET/CT imaging. Clin Nucl Med 39(9):816–818

Conley (2014) Dramatic response to pazopanib in a patient with metastatic malignant granular cell tumor. J Clin Oncol 32(32):e107–e110

D'hulst (2018) 18F-FDG PET/CT and MRI of a mediastinal malignant granular cell tumor with associated recurrent pericarditis. Clin Nucl Med 43(8):589–590

Fletcher (2020) WHO classification of tumours of soft tissue and bone (5th edition)

Moten (2018) Malignant granular cell tumor: clinical features and long-term survival. J Surg Oncol 118(6):891–897

Morita (2015) Pazopanib monotherapy in a patient with a malignant granular cell tumor originating from the right orbit: a case report. Oncol Lett 10(2):972–974

Nasser (2011) Malignant granular cell tumor: a look into the diagnostic criteria. Pathol Res Pract 207(3):164–168

Pérez-González (2015) Primary cutaneous malignant granular cell tumor: an immunohistochemical study and review of the literature. Am J Dermatopathol 37(4):334–340

Quinn (2019) Malignant granular cell tumor of the bile duct. ACG Case Rep J 6(8):e00193

Wei (2015) Whole-genome sequencing of a malignant granular cell tumor with metabolic response to pazopanib. Cold Spring Harb Mol Case Stud 1(1):a000380

Definition

Malignant peripheral nerve sheath tumor (MPNST) is a malignant neoplasm arising from the Schwann cells of a peripheral nerve. It is also referred to as malignant schwannoma, neurofibrosarcoma, and neurogenic sarcoma.

Epidemiology and Presentation

MPNST accounts for about 3–5% of soft tissue sarcomas. It occurs mainly in patients aged 20–50 years, although it may arise in children (particularly those with neurofibromatosis type I).

The tumor most frequently affects the extremities (the sciatic nerve being the is most commonly affected nerve), but trunk and head and neck are also sites of involvement. Visceral and bone cases have been rarely reported.

Clinically, it presents as an asymptomatic (which is palpable or discovered at radiological imaging) or symptomatic (e.g., pain, paresthesia, motor weakness) mass (often greater than 5 cm in size) which originates from a large nerve in about 70% of cases.

Computed tomography and magnetic resonance imaging studies do not show features specific for MPNST, except for the tight relationship with a large nerve. Positron emission tomography is the considered a sensitive technique for the detection of MPNST.

Etiology and Predisposition

About 50% of MPNST cases develop in patients with the hereditary syndrome neurofibromatosis type I (for details on this syndrome → see Chap. 187), and it is estimated that up to 15% of patients with neurofibromatosis type I develop

S. Mocellin, *Soft Tissue Tumors*, https://doi.org/10.1007/978-3-030-58710-9_167

MPNST. Patients with syndromic MPNST are usually younger than those with sporadic MPNST. Among patients with neurofibromatosis type I, those with plexiform neurofibromas (→ see Chap 187) have the highest likelihood of malignant transformation: the presence of an internal plexiform neurofibroma is associated with a 20-fold increased risk of developing an MPNST as compared to the risk in those without a plexiform neurofibroma. Cutaneous MPNST (arising in cutis or subcutis) is rarely associated with neurofibromatosis type I.

It is estimated that 10% of MPNST cases are radiation-induced.

Extremely rarely, MPNST arisen from schwannoma, ganglioneuroblastoma/ganglioneuroma, or pheochromocytoma has been reported.

Pathology

MPNST may show different histopathological appearances and its diagnosis may be challenging. Typical cases are composed of spindle cells (monomorphic serpentine cells) with a fascicular growth pattern, frequently accompanied by a hemangiopericytoma-like branching vascular pattern and alternating hypercellular and hypocellular areas; geographic areas of necrosis may be present; mitotic figures are frequent.

Occasionally, MPNST is pleomorphic and resembles an undifferentiated pleomorphic sarcoma (→ see dedicated section). Heterologous elements (e.g., skeletal muscle, bone, cartilage, or blood vessels) are present in about 15% of cases: in particular, a malignant Triton tumor (→ see dedicated section) is an MPNST with skeletal muscle differentiation.

Glandular MPNST shows glandular differentiation. Melanotic MPNST (also known as pigmented MPNST) is characterized by the presence of melanin in tumor cells and arises more frequently from spinal nerve roots: it may require differential diagnosis with primary melanoma of nerves.

In syndromic MPNST, there may be areas displaying increased cellularity and nuclear atypia without clear features of malignancy: these areas may represent the transition from neurofibroma to MPNST, and the distinction between these "atypical" neurofibromas and low-grade MPNST may be challenging (particularly on a small biopsy specimen).

Epithelioid MPNST is a rare variant (<5% of cases) composed of epithelioid cells with abundant eosinophilic cytoplasm, sometimes embedded in abundant myxoid matrix and characteristically showing a lobulated growth pattern. The epithelioid variant is the most frequent type of MPNST that arises from a benign schwannoma, whereas it is never found in patients with neurofibromatosis type I.

Differential diagnosis may be needed with the following: undifferentiated pleomorphic sarcoma; melanoma (positive for melanoma biomarkers); dedifferentiated liposarcoma (positive for MDM2 amplification); cellular schwannoma (strong positivity for S100); clear cell sarcoma (strong positivity for S100), interdigitating dendritic cell sarcoma (strong positivity for S100); and synovial sarcoma (positive for CD19, TLE1; characterized by the SS18-SSX fusion gene).

Biomarkers

MPNST stains positive for S100 protein in fewer than 50% of cases and is usually focal: diffuse staining for S100 should raise the suspicion of other neoplasm (e.g., cellular schwannoma, melanoma, clear cell sarcoma, interdigitating dendritic cell sarcoma). The exception is epithelioid MPNST which stains strongly and diffusely positive for S100: however, epithelioid MPNST is negative for melanoma markers and sometimes for SMARCB1/INI1 (30–50%), and it may be positive for cytokeratins. Glandular MPNST usually stains positive for cytokeratins, EMA, CEA, and chromogranin. In some cases, no discernable Schwann cell features can be demonstrated at any level.

Most cases of MPNST stain positive for TP53 positive and negative for p16 (encoded by CDKN2A, which is the target of homozygous deletions) and CD19.

Patients with neurofibromatosis type I carry germline inactivating mutations in the NF1 gene (located on chromosome 17q11.2) which codes for the tumor suppressor protein neurofibromin. Biallelic mutations of NF1 are found in a significant portion of MPNSTs. Cytogenetics analysis shows that most MPNSTs carry complex karyotypes with multiple structural and numerical alterations.

In addition to the well-characterized biallelic mutations in NF1 and CDKN2A, MPNST frequently harbors inactivating mutations in SUZ12 or EED genes, resulting in polycomb repressive complex 2 (PRC2) dysfunction and loss of histone H3 lysine 27 trimethylation (H3K27me3), both in sporadic and syndromic tumors. Accordingly, immunohistochemistry for H3K27me3 has become a useful diagnostic biomarker. Considering that H3K27me3 loss may be found also in other tumors (e.g., synovial sarcoma, fibrosarcomatous dermatofibrosarcoma protuberans, and melanoma), it is interesting to note that loss of H3 lysine 27 dimethylation (H3K27me2) has been recently reported to be a superior diagnostic biomarker for MPNST.

Chromosomal translocations leading to the formation of chimeric genes (e.g., EWSR1-VEZF1 fusion gene) have been recently described in MPNST.

Prognosis

MPNST is an aggressive malignancy with a poor prognosis in most cases. The local recurrence rate after surgical resection is about 50%; distant metastatic disease occurs in 30–60% of patients. Truncal location, tumor diameter (>5 cm) and local recurrence are adverse prognostic factors. Although some investigators have associated high-grade with worse prognosis, the use of tumor grading is not recommended for MPNST.

Prognosis of patients with syndromic MPNST appears to be worse than that of patients with sporadic MPNST.

Malignant Triton tumors is more aggressive than "conventional" MPNST.

Therapy

Surgery is the treatment of choice for primary tumor. Nerve grafting is often unfeasible also for the use of postoperative radiation therapy. **Radiotherapy** (adjuvant or neoadjuvant) is generally utilized for patients with large (>5 cm) high-grade lesions to improve local disease control.

As tumor cells tend to grow along the nerve bundles frequently for a long distance, examination of nerve margins is of pivotal importance to guarantee radical exeresis (to this aim, intraoperative frozen section assessment is suggested).

MPNST is poorly sensitive to **chemotherapy**; metastatic MPNST is generally treated with drugs utilized for other soft tissue sarcomas (e.g., doxorubicin). Although MPNST is deemed to be somewhat more sensitive to etoposide plus ifosfamide, this drug combination resulted inferior to epirubicin plus ifosfamide in terms of disease-free survival in a randomized trial of neoadjuvant chemotherapy for soft tissue sarcomas including MPNST (ISG-STS 1001).

Target therapy (e.g., everolimus, bevacizumab) and **immunotherapy** (e.g., pembrolizumab) are being investigated. Exploiting the dependence of malignant genetic programs on BET proteins,[1] BET inhibitors are also being clinically tested.

In the light of the lack of effective systemic treatments, it has been suggested that all cases of MPNST should undergo genomic profiling (e.g., by means of next generation sequencing, NGS) in the search of molecular alterations (e.g., NTRK fusion genes, RET fusion genes, $BRAF_{V600E}$ mutation) druggable with clinically available compounds.

Suggested Readings

Antonescu (2019) Spindle cell tumors with RET gene fusions exhibit a morphologic spectrum akin to tumors with NTRK gene fusions. Am J Surg Pathol 43(10):1384–1391

Benini (2020) Identification of a novel fusion transcript EWSR1-VEZF1 by anchored multiplex PCR in malignant peripheral nerve sheath tumor. Pathol Res Pract 216(1):152760

Chung (2020) Soft tissue sarcoma in neurofibromatosis type 1: a rare case of malignant peripheral nerve sheath tumor of the skin. Arch Plast Surg 47(1):92–96

Cooper (2019) Overcoming BET inhibitor resistance in malignant peripheral nerve sheath tumors. Clin Cancer Res 25(11):3404–3416

---

[1] BET proteins: Epigenetic writers, erasers, and readers are three categories of chromatin regulators for which small-molecule inhibitors have been developed. BET proteins are a family of epigenetic reader: of these, BET bromodomain protein BRD4 has recently emerged as an important chromatin-regulatory protein across multiple cancer types. BET proteins are characterized by two tandem bromodomains (B), which bind acetylated histones to support the recruitment of transcription elongation factor machinery to open chromatin regions, and an extra-terminal domain (ET) that mediates protein-protein interactions. BET proteins often interact with and support the activity of key transcription factors such as c-Myc, c-Jun, and p53. Members of the BET protein family, including BRD4, BRD3, and BRD2, can be potently inhibited pharmacologically with pan-BET bromodomain inhibitors (BET inhibitors) including JQ1, I-BET151, CPI-203, or OTX-015, which competitively bind both bromodomains, perturbing BET protein association with histones and subsequent regulation of gene expression.

Davis (2019) PD-1 inhibition achieves a complete metabolic response in a patient with malignant peripheral nerve sheath tumor. Cancer Immunol Res 7(9):1396–1400

Fletcher (2020) WHO classification of tumours of soft tissue and bone (5th edition)

Gilder (2018) Low-grade malignant peripheral nerve sheath tumor mimicking schwannoma: role and importance of trimethylated H3K27M staining. World Neurosurg 117:178–181

Gronchi (2017) Histotype-tailored neoadjuvant chemotherapy versus standard chemotherapy in patients with high-risk soft-tissue sarcomas (ISG-STS 1001): an international, open-label, randomised, controlled, phase 3, multicentre trial. Lancet Oncol 18(6):812–822

Hornick (2019) Beyond "triton": malignant peripheral nerve sheath tumors with complete heterologous rhabdomyoblastic differentiation mimicking spindle cell rhabdomyosarcoma. Am J Surg Pathol 43(10):1323–1330

James (2016) Malignant peripheral nerve sheath tumor. Surg Oncol Clin N Am 25(4):789–802

Kaplan (2018) Genomic profiling in patients with malignant peripheral nerve sheath tumors reveals multiple pathways with targetable mutations. J Natl Compr Cancer Netw 16(8):967–974

Le Guellec (2016) Malignant peripheral nerve sheath tumor is a challenging diagnosis: a systematic pathology review, immunohistochemistry, and molecular analysis in 160 patients from the French Sarcoma Group database. Am J Surg Pathol 40(7):896–908

Le Guellec (2017) Loss of H3K27 trimethylation is not suitable for distinguishing malignant peripheral nerve sheath tumor from melanoma: a study of 387 cases including mimicking lesions. Mod Pathol 30(12):1677–1687

Lu (2019) H3K27 trimethylation loss in malignant peripheral nerve sheath tumor: a systematic review and meta-analysis with diagnostic implications. J Neuro-Oncol 144(3):433–443

Luzar (2017) Cutaneous malignant peripheral nerve sheath tumor. Surg Pathol Clin 10(2):337–343

Makise (2018) Clarifying the distinction between malignant peripheral nerve sheath tumor and dedifferentiated liposarcoma: a critical reappraisal of the diagnostic utility of MDM2 and H3K27me3 status. Am J Surg Pathol 42(5):656–664

Marchione (2019) Histone H3K27 dimethyl loss is highly specific for malignant peripheral nerve sheath tumor and distinguishes true PRC2 loss from isolated H3K27 trimethyl loss. Mod Pathol 32(10):1434–1446

Martin (2019) Non-cytotoxic systemic treatment in malignant peripheral nerve sheath tumors (MPNST): a systematic review from bench to bedside. Crit Rev. Oncol Hematol 138:223–232

Miettinen (2017) Histopathologic evaluation of atypical neurofibromatous tumors and their transformation into malignant peripheral nerve sheath tumor in patients with neurofibromatosis 1-a consensus overview. Hum Pathol 67:1–10

Schaefer (2015) Malignant peripheral nerve sheath tumor (MPNST) arising in diffuse-type neurofibroma: clinicopathologic characterization in a series of 9 cases. Am J Surg Pathol 39(9):1234–1241

Schaefer (2016) Loss of H3K27 trimethylation distinguishes malignant peripheral nerve sheath tumors from histologic mimics. Mod Pathol 29(1):4–13

Suurmeijer (2019) The histologic spectrum of soft tissue spindle cell tumors with NTRK3 gene rearrangements. Genes Chromosomes Cancer 58(11):739–746

Widemann (2019) Targeting sporadic and neurofibromatosis type 1 (NF1) related refractory malignant peripheral nerve sheath tumors (MPNST) in a phase II study of everolimus in combination with bevacizumab (SARC016). Sarcoma 2019:7656747

168.1 Definition

Malignant Triton tumor is a variant of malignant peripheral nerve sheath tumor ($\rightarrow$ see dedicated section) characterized by a rhabdomyoblastic cell component and a more aggressive behavior (worse prognosis) as compared to conventional MPNST.

This heterologous differentiation occurs in up to in 10% of cases and leads some investigators to consider Triton tumor as a mesenchymoma ($\rightarrow$ see dedicated section).

The name "Triton" refers to experiments performed on salamanders of the genus *Triturus* (also known as Tritons), in which implantation of the cut end of a sciatic nerve into the soft tissue of the back resulted in the growth of a supernumerary limb.

The name includes the term "malignant" to differentiate this malignancy from the so-called benign Triton tumor ($\rightarrow$ see dedicated section), a synonymous of neuromuscular choristoma (a rare benign peripheral nerve lesion in which well-differentiated skeletal muscle fibers are intimately associated or admixed with mature nerve fibers).

Suggested Readings

Bian (2019) A series of 10 malignant triton tumors in one institution. Medicine (Baltimore) 98(36):e16797

Fletcher (2013) WHO classification of tumours of soft tissue and bone (fourth edition)

Hornick (2019) Beyond "triton": malignant peripheral nerve sheath tumors with complete heterologous rhabdomyoblastic differentiation mimicking spindle cell rhabdomyosarcoma. Am J Surg Pathol 43(10):1323–1330

Thakrar (2014) Benign triton tumor: multidisciplinary approach to diagnosis and treatment. Pediatr Dev Pathol 17(5):400–405

Woodruff (1973) Peripheral nerve tumors with rhabdomyosarcomatous differentiation (malignant "Triton" tumors). Cancer 32:426–439

© The Editor(s) (if applicable) and The Author(s), under exclusive license to Springer Nature Switzerland AG 2021
S. Mocellin, *Soft Tissue Tumors*, https://doi.org/10.1007/978-3-030-58710-9_168

The following is the list of mediastinal soft tissue tumors (alphabetical order): for details on each single neoplasm → see dedicated sections.

Soft tissue tumors of the mediastinum should be differentiated from other mediastinal masses, such as thymic tumors (thymoma, thymic carcinoma), germ cell tumors (teratoma, seminoma, non-seminomatous germ cell tumor), lymphomas, parathyroid adenoma, intrathoracic goiter, cystic lesions (bronchogenic, pericardial, enteric), meningocele, as well as neurogenic neoplasms (i.e., paraganglioma, ganglioneuroma, neuroblastoma and ganglioneuroblastoma) that are not covered in this book.

Tumor	Notes
Angiomyolipoma	–
Chordoma	→ See Chap. 92
Hemangioendothelioma	–
Hemangioma	–
Inflammatory myofibroblastic tumor	–
Leiomyosarcoma	–
Lipoma	–
Liposarcoma	–
Lymphangioma	–
Malignant peripheral nerve sheath tumor	–
Meningioma	→ See Chap. 79
Neurofibroma	–
Primitive neuroectodermal tumor	PNET
Rhabdomyosarcoma	–
Schwannoma	–
Solitary fibrous tumor	–
Synovial sarcoma	–

Definition

Melanotic schwannoma is a nerve sheath tumor and is considered a schwannoma variant (→ see Chap. 225). It may (though rarely) metastasize.

Epidemiology and Presentation

Melanotic schwannoma is a rare neoplasm occurring most frequently in adulthood (peak incidence: fourth decade of life), with a slight female predominance.

Approximately 50% of lesions arise from spinal nerves and paraspinal ganglia (most melanotic schwannomas tend to develop in paraspinal and axial sites), especially in the head and neck and thorax; the second most frequent affected site is the gastrointestinal tract. Primary cutaneous presentation is extremely rare.

The lesion presents with pain, sensory abnormality, and the effects of mass compression. Spinal-root tumors may cause bone erosion. In metastatic disease, lungs are the most frequent target, other sites being the gastrointestinal tract, liver, adrenals, and brain.

Most melanotic schwannomas are solitary lesions but may occasionally be multiple and multicentric, especially in the Carney complex (→ see below paragraph).

Etiology and Predisposition

About 50% of patients with melanotic schwannoma have the **Carney complex** (also known as Carney syndrome), a rare cancer predisposition syndrome characterized by the development of several types of tumors and skin pigmentation (e.g., lentigines, especially in the lips, eyes, and genitalia).

S. Mocellin, *Soft Tissue Tumors*, https://doi.org/10.1007/978-3-030-58710-9_170

Signs and symptoms of this condition commonly begin in childhood or early adulthood. Patients are at increased risk of developing the following tumors: myxomas in the heart (cardiac myxoma) and other body sites (e.g., skin and in internal organs); endocrine tumors in adrenal glands, thyroid, testes, ovaries, or hypophysis (which can cause overproduction of hormones such as hypercortisolism); and melanotic schwannoma. Moreover, patients may develop a specific type of adrenal disease called primary pigmented nodular adrenocortical disease (PPNAD), which is a cause of hypercortisolism.

Most cases of Carney complex are due to mutations in the PRKAR1A gene, which encodes a subunit of the protein kinase A (PKA) a protein that can act as an oncogene. Most mutations in the PRKAR1A gene that cause Carney complex result in an abnormal protein that is rapidly degraded, which in turn causes overactivation of PKA. The Carney complex is inherited in an autosomal dominant pattern: in about 80% of cases, a patient inherits the germline mutation from one affected parent; the remaining cases result from new mutations in the PRKAR1A gene and occur in patients without a family history of Carney complex.

Pathology

Macroscopically, the tumor is usually pigmented from brown to black (hence the name).

Microscopically, the lesion appears as a cellular, unencapsulated uniform composition of variably pigmented Schwann cells (plump spindle and epithelioid cells arranged in short fascicles or nests). About 50% of cases contain psammoma bodies (psammomatous melanotic schwannoma), and about 50% of these patients have Carney complex. There are no pathognomonic features of malignancy, but malignant forms often have large vesicular nuclei, mitotic figures, and necrosis.

Differential diagnosis may be needed with melanoma, which stains negative for laminin and collagen type IV and positive for HMB45 and Melan-A.

Biomarkers

The tumor stains diffusely and strongly positive for S100 protein. Laminin and collagen IV are often expressed. HMB45 and Melan-A are not expressed.

Prognosis

Melanotic schwannoma may develop late metastasis; this appears particularly true for patients with Carney complex. Mortality is about 15% for patients having either conventional or psammomatous tumor.

As abovementioned, no histopathological features are currently available to predict malignant behavior, which calls for long follow-up.

Therapy

Surgical excision is the treatment of choice.

Suggested Readings

Alexiev (2018) Pathology of melanotic schwannoma. Arch Pathol Lab Med 142(12):1517–1523

Bakan (2015) Primary psammomatous melanotic schwannoma of the spine. Ann Thorac Surg 99(6):e141–e143

Chatelet (2018) Laparoscopic resection of a giant retroperitoneal melanotic schwannoma. J Surg Case Rep 2018(3):rjy040

Cohen (2020) Melanotic schwannoma of the vulva: a case report and review of the literature. Am J Dermatopathol 42(1):46–51

Fletcher (2020) WHO classification of tumours of soft tissue and bone (5th edition)

Kamilaris (2019) Carney complex. Exp Clin Endocrinol Diabetes 127(2–03):156–164

Definition

Mesenchymal chondrosarcoma (MCS) is a malignant tumor typically involving the bones but that can primarily arise in soft tissues (it is also known as extraskeletal mesenchymal chondrosarcoma).

Epidemiology and Presentation

MCS is a rare tumor accounting for less than 3% of all primary chondrosarcomas. Although it can occur at any age, the peak incidence is in the second to third decade of life, without gender differences.

About 20–30% of cases primarily affect the soft tissues, the meninges being one of the most common sites of extraskeletal involvement (others: orbit, trunk, retroperitoneum, extremities); very rarely, the viscera (e.g., kidney) are affected.

Radiologically, chondroid-type calcifications are often present, and the lesion (size range: 3–30 cm) uptakes contrast medium both on computed tomography and magnetic resonance imaging.

Pathology

Macroscopically, most lesions contain hard mineralized areas, some tumors showing a clearly cartilaginous appearance, foci of necrosis, and hemorrhage. Microscopically, MCS is characterized by a bimorphic pattern that is composed of poorly differentiated small round cells (typically simulating Ewing sarcoma) often with hemangiopericytoma-like appearance and areas of well-differentiated hyaline cartilage.

MCS may be difficult to diagnose with certainty if no clear cartilaginous differentiation is observed, especially in small biopsy specimens.

© The Editor(s) (if applicable) and The Author(s), under exclusive license to Springer Nature Switzerland AG 2021

S. Mocellin, *Soft Tissue Tumors*, https://doi.org/10.1007/978-3-030-58710-9_171

Differential diagnosis may be needed with the following: synovial sarcoma (no cartilaginous component, positivity for cytokeratins, EMA, and TLE1; characteristic chromosomal translocation); solitary fibrous tumor (usually patternless, no cartilaginous component, positive for CD34; immunohistochemical positivity for STAT6 is helpful; characteristic chromosomal translocation); Ewing sarcoma (similar CD99 positivity, but no cartilaginous component; characteristic chromosomal translocation); and other small round blue cell tumors (particularly in biopsy specimens).

Biomarkers

Positivity for SOX9 coupled with negativity for FLI1 in the small cell component may be helpful for differential diagnosis with Ewing sarcoma. Staining for CD99 and desmin may be positive, while for CD45 is generally negative. Recently, MCS has been found to express NKX3-1, an immunohistochemical biomarker also positive in prostate carcinoma and EWSR1-NFATC2 rearranged sarcoma ($\rightarrow$ see Chap. 88) but not in Ewing sarcoma or other soft tissue sarcomas.

MCS is characterized by a recurrent **chromosomal translocation** der(13;21) (q10;q10) leading to the formation of the HEY1-NCOA2 fusion gene,[1] which is found both in bone and extraskeletal tumors; this biomarker can be helpful for the diagnosis of doubtful cases.

Of note, the IDH1 or IDH2 mutations found in conventional bone chondrosarcoma are not detected in mesenchymal chondrosarcoma.

Prognosis

MCS is a highly malignant tumor. The clinical course may be relentless, with distant metastases occurring even after 20 years from primary diagnosis (which calls for long-term follow-up). There is no correlation between prognosis and histological features.

---

[1] HEY1-NCOA2 fusion gene: HEY1 (HES related family BHLH transcription factor with YRPW Motif 1) codes for a nuclear protein that belongs to the hairy and enhancer of split-related (HESR) family of basic helix-loop-helix (bHLH)-type transcriptional repressors; HEY1 expression is triggered by the Notch and c-Jun signal transduction pathways. NCOA2 (nuclear receptor coactivator 2) encodes a protein that functions as a transcriptional coactivator for nuclear hormone receptors (e.g., steroid, thyroid, retinoid, and vitamin D receptors); in various cancers, NCOA2 is involved in chromosomal translocations resulting in fusions with other genes, such as lysine acetyltransferase 6A (KAT6A) gene in acute myeloid leukemia, ETS variant 6 (ETV6) gene in acute lymphoblastic leukemia, and HEY1 gene in mesenchymal chondrosarcoma.

Therapy

Surgery is the treatment of choice for localized primary MCS. Due to the rarity of the disease, the role of both radiotherapy and chemotherapy is unclear in the perioperative setting. As regards advanced/metastatic disease, the tumor appears poorly sensitive to medical therapy.

Suggested Readings

Arora (2018) Extraskeletal mesenchymal chondrosarcoma. Arch Pathol Lab Med 142(11):1421–1424

El Beaino (2018) Mesenchymal chondrosarcoma: a review with emphasis on its fusion-driven biology. Curr Oncol Rep 20(5):37

Fletcher (2020) WHO classification of tumours of soft tissue and bone (5th edition)

Nachawi (2020) A challenging case of mesenchymal chondrosarcoma involving the thyroid and special considerations for diagnosis. Clin Diabetes Endocrinol 6:6

Naumann (2002) Translocation der(13;21)(q10;q10) in skeletal and extraskeletal mesenchymal chondrosarcoma. Mod Pathol 15(5):572–576

Uneda (2020) Intracranial mesenchymal chondrosarcoma lacking the typical histopathological features diagnosed by HEY1-NCOA2 gene fusion. NMC Case Rep J 7(2):47–52

Yoshida (2020). NKX3-1 Is a useful immunohistochemical marker of EWSR1-NFATC2 sarcoma and mesenchymal chondrosarcoma. Am J Surg Pathol. [Epub ahead of print]

Definition

This term refers to soft tissue tumors with two or more lines of differentiation. Both benign mesenchymoma and malignant mesenchymoma cases have been reported. Of note, mesenchymomas of the bone have also been described.

The World Health Organization suggests that this should not be considered a separate nosological entity but rather as a group of neoplasms with a prevalent differentiation with coexistence of additional cell elements of different origin.

Examples are liposarcoma with cartilaginous metaplasia and/or osteogenic areas, malignant peripheral nerve sheath tumor with heterologous elements (which can be observed in about 15% of cases; → see Chap. 244), the (rare) leiomyosarcomas with osteosarcoma-like or rhabdomyosarcomatous zones, and the (rare) embryonal rhabdomyosarcomas presenting with focal cartilage.

Suggested Readings

Argintar (2012) Soft-tissue benign mesenchymoma in a pediatric patient. Am J Orthop (Belle Mead NJ) 41(12):561–564

Brannan (2003) Malignant mesenchymoma of the orbit: case report and review of the literature. Ophthalmology 110(2):314–317

Fletcher (2020) WHO classification of tumours of soft tissue and bone (5th edition)

Gambarotti (2017) Fibrocartilaginous mesenchymoma of bone: a single-institution experience with molecular investigations and a review of the literature. Histopathology 71(1):134–142

Melton (2006) Benign mesenchymoma of the mediastinum: a report and review of the literature. Thorac Surg Sci 3:Doc02

Yang (2017) Primary malignant mesenchymoma of bladder: case report and review of the literature. Medicine (Baltimore) 96(32):e7579

© The Editor(s) (if applicable) and The Author(s), under exclusive license to Springer Nature Switzerland AG 2021

S. Mocellin, *Soft Tissue Tumors*, https://doi.org/10.1007/978-3-030-58710-9_172

Definition

Microvenular hemangioma is a benign vascular tumor of the skin. Also known as microcapillary hemangioma.

Epidemiology and Presentation

Microvenular hemangioma is a very rare type of hemangioma occurring in the skin of young to middle-aged adults (mainly on trunk or extremities). With the term microcapillary hemangioma, it has been associated with young women taking oral contraceptives and pregnancy.

Clinically it presents as a slowly growing, solitary, asymptomatic, purple-red papule or plaque (diameter: 0.5–2 cm).

Pathology

Microvenular hemangioma presents as a well-defined dermal proliferation of small, irregular branching capillaries and venules with inconspicuous lumina. Endothelial cells show no atypia. The stroma is collagenous with variable lymphocytes. Neither fat invasion nor spindle cells are present.

Differential diagnosis may be needed with the following: acquired (tufted) angioma (multiple vascular lobules similar to pyogenic granuloma but more cellular, resembling cannon balls); Kaposi sarcoma, patch stage (irregular vascular spaces are anastomosing but not collapsed and are accompanied by atypical endothelial cells, eosinophilic hyaline globules, plasma cells, and fascicles of spindle cells; spindle cells are HHV8 positive); Kaposiform hemangioendothelioma (it also has slit-like lumina, but they are due to nodules and sheets of compact spindle cells;

it affects the skin or retroperitoneum of infants and children, may be associated with severe coagulopathy); and sclerosing hemangioma (prominent sclerosis).

Biomarkers

Microvenular hemangioma stains positive endothelial cell biomarkers (CD34, CD31, Factor VIII). It stains negative for podoplanin and HHV8.

Prognosis

Microvenular hemangioma is a benign neoplasm.

Therapy

Surgical excision is the treatment of choice.

Suggested Readings

Juan (2018) A microvenular hemangioma with a rare expression of progesterone receptor immunocreativity and a review of the literature. J Cutan Pathol 45(11):847–850
Napekoski (2014) Microvenular hemangioma: a clinicopathologic review of 13 cases. J Cutan Pathol 41(11):816–822

Definition

Myelolipoma is a benign neoplasm composed of both adipose and hematopoietic cells.

Epidemiology and Presentation

Myelolipoma usually occurs in adults older than 40 years, without significant gender differences. It typically locates in the adrenal gland, although it has been rarely described also outside this gland (e.g., in the presacral region or mediastinum). Adrenal myelolipomas are the second most common adrenal incidentalomas (they account for 5–15% of adrenal incidentalomas) after benign adrenal adenomas.

In most cases, myelolipoma is asymptomatic and is incidentally discovered during radiological studies performed for other reasons (incidentaloma). The mass is generally smaller than 5 cm in size, but much larger lesions have been described; larger lesions may become symptomatic.

Computed tomography is the best imaging modality for the diagnosis of adrenal myelolipoma (hypodense well-circumscribed heterogeneous mass; virtually all myelolipomas have some area of fat, although it may be very small).

Etiology and Predisposition

An increased incidence of adrenal myelolipomas is observed in congenital adrenal hyperplasia, which has led to the hypothesis that high levels of ACTH might play a role in the pathogenesis of this disease.

Adrenal myelolipoma has been also associated with conditions like Cushing disease, obesity, hyperlipidemia, hypertension, and diabetes.

Pathology

Myelolipoma is typically composed of mature adipose tissue (no atypia, no lipo-blasts) and mature bone marrow hematopoietic elements (all three lines: myeloid, erythroid, and megakaryocytic).

Differential diagnosis may be needed with the following: extramedullary hema-topoiesis, lipoma, well-differentiated liposarcoma, angiomyolipoma, myeloid sar-coma, and adrenocortical adenoma.

Biomarkers

There is no specific biomarker.

Prognosis

Myelolipoma is a benign neoplasm.

Therapy

Treatment may not be necessary if radiological diagnosis is reasonably certain. In case of uncertain diagnosis (or in symptomatic cases), surgery (adrenalectomy) is a definitive treatment.

Suggested Readings

Adapa (2019) Adrenal incidentaloma: challenges in diagnosing adrenal myelolipoma. J Investig Med High Impact Case Rep 7:2324709619870311

Cochetti (2019) Robotic treatment of giant adrenal myelolipoma: a case report and review of the literature. Mol Clin Oncol 10(5):492–496

Diaz-Perez (2019) Epithelioid hemangioendothelioma arising within mediastinal myelolipoma: a WWTR1-driven composite neoplasm. Int J Surg Pathol 27(6):664–668

Goel (2018) Bilateral posterior mediastinal primary myelolipoma. Ann Thorac Surg 106(5):e235–e237

Sethi (2018) Myelolipoma of the pelvis: a case report and review of literature. Front Oncol 8:251

Hamidi (2020) Clinical course of adrenal myelolipoma: A long-term longitudinal follow-up study. Clin Endocrinol. [Epub ahead of print]

Pakalniskis (2020) Adrenal collision tumour comprised of adrenocortical carcinoma and myeloli-poma in a patient with congenital adrenal hyperplasia. J Med Imaging Radiat Oncol 64(1):67–68

Vigutto (2019) Giant retroperitoneal myelolipoma: an unusual diagnostic GI challenge-case report and review of the literature. Dig Dis Sci 64(12):3431–3435

Definition

Myoepithelial tumors represent a family of lesions with variable terminology, based on anatomic location: pleomorphic adenoma in the salivary gland (where myoepithelioma was first described), benign mixed tumor in the skin, and myoepithelial tumor or parachordoma in the soft tissues.

Myoepithelioma was included in the World Health Organization classification of soft tissue tumors in 2002 and classified as intermediate malignancy tumor of uncertain line of differentiation in 2013; in fact, in contrast to the salivary gland, primary myoepithelial tumors in the soft tissue, bone, and skin have no known normal cellular counterpart.

It is also known as myoepithelioma of soft tissue, ectomesenchymal chondromyxoid tumor, myoepithelial tumor, parachordoma, and myoepithelial carcinoma (the malignant variant).

Some authors believe that parachordoma (which should not be confused with extra-axial chordoma or chordoma periphericium) is a separate entity, although most investigators support the hypothesis that myoepithelioma and parachordoma represent morphological variants of a single tumor type.

Epidemiology and Predisposition

Myoepithelioma of soft tissues is a rare tumor occurring in a wide age range but mainly in young to middle-aged adults (median: 40 years), without gender predilection. Of note, myoepithelial carcinoma predominates in the pediatric population. The body sites most frequently involved are the limbs and limb girdles, trunk, and head and neck; rarely other sites (including bone and viscera) are affected.

Clinically, the lesion typically presents as a palpable painless mass (1–20 cm in diameter; mean: 5 cm) involving the subcutaneous tissue and less frequently deep soft tissues; sometimes the tumor develops primarily in the skin.

Pathology

Macroscopically, most tumors are well circumscribed and nodular, but rarely they have infiltrative margins.

Microscopically, myoepithelioma shows a wide morphological spectrum, in analogy to its salivary counterpart. The tumor shows reticular or trabecular architecture with myxoid stroma and focal areas with nested or solid architecture and hyalinized or chondroid stroma that may predominate in some cases. Myoepithelioma is composed exclusively (or predominantly) of myoepithelial cells, as opposed to mixed tumors which also show ductal differentiation. Plasmacytoid "hyaline cell," spindle, epithelioid, clear cell, and mixed tumor cell variants of myoepithelioma have been described.

Differential diagnosis may be needed with the following: extraskeletal myxoid chondrosarcoma(NR4A3 rearrangement); malignant mixed tumor (malignant cartilage or bone are present); neurothekeoma (nested architecture, sclerotic dermal collagen; negative for S100, EMA, and cytokeratins); epithelioid benign fibrous histiocytoma (plump and often binucleate epithelioid cells; negative for cytokeratins and S100); epithelioid sarcoma (it develops in distal extremities of young adults; S100 and GFAP negative); and Spitz nevus (large epithelioid melanocytes, junctional component, HMB45 and S100 positive; EMA and cytokeratin negative).

Biomarkers

More than 90% of cases stain positive for cytokeratins, S100, and calponin. Desmin, CD34, and brachyury are consistently negative.

Chromosomal translocations leading to the formation of EWSR1-based[1] gene fusions have been reported in about 45% of cases: EWSR1-POU5F1 fusion gene (from t(6;22)(p21;q12)), EWSR1-ZNF444 fusion gene (from t(19;22)(q13;q12)), EWSR1-PBX1 fusion gene (from t(1;22)(q23;q12)), EWSR1-PBX3 fusion gene (from t(9;22)(q33;q12)), and EWSR1-KLF17 fusion gene (from t(1;22)(p34;q12)).

In mixed tumors, PLAG1 is frequently expressed, which correlates with PLAG1 gene rearrangement.

---

[1] EWSR1 (Ewing Sarcoma Breakpoint Region 1) encodes a multifunctional protein that is involved in various cellular processes, including gene expression, cell signaling, and RNA processing and transport. EWSR1 is a "promiscuous" gene because it can fuse with different partner genes in phenotypically similar neoplasms or with the same genes in morphologically and behaviorally different tumors. In fact, EWSR1-based chimeric genes can be found not only in Ewing and Ewing-like sarcomas but also in other tumors such as angiomatoid fibrous histiocytoma, clear cell sarcoma, low-grade fibromyxoid sarcoma, sclerosing epithelioid fibrosarcoma, hemangioma of bone, desmoplastic small round cell tumor, extraskeletal myxoid chondrosarcoma, myoepithelial tumor of soft tissue, and myxoid liposarcoma.

It must be underscored that fluorescence in situ hybridization (FISH) analysis has a significant risk of false-negative results, making next-generation sequencing (NGS)-based diagnostic tools more sensitive for detecting EWSR1 rearrangements.

Prognosis

Myoepithelial tumors of soft tissue are classified as benign (myoepithelioma and mixed tumor/chondroid syringoma) and malignant (myoepithelial carcinoma).

Most myoepitheliomas are benign tumors. The only reliable criterion for malignancy is cytologic atypia (moderate to severe nuclear atypia), which is in contrast to salivary tumors for which malignancy is defined by the presence of capsular invasion and infiltrative growth. Benign tumors are referred to as "myoepitheliomas," which overall lack cytologic atypia (if present, it is at most mild). Necrosis and increased mitotic activity alone are not predictive of malignant behavior.

Histologically benign tumors have been associated with a 20% local recurrence rate and rarely metastasize. In contrast, myoepithelial carcinoma recur and metastasize in about 50% of cases (mainly to lungs, lymph nodes, bone, and soft tissues).

Therapy

The primary treatment modality of soft tissue myoepithelioma is complete excision. Some data support the use of perioperative radiation therapy in the management of myoepithelial carcinoma. Metastatic disease is poorly to moderately sensitive to systemic chemotherapy (e.g., doxorubicin).

Suggested Readings

Chamberlain (2019) Adult soft tissue myoepithelial carcinoma: treatment outcomes and efficacy of chemotherapy. Med Oncol 37(2):13

Fletcher (2020) WHO classification of tumours of soft tissue and bone (5th edition)

Jo (2020) Soft tissue special issue: myoepithelial neoplasms of soft tissue: an updated review with emphasis on diagnostic considerations in the head and neck. Head Neck Pathol 14(1):121–131

Koyama (2020) Metachronous pancreatic and thyroid metastases from primary soft-tissue myoepithelioma in the clavicular region: a case report of a long-term survivor. Am J Case Rep 21:e920702

Kravtsov (2017) Myoepithelioma of soft tissue: a cytological-pathological correlation with literature review. Ann Diagn Pathol 27:14–17

Rastrelli (2019) Myoepithelioma of the soft tissue: a systematic review of clinical reports. Eur J Surg Oncol 45(9):1520–1526

Verma (2017) Myoepithelial tumor of soft tissue and bone: a current perspective. Histol Histopathol 32(9):861–877

Definition

Myofibroblastoma (MFB) is a benign neoplasm classified among fibroblastic-myofibroblastic tumors. When the location is extra-mammary, the neoplasm is also known as mammary-type myofibroblastoma.

Epidemiology and Presentation

MFB is a rare tumor developing in adults (age range: 35–85 years) with equal gender distribution. It locates in the breast, but extra-mammary locations have been reported (mainly in the inguinal/groin region and paratesticular-vulvovaginal areas, less frequently perianal region, buttock, abdominal wall, back, neck, and popliteal fossa).

Incidence seems to be higher along the anatomical "milk line" (extending from axilla to groin). The lesion presents as a painless subcutaneous well-circumscribed mass that ranges from 1 to 10 cm in diameter and can be present for years before the diagnosis. Radiological appearance is not specific.

Pathology

MFB is composed of spindled cells with features of myofibroblasts, embedded in a stroma that contains coarse bands of hyalinized collagen and scattered mast cells, admixed with a variable amount of adipose tissue. MFB is believed to be part of a spectrum of lesions encompassing spindle cell lipoma and cellular angiofibroma (→ see dedicated sections). The blood vessels are generally small and show a perivascular lymphocytic infiltrate. Mitotic figures are infrequent. Histopathological variants such as classic, cellular, collagenous/fibrous, lipomatous, infiltrative, myxoid, and epithelioid have been reported, as well as cases with nuclear atypia.

Differential diagnosis may be necessary with the following: cellular angiofibroma (medium to large hyalinized vessels, focal to absent myogenic marker expression); metaplastic (spindle cell) breast carcinoma (usually infiltrative rather than circumscribed, cytokeratin positive); spindle cell lipoma (adipocytic component usually predominates, focal to absent myogenic marker expression); lipomatous solitary fibrous tumor (larger ectatic vessels with adjacent sclerosis, no myofibroblastic spindle cells); fibromatosis (not circumscribed, more diffuse fibrosis); low-grade myofibroblastic sarcoma (marked cellular pleomorphism, infiltrating margins and high mitotic rate); myoepithelioma (S100 positive, cytokeratin positive); and nodular fasciitis (more infiltrative, mucoid stroma).

Biomarkers

MFB coexpresses desmin and CD34 in the spindle cells (which are S100 and cytokeratin negative). Expression of CD10, estrogen receptor, and progesterone receptor has been reported.

Prognosis

This is a benign tumor with an excellent prognosis.

Therapy

Surgical excision is the treatment of choice.

Suggested Readings

Akrami (2019) A case report of a mammary myofibroblastoma in a male and literature review of radiologic and pathologic features of breast myofibroblastoma. Clin Case Rep 7(10):1968–1971

Fletcher (2020) WHO classification of tumours of soft tissue and bone (5th edition)

Jung (2020) Myofibroblastoma of the breast in postmenopausal women: Two case reports with imaging findings and review of the literature. J Clin Ultrasound 48(5):279–282

Metry (2016) Myofibroblastoma of the breast: literature review and case report. Case Rep Oncol Med 2016:1714382

Ross (2019) Myxoid myofibroblastoma of the breast with atypical cells. Int J Surg Pathol 27(4):446–449

Salemis (2012) Rapidly growing myofibroblastoma of the breast diagnosed in a premenopausal woman: management and review of the literature. Breast Dis 34(1):29–34

Definition

Myofibroma is a benign tumor classified among perivascular (pericytic) soft tissue tumors (along with myopericytoma, angioleiomyoma, and glomus tumor, → see dedicated sections).

It is also known as infantile myofibroma, myofibromatosis, infantile myofibromatosis, and infantile hemangiopericytoma.

Epidemiology and Presentation

Myofibroma may be present at birth (about half cases) or develop in the first 2 years of life; it rarely occurs in adults; it is characterized by a male predominance.

Clinically, this neoplasm presents as a solitary (myofibroma, more common) or multiple (myofibromatosis, less common) lesion. Myofibromatosis is the most common fibrous tumor in childhood. The majority of myofibromas occur in dermal and subcutaneous tissues, the extremities, head and neck region, and trunk being the usual sites. Myofibromatosis involves soft tissue and bone, more frequently occurs in deep soft tissues and may involve viscera.

Cutaneous lesions present as purple macules and resemble a vascular neoplasm; subcutaneous lesions present as painless freely mobile masses.

Etiology and Predisposition

A subset of solitary and multiple (non-visceral) forms of infantile myofibromatosis are familial. Familial infantile myofibromatosis appears to be inherited according to an autosomal dominant pattern with variable penetrance. Gain-of-function germline mutations in the PDGFRB gene have been reported as the cause of this inherited disease.

Pathology

Myofibroma is a nodular, well-circumscribed neoplasms, characterized by a biphasic growth of immature-appearing, plump spindled tumor cells associated with numerous thin-walled, branching solitary fibrous tumor-like vessels associated with more mature, spindled tumor cells arranged in bundles. The background is represented by a collagenous stroma with often characteristic myxohyaline changes. Mitoses are variable in number and necrosis may be present.

Although myofibroma, angioleiomyoma, glomus tumor, and myopericytoma are currently considered separate clinicopathological entities, the occurrence of hybrid cases and the presence of shared morphological and immunohistochemical features underscore the existence of a continuous spectrum of perivascular myoid neoplasms.

Differential diagnosis may be needed with the following: inflammatory myofibroblastic tumor (prominent inflammation with plasma cells, no primitive cells with hemangiopericytic vascular pattern, no zonation); myopericytoma (predominant growth pattern is concentric perivascular arrangement of plump spindle cells); and smooth muscle tumor (single lesion, no zonation, minimal fibrous tissue with trichrome stain).

Biomarkers

Tumor cells in both components of myofibroma stain positive for SMA[1] and vimentin, while h-caldesmon S100, cytokeratin, desmin, and EMA[2] are negative.

Infantile myofibromatosis is negative for the ETV6-NTRK3 fusion gene associated with infantile fibrosarcoma (→ see dedicated section).

Recurrent somatic mutations of PDGFRB[3] have been reported in myofibroma (as well as in myopericytoma, → see dedicated section).

Finally, the presence of SRF-based[4] fusion genes (e.g., SRF-RELA fusion gene and SRF-ICA1L fusion gene) has been recently described in a group of cellular spindle cell neoplasms with histologic features reminiscent of cellular myofibroma or cellular myopericytoma.

---

[1] SMA: smooth muscle actin.

[2] EMA: epithelial membrane antigen.

[3] PDGFRB: platelet-derived growth factor receptor beta encodes a cell surface tyrosine kinase receptor for members of the platelet-derived growth factor family. These growth factors are mitogens for cells of mesenchymal origin. The type of growth factor bound to a receptor monomer determines whether the receptor homodimerizes (PDGFB or PDGFD) or heterodimerizes (PDGFA and PDGFB) with PDGFRA.

[4] SRF: serum response factor encodes a ubiquitous nuclear protein that stimulates both cell proliferation and differentiation. SRF is a member of the MADS (MCM1, agamous, deficiens, and SRF) box superfamily of transcription factors. SRF binds to the serum response element (SRE) in the promoter region of target genes such as c-Fos and thus plays a role in cell cycle, apoptosis, cell growth, and differentiation. SRF is the downstream target of many pathways such as the mitogen-activated protein kinase (MAPK) pathway.

Prognosis

Myofibroma is a benign tumor with an overall excellent prognosis (<10% of myofibromas recur and are cured by local re-excision), although complications of visceral cases may be fatal. Of note, myofibroma spontaneous regression has been reported.

Therapy

Surgical excision is the mainstay of treatment. Clinical efficacy of PDGFR inhibitors (e.g., imatinib) has been recently reported for myofibromatosis.

Suggested Readings

Agaimy (2017) Recurrent somatic PDGFRB mutations in sporadic infantile/solitary adult myofibromas but not in angioleiomyomas and myopericytomas. Am J Surg Pathol 41:195–203

Antonescu (2017) Recurrent SRF-RELA fusions define a novel subset of cellular myofibroma/myopericytoma: a potential diagnostic pitfall with sarcomas with myogenic differentiation. Am J Surg Pathol 41:677–684

Arts (2017) PDGFRB gain-of-function mutations in sporadic infantile myofibromatosis. Hum Mol Genet 26(10):1801–1810

Dachy (2019) Association of PDGFRB mutations with pediatric myofibroma and myofibromatosis. JAMA Dermatol. [Epub ahead of print]

Fletcher (2020) WHO classification of tumours of soft tissue and bone (5th edition)

Hassan (2019) Novel PDGFRB rearrangement in multifocal infantile myofibromatosis is tumorigenic and sensitive to imatinib. Cold Spring Harb Mol Case Stud. 5(5). pii: a004440

Pond (2018) A patient with germ-line gain-of-function PDGFRB p.N666H mutation and marked clinical response to imatinib. Genet Med 20(1):142–150

Rastogi (2019) Myofibromatosis. Fetal Pediatr Pathol. [Epub ahead of print]

Suurmeijer (2019) Novel SRF-ICA1L fusions in cellular myoid neoplasms with potential for malignant behavior. Am J Surg Pathol. [Epub ahead of print]

Weller (2019) PDGRFB mutation-associated myofibromatosis: Response to targeted therapy with imatinib. Am J Med Genet A 179(9):1895–1897

Definition

Myolipoma of soft tissue is a benign neoplasm classified by the World Health Organization as a variant of lipoma of extrauterine sites, thereby being distinguished from uterine lipoleiomyoma (→ see Chap. 249).

Epidemiology and Presentation

Myolipoma of soft tissue is a very rare tumor more often occurring in adults with a female predominance. It most often arises in deep-seated locations (e.g., retroperitoneum, pelvis, and other intra-abdominal sites) and tends to be large (usually 20 cm in size); it less frequently develops in the subcutis of the trunk wall or extremities.

Pathology

Myolipoma is characterized by the admixture of mature adipocytes and well-differentiated smooth muscle cells. Thin fascicles of bland smooth muscle traverse mature fat within a relatively well-circumscribed or encapsulated lesion.

Biomarkers

This tumor stains positive for desmin and SMA. Staining for HMB45 is negative.

Prognosis

Myolipoma of soft tissue is a benign tumor.

Therapy

Surgical resection is curative.

Suggested Readings

Fletcher (2020) WHO classification of tumours of soft tissue and bone (5th edition)
Fukushima (2017) Myolipoma of soft tissue: clinicopathologic analysis of 34 cases. Am J Surg
    Pathol 41(2):153–160

Definition

Myopericytoma is a (almost always) benign tumor classified among perivascular (pericytic) soft tissue tumors (along with myofibroma, angioleiomyoma, and glomus tumor, → see dedicated sections).

It is also known as hemangiopericytoma, perivascular myoid tumor, pericytoma, myopericytomatosis, glomangiopericytoma, and solitary myofibroma.

Epidemiology and Presentation

Myopericytoma occurs at any age, but it is most frequently observed in adults (males: 60%). An association between myopericytoma and EBV has been reported in patients with AIDS.

This tumor generally develops in dermal or subcutaneous tissue (mainly distal extremities, followed by proximal extremities, neck, and trunk), the involvement of deep soft tissues and viscera being rare.

Clinically, the tumor commonly presents as a painless, slow-growing, superficially located, and well-circumscribed nodule (typically less than 2 cm in diameter) that can be present for years. The lesion is usually solitary, but multiple lesions have been described.

Pathology

The lesion is composed of cytologically uniform oval- to spindle-shaped myoid cells showing a typical multilayer, perivascular, concentric growth. Lesional blood vessels are numerous and variable in size; branching vascular structures with a solitary fibrous tumor-like appearance can be observed. In some cases, a more prominent fascicular arrangement of tumor cells is present, mimicking myofibroma or

© The Editor(s) (if applicable) and The Author(s), under exclusive license to
Springer Nature Switzerland AG 2021
S. Mocellin, *Soft Tissue Tumors*, https://doi.org/10.1007/978-3-030-58710-9_179

angioleiomyoma. In other cases, a cellular component with glomus cell-like features is present: for these hybrid cases, the term glomangiopericytoma has been utilized.

The very rare cases of malignant myopericytoma are characterized by infiltrative growth composed of atypical, perivascular myoid tumor cells with evident proliferative activity.

Differential diagnosis may be needed with the other members of the perivascular (pericytic) soft tissue tumor family (myofibroma, angioleiomyoma, and glomus tumor).

Of note, hemangiopericytoma (along with fibrosarcoma) in the past represented one of the most common diagnoses in soft tissue pathology, whereas it is now rarely diagnosed mainly because many cases are currently classified otherwise (e.g., solitary fibrous tumor).

Biomarkers

Myopericytoma stains positive for SMA[1] and h-caldesmon. In contrast, tumor cells are negative for desmin, S100, and cytokeratins.

A subgroup of tumors considered to fall within the myopericytic category carry the **chromosomal translocation** t(7;12)(p22;q13), which leads to the formation of the ACTB-GLI1 fusion gene[2]; in the international literature, this tumor subtype is also called pericytoma with t(7;12). SRF-based rearrangements[3] leading to the formation of SRF-RELA fusion gene or SRF-ICA1L fusion gene has been recently described in a group of cellular spindle cell neoplasms with histologic features reminiscent of cellular myofibroma or cellular myopericytoma.

Finally, recurrent **somatic mutations** of PDGFRB[4] have been reported in myopericytoma (as well as in myofibroma, → see dedicated section).

---

[1] SMA: smooth muscle actin.

[2] ACTB-GLI1 fusion gene: ACTB (actin beta) encodes one of six different actin proteins, which are highly conserved proteins involved in cell motility, structure, integrity, and intercellular signaling. GLI1 (GLI family zinc finger 1) encodes a member of the Kruppel family of zinc finger proteins; the encoded transcription factor is activated by the sonic hedgehog signal transduction pathway and regulates stem cell proliferation (the activity and nuclear localization of GLI1 is negatively regulated by p53).

[3] SRF: serum response factor encodes a ubiquitous nuclear protein that stimulates both cell proliferation and differentiation. SRF is a member of the MADS (MCM1, agamous, deficiens, and SRF) box superfamily of transcription factors. SRF binds to the serum response element (SRE) in the promoter region of target genes such as c-Fos and thus plays a role in cell cycle, apoptosis, cell growth, and differentiation. SRF is the downstream target of many pathways such as the mitogen-activated protein kinase (MAPK) pathway.

[4] PDGFRB: platelet-derived growth factor receptor beta encodes a cell surface tyrosine kinase receptor for members of the platelet-derived growth factor family. These growth factors are mitogens for cells of mesenchymal origin. The type of growth factor bound to a receptor monomer determines whether the receptor homodimerizes (PDGFB or PDGFD) or heterodimerizes (PDGFA and PDGFB) with PDGFRA.

Prognosis

Most cases of myopericytoma are benign and do not tend to recur even if incompletely excised. Very rare cases of malignant myopericytoma have been reported, mostly seen in deep soft tissues: the prognosis of these cases is very poor.

Therapy

Surgical excision is the treatment of choice.

Suggested Readings

Antonescu (2017) Recurrent SRF-RELA fusions define a novel subset of cellular myofibroma/myopericytoma: a potential diagnostic pitfall with sarcomas with myogenic differentiation. Am J Surg Pathol 41:677–684

Fletcher (2020) WHO classification of tumours of soft tissue and bone (5th edition)

Folpe (2019) "Hey!—Whatever happened to hemangiopericytoma and fibrosarcoma?" An update on selected conceptual advances in soft tissue pathology which have occurred over the past 50 years. Hum Pathol. [Epub ahead of print]

Hung (2017) Myopericytomatosis: clinicopathologic analysis of 11 cases with molecular identification of recurrent PDGFRB alterations in myopericytomatosis and myopericytoma. Am J Surg Pathol 41:1034–1044

Kerr (2019) Pericytoma with t(7;12) and ACTB-GLI1 fusion: reevaluation of an unusual entity and its relationship to the spectrum of GLI1 fusion-related neoplasms. Am J Surg Pathol 43(12):1682–1692

Suurmeijer (2019) Novel SRF-ICA1L fusions in cellular myoid neoplasms with potential for malignant behavior. Am J Surg Pathol. [Epub ahead of print]

Definition

Myositis ossificans is a benign lesion classified among the fibroblastic and myofibroblastic soft tissue tumors.

It is usually considered together with fibro-osseous pseudotumor of digits (FOPD), which mainly differ for localization. They are also known as pseudomalignant osseous tumor of soft tissue, myositis ossificans circumscripta, and myositis ossificans traumatica.

Epidemiology and Presentation

Like FOPD, myositis ossificans can occur at any age, although most cases are described in young adults (mean age: 30 years), with a male prevalence (M/F = 3:2). Soft tissue injury (including surgical trauma) is the initiating event in most cases. Unlike FOPD (which occurs exclusively in the fingers and less frequently the toes), myositis ossificans can arise anywhere in the body, although most cases develop in areas (e.g., elbow, thigh, buttock, and shoulder) more susceptible to trauma (both acute and chronic). As opposed to FOPD (which develops in the subcutaneous tissue), myositis ossificans locates in skeletal muscle (similar lesions occurring in the subcutis, tendons, or fascia should be classified as panniculitis ossificans and fasciitis ossificans, respectively).

Both myositis ossificans and FOPD present as a rapidly growing lesion, which is initially painful and can limit the range of motion of the affected body segment.

The lesion appears hyperintense on T2-weighted magnetic resonance imaging; upon plain X-rays, calcifications become evident only after 2–6 weeks.

© The Editor(s) (if applicable) and The Author(s), under exclusive license to
Springer Nature Switzerland AG 2021
S. Mocellin, *Soft Tissue Tumors*, https://doi.org/10.1007/978-3-030-58710-9_180

Pathology

Both myositis ossificans and FOPD are localized self-limiting lesions composed of hypercellular fibrous tissue and metaplastic bone. Myositis ossificans is a well-demarcated lesion which can be up to 10 cm in diameter (FOPD is smaller and less demarcated). Microscopically, the cellular component may resemble nodular fasciitis and is composed of proliferating fibroblasts oriented randomly or in intersecting fascicles. Mitoses may be numerous, but they are normal. At the periphery, the fibroblastic component is enriched with osteoblasts and merges with sheets of bone. Zonation is the typical appearance of these lesions.

The rapid clinical growth together with hypercellularity and mitotic activity makes both myositis ossificans and FOPD classic examples of pseudosarcoma (i.e., a lesion that histologically mimics a sarcoma).

Differential diagnosis may be needed with extraosseous osteosarcoma and juxtacortical osteosarcoma (malignant cytology with atypical mitotic figures, no or reverse zonation, may have necrosis) and aneurysmal bone cyst of soft tissue (more protracted clinical course).

Biomarkers

Fibroblasts and myofibroblasts may express vimentin, SMA,[1] and desmin. Osteoclasts express vimentin.

The **chromosomal translocation** t(17;22)(p13;q12) leading to the formation of the MYH9-USP6 fusion gene[2] is a frequent event in myositis ossificans (establishing its clonal neoplastic nature). Also nodular fasciitis and aneurysmal bone cyst of soft tissue often carry this chromosomal rearrangement, providing evidence that these three entities are genetically related.

Prognosis

Prognosis is excellent and recurrence is exceptional after surgery.

Therapy

If conservative treatment (i.e., physical therapy) does not relieve pain or restore the range of motion, surgical excision is the treatment of choice.

---

[1] SMA: smooth muscle actin.

[2] MYH9-USP6 fusion gene: MYH9 (ayosin heavy chain 9) encodes a non-muscle myosin which is involved in cytokinesis, cell motility, and maintenance of cell shape. USP6 (ubiquitin-specific peptidase 6) encodes a deubiquitinase with an ATP-independent isopeptidase activity, cleaving at the C-terminus of the ubiquitin moiety.

Suggested Readings

Bekers (2018) Myositis ossificans—another condition with USP6 rearrangement, providing evidence of a relationship with nodular fasciitis and aneurysmal bone cyst. Ann Diagn Pathol 34:56–59

de Smet (2020) Surgical excision of post-traumatic myositis ossificans of the adductor longus in a football player. BMJ Case Rep 13(3):e233504

Devilbiss (2018) Myositis ossificans in sport: a review. Curr Sports Med Rep 17(9):290–295

Fletcher (2020) WHO classification of tumours of soft tissue and bone (5th edition)

Schmitz (2019) Myositis ossificans mimicking metaplastic breast cancer on core needle biopsy. Hum Pathol 93:97–102

Sferopoulos (2017) Myositis ossificans in children: a review. Eur J Orthop Surg Traumatol 27(4):491–502

Walczak (2015) Myositis ossificans. J Am Acad Orthop Surg 23(10):612–622

Zhang (2020) Myositis ossificans-like soft tissue aneurysmal bone cyst: a clinical, radiological, and pathological study of seven cases with COL1A1-USP6 fusion and a novel ANGPTL2-USP6 fusion. Mod Pathol. [Epub ahead of print]

Zubler (2020) Diagnostic utility of perilesional muscle edema in myositis ossificans. Skelet Radiol 49(6):929–936

Definition

Myxofibrosarcoma (MFS) includes a range of malignant fibroblastic lesions with myxoid stroma, cell pleomorphism, and distinctive curvilinear vessels. In the past it was known as myxoid malignant fibrous histiocytoma.

Epidemiology and Presentation

MFS is one of the most common sarcomas in the elderly, its incidence peaking between 60 and 80 years (it is very rare under the age of 20 years).

Most MFS arise in the extremities and girdles, with lower limbs being more frequently affected. Approximately 50% of cases arise in dermis or subcutis, the other 50% developing underneath the muscular fascia.

Rarely observed on the trunk, head and neck, and hands/feet, it is extremely rare in the retroperitoneum and in the abdominal cavity where it might represent a misdiagnosed dedifferentiated liposarcoma.

Pathology

Myxofibrosarcoma displays a wide range of cellularity, pleomorphism, and proliferative activity; nonetheless, all cases share some morphological features, such as myxoid stroma and multinodular growth with incomplete fibrous septa. Superficial MFS generally has very infiltrative margins which often extend beyond what can be clinically detected.

Low-grade lesions are characterized by hypocellularity with only a few noncohesive, plump spindled cells with atypical nuclei, mitotic figures being infrequent; a typical feature is the presence of prominent elongated, curvilinear, blood vessels with perivascular accumulation of tumor cells; moreover, so-called pseudolipoblasts (vacuolated neoplastic fibroblastic cells with cytoplasmic acid mucin) are often noted.

In high-grade MFS, solid sheets and cellular fascicles of spindled and pleomorphic malignant cells are present, with numerous (often atypical) mitoses, areas of hemorrhage, and necrosis.

Intermediate-grade MFS is more cellular and pleomorphic than low-grade MFS but lack prominent solid areas, pronounced cellular pleomorphism and necrosis.

Differential diagnosis may be needed with the following: low-grade fibromyxoid sarcoma (nonpleomorphic spindle cells set in alternating myxoid and fibrous background, usually with whorled pattern and sometimes collagen rosettes; it lacks prominent curvilinear vascular structures and cellular atypia of MFS); myxoid liposarcoma (lipoblasts with clear cytoplasmic vacuoles, plexiform vasculature, monotonous nuclei usually with no pleomorphism); myxoma (no atypia, less prominent vasculature, no perivascular condensation of tumor cells, few mitotic figures, normal karyotype); nodular fasciitis (no atypical cells, no atypical mitotic figures); and undifferentiated pleomorphic sarcoma (differential diagnosis may be difficult especially in the case of high-grade MFS).

The rare variant known as epithelioid myxofibrosarcoma is composed mainly of atypical epithelioid neoplastic cells arranged in small clusters in the myxoid areas or forming sheets in the hypercellular areas, thus resembling metastatic carcinoma, melanoma, or malignant myoepithelioma of soft tissues.

Biomarkers

No specific stains exist; staining for desmin and histiocyte-specific markers is negative.

Typically, karyotypes are highly complex (aneuploidy) with pronounced intratumoral heterogeneity: these cytogenetic features occur regardless of tumor grading, although chromosomal aberrations increase with grade. No specific cytogenetic aberration has been identified. MFS has recently been shown to commonly harbor copy number alterations or mutations in the tumor suppressor genes RB1 and TP53.

As opposed to intramuscular myxoma (→ see dedicated section), no activating mutations of the GNAS géne[1] have been observed in MFS.

---

[1] GNAS: alternative splicing of downstream exons of this gene (also named GNAS complex locus and guanine nucleotide-binding protein alpha stimulating activity polypeptide 1) results in different forms of the stimulatory G protein alpha subunit, a key element of the classical signal transduction pathway linking G protein-coupled receptors (GPCR) with the activation of adenylyl cyclase and ultimately a variety of cell activities.

Prognosis

Local recurrence, independently of histological grade, occurs in up to 60% of cases. In addition to pulmonary and osseous metastases, lymph node metastasis may occur in a small but non-negligible number of cases.

Metastases and tumor-related mortality are closely related to tumor grading. In fact, no low-grade MFS metastasizes, whereas intermediate-grade and high-grade MFS do so in about 30% of cases.

Early (<12 months) local relapse increases disease specific mortality, which suggests that optimal local control may translate into a survival advantage. Besides tumor grade, also tumor size and margins are statistically significantly associated with patient survival.

Notably, low-grade MFS may progress into higher-grade lesions when they recur (and thus the prognosis worsens).

Therapy

Surgical wide excision is the treatment of choice for primary MFS. Adjuvant radiotherapy may be indicated to improve local control in higher risk lesions (larger, deeper, higher grade).

Suggested Readings

Fletcher (2020) WHO classification of tumours of soft tissue and bone (5th edition)

Fujiwara (2019) What is an adequate margin for infiltrative soft-tissue sarcomas? Eur J Surg Oncol. [Epub ahead of print]

Look Hong (2013) Prognostic factors and outcomes of patients with myxofibrosarcoma. Ann Surg Oncol 20(1):80–86

Li (2020) Rb and p53-deficient myxofibrosarcoma and undifferentiated pleomorphic sarcoma require skp2 for survival. Cancer Res. [Epub ahead of print]

Mühlhofer (2019) Prognostic factors and outcomes for patients with myxofibrosarcoma: a 13-year retrospective evaluation. Anticancer Res 39(6):2985–2992

Teurneau (2019) High recurrence rate of myxofibrosarcoma: the effect of radiotherapy is not clear. Sarcoma 2019:8517371

Widemann (2018) Biology and management of undifferentiated pleomorphic sarcoma, myxofibrosarcoma, and malignant peripheral nerve sheath tumors: state of the art and perspectives. J Clin Oncol 36(2):160–167

Yoshimoto (2020) Retroperitoneal myxofibrosarcoma: a controversial entity. Pathol Res Pract. [Epub ahead of print]

Yoshimoto (2020) Comparative study of myxofibrosarcoma with undifferentiated pleomorphic sarcoma: histopathologic and clinicopathologic review. Am J Surg Pathol 44(1):87–97

Definition

Myxoid/round cell liposarcoma (MRLS) is a malignant tumor of adipocytic origin. This entity is also known as myxoid liposarcoma and includes the more cellular neoplasm formerly known as round cell liposarcoma.

For general information on liposarcomas → see Chap. 155. As regards the other types of liposarcomas (i.e., well-differentiated liposarcoma, dedifferentiated liposarcoma, pleomorphic liposarcoma) → see dedicated sections.

Epidemiology and Presentation

MRLS accounts for 20–30% of all liposarcomas and about 5% of all soft tissue sarcomas in adulthood. It occurs mainly in young adults (peak incidence: 30–50 years) and may occur in childhood/adolescence (although rare, it is the most frequent type of liposarcoma in this population). No significant gender differences have been reported.

The most common sites of involvement are the deep soft tissues of the extremities (about 70% within the thigh musculature). MRLS rarely localizes in the retroperitoneum or subcutis. Some visceral cases have been reported. Clinically, it presents as a large painless mass. The disease may sometimes be multifocal (both synchronous or metachronous).

Pathology

Macroscopically, MRLS typically presents as a well-circumscribed, multinodular intramuscular lesion, which shows a gelatinous cut surface in the low-grade myxoid version of this neoplasm or fleshy tan appearance in higher-grade areas.

Microscopically, it is composed of uniform round to oval non-lipogenic cells and a variable number of small signet ring lipoblasts in a prominent myxoid stroma (hence the name; the extracellular mucin forms large pools leading to a microcystic lymphangioma-like growth pattern) with a typical branching vascular pattern ("chicken wire" capillary vasculature). Cells display a nodular growth pattern, with higher cellularity at the periphery. Classically, MRLS lacks nuclear pleomorphism and giant tumor cells; mitotic activity is generally low and necrosis absent. This low-grade presentation is also known as myxoid liposarcoma.

A subgroup of MRLS displays a histological shift to hypercellular round cell morphology (which is linked to a worse prognosis). The high-grade ("round cell") areas are characterized by solid sheets of round cells with a high nucleus-to-cytoplasm ratio, frequent mitotic figures, and lack of interposing myxoid stroma. This high-grade round cell liposarcoma is also known as poorly differentiated myxoid liposarcoma. The presence of a gradual transition from myxoid to round cell areas supports the hypothesis that myxoid and round cell liposarcoma represent a histological continuum of the same nosological entity (which is confirmed by the fact that both subtypes carry the same chromosomal translocation; see below paragraph). There is general agreement on considering high-grade round cell liposarcoma the lesions showing more than 5% of round cell component.

Differential diagnosis may be needed with the following: Ewing sarcoma/ PNET (neuroendocrine morphology, CD99 positivity, translocations involving the EWS gene); lymphoma (positive for B-cell biomarkers such as CD20 and CD79a or T-cell biomarkers such as CD3 and CD4); melanoma (positive for S100 and HMB45); metastatic carcinoma (clinical history, cytokeratin positivity).

Biomarkers

S100 immunostaining is variably positive in lipoblasts of the high-grade component. CD31 and CD34 can highlight the vasculature. However, due to the typical appearance, in many cases immunohistochemistry is not needed to make a diagnosis.

In doubtful cases, detection of typical **chromosomal translocation** is the best diagnostic tool. In fact, most cases of MRLS are characterized by the translocation t(12;16)(q13;p11), which leads to the formation of the FUS-DDIT3 fusion gene[1] (about 95% of cases); the remaining cases carry the t(12;22)(q13;q12) translocation, which leads to the formation of the EWSR1-DDIT3 fusion gene. The presence

---

[1] FUS-DDIT3 fusion gene: FUS (fused in sarcoma; also known as translocated in liposarcoma, TLS) encodes for a protein belonging to the FET family of RNA-binding proteins (implicated in regulation of gene expression and mRNA/microRNA processing). DDIT3 (DNA damage inducible transcript 3; also known as C/EBP-homologous protein, CHOP) encodes a member of the CCAAT/enhancer-binding protein (C/EBP) family of transcription factors. The FUS-DDIT3 fusion protein is believed to confer tumorigenicity through dysregulation of adipocyte differentiation, leading to unchecked proliferation of immature lipoblasts that are incapable of differentiating. FUS is involved also in the FUS-DDIT3 fusion gene, which is characteristic of myxoid liposarcoma.

of the FUS-DDIT3 fusion is highly accurate for the diagnosis of MRLS as it is absent in morphological mimics such as low-grade myxoid liposarcoma, dedifferentiated liposarcoma, and myxofibrosarcoma.

Activating mutations of PIK3CA (which increase the activity of the AKT signaling pathway) have been observed in 15% of MRLS cases, which makes this fraction of the disease theoretically targetable with PI3K inhibitors (e.g., alpelisib) already approved for the treatment of other cancers (e.g., breast carcinoma).

Prognosis

MRLS is a malignant neoplasm with different prognosis mainly depending upon histological grading (low-grade versus high-grade, the cutoff being 5% of round cell component). Patients with high-grade tumors are at higher risk of local recurrence, metastasis, and tumor-related death. Low-grade myxoid liposarcoma is associated with a metastatic risk lower than 10%, whereas in patients with high-grade round cell liposarcoma, the risk is up to 40%. Presence of necrosis, primary size, and p53 overexpression are other prognostic factors. The different isoforms of the FUS-DDIT3 fusion transcripts do not correlate with clinical outcome.

As opposed to other sarcomas, MRLS tends to metastasize to unusual locations such as soft tissues (e.g., retroperitoneum, opposite extremity, axilla), bone (with special regard to the spine), or serosal surfaces (e.g., peritoneum) even before spreading to the lungs, which justifies the use of thoraco-abdominal radiological imaging for staging purposes. Finally, the presence of apparently primary MRLS in unusual locations must raise the suspicion of metastatic MRLS.

Therapy

Surgery is the treatment of choice for **localized primary tumors**. Importantly, MRLS is typically both radiosensitive and chemosensitive, with tumor responses in up to 70% of cases. As regards extremity tumors (which represent the majority of all cases), (A) myxoid liposarcoma (low-grade tumor) can be managed with surgery alone; however, if morbid surgery is needed to obtain wide resection margins, then neoadjuvant radiotherapy with or without chemotherapy is indicated to downsize the neoplasm and allow for less demolitive surgery; (B) round cell liposarcoma (high-grade tumor) can be treated with surgery alone if the primary tumor is <5 cm; if larger than 5 cm, neoadjuvant chemotherapy with neoadjuvant or adjuvant radiotherapy is recommended.

Although high-grade MRLS is deemed to be somewhat more sensitive to trabectedin, this drug yielded results overlapping to those of epirubicin plus ifosfamide in terms of disease-free survival in a randomized trial of neoadjuvant chemotherapy (ISG-STS 1001).

For patients with **locally advanced/unresectable or metastatic disease**, anthracycline-based chemotherapy remains the standard first-line treatment. As second-line treatment, gemcitabine plus docetaxel and high-dose ifosfamide mono-therapy can be used. More recently, trabectedin and eribulin have been approved for the treatment of patients with metastatic liposarcoma who failed anthracycline-based first-line chemotherapy.

Suggested Readings

Antonescu (2001) Prognostic impact of P53 status, TLS-CHOP fusion transcript structure, and histological grade in myxoid liposarcoma: a molecular and clinicopathologic study of 82 cases. Clin Cancer Res 7(12):3977–3987

Assi (2019) A comprehensive review of the current evidence for trabectedin in advanced myxoid liposarcoma. Cancer Treat Rev 72:37–44

Chowdhry (2018) Myxoid liposarcoma: treatment outcomes from chemotherapy and radiation therapy. Sarcoma 2018:8029157

Chung (2009) Radiosensitivity translates into excellent local control in extremity myxoid liposarcoma: a comparison with other soft tissue sarcomas. Cancer 115(14):3254–3261

Crago (2016) Liposarcoma: multimodality management and future targeted therapies. Surg Oncol Clin N Am 25(4):761–773

Fletcher (2020) WHO classification of tumours of soft tissue and bone (5th edition)

Gorelik (2018) Early detection of metastases using whole-body MRI for initial staging and routine follow-up of myxoid liposarcoma. Skelet Radiol 47(3):369–379

Gouin (2019) Early detection of multiple bone and extra-skeletal metastases by body magnetic resonance imaging (BMRI) after treatment of Myxoid/Round-Cell Liposarcoma (MRCLS). Eur J Surg Oncol 45(12):2431–2436

Gronchi (2017) Histotype-tailored neoadjuvant chemotherapy versus standard chemotherapy in patients with high-risk soft-tissue sarcomas (ISG-STS 1001): an international, open-label, randomised, controlled, phase 3, multicentre trial. Lancet Oncol 18(6):812–822

Grosso (2007) Efficacy of trabectedin (ecteinascidin-743) in advanced pretreated myxoid liposarcomas: a retrospective study. Lancet Oncol 8(7):595–602

Jones (2005) Differential sensitivity of liposarcoma subtypes to chemotherapy. Eur J Cancer 41(18):2853–2860

Muratori (2018) Myxoid liposarcoma: prognostic factors and metastatic pattern in a series of 148 patients treated at a single institution. Int J Surg Oncol 2018:8928706

Pollack (2020) Clinical outcomes of patients with advanced synovial sarcoma or myxoid/round cell liposarcoma treated at major cancer centers in the United States. Cancer Med. [Epub ahead of print]

Sonoda (2019) Giant myxoid liposarcoma of the stomach: report of a case. Int J Surg Case Rep 60:234–238

Tornin (2018) FUS-CHOP promotes invasion in myxoid liposarcoma through a SRC/FAK/RHO/ROCK-dependent pathway. Neoplasia 20(1):44–56

Trautmann (2017) FUS-DDIT3 fusion protein-driven IGF-IR signaling is a therapeutic target in myxoid liposarcoma. Clin Cancer Res 23(20):6227–6238

Trautmann (2019) Phosphatidylinositol-3-kinase (PI3K)/Akt signaling is functionally essential in myxoid liposarcoma. Mol Cancer Ther 18(4):834–844

Definition

Myxoinflammatory fibroblastic sarcoma (MIFS) is a neoplasm of intermediate biological aggressiveness and is classified among fibroblastic-myofibroblastic tumors.

It is also known as atypical myxoinflammatory fibroblastic tumor, acral myxoinflammatory fibroblastic sarcoma, inflammatory myxohyaline tumor of the distal extremities with virocyte/Reed-Sternberg-like cells, and inflammatory myxoid tumor of the soft parts with bizarre giant cells.

Epidemiology and Presentation

MIFS typically develops in middle-aged subjects without gender prevalence. The great majority of lesions arise in the distal extremities (80% in the hands, mainly in the fingers, hence the name acral MIFS).

In most patients the tumor presents as a slow-growing mass (usually <5 cm) that can be misdiagnosed with a benign condition (e.g., tenosynovitis or ganglion cyst).

Pathology

Macroscopically, most MIFS show a multinodular appearance with fibrous and myxoid zones, with the tumor periphery being ill-defined, which makes complete excision difficult.

Microscopically the tumor is characterized by the presence of epithelioid fibroblasts interspersed with a prominent mixed inflammatory infiltrate and a variable myxoid matrix. The lesion typically involves the tenosynovial structures, with extension into the subcutis and rarely into bone. MIFS shows Touton-type giant cells and a mononuclear cell background (ranging from relatively bland to bizarre epithelioid cells with inclusion-like nucleoli, sometimes resembling virocytes or

© The Editor(s) (if applicable) and The Author(s), under exclusive license to $\qquad$ 585
Springer Nature Switzerland AG 2021
S. Mocellin, *Soft Tissue Tumors*, https://doi.org/10.1007/978-3-030-58710-9_183

Reed-Sternberg cells) with varying degrees of nuclear atypia. Lipoblast-like cells can also be present.

Differential diagnosis may be needed with the following: epithelioid sarcoma (most cells are round with dense eosinophilic cytoplasm; strong positivity for cytokeratins; loss of INI1/SMARCB); Hodgkin lymphoma (it lacks giant cells and lipoblast-like cells; tumor cells have different staining patterns); myxofibrosarcoma (rare in soft tissues of hands and feet; more frequent mitotic figures with atypical forms; no inflammatory infiltrate); pleomorphic liposarcoma (true pleomorphic lipoblasts, rare in soft tissues of hands and feet, more frequent mitotic figures with atypical forms, no inflammatory infiltrate); Rosai-Dorfman disease (emperipolesis but no intranuclear viral-like inclusions; S100 positive; usually not myxoid); and tenosynovitis (no enlarged atypical cells).

Biomarkers

Positivity for CD68, CD34, vimentin, and SMA[1] is variable; of note, lymphoid markers (e.g., CD30, CD45) are negative.

In a subset of cases, the **chromosomal translocation** t(1;10)(p22;q24) leads to the formation of the TGFBR3-MGEA5 fusion gene[2] (whose functional effect appears to be the transcriptional upregulation of the FGF8 gene, located close to MGEA5 on chromosome 10), which has been described also in pleomorphic hyalinizing angiectatic tumor ($\rightarrow$ see dedicated section) and hemosiderotic fibrolipomatous tumor ($\rightarrow$ see dedicated section). A mutually exclusive chromosomal rearrangement t(17;7)(p11;q34) leads to the formation of the TOM1L2-BRAF fusion gene[3] in another subset of MIFS. VGLL3 gene amplification can coexist with both t(1;10) and t(17;7) in some MIFS.

---

[1] SMA: smooth muscle actin.

[2] TGFBR3-MGEA5 fusion gene: TGFBR3 (transforming growth factor beta receptor 3) encodes a receptor which is a membrane proteoglycan that often functions as a co-receptor with other TGF-beta receptor superfamily members. MGEA5 (also known as OGA, O-GlcNAcase): the modification of cytoplasmic and nuclear proteins by O-linked N-acetylglucosamine (O-GlcNAc) addition and removal on serine and threonine residues is catalyzed by OGT (which adds O-GlcNAc) and MGEA5, a glycosidase that removes O-GlcNAc modifications.

[3] TOM1L2-BRAF fusion gene: TOM1L2 (target Of Myb1 like 2 membrane trafficking protein) encodes a protein which belongs to a small family whose members have an N-terminal VHS domain followed by a GAT domain, which typically participate in vesicular trafficking. The BRAF proto-oncogene encodes a protein belonging to the RAF family of serine/threonine protein kinases; this protein plays a key role in the MAPK/ERK signaling pathway, which affects cell division, differentiation, and secretion; mutations in this gene (mainly V600E mutation) are frequently encountered in melanoma as well as non-Hodgkin lymphoma, colorectal cancer, thyroid carcinoma, non-small cell lung carcinoma, hairy cell leukemia, and adenocarcinoma of lung.

Prognosis

MIFS is classified as an intermediate aggressive tumor. The reported rates of local recurrence range from 20% to 70%. Multiple disease relapses can lead to limb amputation. Regional lymph node metastases and local bone invasion occasionally occur. Distant metastasis is very rare. Currently, no prognostic factors can reliably predict the clinical behavior.

Therapy

Wide surgical excision is the treatment of choice.

Suggested Readings

Fletcher et al (2020) WHO classification of tumours of soft tissue and bone, 5th edn
Kao et al (2017) Recurrent BRAF gene rearrangements in myxoinflammatory fibroblastic sarcomas, but not hemosiderotic fibrolipomatous tumors. Am J Surg Pathol 41(11):1456–1465
Liu et al (2019) The t(1;10)(p22;q24) TGFBR3/MGEA5 translocation in pleomorphic hyalinizing angiectatic tumor, myxoinflammatory fibroblastic sarcoma, and hemosiderotic fibrolipomatous tumor. Arch Pathol Lab Med 143(2):212–221

Different soft tissue tumors include the term "myxoma" in their names, such as the following:

- Acral fibromyxoma
- Angiomyxoma (with deep and superficial subtypes)
- Cardiac myxoma (also known as heart myxoma)
- Dermal nerve sheath myxoma
- Intramuscular myxoma
- Juxta-articular myxoma
- Superficial angiomyxoma

For details on each single neoplasm → see dedicated sections.

Definition

Nasal glial heterotopia (NGH) is a benign lesion classified by the World Health Organization among nerve sheath tumors, although it is not a neoplasm (but rather a heterotopia).

It is also known as nasal glioma and facial glioma (these terms should be abandoned since this is not a tumor), neuroglial heterotopia, glial choristoma, nasal atretic cephalocele, and ectopic glial tissue.

Epidemiology and Presentation

NGH is a rare congenital non-hereditary malformation diagnosed almost always before the age of 2 years, without gender differences. The lesion (usually polypoid in shape and 1–3 cm in size) is located most often close to or within the nose, other sites being paranasal sinuses, nasopharynx, pharynx, tongue, palate, tonsil, and orbit.

Since there is no connection of the mass with the cerebrospinal fluid system, the Furstenberg test is negative (the lesion does not enlarge with Valsalva maneuver or jugular vein compression).

Computed tomography scan or magnetic resonance imaging shows a soft tissue mass without an intracranial component or bony defect: if a defect is present, then an encephalocele is more likely to be diagnosed.

Pathology

NGH is a unencapsulated mass of mature, heterotopic neuroglial tissue (where cells are astrocytes) organized in islands separated by bands of vascularized fibrous connective tissue. Mitoses are absent. NGH should be differentiated from nasal encephalocele and fibrosed nasal polyp.

© The Editor(s) (if applicable) and The Author(s), under exclusive license to   591
Springer Nature Switzerland AG 2021
S. Mocellin, *Soft Tissue Tumors*, https://doi.org/10.1007/978-3-030-58710-9_185

Biomarkers

The glial tissue can be confirmed by a trichrome stain (glial tissue is blue, fibrosis is red) or by immunoreactivity for GFAP,[1] NSE,[2] or S100 protein.

Prognosis

NGS is a benign lesion. It has been reported to develop in association with sinonasal undifferentiated carcinoma.

Therapy

Surgical excision is the treatment of choice.

Suggested Reading

Fletcher et al (2013) WHO classification of tumours of soft tissue and bone, 4th edn

---

[1] GFAP: glial fibrillary acidic protein.
[2] NSE: neuron specific enolase.

Definition

Nasopharyngeal angiofibroma (NAF) is a benign vascular lesion arising from erectile-like fibrovascular stroma in the posterolateral wall of the nasal roof. It belongs to the angiofibroma family of tumors ($\rightarrow$ see Chap. 17).

NAF is also known as juvenile nasopharyngeal angiofibroma, juvenile angiofibroma, and angiofibromatous hamartoma of the nasal cavity.

Epidemiology and Presentation

NAF is a rare lesion that occurs almost exclusively in adolescent/young adult males and accounts for approximately 0.1–0.5% of all the head and neck masses.

Computed tomography and magnetic resonance imaging can be used to suspect the diagnosis, but final diagnosis needs a biopsy performed during an epypharyngoscopy.

Although arising in the posterolateral wall of the nasal roof, it may grow into the nasopharynx, orbit, or cranial cavity. NAF may regress after puberty, especially after incomplete surgical excision or radiotherapy.

Clinically, it presents as a well-circumscribed polypoid lesion, which easily bleeds upon manipulation and biopsy; it may occlude the nares; spontaneous bleeding can be a complication.

Pathology

Macroscopically, NAF is a well-circumscribed but unencapsulated polypoid fibrous mass with a spongy cut surface.

Microscopically NAF is a histologically benign hypervascular tumor composed of a mixture of stellate and staghorn blood vessels with variable vessel wall thickness. The irregular fibrous stroma is composed of stellate fibroblasts; multinucleated stromal cells are frequently observed. Mitotic figures are rare. Overall, NAF shows an erectile tissue appearance.

Differential diagnosis may be needed with capillary hemangioma (less fibrous tissue; the vessels lack erectile tissue appearance).

Biomarkers

Androgen receptor is expressed in 75% of cases (neither estrogen nor progesterone receptors are expressed).

Prognosis

Although NAF is considered a benign entity, it recurs in 40% of cases (especially if not completely removed) and often shows aggressive features with invasion into the nasal turbinates, nasal septum, and medial pterygoid lamina; it frequently extends into the nasal cavity, nasopharynx, and pterygopalatine fossa, with larger lesions extending into the sphenoid, maxillary, and ethmoid sinuses. Severe disease with orbital and intracranial involvement can be observed in up to 30% of cases.

Rare sarcomatous transformation after radiation therapy has been described.

Use of target therapy (e.g., sirolimus, an mTOR inhibitor) is in its infancy.

Therapy

Surgery is the treatment of choice, but NAF is difficult to be completely excised (due to anatomic restraints); preoperative arterial embolization (through angiography and catheterization of its primary arterial supply, the internal maxillary artery, a branch of the external carotid artery) or antiandrogen therapy has been suggested to improve the results of surgery. Radiotherapy and (less frequently) chemotherapy have been advocated for advanced or aggressive disease not amenable to other treatments.

Suggested Readings

Bertazzoni et al (2019) Contemporary management of juvenile angiofibroma. Curr Opin Otolaryngol Head Neck Surg 27(1):47–53
Doody et al (2019) The genetic and molecular determinants of juvenile nasopharyngeal angiofibroma: a systematic review. Ann Otol Rhinol Laryngol 128(11):1061–1072
Fernández et al (2020) Sirolimus for the treatment of juvenile nasopharyngeal angiofibroma. Pediatr Blood Cancer 67(4):e28162

Rupa et al (2018) Management and outcome in patients with advanced juvenile nasopharyngeal angiofibroma. J Neurol Surg B Skull Base 79(4):353–360

Suroyo et al (2020) The role of diagnostic and interventional radiology in juvenile nasopharyngeal angiofibroma: a case report and literature review. Radiol Case Rep 15(7):812–815

Yu et al (2020) Juvenile nasopharyngeal angiofibroma outcomes and cost: analysis of the kids' inpatient database. Ann Otol Rhinol Laryngol 129(5):498–504

Definition

Neurofibroma is a benign peripheral nerve sheath tumor.

Five macroscopic subtypes are recognized: (1) localized cutaneous neurofibroma (also known as solitary neurofibroma), (2) diffuse cutaneous neurofibroma, (3) localized intraneural neurofibroma, (4) plexiform intraneural neurofibroma, and (5) diffuse plexiform neurofibroma (also known as massive soft tissue neurofibroma or elephantiasis neurofibromatosis).

Epidemiology and Presentation

Neurofibroma (along with schwannoma → see dedicated section) is the most common type of peripheral nerve sheath tumor and most often occurs sporadically as a solitary lesion (localized cutaneous neurofibroma). Less frequently it presents as multiple tumors, typically in individuals with neurofibromatosis type 1 (→ see below paragraph). All ages may be affected (although most cases occur during the second to fourth decades of life), without gender differences. The commonest site of development is the skin, where the neoplasm is associated with a single small nerve (cutaneous neurofibroma is also called dermal neurofibroma). More deeply situated larger nerves (including spinal nerve roots or cranial nerves) are less frequently involved. Mucous membranes (e.g., oral mucosa) may also be affected (though rarely).

Patients with neurofibromas are often asymptomatic; however, irritation, mild pruritus, pain, or paresthesia can occur. The presentation may vary by type of neurofibroma, but the most common chief complaint is cosmetic appearance (which can reach disfiguration in multiple lesions proper of neurofibromatosis). Paraspinal neurofibromas can cause spinal cord compression.

Cutaneous neurofibroma (localized or diffuse) usually presents as a soft mobile asymptomatic lesion (rarely painful) which is usually skin-colored in sporadic

© The Editor(s) (if applicable) and The Author(s), under exclusive license to   597
Springer Nature Switzerland AG 2021
S. Mocellin, *Soft Tissue Tumors*, https://doi.org/10.1007/978-3-030-58710-9_187

forms and hyperpigmented in neurofibromatosis type 1. In contrast, deeper tumors frequently are firm and present with motor or sensory signs and symptoms in the distribution of the affected nerve (signs and symptoms of compression of the spinal cord may coexist). In the least common situation, the lesion presents as a plaque-like cutaneous and subcutaneous mass (especially in the head and neck), or as a massive soft tissue enlargement of a body region (e.g., the shoulder or pelvic girdle).

Specific aspects of presentation of the five subtypes are the following:

1. Localized cutaneous neurofibroma is a nodular or polypoid lesion (up to 2 cm in size) which is most often sporadic, only a small minority being associated with neurofibromatosis type 1 syndrome; the lesion is associated with the so-called buttonhole sign where on palpation the tumor retracts into the subcutis and reappears on pressure release.
2. Diffuse cutaneous neurofibroma is a plaque-like lesion which may extend into the subcutis; it is an uncommon variant of neurofibroma and is associated with neurofibromatosis type 1 in about 60% of cases; malignant transformation is extremely rare.
3. Localized intraneural neurofibroma is a solitary segmental fusiform enlargement of a sizeable nerve.
4. Plexiform intraneural neurofibroma presents as a series of lumpy masses involving a nerve or a nerve plexus and can become large; the term "plexiform" refers to the complex way of growing in the form of a plexus or network; if superficial it presents as a skin-colored or hyperpigmented nodular swelling. Deeper lesions may become irregular and tortuous (wormlike growth) and present with pain, numbness, paresthesias, mass effect, and sequelae of spinal nerve compression; plexiform neurofibroma almost always develops during childhood.
5. Diffuse plexiform neurofibroma may present as a relatively uniform regional soft tissue enlargement or as a pendulous bag-like mass with hyperpigmentation of the overlying skin.

A neurofibroma involving a nerve encased in bone may result in bone erosion, which can be appreciated upon X-ray-based imaging. On magnetic resonance imaging (MRI), neurofibroma appears as a T1 hypointense and T2 hyperintense lesion with heterogeneous contrast enhancement (MRI does not reliably differentiate between neurofibroma and schwannoma). As up to 50% of individuals with neurofibromatosis type 1 have internal neurofibromas, volumetric whole-body MRI is used in some centers to assess and follow up the tumor burden and growth, although this is not recommended as a routine strategy.

Etiology and Predisposition

Whereas 90% of neurofibromas are sporadic, in 10% of cases, the tumor develops within the frame of a cancer predisposition syndrome known as **neurofibromatosis type 1** (also called von Recklinghausen disease), a condition characterized by skin pigmentation and the growth of different tumor types (signs and symptoms varying widely across affected patients). The incidence of neurofibromatosis type 1 is about one in 3000 people worldwide. The life expectancy is reduced by 10–20 years compared with the general population, the most common cause of early death being malignant neoplasm (whose lifetime risk is about 60%).

Beginning in early childhood, almost all people with neurofibromatosis type 1 have multiple café-au-lait spots (milk-and-coffee spots, cutaneous flat patches of hyperpigmentation) which increase in size and number with age. Freckles in the underarms and groin typically develop later in childhood. Most adults with neurofibromatosis type 1 develop multiple neurofibromas especially (but not exclusively) on the skin. Plexiform neurofibroma is almost pathognomonic of neurofibromatosis type 1 (plexiform neurofibromas in the absence of neurofibromatosis type 1 are extremely rare) and is present in about 20% of cases. Some patients (5–15%) develop malignant peripheral nerve sheath tumor (MPNST), usually in adolescence or adulthood: most cases are the result of malignant transformation of a preexisting plexiform neurofibroma. People with neurofibromatosis type 1 also have an increased risk of developing brain (glioblastoma), breast, and hematological cancers. During childhood, benign lesions called Lisch nodules often appear in the iris, which do not affect vision. Some affected people develop optic nerve glioma (the most common central nervous system tumor in these patients), which may lead to vision alteration or loss. Skeletal abnormalities (e.g., bone dysplasia, scoliosis) and learning disabilities can also occur. Rarer manifestations include juvenile xanthogranuloma, pheochromocytoma, and gastrointestinal stromal tumor.

Inactivating mutations in the NF1 tumor suppressor gene[1] are the cause of neurofibromatosis type 1. The NF1 gene encodes protein called neurofibromin, which is produced in many cells (including oligodendrocytes and Schwann cells) and acts as an inhibitor of the RAS oncogene: in fact, neurofibromatosis type 1 is considered a RASopathy along with Noonan syndrome, cardiofaciocutaneous syndrome, and Costello syndrome. Neurofibromatosis type 1 has an autosomal dominant pattern of inheritance. In about 50% of cases, the germline mutation is inherited from an affected parent; the remaining cases result from new mutations in the NF1 gene and occur in people without a family history of the syndrome. Two copies of the NF1 gene must be altered to trigger tumor formation in neurofibromatosis type 1: the inactivation of the second allele occurs as a somatic mutation during patient's life (according to the classical "two-hit hypothesis"). Additional genetic alterations (e.g., TP53 inactivating mutations) are required for the formation of MPNST.

Diagnostic criteria of neurofibromatosis type 1 are met if two or more of the following are present: (1) ≥6 café-au-lait patches > 0.5 cm in prepubertal

---

[1] NF1: this gene encodes neurofibromin 1, a negative regulator of the RAS signal transduction pathway. Neurofibromin acts by accelerating the conversion of active GTP-bound RAS to its inactive GDP-bound form. The RAS signaling can be activated by receptor tyrosine kinases following the binding of growth factors, which results in increased AKT and/or MEK activity. In addition, RAS controls the generation of cyclic AMP (cAMP) through protein kinase C (PKC) following the activation of a G protein-coupled receptor (GPCR).

individuals or >1.5 cm in postpubertal individuals; (2) ≥2 neurofibromas of any type or 1 plexiform neurofibroma; (3) axillary or inguinal freckling; (4) ≥2 Lisch nodules; (5) optic glioma; (6) sphenoid dysplasia or thinning of the long bone cortex with or without pseudoarthrosis; and (7) first-degree relative diagnosed with neurofibromatosis type 1. In doubtful cases, genetic test for NF1 heterozygous pathogenetic mutations is recommended.

As regards the development of MPNST, the presence of a symptomatic or large neurofibroma, the diagnosis of plexiform neurofibroma, previous treatment with radiotherapy, and a personal or family history of MPNST are considered risk factors: however, serial screening with MRI or positron emission tomography (PET) is not recommended. MPNST should be suspected in rapidly growing neurofibromas that cause persistent or nocturnal pain, or a neurological deficit: in these cases, PET is the most sensitive and specific imaging technique to confirm the suspect, and then guided biopsy should be obtained to confirm the diagnosis.

Pathology

Neurofibroma is composed of loosely arranged differentiated Schwann cells, perineurial-like cells, fibroblasts, and mast cells in a variably myxoid background. In most cutaneous neurofibromas, nerves within the tumor are infrequent and small. In intraneural neurofibromas (solitary or plexiform), nerve fascicles are expanded by neoplastic cells dispersed in abundant myxoid matrix. Massive soft tissue neurofibromas may infiltrate skeletal muscle as well as fibroadipose tissue. Nuclear atypia (focal or diffuse) may be encountered; low-grade malignant peripheral nerve sheath tumor may be diagnosed if there is diffuse nuclear atypia, high cellularity, and low-level mitotic activity.

Several neurofibroma variants have been described: cellular neurofibroma (increased cellularity, with or without atypia, no significant increase in mitotic activity); pigmented neurofibroma (histologically and immunohistochemically shows melanin production); atypical neurofibroma (hypercellularity and atypical nuclei, but few mitoses and no necrosis); epithelioid neurofibroma (nests of epithelioid tumor cells); granular cell neurofibroma (granular cells, eosinophilic and similar in appearance to those of granular cell tumors); lipomatous neurofibroma (diffusely scattered adipocytes, intrinsic to the tumor); and dendritic cell neurofibroma (dendritic cell morphology with pseudorosettes). A variant called neurofibroma/schwannoma hybrid nerve sheath tumor has also been described, which is associated with larger nerves and occurs either sporadically or in the context of schwannomatosis or neurofibromatosis type 1 or 2 (→ see Chap. 128).

Differential diagnosis may be needed with the following: neurofibroma (→ see Table 187.1); malignant peripheral nerve sheath tumor (→ see Table 187.2); desmoplastic melanoma (it occurs in sun-damaged skin; atypical junctional melanocytic hyperplasia or dysplasia; "packeted" hyperchromatic cell pattern of growth, dense fibrosis, and deep nodular lymphoid aggregates; negative for melanocytic biomarkers HMB45, melan-A, tyrosinase; CD34 usually negative); neurothekeoma;

Table 187.1 Differential diagnosis between schwannoma and neurofibroma: clinicopathological features

	Schwannoma	Neurofibroma
Epidemiology	Age: 20–50 years Gender: M = F	Age: 20–40 years Gender: M = F
Etiology	Sporadic but may occur in NF2 > NF1	Sporadic, some in NF1
Pathology	Typically encapsulated; Antoni A and Antoni B areas (alternating hypercellular and hypocellular areas)	Usually no capsule; spindle cells, shredded carrot collagen, mast cells; hypocellular, myxoid areas without hypercellular areas
Plexiform variant	Less common	More common
Biomarkers	S100: strong and diffuseCalretinin: strongerCD34: scattered Factor XIIIa: negative/focal	S100: weaker Calretinin: focalCD34: strongerFactor XIIIa: stronger
Malignant potential	Malignant transformation: extremely rare	Malignant transformation occurs in 5–15% of patients with neurofibromatosis type 1

Table 187.2 Differential diagnosis between neurofibroma and malignant peripheral nerve sheath tumor (MPNST): histopathological features

	Neurofibroma	MPNST
Pathology	Smaller nuclear size, minimal hyperchromasia, wavy nuclei, abundant shredded carrot-type collagen, rare fascicular growth pattern, no necrosis, rare mitoses	Larger nuclear size, marked hyperchromasia, less evident wavy nuclei, rare shredded carrot-type collagen, obvious fascicular growth pattern,shows necrosis and conspicuous mitosis
S100	+++/++	++/+
Collagen type IV	+++/++	++/+
EMA	+	–
CD34	+++	++
Neurofilament	++	+++/+
Podoplanin	+	+
SOX10	+++	++/+
Hyaluronan	Lower levels	Higher levels

plexiform schwannoma; palisaded encapsulated neuroma (moderately cellular lesion with delicate EMA positivity at the periphery; neurotized nevus (S100 positive but usually positive for Melan-A and negative for factor XIIIa); nerve sheath myxoma (hypocellular with abundant mucopolysaccharides); perineurioma (rare, benign mesenchymal tumor comprised of perineurial cells; no definitive association with neurofibromatosis; positive for EMA, claudin-1 and GLUT1, negative for S100); dermatofibroma (benign proliferation of fibroblasts and histiocytes within the dermis; positive for factor XIIIa, CD163, and CD68, negative for CD34); dermatofibrosarcoma protuberans (positive for CD34 and COL1A1-PDGFB fusion gene, negative for S100 and factor XIIIa); superficial leiomyoma (benign dermal smooth muscle neoplasm; positive for SMA, MSA, and desmin); ganglioneuroma (benign tumor of neural crest origin, comprised of ganglion cells arising from nerves; most commonly found in the posterior mediastinum and retroperitoneum; Schwann cells are S100 positive, ganglion cells are synaptophysin positive); plexiform fibrohistiocytic tumor (infiltrative mesenchymal neoplasm, most commonly at the dermal-subcutaneous junction, comprised of fibroblasts and histiocytes; SMA positive, S100 negative).

Biomarkers

Neurofibroma always stains positive for S100 (although only 50% of cells are stained). Also SOX10 results are strongly expressed. Positivity for collagen IV is frequent. Perineurial-like cells are positive for EMA and GLUT1, whereas stromal cells are CD34 positive. Positivity for neurofilament proteins shows the presence of axons, especially in plexiform variants. The tumor is instead negative for cytokeratins, SMA, and desmin. Neurofibromas (including sporadic forms) are characterized (and caused) by a biallelic inactivation of the tumor suppressor gene NF1 (which is located on 17q11.2).

Prognosis

All types of neurofibroma are benign. Local recurrence is extremely rare after complete excision of the lesion. Overall, the risk of malignant transformation is exceedingly low. Localized cutaneous neurofibroma never undergoes transformation. In contrast, plexiform neurofibroma and solitary intraneural neurofibroma arising in sizeable nerves are considered potential precursor lesions of MPNST. The lifetime risk for MPNST in patients with neurofibromatosis type 1 is up to 15%. Patients with plexiform neurofibromas and those with multiple localized neurofibromas should be submitted to further neurofibromatosis testing.

Hypercellularity of otherwise unremarkable neurofibroma cells, atypical tumor cells with hyperchromatic nuclei, or mitotic activity (alone or together) do not necessarily indicate malignant change ("atypical neurofibroma").

Therapy

Asymptomatic lesions can be just followed up, as long as no MPNST (or other malignancies) is suspected. **Surgery** is the treatment of choice and is curative in most cases. Sometimes complete excision requires nerve sacrifice (with subsequent neurological deficit, which must be balanced against excision). Diffuse or plexiform neurofibromas may not be suitable for complete surgical excision due to their extension and/or type of growth (ill-defined): thus surgery may be followed by disease recurrence. Laser ablation can be used for superficial (dermal) neurofibromas. Since no specific therapy exists for neurofibromatosis type 1, the aim of management of these patients is the early detection of potential treatable complications.

Radiotherapy is contraindicated in patients with cancer predisposition syndrome neurofibromatosis type 1 due to the risk of malignant transformation.

Although pain management and the excision of surgically amenable neurofibromas are the mainstay of treatment for associated morbidity or tumor progression, several **targeted therapy** drugs have been tested either to avoid/postpone surgery or in the neoadjuvant setting (to downsize the tumor and ease surgical exeresis): farnesyltransferase inhibitors[2] (e.g., tipifarnib) and anti-fibrotic agents (e.g., pirfenidone) have failed to show clinical activity, and mTOR inhibitors (e.g., everolimus) have provided inconsistent results, while multikinase inhibitor imatinib,[3] cytokines (e.g., interferon-alpha), and anti-MEK inhibitors (e.g., selumetinib) have demonstrated some therapeutic effects. Of note, selumetinib has been found to be effective also against another manifestation of neurofibromatosis type 1 such as low-grade glioma.

Suggested Readings

Cimino et al (2018) Neurofibromatosis type 1. Handb Clin Neurol 148:799–811

Dombi et al (2017) Activity of selumetinib in neurofibromatosis type 1-related plexiform neurofibromas. N Engl J Med 375:2550–2560

Evans et al (2006) Malignant transformation and new primary tumours after therapeutic radiation for benign disease: substantial risks in certain tumour prone syndromes. J Med Genet 43(4):289–294

Fangusaro et al (2019) Selumetinib in paediatric patients with BRAF-aberrant or neurofibromatosis type 1-associated recurrent, refractory, or progressive low-grade glioma: a multicentre, phase 2 trial. Lancet Oncol 20(7):1011–1022

Fletcher et al (2020) WHO classification of tumours of soft tissue and bone, 5th edn

Gutmann et al (2017) Neurofibromatosis type 1. Nat Rev Dis Primers 3:17004

Jakacki et al (2017) Phase II trial of pegylated interferon alfa-2b in young patients with neurofibromatosis type 1 and unresectable plexiform neurofibromas. Neuro-Oncology 19(2):289–297

Lee et al (2020) Intramuscular peripheral nerve sheath tumors: schwannoma, ancient schwannoma, and neurofibroma. Skelet Radiol 49(6):967–975

Ly et al (2019) The diagnosis and management of neurofibromatosis type 1. Med Clin North Am 103(6):1035–1054

Passos et al (2020) Dramatic improvement of a massive plexiform neurofibroma after administration of selumetinib. Pediatr Neurol 105:69–70

Robertson et al (2012) Imatinib mesylate for plexiform neurofibromas in patients with neurofibromatosis type 1: a phase 2 trial. Lancet Oncol 13(12):1218–1224

Ronellenfitsch et al (2020) Targetable ERBB2 mutations identified in neurofibroma/schwannoma hybrid nerve sheath tumors. J Clin Invest 130(5):2488–2495

---

[2] Farnesyltransferase inhibitors: after translation, RAS undergoes multiple posttranslational modifications including farnesylation by the enzyme farnesyltransferase: the farnesyl group is necessary to attach RAS to the cell membrane, and without attachment to the cell membrane, RAS cannot mediate signal transduction from membrane receptors into the cell.

[3] Imatinib: tyrosine kinase inhibitor targeting the following: KIT, ABL, RET, PDGFR.

Schaefer et al (2015) Malignant peripheral nerve sheath tumor (MPNST) arising in diffuse-type neurofibroma: clinicopathologic characterization in a series of 9 cases. Am J Surg Pathol 39(9):1234–1241

Slopis et al (2018) Treatment of disfiguring cutaneous lesions in neurofibromatosis-1 with everolimus: a phase II, open-label, single-arm trial. Drugs R D 18(4):295–302

Widemann et al (2014a) Phase II trial of pirfenidone in children and young adults with neurofibromatosis type 1 and progressive plexiform neurofibromas. Pediatr Blood Cancer 61(9):1598–1602

Widemann et al (2014b) Phase 2 randomized, flexible crossover, double-blinded, placebo-controlled trial of the farnesyltransferase inhibitor tipifarnib in children and young adults with neurofibromatosis type 1 and progressive plexiform neurofibromas. Neuro-Oncology 16(5):707–718

Zehou et al (2019) Absence of efficacy of everolimus in neurofibromatosis 1-related plexiform neurofibromas: results from a phase 2a trial. J Invest Dermatol 139(3):718–720

Definition

Neuromas are benign tumors of the nervous system most frequently arising from nonneural nervous tissue. They are a family of lesions including true neoplasms (e.g., acoustic neuroma and solitary circumscribed neuroma → see dedicated sections), traumatic neuroma (described in this section), and neuroma within the frame of a genetic syndrome (also briefly described in this section).

Epidemiology and Presentation

Traumatic neuroma develops as a consequence of an injured nerve (the proximal nerve regenerates into a tangled mass of nerve fibers if it does not meet the distal end of the same nerve). Traumatic neuromas arise after blunt or sharp trauma or traction injury as well after elective surgery (with special regard to hand surgery and knee arthroplasty; especially susceptible are the superficial radial nerve and the saphenous nerve). A neuroma developing after amputation is called stump neuroma (the symptoms it produces should not be confused with phantom limb pain); after digital amputation, about 6% of patients develop a neuroma. The so-called Morton neuroma is an interdigital lesion of the foot (typically occurring in the third metatarsal interspace) often affecting in women due to poorly fitting shoes. Surgery-related neuromas can develop also in deep tissues (e.g., the bile duct, breast).

The key symptom is pain: its severity may lead to significant impairment of quality of life. On examination, a well-defined hard nodule is usually palpable; on pressure, the pain can be exacerbated (electric shock sensation).

Diagnosis is usually suspected clinically: the surgical specimen is then sent for pathology examination to confirm the diagnosis.

If there is no history of trauma, the lesion should be differentiated from syndromic neuroma and true neoplasms.

Etiology and Predisposition

Traumatic neuroma should not be confused with mucosal neuroma, typically presenting in the oral cavity (especially the tongue): this syndromic neuroma can be found as part of a syndrome known as multiple endocrine neoplasia type 2B (MEN2B). MEN2B patients are at risk of developing multiple mucosal neuromas, medullary thyroid carcinoma, and pheochromocytoma. MEN2B is a hereditary genetic condition due to the germline activating mutation of the RET oncogene and transmitted in an autosomal dominant fashion.

Pathology

Neuroma is an overgrowth of nerve fibers and Schwann cells. Myofibroblasts are frequently part of the scar tissue (as more collagen is laid down, their number diminishes). With time, fibrosis is found around and within the affected nerve.

Therapy

Prevention is essential: for instance, during elective surgery if a nerve is transected, the surgeon should reconnect the two nerve endings whenever feasible; if the two ends cannot be rejoined (e.g., amputation), the nerve can be buried onto a muscle to prevent neuroma formation (targeted muscle reinnervation).

For an already existing neuroma, there is no consensus on the optimal treatment. Medical therapy (oral painkillers; local anesthetic or dehydrated alcohol or steroid intralesional injections) is often unsuccessful. Surgery is often utilized when medical treatments fail, although recurrence rates are high (15–50%).

Suggested Readings

Alotaiby et al (2019) Demographic, clinical and histopathological features of oral neural neoplasms: a retrospective study. Head Neck Pathol 13(2):208–214

Crosio et al (2020) Prevention of symptomatic neuroma in traumatic digital amputation: a RAND/UCLA appropriateness method consensus study. Injury. https://doi.org/10.1016/j.injury.2020.03.018

Erian et al (2019) Post-traumatic neuroma of the breast in a 52-year-old female with a remote history of breast augmentation and explantation. Breast J 25(3):493–494

Lalchandani et al (2019) Traumatic bile duct neuroma presenting with acute cholangitis: a case report and review of literature. Ann Hepatobiliary Pancreat Surg 23(3):282–285

Oliveira et al (2018) Time course of traumatic neuroma development. PLoS One 13(7):e0200548

Scott et al (2019) Mucosal neuromas. N Engl J Med 381(3):e5

Vlot et al (2018) Symptomatic neuroma following initial amputation for traumatic digital amputation. J Hand Surg [Am] 43(1):86.e1–86.e8

Definition

Neurothekeoma is a benign of unknown histogenesis, although fibrohistiocytic derivation has been suggested (it was once believed to derive from the nerve sheath). The name derives from the appearance of tumor cells, which resemble Schwann cells on electron microscopy (spindle-shaped and surrounded by a basement membrane without myofilament or melanosomes).

Epidemiology and Presentation

Neurothekeoma is a rare soft tissue tumor of the skin. It usually occurs in young people (mean age, 15 years; range, 2–85 years), with a female prevalence. The lesion typically presents as a solitary, superficial, slow-growing, painless mass (up to 2 cm) located on the head, upper extremities, or shoulder girdle.

The clinical differential diagnoses for these lesions include Spitz nevi, keloid, juvenile xanthogranuloma, cutaneous lymphoid hyperplasia, and lymphomatoid papulosis.

Pathology

Neurothekeoma is a cutaneous tumor (involves the dermis or subcutis) with different histologic patterns including myxoid, cellular, or mixed-type based mainly on the amount of myxoid matrix. It presents as a multinodular lesion with myxoid matrix and peripheral fibrosis; spindled and epithelioid mononuclear cells with abundant cytoplasm are arranged in whorled or fascicular patterns; occasional multinucleated giant cells may be present. Variable nuclear atypia and mitoses (median: 4/25 HPF) are present: accurate diagnosis of these lesions is crucial, as they can be mistaken for malignancy (leading to unnecessary treatment).

© The Editor(s) (if applicable) and The Author(s), under exclusive license to
Springer Nature Switzerland AG 2021
S. Mocellin, *Soft Tissue Tumors*, https://doi.org/10.1007/978-3-030-58710-9_189

Differential diagnosis should be made with nerve sheath myxoma (it stains positive for S100), granular cell tumor, neurofibroma, schwannoma, benign fibrous histiocytoma, and melanocytic lesions (e.g., Spitz nevus and melanoma).

Biomarkers

Neurothekeoma usually stains positive for vimentin, NKI-C3, CD10, and MITF, whereas it stains negative for S100 (regardless of the histologic pattern), GFAP, and Melan-A.

Prognosis

Neurothekeoma is a benign tumor. Cellular neurothekeoma can be locally invasive with perineural and vascular invasion and occasional local recurrence.

Therapy

Surgical excision is the treatment of choice.

Suggested Readings

Cavicchini et al (2018) Neurothekeoma, a hard to diagnose neoplasm among red nodules. Australas J Dermatol 59(4):e280–e282

Fox et al (2012) Expression of MiTF may be helpful in differentiating cellular neurothekeoma from plexiform fibrohistiocytic tumor (histiocytoid predominant) in a partial biopsy specimen. Am J Dermatopathol 34(2):157–160

Murphrey et al (2020) Pediatric cellular neurothekeoma: seven cases and systematic review of the literature. Pediatr Dermatol 37(2):320–325

Tran et al (2018) Atypical cellular neurothekeoma: a potential diagnostic pitfall for benign and malignant spindle cell lesions in skin. J Cutan Pathol 45(8):619–622

Definition

The nevus lipomatosus superficialis (NLS) is a benign mesenchymal tumor of the skin. It is unclear if NLS should be considered a hamartoma rather than a tumor. NLS is also known as dermolipoma and nevus lipomatosus cutaneous superficialis.

Epidemiology and Presentation

This is an uncommon cutaneous lesion presenting as a solitary (more common) or multiple lesion.

Multiple NLS presents as groups of multiple, soft, non-tender, pedunculated or sessile, skin-colored or yellow papules, nodules, or plaques that commonly develop at birth or within the first two decades of life; these lesions are slowly growing, have a smooth or cerebriform surface, and may grow larger if untreated; the distribution is usually linear or along the skinfolds, with a preference for the pelvic girdle, most commonly the buttock, sacrococcygeal region, and upper portion of the posterior thigh.

Solitary NLS is less common and typically occurs later as compared to the multiple type (between the third and the sixth decade of life); the lesion generally presents as a soft, dome-shaped or sessile, skin-colored papule or nodule mimicking a skin tag; there is no site predilection for this type.

S. Mocellin, *Soft Tissue Tumors*, https://doi.org/10.1007/978-3-030-58710-9_190

Pathology

NLS presents with mature ectopic adipocytes that proliferate in the reticular dermis with possible extension to the papillary dermis and intermingled with collagen bundles. No encapsulation or connection with subcutaneous fat is present. No distinct epidermal changes are observed.

Differential diagnosis may be needed with the following: fibroepithelial polyp, neurofibroma, and nevus sebaceous.

Biomarkers

None is specific.

Prognosis

NLS is a benign lesion.

Therapy

Surgical and laser excision (mainly for cosmetic reasons) are the treatments of choice.

Suggested Readings

Ancer-Arellano et al (2019) Electrodissection for nevus lipomatosus cutaneous superficialis removal. J Am Acad Dermatol 81(5):e127–e128
Kim et al (2014) Nevus lipomatosus superficialis. Dermatol Online J 20(12) pii: 13030/qt2cb3c5t3
Lima et al (2017) Nevus lipomatosus cutaneous superficialis. An Bras Dermatol 92(5):711–713
Sardana et al (2017) Treatment of Nevus lipomatosus cutaneous superficialis with CO_2 laser. J Cosmet Dermatol 16(3):333–335

Definition

Nodular fasciitis is a benign fibrous tumor classified among the fibroblastic/myofibroblstic tumors. It is also known as pseudosarcomatous fasciitis.

Epidemiology and Presentation

It is relatively common and can occur at any age but more often in young adults. It generally develops in the subcutaneous tissue; intravascular fasciitis and cranial fasciitis are rare (cranial fasciitis develops predominantly in infants aged less than 2 years).

Nodular fasciitis typically develops from the surface of fascia and extends into the subcutis, although occasional cases are intramuscular. Although any part of the body can be involved, the upper extremity, trunk, and head and neck are most frequently affected.

Intravascular fasciitis is usually subcutaneous and occurs in small- to medium-sized vessels, predominantly the veins. Cranial fasciitis typically involves the outer table of the skull and contiguous soft tissue of the scalp.

Nodular fasciitis typically grows rapidly and has a preoperative duration in most cases of not more than 2–3 months. Soreness or tenderness may be present. It usually measures 2 cm or less and almost always <5 cm. When the skull is involved, X-ray imaging may demonstrate a lytic defect frequently with a sclerotic rim.

Pathology

Nodular fasciitis appears as a reactive appearing proliferation of fibroblasts and myofibroblasts in myxoid stroma with granulation tissue-like vascular proliferation. It is composed of plump but uniform spindle-shaped fibroblasts (or myofibroblasts) lacking nuclear hyperchromasia and pleomorphism and displaying a loose or tissue culture-like growth pattern. Mitotic figures may be numerous, but not atypical. Osteoclast-like giant cells are frequently present. The lesion border is typically (at least focally) infiltrative, although it may be well delineated; peripheral extension is often seen between fat cells in the subcutis and between muscle cells in intramuscular locations.

Because of its rapid growth, cellularity, prominent mitotic activity, and locally infiltrative growth pattern, nodular fasciitis can be misdiagnosed as a sarcoma (it is a typical example of so-called pseudosarcoma).

Differential diagnosis may be needed with the following: benign fibrous histiocytoma (based in the dermis, storiform pattern, often Touton giant cells); fibromatosis (usually large tumor that infiltrates surrounding soft tissue, spindled cells are parallel and separated by abundant collagen and arranged in broad sweeping fascicles, no loose tissue culture appearance); inflammatory myofibroblastic tumor (larger tumor size, mixed inflammatory infiltrate, 50% ALK expression; no rapid growth); myositis ossificans (centered in the muscle, calcifications); myxofibrosarcoma (large, regularly arborizing vessels, atypia and pleomorphism); and other sarcomas (nuclear atypia is prominent, it may have necrosis, larger size usually).

Biomarkers

Nodular fasciitis stains usually strongly and diffusely positive for SMA[1] and MSA,[2] while desmin is generally negative. CD68 staining is present in the osteoclast-like giant cells. Staining for keratin and S100 protein is typically negative.

Immunohistochemical expression of HMGA2 is present in about 90% of cases and is considered a useful biomarker.

The identification of the MYH9-USP6 fusion gene[3] (resulting from the **chromosomal translocation** t(17;22)(p13;q12) as a frequent event in nodular fasciitis) has definitely established its previously disputed clonal neoplastic nature. Also myositis ossificans and aneurysmal bone cyst of soft tissue often carry this chromosomal rearrangement, providing evidence that these three entities are genetically related.

Prognosis

This is a benign tumor. Recurrence after excision is rare, but it is occasionally observed after incomplete excision.

---

[1] SMA: smooth muscle actin.

[2] MSA: muscle-specific actin.

[3] MYH9-USP6 fusion gene: MYH9 (myosin heavy chain 9) encodes a non-muscle myosin which is involved in cytokinesis, cell motility, and maintenance of cell shape. USP6 (ubiquitin-specific peptidase 6) encodes a deubiquitinase with an ATP-independent isopeptidase activity, cleaving at the C-terminus of the ubiquitin moiety.

Therapy

Surgical excision is the treatment of choice (if needed for diagnostic purposes or desired by the patient).

Suggested Readings

Bekers et al (2018) Myositis ossificans—another condition with USP6 rearrangement, providing evidence of a relationship with nodular fasciitis and aneurysmal bone cyst. Ann Diagn Pathol 34:56–59

Dreux et al (2010) Value and limitation of immunohistochemical expression of HMGA2 in mesenchymal tumors: about a series of 1052 cases. Mod Pathol 23(12):1657–1666

Fletcher et al (2020) WHO classification of tumours of soft tissue and bone, 5th edn

Jebastin et al (2018) Pseudosarcomatous myofibroblastic proliferations of the genitourinary tract are genetically different from nodular fasciitis and lack USP6, ROS1 and ETV6 gene rearrangements. Histopathology 73(2):321–326

Lenz et al (2020) Novel EIF5A-USP6 gene fusion in nodular fasciitis associated with unusual pathologic features: a report of a case and review of the literature. Am J Dermatopathol 42(7):539–543

Maloney et al (2019) Superficial nodular fasciitis with atypical presentations: report of 3 cases and review of recent molecular genetics. Am J Dermatopathol 41(12):931–936

Naso et al (2019) Benign spindle cell lesions of the breast: a diagnostic approach to solitary fibrous tumour, nodular pseudoangiomatous stromal hyperplasia and nodular fasciitis. J Clin Pathol 72(6):438–442

Oliveira et al (2014) USP6-induced neoplasms: the biologic spectrum of aneurysmal bone cyst and nodular fasciitis. Hum Pathol 45(1):1–11

Definition

Nuchal-type fibroma (NTF) is a benign lesion classified among the fibroblastic-myofibroblastic tumors.

It is also known as nuchal fibroma and collagenosis nuchae.

Epidemiology and Presentation

NTF is a rare tumorlike lesion which presents as a hard consistency nodule (mean diameter: 3 cm) and occurs more frequently in men, with a peak incidence between the third and the fifth decade of life. It characteristically involves the posterior neck (hence the name), but can also develop elsewhere (the upper back, face, extremities).

Etiology and Predisposition

Nuchal-type fibroma has been associated with Gardner syndrome ($\rightarrow$ see Chap. 105) and (chronic) trauma.

There is a clear association with diabetes mellitus; interestingly, diabetic scleredema (another tumorlike change in soft tissues found in patients with diabetes mellitus) has a histological appearance identical to NTF.

Pathology

NTF is an unencapsulated, ill-circumscribed, hypocellular lesion composed of thick, haphazardly arranged collagen fibers. It shows an expansion of collagenized dermis with entrapment of adnexa and adipocytes and extension into the underlying skeletal muscle.

© The Editor(s) (if applicable) and The Author(s), under exclusive license to
Springer Nature Switzerland AG 2021
S. Mocellin, *Soft Tissue Tumors*, https://doi.org/10.1007/978-3-030-58710-9_192

Differential diagnosis may be needed with the following: elastofibroma (prominent abnormal elastic fibers, subscapular location); fibrolipoma (circumscribed, different location); fibromatosis (deep soft tissue, not back of neck, more cellular with broad fascicles of fibroblasts); Gardner fibroma (same histologic features but extra-nuchal location); and solitary fibrous tumor (patternless pattern, more cellular, staghorn-type vessels).

Biomarkers

Cells stain positive for CD34, CD99, and vimentin and negative for actins and desmin. S100 may be positive when nerves are entrapped.

Prognosis

Despite its benign nature, NTF often locally recurs.

Therapy

Surgical excision is the treatment of choice.

Suggested Readings

Fletcher et al (2020) WHO classification of tumours of soft tissue and bone, 5th edn
Gong et al (2016) Nuchal-type fibroma of the shoulder: a case report and review of the literature. Oncol Lett 11(6):4152–4154
Linos et al (2011) Extra nuchal-type fibroma associated with elastosis, traumatic neuroma, a rare APC gene missense mutation, and a very rare MUTYH gene polymorphism: a case report and review of the literature. J Cutan Pathol 38(11):911–918
Zamecnik et al (2001) Nuchal-type fibroma is positive for CD34 and CD99. Am J Surg Pathol 25(7):970

Definition

Ossifying fibromyxoid tumor (OFT) is a soft tissue neoplasm on uncertain differentiation and intermediate malignant potential.

Epidemiology and Presentation

This very rare tumor develops as a slow-growing painless nodule (typically 3–5 cm in diameter) in the subcutis of adults (mean age: 50 years). OFT mainly arises in the lower limbs (approximately 50% of cases).

Pathology

This mesenchymal tumor is composed of cords and trabeculae of ovoid cells embedded in a fibromyxoid matrix, usually surrounded by a peripheral partial shell of lamellar bone (hence, the typical radiologically finding of a well-circumscribed nodule surrounded by an incomplete ring of calcification).

The neoplastic cells are monomorphous with round to ovoid nuclei and a scant amount of pale eosinophilic cytoplasm. Mitotic activity is usually less than 1 per 10 HPF,[1] but cases with a higher mitotic count have been reported.

Biomarkers

OFT typically stains positive for S100 in most cases (>90%), and for desmin in half cases.

---

[1] HPF: high-power field.

The genetic hallmark of OFT is the **chromosomal translocation** leading to rearrangements of the PHF1 gene,[2] which are found in up to 80% of cases. The most common PHF1 fusion partner is EP400 (about 50% of cases) within the frame of the chromosomal translocation t(6;12)(p21;q24.3); other fusion partners are MEAF6 and EPC1. Recently described fusion partner TFE3 appears to confer malignant potential.

Prognosis

OFT is known for the ability to recur (up to 20% of cases), even after many years. Higher mitotic activity has been associated with the likelihood to relapse. Distant metastasis has been very rarely described.

Therapy

Surgical excision is the treatment of choice.

Suggested Readings

Bakiratharajan, Rekhi (2016) Ossifying fibromyxoid tumor: an update. Arch Pathol Lab Med 140(4):371–375
Buehler, Weisman (2017) Soft tissue tumors of uncertain histogenesis: a review for dermatopathologists. Clin Lab Med 37(3):647–671
Carter, Patel (2019) Ossifying fibromyxoid tumor: a review with emphasis on recent molecular advances and differential diagnosis. Arch Pathol Lab Med 143(12):1504–1512
Fletcher et al (2020) WHO classification of tumours of soft tissue and bone, 5th edn
Kumari et al (2020) Ossifying fibromyxoid tumor: fine-needle aspiration cytology findings of a rare soft tissue neoplasm. Diagn Cytopathol 48(4):396–400
Suurmeijer et al (2019) Novel recurrent PHF1-TFE3 fusions in ossifying fibromyxoid tumors. Genes Chromosom Cancer 58(9):643–649

---

[2] PHF1: PHD finger protein 1 encodes a polycomb group protein that acts as a component of a histone H3 lysine-27 (H3K27)-specific methyltransferase complex and functions in transcriptional repression of homeotic genes.

Definition

Ovarian fibroma is a benign neoplasm classified among the pure stromal tumors (along with sclerosing stromal tumor, thecoma, Leydig cell tumor, and steroid cell tumor), which in turn belong to the family of sex cord-stromal tumors (which include pure sex cord tumors and mixed sex cord-stromal tumors).

Epidemiology and Presentation

Ovarian fibroma accounts for 4% of all ovarian neoplasms, but it is the most common among the sex cord-stromal ovarian tumors (which account for 7% of all ovarian tumors). This tumor can occur at all ages but is most frequently observed in middle-aged women.

Unlike most other sex cord-stromal tumors (e.g., granulosa cell tumor and techoma which produce estrogens), ovarian fibroma is hormonally inactive. It can reach several centimeters in diameter before the diagnosis, when it becomes symptomatic due to space occupation; the clinical presentation can be acute only in case of ovarian torsion.

Meigs syndrome is defined as the triad of a benign ovarian tumor with ascites and pleural effusion (which resolve after resection of the tumor): ovarian fibroma is the most frequent neoplasm observed in this syndrome. Obviously, to make diagnosis of Meigs syndrome, ovarian carcinoma (which is often associated with ascites and possibly pleural effusion) must be ruled out.

© The Editor(s) (if applicable) and The Author(s), under exclusive license to
Springer Nature Switzerland AG 2021
S. Mocellin, *Soft Tissue Tumors*, https://doi.org/10.1007/978-3-030-58710-9_194

Etiology and Predisposition

Gorlin syndrome, also known as **nevoid basal cell carcinoma syndrome** (NBCCS), is a rare multisystem disease inherited with an autosomal dominant pattern. Its prevalence is estimated to be 1/50,000–1/250,000 people.

It is characterized by multiple basal cell carcinomas, multiple odontogenic keratocysts, skeletal abnormalities, and ovarian fibroma (often bilateral), among other disorders. It generally appears in the adolescence, without difference in prevalence between males and females.

Germline mutations of the PTCH1 tumor suppressor gene (located on chromosome 9 and encoding the receptor of the sonic hedgehog ligand) are believed to be responsible for the majority of NBCCS cases.

Pathology

The neoplasm is composed of thin spindle cells in a whorled arrangement with a variable amount of extracellular collagen. Cytologic atypia is rare and mitoses can be up to 3 per 10 HPF.

In 10% of cases, the tumor is hypercellular (containing little intercellular collagen) and is known as cellular fibroma. Cellular fibroma can mimic a granulosa cell tumor (which is often hormonally active and stains negative for reticulin).

When an otherwise typical cellular fibroma shows more than 4 mitoses per 10 HPF, the tumor is named mitotically active cellular fibroma (MACF), which should be distinguished from fibrosarcoma (exceptionally rare in the ovary, usually characterized by marked cellular atypia).

Another differential diagnosis might be needed with endometrial stromal sarcoma (CD10 positive, shows JAZF1-SUZ12 fusion gene but only present in 75% of endometrial stromal nodules and 50% of low-grade endometrial stromal sarcomas, so a negative result may be inconclusive).

Biomarkers

Ovarian fibroma stains positive for reticulin, WT1, SF1, and FOXL2; it stains negative for CD10.

Trisomy 12 is a common cytogenetic abnormality associated with ovarian fibroma.

Prognosis

This is a benign tumor. However, both cellular fibroma and MACF should be followed up due to the reported possibility of local recurrence.

Therapy

Surgical excision is the treatment of choice.

Suggested Readings

Aram, Moghaddam (2009) Bilateral ovarian fibroma associated with Gorlin syndrome. J Res Med Sci 14(1):57–61

Hanley et al (2019) Practical review of ovarian sex cord-stromal tumors. Surg Pathol Clin 12(2):587–620

Irving et al (2006) Cellular fibromas of the ovary: a study of 75 cases including 40 mitotically active tumors emphasizing their distinction from fibrosarcoma. Am J Surg Pathol 30(8):929–938

Macciò et al (2014) Large twisted ovarian fibroma associated with Meigs' syndrome, abdominal pain and severe anemia treated by laparoscopic surgery. BMC Surg 14:38

Shen et al (2018) Ovarian fibroma/fibrothecoma with elevated serum CA125 level: a cohort of 66 cases. Medicine (Baltimore) 97(34):e11926

Sofoudis et al (2016) Enormous ovarian fibroma with elevated Ca-125 associated with Meigs' syndrome. Presentation of a rare case. Eur J Gynaecol Oncol 37(1):142–143

Definition

Ovarian sclerosing stromal tumor (OSST) is a benign neoplasm classified among the pure stromal tumors (along with ovarian fibroma, thecoma, Leydig cell tumor, and steroid cell tumor), which in turn belong to the family of sex cord-stromal tumors (which include pure sex cord tumors and mixed sex cord-stromal tumors).

Epidemiology and Presentation

OSST accounts for less than 5% of ovarian sex cord-stromal tumors. Unlike ovarian fibroma, thecoma, and adult granulosa cell tumor, OSST is more likely to occur in young women (approximately 80% of cases are under 30 years of age).

Typically, OSST presents as an unilateral mass which can be asymptomatic or cause pelvic pain and menstrual irregularities. OSST is hormonally inactive, although some hormonally active cases (producing androgens and/or estrogens) have been reported. OSST is rarely associated with the Meigs syndrome (the triad of a benign ovarian tumor with ascites and pleural effusion which resolve after resection of the tumor). Serum levels of tumor marker CA-125 are usually (but not always) within normal limits.

Clinically, OSST must be differentiated from other ovarian masses (both benign and malignant): in this regard, radiological imaging is generally insufficient, and the diagnosis is made upon pathological evaluation of the surgical specimen.

Pathology

OSST is characterized by a pseudolobular appearance resulting from alternating cellular and hypocellular areas: pseudolobules contain a haphazard arrangement of epithelioid (lutein) and spindled cells. Hemangiopericytoma-like vessels are

© The Editor(s) (if applicable) and The Author(s), under exclusive license to
Springer Nature Switzerland AG 2021
S. Mocellin, *Soft Tissue Tumors*, https://doi.org/10.1007/978-3-030-58710-9_195

prominent in both components. Hypocellular areas can be edematous, collagenous, or myxoid. Cytologic atypia is minimal or absent; mitoses are infrequent (rarely higher than 10 per 10 HPF), without atypical forms.

Differential diagnosis may be needed with the following: thecoma (typically postmenopausal; estrogenic manifestations in 50% of cases; no staghorn vessels); steroid cell tumor (hormonal manifestations in 50% of cases; no staghorn vessels); ovarian fibroma (peri- or postmenopausal tumor; no staghorn vessels; no pseudol-obules); metastatic signet ring cell carcinoma (also known as Krukenberg tumor; bilateral in >50% of cases, often with extraovarian disease at presentation; no stag-horn vessels; presence of glands, nests, or cords of malignant cells; cytokeratin positive); and solitary fibrous tumor (patternless architecture; no epithelioid cells; STAT6 positive, inhibin negative).

Biomarkers

OSST stains positive for sex cord biomarkers such as inhibin, calretinin, SF1, and FOXL2. Moreover, this tumor expresses estrogen receptor, progesterone receptor, CD10, vimentin, and SMA.[1] It stains negative for cytokeratins and EMA.[2]

Recently, **chromosomal translocations** leading to GLI2[3] based fusion genes (most frequent fusion partner: FHL2) have been reported to be present in about 80% of cases (none of these gene rearrangements have been detected in other types of sex cord-stromal tumors or other common cancer types).

Prognosis

OSST is a benign tumor.

Therapy

Surgery is the treatment of choice.

---

[1] SMA: smooth muscle actin.

[2] EMA: epithelial membrane antigen.

[3] GLI2: GLI family zinc finger 2 encodes a protein belonging to the C2H2-type zinc finger protein subclass of the Gli family, which includes transcription factors that bind DNA through zinc finger motifs. Gli family zinc finger proteins are mediators of Sonic hedgehog (Shh) signaling and act as potent oncogenes in the embryonal carcinoma cell. GLI2 protein localizes to the cytoplasm and activates patched *Drosophila* homolog (PTCH) gene expression.

Suggested Readings

Kim et al (2020) Identification of recurrent FHL2-GLI2 oncogenic fusion in sclerosing stromal tumors of the ovary. Nat Commun 11(1):44

Park et al (2017) Clinicopathological characteristics of ovarian sclerosing stromal tumor with an emphasis on TFE3 overexpression. Anticancer Res 37(10):5441–5447

Young et al (2018) Ovarian sex cord-stromal tumours and their mimics. Pathology 50(1):5–15

Zhao et al (2018) The value of MRI for differentiating benign from malignant sex cord-stromal tumors of the ovary: emphasis on diffusion-weighted MR imaging. J Ovarian Res 11(1):73

Definition

Palmar/plantar fibromatosis is a neoplasm with intermediate biological behavior classified among the fibroblastic-myofibroblastic tumors. Palmar fibromatosis is also known as Dupuytren disease; plantar fibromatosis is also known as Ledderhose disease.

They belong to the family of superficial fibromatosis, which include also penile fibromatosis (also known as Peyronie disease and induratio penis plastica), knuckle pads (also known as Garrod's pads), pachydermodactyly, and infantile digital fibromatosis (also known as Reye's tumor, multiple hyaline fibromatosis).

For deep fibromatosis → see Chap. 69.

Epidemiology and Presentation

Palmar/plantar fibromatosis develops most frequently in adults (although plantar fibromatosis can be found in children as well), with a male predominance. Some 10–20% of cases present with both palmar and plantar localizations.

Palmar fibromatosis is the most frequent type of superficial fibromatosis affecting 1–2% of the general population (it is rare in Asian and African populations but frequent in the Northern European countries); patients are typically over 65 years of age (the disease is rarely observed in children), with males being affected three to four times more often than females; the lesion occurs on the volar surface of the hand and is bilateral in 50% of cases; the disease presents as an isolated firm asymptomatic ill-defined small palmar nodule, but ultimately cord-like lesions and multiple nodules occur, which leads to puckering of the overlying skin and flexion contractures, especially in the fourth and fifth digit. Ultimately, the disease can lead to debilitating functional impairment.

Plantar fibromatosis occurs less frequently than the palmar counterpart, with an annual incidence of 0.23%; although the lesion can occur in children, incidence increases with age; men are affected twice as often as females, and lesions are bilateral in 20–50% of cases; the disease presents as a firm subcutaneous ill-defined small nodule or thickening (70–80% of cases arise in the medial aspect of the plantar arch) which adheres to the skin and is generally asymptomatic (although some patients complain of aching pain after walking or standing for long periods of time) and rarely results in contraction of the toes; palmar fibromatosis is present in 10–65% of patients with plantar fibromatosis. Although the lesion is usually painless, patients may experience pain when the nodule rubs on the shoe. Ultimately, the disease can lead to debilitating functional impairment.

Both ultrasonography and magnetic resonance imaging can be useful to support the diagnosis of palmar/plantar fibromatosis.

Etiology and Predisposition

Both genetic (many patients have a family history of this disease) and environmental factors (e.g., trauma) contribute to the pathogenesis. An association with diabetes mellitus and alcoholism has been reported.

Pathology

The lesion, which is intimately associated with aponeurosis (fascia) and subcutaneous fat, is composed of a fibroblastic proliferation featuring an infiltrative growth. Cells are homogeneous, without atypia and with infrequent mitotic figures. Older lesions are significantly less cellular and often more densely collagenized.

Differential diagnosis may be needed with the following: fibrosarcoma (single large mass of deep soft tissue with intersecting bundles of cells with atypia); epithelioid sarcoma (common in hands, but some cells have distinctive epithelioid appearance with abundant bright eosinophilic cytoplasm, necrosis, cytokeratin positive, CD34 positive); desmoid tumors (rare in hand, dominant mass infiltrates skeletal muscle; CTNNB1 gene mutations); calcifying aponeurotic fibroma (plump or epithelioid fibroblasts palisading around cartilage and spotty calcification); and monophasic synovial sarcoma (uniformly hypercellular, often staghorn vascular pattern; typical fusion genes).

Biomarkers

The cells stain variably positive for vimentin, SMA,[1] and MSA.[2] At least 50% may stain positive for nuclear beta-catenin (without mutation in the CTNNB1 gene). The cells stain negative for CD34 and cytokeratin.

---

[1] SMA: smooth muscle actin.

[2] MSA: muscle-specific actin.

Prognosis

Palmar/plantar fibromatosis is characterized by a risk of local recurrence, but it never metastasizes. Disease recurrence relates to the extent of surgical excision (dermofasciectomy followed by skin grafting is associated with the lowest rate of local recurrence).

Therapy

For palmar fibromatosis, wide surgical excision is the most effective treatment.

The treatment of plantar fibromatosis is often conservative and consists of footwear modifications in order to relieve symptoms, whereas surgical resection is reserved for large lesions causing significant disability and refractory to other approaches.

In both diseases, surgical treatment consisting of simple excision results in high rates of local recurrence.

Radiotherapy has been proposed as an effective therapy to stabilize or improve symptoms.

Suggested Readings

Fetsch et al (2005) Palmar-plantar fibromatosis in children and preadolescents: a clinicopathologic study of 56 cases with newly recognized demographics and extended follow-up information. Am J Surg Pathol 29(8):1095–1105

Fletcher et al (2020) WHO classification of tumours of soft tissue and bone, 5th edn

Fuiano et al (2019) Current concepts about treatment options of plantar fibromatosis: a systematic review of the literature. Foot Ankle Surg 25(5):559–564

Kelenjian et al (2019) Clinical features and management of superficial fibromatoses. J Dtsch Dermatol Ges 17(4):393–397

Morris et al (2019) Ultrasound features of palmar fibromatosis or dupuytren contracture. J Ultrasound Med 38(2):387–392

Okano et al (2020) Bilateral plantar fibromatosis complicated by Dupuytren's contracture. J Surg Case Rep 2020(2):rjz402

Schuster et al (2015) Patient-reported outcomes after electron radiation treatment for early-stage palmar and plantar fibromatosis. Pract Radiat Oncol 5(6):e651–e658

Definition

Papillary intralymphatic angioendothelioma (PILA) is a lymphatic vascular tumor of intermediate aggressiveness.

It is also known as Dabska tumor, malignant endothelial papillary angioendothelioma, and hobnail hemangioendothelioma; the last synonym is shared with that of retiform hemangioendothelioma, and the two entities are considered to be related.

Epidemiology and Presentation

PILA is a very rare neoplasm occurring more commonly in infants and children (75% of cases), without gender predilection. Most cases involve the skin of the extremities, but cases arising in other parts of the skin and in deeply located body regions (including viscera and bones) have been described.

PILA presents as a slow-growing painless skin plaque (which can reach several centimeters in diameter) with unremarkable overlying skin.

Pathology

PILA is composed of the proliferation of lymphatic channels with intraluminal proliferations of columnar/hobnail endothelial cells. Necrosis, cytological atypia, and mitotic activity are typically absent.

Biomarkers

Tumor cells are positive for both endothelial (CD31 and CD34) and lymphatic biomarkers (podoplanin and VEGFR3).

Prognosis

PILA is a rarely metastasizing neoplasm, lymph nodes being the most frequent metastatic site.

Therapy

Surgical wide excision is the treatment of choice.

Suggested Readings

Fanburg-Smith et al (1999) Papillary intralymphatic angioendothelioma (PILA): a report of twelve cases of a distinctive vascular tumor with phenotypic features of lymphatic vessels. Am J Surg Pathol 23(9):1004–1010

Fletcher et al (2020) WHO classification of tumours of soft tissue and bone, 5th edn

Gambarotti et al (2018) Intraosseous papillary intralymphatic angioendothelioma (PILA): one new case and review of the literature. Clin Sarcoma Res 8:1

Silva et al (2020) Papillary intralymphatic angioendothelioma: dabska tumor. An Bras Dermatol 95(2):214–216

Definition

The term perivascular epithelioid cell tumor (PEComa) encompasses a family of mesenchymal tumors of variable malignant potential and characterized by perivascular epithelioid cell (PEC) differentiation. The PEComa family is also known as myomelanocytoma family.

No normal counterpart for PEC is known, and thus PEComa is currently classified among soft tissue tumors of uncertain differentiation.

The PEComa family includes the following nosological entities:

1. Angiomyolipoma (mainly of the kidney) (AML → see dedicated section).
2. Clear cell sugar tumor (mainly of the lung) (CCST → see dedicated section).
3. Lymphangioleiomyomatosis (mainly of the lung) (LAM → see dedicated section).
4. PEComa NOS (not otherwise specified): a group of neoplasms arising from a variety of soft tissue and visceral sites (covered in this section); this subset has been previously named also: clear cell sugar tumor, primary extrapulmonary sugar tumor, abdominopelvic sarcoma of perivascular epithelioid cells, and clear cell myomelanocytic tumor.

Epidemiology and Presentation

PEComa NOS is very rare. It is much more frequently observed in females (F:M = 6:1), with a wide age range and an incidence peak in young to middle-aged adults.

PEComa NOS can arise from a variety of anatomical sites, but most frequently arises in the retroperitoneum, abdominopelvic region, uterus, and gastrointestinal tract.

Etiology and Predisposition

While AML and LAM are known to be associated with the tuberous sclerosis complex (TSC), the relationship between this syndrome and PEComa NOS is less clear.

TSC is a neurocutaneous autosomal dominant genetic disease with an estimated prevalence of 1/15,000 and is due to due to inactivating mutations of tumor suppressor genes TSC1 (9q34) and TSC2 (16p13.3), which encode proteins that inhibit the mTOR pathway. One copy of the mutated gene is sufficient to increase the risk of developing this cancer predisposition syndrome; in approximately one third of cases, an affected person inherits the mutated gene from a parent who has the disorder. The remaining two thirds of patients with TSC are born with new mutations in the TSC1 or TSC2 gene: these cases are described as sporadic and occur in people with no history of TSC in their family. TSC1 mutations appear to be more common in familial cases of TSC, whereas TSC2 mutations are more frequent in sporadic cases.

Clinically, TSC is characterized by hamartomas, most commonly affecting the skin, brain, kidney, lung, and heart. Skin involvement includes the following: hypomelanotic macules (ash leaf), angiofibromas ($\rightarrow$ see dedicated section), ungual fibromas, cephalic and lumbar (shagreen patch) fibrous plaques, and "confetti" skin lesions. The brain is almost always involved with different neuropathological lesions (e.g., cortico-/subcortical tubers and subependymal giant cell astrocytoma—SEGA—which can cause hydrocephalus). Early-onset epilepsy is present in 85% of patients. Renal AML develops during childhood and grows during adolescence and adulthood manifesting with pain, hematuria, retroperitoneal hemorrhage, abdominal masse, hypertension, and renal failure. LAM, multifocal micronodular pneumocyte hyperplasia (MMPH), and pulmonary cysts develop during adulthood and manifest with dyspnea, pneumothorax, or chylothorax. TSC patients are at higher risk also of cardiac rhabdomyoma, which appears during the fetal period and may become symptomatic during infancy and childhood (outflow tract obstruction or valvular dysfunction).

Pathology

PEComas typically show a nested architecture and are usually composed of clear to granular eosinophilic epithelioid cells that express melanocytic and smooth muscle markers and show a focal association with blood vessel walls (the nests are typically surrounded by thin-walled capillary vessels).

Malignant PEComas are characterized by mitotic activity, necrosis, marked nuclear atypia, and pleomorphism.

About 15% of PEComas are composed of cords of cells in a densely collagenous stroma (sclerosing PEComas). The epithelioid shape is sometimes replaced by a spindle shape, which can call for differential diagnosis with other spindle cell neoplasms.

Differential diagnosis may be needed with the following: melanoma (S100 positive); adrenal carcinoma (inhibin positive); leiomyosarcoma (negative for melanoma markers); clear cell renal carcinoma (cytokeratin positive); GIST (CD117/c-Kit positive); TFE3-positive renal cell carcinoma (PAX8 positive); alveolar soft part sarcoma (TFE3 positive, rod-shaped cytoplasmic inclusions; negative for melanoma markers); clear cell sarcoma (translocation involving the EWSR1 gene); and epithelioid sarcoma (cytokeratin positive).

Biomarkers

PEComas are biphenotypic tumors that typically coexpress melanocytic markers such as HMB45 (the most sensitive), Melan-A and MITF,[1] and smooth muscle markers such as SMA[2] (the most sensitive) and calponin, which defines a myomelanocytic differentiation. PEComas are typically cytokeratin negative, and S100 is rarely expressed.

Although PEComa NOS is rarely associated with TSC, most PEComa NOS show loss of function in TSC1 or TSC2 (usually as a result of loss of heterozygosity, LOH), the two tumor suppressor genes involved in the pathogenesis of TSC. The decreased function of these genes leads to overactivation of mTORC1 signaling, which in turn favors cell growth.

Up to 20% of PEComas show strong nuclear staining for TFE3 due to the presence of a **chromosomal translocation** leading to the formation of a TFE3-based[3] fusion genes (TFE3 is located on chromosome Xp11).

While 80% of TFE3 fusion-negative PEComas have been shown to harbor TSC2 mutations, PEComas harboring TFE3 gene rearrangements are thought to form a distinct subset as they lack the TSC2 alterations characteristic of conventional PEComas.

Prognosis

PEComa NOS clinical behavior can vary from benign to highly malignant. Clinically malignant PEComas (approximately 30% of all reported cases) are typically large (>5 cm), with infiltrative margins, and show mitotic activity, necrosis, marked

---

[1] MITF: melanocyte-Inducing transcription factor (also known as microphthalmia-associated transcription factor).

[2] SMA: smooth muscle actin.

[3] TFE3: transcription factor binding to IGHM enhancer three encodes a transcription factor that binds MUE3-type E-box sequences in the promoter of genes. In particular, this protein enhances the expression of genes downstream of transforming growth factor beta (TGF-beta) signaling. This gene is involved in chromosomal translocations in renal cell carcinomas and other cancers; fusion partners include PRCC (papillary renal cell carcinoma), NONO (non-POU domain-containing, octamer-binding), and ASPSCR1 (alveolar soft part sarcoma chromosome region, candidate 1), among others.

Table 198.1 PEComa prognostic classification according to Folpe (published in Bleeker et al 2012)

High-risk features	
Size	>5 cm
Growth pattern	Infiltrative
Nuclear grade	High
Mitotic rate	>1/50 HPF
Necrosis	Present
Vascular invasion	Present
Risk category	
Benign	<2 high-risk features with size <5 cm
Uncertain behavior	Size >5 cm OR nuclear polymorphism
Malignant	2 or more high-risk features

HPF high-power field

nuclear atypia, and pleomorphism: they are usually characterized by a poor prognosis. The most common metastatic sites are the liver, lymph nodes, lungs, and bone.

A three-category (benign, uncertain behavior, malignant) classification has been proposed (→ see Table 198.1), although it is not universally accepted.

Therapy

Surgery appears to be the only potentially curative approach, when feasible. The role of chemotherapy and radiotherapy is unclear.

Due to the frequent overactivation of the mTORC1 pathway, mTOR inhibitors (such as sirolimus) have been tested with some encouraging results.

Suggested Readings

Agrawal et al (2020) Uterine PEComa—a group of rare mesenchymal tumors. J Minim Invasive Gynecol 27(4):803–804

Bleeker et al (2012) "Malignant" perivascular epithelioid cell neoplasm: risk stratification and treatment strategies. Sarcoma 2012:541626

Dickson et al (2013) Extrarenal perivascular epithelioid cell tumors (PEComas) respond to mTOR inhibition: clinical and molecular correlates. Int J Cancer 132(7):1711–1717

Fletcher et al (2020) WHO classification of tumours of soft tissue and bone, 5th edn

Gao et al (2016) Combination targeted therapy of VEGFR inhibitor, sorafenib, with an mTOR inhibitor, sirolimus induced a remarkable response of rapid progressive Uterine PEComa. Cancer Biol Ther 17(6):595–598

Gondran et al (2019) First pancreatic perivascular epithelioid cell tumor (PEComa) treated by mTOR inhibitor. Pancreatology 19(4):566–568

Hamza et al (2020) Perivascular epithelioid cell tumor of the urinary bladder: a systematic review. Int J Surg Pathol 28(4):393–400

Raimondi et al (2018) Prolonged activity and toxicity of sirolimus in a patient with metastatic renal perivascular epithelioid cell tumor: a case report and literature review. Anti-Cancer Drugs 29(6):589–595

Starbuck et al (2016) Treatment of advanced malignant uterine perivascular epithelioid cell tumor with mTOR inhibitors: single-institution experience and review of the literature. Anticancer Res 36(11):6161–6164

Thway, Fisher (2015) PEComa: morphology and genetics of a complex tumor family. Ann Diagn Pathol 19(5):359–368

Torres Luna et al (2020) A primary adrenal epithelioid angiomyolipoma (PEComa) in a patient with tuberous sclerosis complex: report of a case and review of the literature. Case Rep Med 2020:5131736

Uhlenhopp et al (2020) Rapidly enlarging malignant abdominal PEComa with hepatic metastasis: a promising initial response to sirolimus following surgical excision of primary tumor. Oxf Med Case Rep 2020(3):omaa013

Wagner et al (2010) Clinical activity of mTOR inhibition with sirolimus in malignant perivascular epithelioid cell tumors: targeting the pathogenic activation of mTORC1 in tumors. J Clin Oncol 28(5):835–840

Xu et al (2019) Gastric perivascular epithelioid cell tumor (PEComa). Am J Clin Pathol 152(2):221–229

Definition

Perineurioma is a nerve sheath tumor classified among benign neoplasms, although an exceedingly rare malignant perineurioma variant exists (also known as perineurial malignant peripheral nerve sheath tumor). Other variants are intraneural perineurioma and mucosal perineurioma.

Epidemiology and Presentation

Perineurioma is a very rare soft tissue tumor occurring over a wide age range, without remarkable gender differences. This tumor most commonly arises on the lower limbs, followed by the upper limbs and trunk; other sites (including viscera) are very rarely involved.

Clinically it presents as a painless well-circumscribed nodule/mass (range: from 1 to 20 cm), usually located in the dermis/subcutis, more rarely in deeper soft tissues. Usually it is not associated with a detectable nerve.

Pathology

Perineurioma is composed entirely of perineurial cells (slender spindle cells with characteristic delicate bipolar cytoplasmic processes) with a predominantly storiform growth pattern. The stroma is usually collagenous, with about 20% of cases containing myxoid matrix. Mitotic activity is typically scarce or absent. Occasionally, nuclear atypia (including pleomorphic and multinucleate cells) is present.

Sclerosing perineurioma is a variant composed of cords of small epithelioid to spindle cells in a dense collagenous stroma. Reticular perineurioma is a variant composed of anastomosing cords of elongated spindle cells with reticular architecture. The very rare malignant perineurioma displays the features of benign perineuriomas along with hypercellularity, nuclear atypia, and a high mitotic rate.

Biomarkers

As it occurs in normal perineurial cells, perineurioma tumor cells usually (but not necessarily) variably express EMA. Claudin-1 and GLUT1 are also usually expressed. Staining for CD34 is positive in about 50% of cases. Staining for S100 and GFAP is negative.

Chromosome 22 (containing the NF2 tumor suppressor gene) deletions and monosomies are found in many perineuriomas, but this alteration is not diagnostically helpful since it is found also in other soft tissue tumors (e.g., benign schwannoma). NF2 mutations have been detected in both conventional and sclerosing perineuriomas.

Prognosis

Conventional perineuriomas (including sclerosing and reticular variants) including those with nuclear atypia are benign neoplasms and rarely relapse. Malignant perineurioma may metastasize, but shows a less aggressive behavior than conventional MPNST (→ see dedicated section).

Therapy

Surgery is the treatment of choice.

Suggested Readings

Fletcher et al (2020) WHO classification of tumours of soft tissue and bone, 5th edn
Grech et al (2020) Spindle cell proliferations of the sigmoid colon, rectum and anus: a review with emphasis on perineurioma. Histopathology 76(3):342–353
McMillan et al (2016) Diagnosis and outcome of childhood perineurioma. Childs Nerv Syst 32(8):1555–1560
Weaver et al (2020) Endoscopic mucosal resection of a gastric perineurioma. ACG Case Rep J 7(2):e00332
White et al (2020) Intraneural perineurioma in neurofibromatosis type 2 with molecular analysis. Clin Neuropathol 39(4):167–171

Definition

Primitive neuroectodermal tumor (PNET) is a family of small round cell malignancies originating from primitive neuroectodermal (hence the name) cells including the following entities: peripheral primitive neuroectodermal tumor (peripheral PNET, pPNET), central PNET (or PNET of the central nervous system, cPNET; in the past it included medulloblastoma), and PNET of the autonomic nervous system (i.e., neuroblastoma).

This section covers exclusively pPNET.

Of note, due to common morphological and molecular features, the term pPNET is often used to refer to a range of tumors belonging to the Ewing family of tumors which includes Ewing sarcoma (including both osseous and extraosseous Ewing sarcomas → see dedicated section) and the Ewing-like sarcoma family (→ see dedicated section). However, it should be noted that Ewing sarcoma is more common in bone, while pPNET is more common in soft tissues.

pPNET is also known as peripheral neuroepithelioma.

Epidemiology and Presentation

pPNET is a very rare disease accounting for 5–15% of all pediatric soft tissue tumors, although its incidence is likely underestimated because only recently the diagnostic advances have allowed pathologists to distinguish this entity from other small, poorly differentiated, round cell tumors. pPNET usually presents in the second decade of life, with a slight male predominance.

pPNET arises in soft tissues and less frequently in bones. Virtually any body site may be affected, but the trunk is the most frequent location; visceral cases have been also described.

Clinical symptoms depend on the site of presentation but often include pain and swelling of the surrounding structures due to mass effect.

© The Editor(s) (if applicable) and The Author(s), under exclusive license to
Springer Nature Switzerland AG 2021
S. Mocellin, *Soft Tissue Tumors*, https://doi.org/10.1007/978-3-030-58710-9_200

Pathology

pPNET appears as a monotonous collection of small, round, darkly stained cells. Differential diagnosis may be needed with other small and poorly differentiated round cell tumors such as lymphoma, rhabdomyosarcoma, neuroblastoma, and so on.

For more details → see Chap. 93.

Biomarkers

Immunohistochemistry can be used to detect FLI1 expression (as a result of the EWSR1-FLI1 fusion gene, see below). CD99 (also known as MIC2) expression consistently identifies both Ewing sarcoma and pPNET (in contrast, central PNET and neuroblastoma uniformly lack CD99 expression). Furthermore, pPNET typically coexpresses CD99 and vimentin.

Cytogenetic analyses of pPNET consistently show **chromosomal translocations** leading to the generation of the EWSR1-FLI1 fusion gene[1] from t(11;22) (q24;q12) in about 85% of cases, and EWSR1-ERG fusion gene from t(21;22) (q22;q12) in other cases, which reveals the close relationship with Ewing sarcoma.

Testing for urinary catecholamines and their metabolites is positive in patients with neuroblastoma but negative in patients with pPNET.

Prognosis

pPNET often exhibits aggressive clinical behavior (with metastatic disease at presentation in 20–30% of patients), with worse outcomes than other small, round cell tumors.

Prognostic factors of pPNET include site (with abdominopelvic disease faring worse than thoracoabdominal wall and head and neck disease), tumor size, and the

---

[1] EWSR1-FLI1 fusion gene: EWSR1 (Ewing sarcoma breakpoint region 1) encodes a multifunctional protein that is involved in various cellular processes, including gene expression, cell signaling, and RNA processing and transport. FLI1 (friend leukemia integration 1) encodes a transcription factor containing an ETS DNA-binding domain. EWSR1-FLI1 chimeric protein is believed to act as an oncoprotein playing a key role in Ewing sarcoma pathogenesis; for instance, its activity leads to upregulation of c-Myc and GLI expression and inhibition of the transcriptional activity of p53, as well as blockage of the ability of Runx2 to induce osteoblast differentiation. Of note, EWSR1 is a "promiscuous" gene because it can fuse with different partner genes in phenotypically similar neoplasms or with the same genes in morphologically and behaviorally different tumors. In fact, EWSR1-based chimeric genes can be found not only in Ewing and Ewing-like sarcomas but also in other tumors such as angiomatoid fibrous histiocytoma, clear cell sarcoma, low-grade fibromyxoid sarcoma, sclerosing epithelioid fibrosarcoma, hemangioma of the bone, desmoplastic small round cell tumor, extraskeletal myxoid chondrosarcoma, myoepithelial tumor of soft tissue, and myxoid liposarcoma. It must be underscored that fluorescence in situ hybridization (FISH) analysis has a significant risk of false-negative results, making next-generation sequencing (NGS)-based diagnostic tools more sensitive for detecting EWSR1 rearrangements.

presence of metastasis. Using reverse transcription polymerase chain reaction (RT-PCR) technology, micrometastatic disease can be detected in the bone marrow of up to 30% of patients thought to have a localized disease. The most common sites of pPNET metastases include the lung, bone, and bone marrow.

Disease staging requires extensive workup with computed tomography (CT) scanning and magnetic resonance imaging (MRI), bone marrow biopsy, bone scan (skeletal scintigraphy), or positron emission tomography (PET) scan.

Therapy

For details on treatment → see Chap. 93.

Suggested Readings

Chao et al (2019) Ovarian primary primitive neuroectodermal tumor: a review of cases at PUMCH and in the published literature. Orphanet J Rare Dis 14(1):147

Gao et al (2019) Peripheral primitive neuroectodermal tumors: a retrospective analysis of 89 cases and literature review. Oncol Lett 18(6):6885–6890

Xiao et al (2019) ZBTB16: a new biomarker for primitive neuroectodermal tumor element/Ewing sarcoma. Pathol Res Pract 215(10):152536

Yagnik et al (2019) Extraskeletal Ewing's sarcoma/peripheral primitive neuroectodermal tumor of the small bowel presenting with gastrointestinal perforation. Clin Exp Gastroenterol 12:279–285

Definition

Phosphaturic mesenchymal tumor (PMT) is a potentially malignant neoplasm of uncertain differentiation.

It is also referred to as malignant phosphaturic mesenchymal tumor (malignant type).

Epidemiology and Presentation

PMT is a very rare neoplasm occurring most commonly in middle-aged adults that characteristically causes tumor-induced osteomalacia (TIO, also called oncogenic osteomalacia) in most affected patients, usually by the production of fibroblast growth factor 23 (FGF23, which leads to increased loss of phosphate in the urine resulting in phosphaturic hypophosphatemia, hence the name). PMT may locate in virtually any soft tissue, may be found in the bone, and is extremely rare in the retroperitoneum, mediastinum, and viscera.

Clinically, the lesion presents as a small nodule (diameter range: 2–14 cm) that may be difficult to locate. A long history of osteomalacia is often (but not always) present.

Pathology

PMT is typically composed of very bland, spindle to stellate cells producing a hyalinized to smudgy matrix. This matrix calcifies with a grungy or flocculent appearance, sometimes forming "flower-like" crystals sometimes resembling cartilage or osteoid. A well-developed capillary network is characteristically found.

© The Editor(s) (if applicable) and The Author(s), under exclusive license to
Springer Nature Switzerland AG 2021
S. Mocellin, *Soft Tissue Tumors*, https://doi.org/10.1007/978-3-030-58710-9_201

Mitotic activity and necrosis are absent. Malignant PMT (which accounts for about 10% of cases) most often develops from a lesion that has recurred locally and displays obviously sarcomatous features.

Differential diagnosis may be needed with giant cell tumor, hemangiopericytoma, and osteosarcoma.

Biomarkers

The immunophenotype is not specific. The blood vessels often have a lymphatic phenotype. Expression of FGF23 has been reported in some tumors. Elevated serum levels of FGF23 can be demonstrated in patients with PMT-associated TIO.

Prognosis

Most PMT cases (about 90%) are histologically and clinically benign: they frequently recur locally, but are cured with complete excision with resolution of osteomalacia. Disease relapse is a risk factor for malignant transformation. Malignant PMT may metastasize.

Therapy

Surgical excision is the treatment of choice.

Suggested Readings

Ding et al (2018) Recurrent/residual intracranial phosphaturic mesenchymal tumor revealed on 68Ga-DOTATATE PET/CT. Clin Nucl Med 43(9):674–675

Fletcher et al (2020) WHO classification of tumours of soft tissue and bone, 5th edn

Liu et al (2020) Surgical treatment of recurrent spinal phosphaturic mesenchymal tumor-induced osteomalacia: a case report. Medicine (Baltimore) 99(4):e18603

Oyama et al (2020) Malignant transformation of phosphaturic mesenchymal tumor: a case report and literature review. Clin Pediatr Endocrinol 29(2):69–75

Saba et al (2019) Genetic profiling of a chondroblastoma-like osteosarcoma/malignant phosphaturic mesenchymal tumor of bone reveals a homozygous deletion of CDKN2A, intragenic deletion of DMD, and a targetable FN1-FGFR1 gene fusion. Genes Chromosom Cancer 58(10):731–736

Wasserman et al (2016) Phosphaturic mesenchymal tumor involving the head and neck: a report of five cases with FGFR1 fluorescence in situ hybridization analysis. Head Neck Pathol 10(3):279–285

Yavropoulou et al (2018) Distant lung metastases caused by a histologically benign phosphaturic mesenchymal tumor. Endocrinol Diabetes Metab Case Rep 2018:18-0023

Definition

Pleomorphic dermal sarcoma (PDS) is a malignant tumor of the skin with uncertain differentiation.

It is also known as undifferentiated pleomorphic sarcoma of the skin and cutaneous undifferentiated pleomorphic sarcoma (the term superficial malignant fibrous histiocytoma should no longer be used).

Epidemiology and Presentation

PDS is one of the most common skin sarcomas. It resembles atypical fibroxanthoma (→ see dedicated section) as it usually affects elderly patients (peak incidence: eight decade of life); it is more frequent in males and typically affects areas of sun-damaged skin (with special regard to the scalp).

Clinically, the lesion typically presents as rapidly growing nodules or plaques, often >2 cm; ulceration may be present.

Pathology

PDS is an undifferentiated pleomorphic tumor centered in the dermis that histologically resembles atypical fibroxanthoma; it is often associated with extensive involvement of deeper tissue (the subcutis, skeletal muscle, fascia), necrosis, and perineural and/or lymphovascular invasion. Pleomorphism is consistent. Cells can be spindled or epithelioid, arranged in sheets and fascicles, often with admixed multinucleated giant cells.

Differential diagnosis may be needed with the following: atypical fibroxanthoma (it may be microscopically identical, particularly if a superficial shave biopsy is performed; it tends to have a well-circumscribed border with less infiltration into deep soft tissues; necrosis as well as perineural invasion and lymphovascular invasion are typically absent); cutaneous leiomyosarcoma (it is dermal based and composed of intersecting fascicles of spindled cells with eosinophilic cytoplasm; typically positive for smooth muscle markers such as desmin, caldesmon, and SMA, but SMA expression alone is not sufficient to diagnose leiomyosarcoma); sarcomatoid squamous cell carcinoma (positive for cytokeratins); and cellular neurothekeoma (it can develop in the head and neck region but occurs in young females instead of elderly males; microscopically it is composed of sheets and nest of spindled and epithelioid cells with cytological atypia and mitoses; usually variably positive for CD10, MITF, and SMA).

Biomarkers

PDS usually stains positive for CD10 and SMA; it stains negative for cytokeratins, desmin, S100, SOX10, and melan-A. Mutations in TERT, NOTCH, and TP53 are found in most cases.

Prognosis

PDS is a high-grade sarcoma with higher rate of local recurrence and metastasis as compared to atypical fibroxanthoma. Local recurrence rate is reported to range between 20% and 30% (median time to recurrence: 10 months). The metastatic rate ranges between 10% and 20%.

The prognosis is better than that of undifferentiated pleomorphic sarcoma arising outside the skin (→ see Chap. 246).

Therapy

Surgery is the mainstay of treatment. Adjuvant radiotherapy is utilized in case of close margins when redo surgery is contraindicated or refused by the patient.

Currently, limited treatment options exist for advanced/metastatic disease; immunotherapy with pembrolizumab (an anti-PD1 monoclonal antibody) has been utilized with efficacy in a few patients.

Suggested Readings

Griewank et al (2018) Atypical fibroxanthoma and pleomorphic dermal sarcoma harbor frequent NOTCH1/2 and FAT1 mutations and similar DNA copy number alteration profiles. Mod Pathol 31(3):418–428

Klein et al (2019) First report on two cases of pleomorphic dermal sarcoma successfully treated with immune checkpoint inhibitors. Oncoimmunology 8(12):e1665977

Koelsche et al (2019) Genome-wide methylation profiling and copy number analysis in atypical fibroxanthomas and pleomorphic dermal sarcomas indicate a similar molecular phenotype. Clin Sarcoma Res 9:2

Kohlmeyer et al (2017) Cutaneous sarcomas. J Dtsch Dermatol Ges 15(6):630–648

Llombart et al (2019) Leiomyosarcoma and pleomorphic dermal sarcoma: guidelines for diagnosis and treatment. Actas Dermosifiliogr 110(1):4–11

Lonie et al (2020) Management of pleomorphic dermal sarcoma. ANZ J Surg. https://doi.org/10.1111/ans.15909

Soleymani et al (2019) Atypical fibroxanthoma and pleomorphic dermal sarcoma: updates on classification and management. Dermatol Clin 37(3):253–259

Winchester et al (2018) Undifferentiated pleomorphic sarcoma: factors predictive of adverse outcomes. J Am Acad Dermatol 79(5):853–859

Definition

Pleomorphic fibroma is a benign skin neoplasm of unclear differentiation.

Epidemiology and Presentation

Pleomorphic fibroma of the skin is a rare tumor typically occurring as a solitary and asymptomatic lesion. It generally appears as a circumscribed, flesh-colored, dome-shaped, or polypoid lesion, measuring 5–15 mm and arising mainly on the trunk or proximal extremity of adults.

Pathology

Histologically, the lesion is intradermal and generally well circumscribed. It is composed of dense collagen fibers with sparsely cellular proliferations of oval or polygonal to spindled cells with characteristic large, pleomorphic, hyperchromatic nuclei and scattered multinucleated giant cells with multilobated nuclei. Mitotic figures are rare or absent.

Pleomorphic fibroma may exhibit marked variability in stromal alteration, ranging from sclerotic to fibrotic to myxoid. In cases with exuberant sclerosis, overlap can occur with sclerotic fibroma (sclerotic pleomorphic fibroma). Independent of the stromal type, some cases of pleomorphic fibroma may have cytologically bland, mature adipocytes within the dermal compartment (which might represent adipocytes secondarily entrapped within the mesenchymal proliferation, or, alternatively, adipocytic metaplasia).

Differential diagnosis may be needed with many other cutaneous lesions. The presence of atypical giant cells may recall other diagnoses, such as giant cell collagenoma, atypical (or monster cell) dermatofibroma, giant cell fibroblastoma,

© The Editor(s) (if applicable) and The Author(s), under exclusive license to
Springer Nature Switzerland AG 2021
S. Mocellin, *Soft Tissue Tumors*, https://doi.org/10.1007/978-3-030-58710-9_203

atypical lipomatous tumor, and pleomorphic lipoma. Tumors of the skin such as atypical fibroxanthoma and pleomorphic dermal sarcoma have tumor cells with similar atypia: these entities typically exhibit higher cellularity with fascicular to storiform arrangement, which is in contrast to the low cellularity of pleomorphic fibroma. Atypical fibroxanthoma and pleomorphic dermal sarcoma often contain xanthomatous cells and frequent mitotic figures, including atypical forms. As regards atypical fibrous histiocytoma, the higher cellularity and the presence of both foam cells and hemosiderin-laden macrophages are useful features to distinguish the two entities. Atypical dermatofibroma (dermatofibroma with atypical cells or "monster" cells) shares characteristics with pleomorphic fibroma (e.g., multinucleated giant cells): however, atypical dermatofibroma typically differs due to hypercellularity as well as the presence of foam cells and hemosiderin-laden macrophages. Like pleomorphic fibroma, giant cell fibroblastoma also has atypical fibroblastic cells: nevertheless, it displays variably myxoid background with infiltrative growth pattern. Melanocytic tumors (e.g., desmoplastic melanoma and desmoplastic Spitz nevus), as well as benign nerve sheath tumors with atypical features (e.g., neurofibroma with atypia and schwannomas with ancient changes), may need to be differentiated from pleomorphic fibroma: lack of S100 expression by pleomorphic fibroma should help make the correct diagnosis. Some cases of sclerotic lipoma reveal bizarre multinucleated giant cells which resemble those found in pleomorphic lipoma and pleomorphic fibroma: unlike pleomorphic fibroma, spindled-shaped cells as well as adipocytes stain positive for S100. Finally, spindle cell and pleomorphic lipoma might be considered in the differential diagnosis: unlike pleomorphic fibroma, they are composed of cytologically bland CD34-positive, spindle-shaped cells, multinucleated giant cells, and mature adipocytes within a background of ropy bundles of collagen and myxoid stroma.

Biomarkers

The tumor stains positive for vimentin, SMA, and CD34, whereas it stains negative for S100 and macrophage marker CD68.

Prognosis

Despite the cytological atypia, pleomorphic fibroma has a benign clinical course.

Therapy

Surgical excision is the treatment of choice.

Suggested Readings

Al-Zaid et al (2013) Dermal pleomorphic liposarcoma resembling pleomorphic fibroma: report of a case and review of the literature. J Cutan Pathol 40(8):734–739

Hinds et al (2017) Loss of retinoblastoma in pleomorphic fibroma: an immunohistochemical and genomic analysis. J Cutan Pathol 44(8):665–671

Mahmood et al (2003) Solitary sclerotic fibroma of skin: a possible link with pleomorphic fibroma with immunophenotypic expression for O13 (CD99) and CD34. J Cutan Pathol 30(10):631–636

Tashakori et al (2018) Pleomorphic fibroma of the skin with MDM2 immunoreactivity: a potential diagnostic pitfall. J Cutan Pathol 45(1):59–62

Definition

Pleomorphic hyalinizing angiectatic tumor (PHAT) of soft parts is a benign soft tissue tumor of uncertain differentiation. PHAT is considered related to hemosiderotic fibrolipomatous tumor ($\rightarrow$ see dedicated section).

Epidemiology and Presentation

This very rare tumor usually arises in the subcutis of the lower extremity (very rarely localizes in deep soft tissues). It typically presents as a slowly growing tan to maroon mass, which can be clinically mistaken for a hematoma.

Pathology

PHAT presents as an unencapsulated lesion with infiltrative margins and consists of spindled and pleomorphic cells, clusters of ectatic fibrin-lined vessels, and inflammatory cells (abundant mast cells). Mitotic activity is low to absent.

Biomarkers

PHAT stains positive for CD34 and negative for S100 protein.

The **chromosomal translocation** t(1;10)(p22;q24) leading to the generation of the TGFBR3-MGEA5 fusion gene[1] or TGFBR3-FBXW4 fusion gene has been reported.

Prognosis

Although classified as a benign tumor, PHAT is locally aggressive and relapses in up to 30–50% of cases (generally well controlled with redo surgery).

Therapy

Surgical excision is the treatment of choice.

Suggested Readings

Fletcher et al (2020) WHO classification of tumours of soft tissue and bone, 5th edn
Liu et al (2019) The t(1;10)(p22;q24) TGFBR3/MGEA5 translocation in pleomorphic hyalinizing angiectatic tumor, myxoinflammatory fibroblastic sarcoma, and hemosiderotic fibrolipomatous tumor. Arch Pathol Lab Med 143(2):212–221
Rougemont et al (2019) Targeted RNA-sequencing identifies FBXW4 instead of MGEA5 as fusion partner of TGFBR3 in pleomorphic hyalinizing angiectatic tumor. Virchows Arch 475(2):251–254
Rush et al (2018) Treatment modalities and outcomes of pleomorphic hyalinizing angiectatic tumor: a systematic review of the literature. Musculoskelet Surg 102(3):213–221

---

[1] TGFBR3-MGEA5 fusion gene: TGFBR3 (transforming growth factor beta receptor 3) encodes a receptor which is a membrane proteoglycan that often functions as a co-receptor with other TGF-beta receptor superfamily members. MGEA5 (also known as OGA, O-GlcNAcase): the modification of cytoplasmic and nuclear proteins by O-linked N-acetylglucosamine (O-GlcNAc) addition and removal on serine and threonine residues is catalyzed by OGT (which adds O-GlcNAc) and MGEA5, a glycosidase that removes O-GlcNAc modifications.

See Chap. 236.

Definition

Pleomorphic liposarcoma (PLS) is a malignant neoplasm with adipocytic differentiation.

For general information on liposarcomas → see Chap. 155.

As regards the other types of liposarcomas (i.e., well-differentiated liposarcoma, dedifferentiated liposarcoma, myxoid/round cell liposarcoma) → see dedicated sections.

Epidemiology and Presentation

PLS is the least frequent type of liposarcoma accounting for about 5–10% of all liposarcomas. Most cases occur in adulthood (peak incidence: 60–70 years), without remarkable gender differences. PLS arises mainly (two thirds of cases) in the extremities (lower > upper limbs); the trunk wall, retroperitoneum, and spermatic cord are less commonly involved. Rarely, cases in the mediastinum, heart, pleura, breast, scalp, colon, and orbit have been reported. Although most cases develop in deep soft tissues, about 25% of PLS develop in the subcutis (dermal cases are extremely rare).

Clinically, the lesion usually presents as an asymptomatic but rapidly growing mass (median size: 10 cm); pain and other signs/symptoms due to compression of adjacent organs/structures may be present.

Pathology

Macroscopically, the lesion is well demarcated (but not encapsulated), although it may be ill-defined and infiltrative. On sectioning, most lesions are white to yellow, with myxoid changes and necrosis being frequently present. Microscopically, most cases have infiltrative margins. PLS is a pleomorphic, high-grade neoplasm containing a variable number of pleomorphic lipoblasts: the presence of lipoblasts is needed to make this diagnosis, and their variable number underscores the importance of adequate sampling. No areas of well-differentiated liposarcoma or other types of differentiation are present.

In most lesions, the non-lipogenic component resembles undifferentiated pleomorphic sarcoma (→ see dedicated section) with spindle and multinucleate giant cells arranged in short fascicles. A myxofibrosarcoma-like component may be present in other cases. Epithelioid morphology may be present in others with areas mimicking poorly differentiated carcinoma, renal clear cell carcinoma, adrenocortical carcinoma, or melanoma. Areas resembling hemangiopericytoma, round cell liposarcoma, or spindle cell liposarcoma may be observed. The mitotic rate is variable but generally high (median: 20–25 mitoses per 10 HPF). Necrosis is observed in more than 50% of cases.

Differential diagnosis may be needed with the following: dedifferentiated liposarcoma (well-differentiated component; MDM2/CDK4 amplification); metastatic carcinoma (cytokeratin positivity or other evidence of epithelial differentiation; no liposarcomatous differentiation); undifferentiated pleomorphic sarcoma (no definite lipoblasts); and pleomorphic rhabdomyosarcoma (skeletal muscle differentiation).

Biomarkers

Lipoblasts stain positive for S100 in fewer than 50% of cases. PLS is positive for SMA[1] and CD34 in about 50% of cases. PLS may stain positive also for cytokeratins, EMA,[2] desmin, and HMGA2. Staining for MDM2 and CDK4 is negative.

PLS cytogenetics resembles more that of other pleomorphic sarcomas than that of well-differentiated liposarcoma, dedifferentiated liposarcoma, or myxoid/round cell liposarcoma. In particular, PLS is characterized by complex karyotypes with high chromosomal counts and complex structural rearrangements. Chromosomal losses frequently involve regions encoding tumor suppressor genes such as RB1 and TP53. No pathognomonic genetic rearrangement has been so far identified.

Prognosis

PLS is a high-grade aggressive malignancy associated with a 30–50% local recurrence rate, a 50% distant metastatic rate, and an overall 5-year survival of about 50%. Distant metastasis occurs mainly in the lungs.

---

[1] SMA: smooth muscle actin.
[2] EMA: epithelial membrane antigen.

Therapy

Surgery (wide excision) is the mainstay of treatment. Neoadjuvant or adjuvant **radiotherapy** is recommended for extremity lesions (particularly if diameter >5 cm). The only randomized controlled trial (STRASS) so far available on neoadjuvant radiotherapy for retroperitoneal sarcomas has not demonstrated an abdominal recurrence-free survival advantage over surgery alone in patients with histologically proven localized and resectable primary soft tissue malignancies (although subgroup analysis shows a significant benefit for the liposarcoma subset).

For locally recurrent disease, surgery remains the best option (when feasible), but the prognosis is dismal (especially for retroperitoneal disease).

As regards **chemotherapy**, PLS shows a variable sensitivity. For patients with locally advanced/unresectable or metastatic disease, anthracycline-based chemotherapy remains the standard first-line treatment. As second-line treatment, gemcitabine plus docetaxel and high-dose ifosfamide monotherapy can be used. More recently, trabectedin and eribulin have been approved for the treatment of patients with metastatic liposarcoma who failed anthracycline-based first-line chemotherapy. Identification of molecular targets druggable by clinically available compounds should be pursued in these patients.

Suggested Readings

Anderson et al (2019) Pleomorphic liposarcoma: updates and current differential diagnosis. Semin Diagn Pathol 36(2):122–128

Bonvalot et al (2009) Primary retroperitoneal sarcomas: a multivariate analysis of surgical factors associated with local control. J Clin Oncol 27:31–37

Bonvalot et al (2019) STRASS (EORTC 62092): a phase III randomized study of preoperative radiotherapy plus surgery versus surgery alone for patients with retroperitoneal sarcoma. J Clin Oncol 37(15_suppl):11001

Crago et al (2016) Liposarcoma: multimodality management and future targeted therapies. Surg Oncol Clin N Am 25(4):761–773

Demetri et al (2016) Efficacy and safety of trabectedin or dacarbazine for metastatic liposarcoma or leiomyosarcoma after failure of conventional chemotherapy: results of a phase III randomized multicenter clinical trial. J Clin Oncol 34(8):786–793

Fletcher et al (2020) WHO classification of tumours of soft tissue and bone, 5th edn

Gronchi et al (2009) Aggressive surgical policies in a retrospectively reviewed single-institution case series of retroperitoneal soft tissue sarcoma patients. J Clin Oncol 27:24–30

Kiyuna et al (2018) Doxorubicin-resistant pleomorphic liposarcoma with PDGFRA gene amplification is targeted and regressed by pazopanib in a patient-derived orthotopic xenograft mouse model. Tissue Cell 53:30–36

Lee et al (2017) Clinical and molecular spectrum of liposarcoma. J Clin Oncol 36:151–159

Lee et al (2020) Primary anatomical site as a prognostic factor for pleomorphic liposarcoma. J Cancer Res Clin Oncol 146(6):1501–1508

Nennstiel et al (2014) Small bowel pleomorphic liposarcoma: a rare cause of gastrointestinal bleeding. Case Rep Gastrointest Med 391871:2014

Ramírez-Bellver et al (2017) Primary dermal pleomorphic liposarcoma: utility of adipophilin and MDM2/CDK4 immunostainings. J Cutan Pathol 44(3):283–288

Schöffski et al (2016) Eribulin versus dacarbazine in previously treated patients with advanced liposarcoma or leiomyosarcoma: a randomised, open-label, multicentre, phase 3 trial. Lancet 387(10028):1629–1637

Definition

Pleomorphic rhabdomyosarcoma (PRMS) is a malignancy that displays skeletal (striated) muscle differentiation.

It is one of the four subtypes of rhabdomyosarcoma (→ see Chap. 224 for further details) along with embryonal (ERMS), alveolar (ARMS), and spindle cell/sclerosing (SRMS) rhabdomyosarcoma (→ see dedicated sections).

Epidemiology and Presentation

PRMS is a rare type of rhabdomyosarcoma and occurs almost exclusively in adults (mainly sixth to seventh decades of life), with a male predominance (70% of cases).

The tumor arises in the deep soft tissues, most frequently in the lower extremity; other sites are the chest/abdominal wall, upper extremity, abdomen/retroperitoneum, and head and neck.

The lesion typically presents as a rapidly growing mass (often painful) which can reach 5–15 cm in diameter.

Pathology

The tumor is composed of sheets of large, atypical, and frequently multinucleated polygonal eosinophilic cells or of undifferentiated round to spindle cells, without embryonal or alveolar components.

Differential diagnosis may be needed with the following: embryonal or alveolar rhabdomyosarcoma (evidence of embryonal or alveolar components); undifferentiated pleomorphic sarcoma (diagnosis of exclusion, no evidence of skeletal muscle differentiation); and pleomorphic liposarcoma (no evidence of skeletal muscle differentiation).

© The Editor(s) (if applicable) and The Author(s), under exclusive license to
Springer Nature Switzerland AG 2021
S. Mocellin, *Soft Tissue Tumors*, https://doi.org/10.1007/978-3-030-58710-9_207

Biomarkers

PRMS may express desmin, MyoD1, myosin, and myogenin. It stains negative for cytokeratins, synaptophysin, EMA, placental-like alkaline phosphatase, and chromogranin.

The tumor is characterized by complex karyotypes with numerical and unbalanced structural chromosomal changes; however, no recurrent structural alterations have been identified.

Prognosis

PRMS is a high-grade sarcoma with an overall poor prognosis.

For more details on staging and prognosis → see Chap. 224

Therapy

PRMS is often chemoresistant. For details on treatment of rhabdomyosarcoma → see dedicated section ("Therapy" paragraph).

Suggested Readings

Alavi (2017) Pleomorphic rhabdomyosarcoma of the uterus—case report and a systematic review of the literature. Anticancer Res 37(5):2509–2514

Fletcher (2020) WHO classification of tumours of soft tissue and bone, 5th edn

Kam (2018) Rapidly growing massive pleomorphic rhabdomyosarcoma of the bladder presenting with bladder outlet obstruction. ANZ J Surg 88(3):E208–E209

Noujaim (2015) Adult pleomorphic rhabdomyosarcoma: a multicentre retrospective study. Anticancer Res 35(11):6213–6217

Okazaki (2020) Pleomorphic rhabdomyosarcoma of the liver in an adult: a rare case report. BMC Surg 20(1):81

Pappo (2018) Rhabdomyosarcoma, Ewing sarcoma, and other round cell sarcomas. J Clin Oncol 36(2):168–179

Skapek (2019) Rhabdomyosarcoma. Nat Rev Dis Primers 5(1):1

Tlemsani (2020) Chemoresistant pleomorphic rhabdomyosarcoma: whole exome sequencing reveals underlying cancer predisposition and therapeutic options. J Med Genet 57(2):104–108

Definition

Pleuropulmonary blastoma (PPB) is a malignant mesenchymal tumor of the thorax. Its cell origin is uncertain (probably a mesenchymal stem cell).

It is also known as pneumoblastoma, mesenchymal cystic hamartoma, cystic mesenchymal hamartoma, pulmonary rhabdomyosarcoma, and pediatric pulmonary blastoma.

PPB is a rare neoplasm developing in the thorax of young children (very rarely in adults), mostly in the first years of life (90% of cases occur between 0 and 2 years of age). Though rare, PPB is the most common primary lung cancer in children. The tumor may arise in the lung parenchyma, mediastinum, and pleura. Patients usually present with shortness of breath, pneumonitis, coughing, or atelectasis.

PPB is classified as follows (with a growing malignant potential):

- Type I: the tumor is composed of cysts (multicystic disease).
- Type II: the tumor contains both cysts and solid nodules.
- Type III: the tumor is solid and can fill a large portion of the chest.

PPB type I is currently believed to be the same nosological entity as congenital pulmonary airway malformation (CPAM) type IV. PPB types II and III can metastasize. PPB can cause pneumothorax due to the rupture of cysts.

Although computed tomography and magnetic resonance imaging can be suggestive, biopsy is advocated to make a definitive diagnosis.

Etiology and Predisposition

DICER1 syndrome, a rare genetic disease inherited in an autosomal dominant manner and due to germline mutations of the gene DICER1 (located at chromosome 14q23.13), whose protein product is involved in the metabolism of microRNA:

most mutations found in this syndrome lead to an abnormally short Dicer protein that is unable to correctly regulate the production of miRNA. DICER1 syndrome is the genetic cause of the majority of PPB cases.

Patients with this cancer predisposition syndrome most commonly develop PPB (which is the hallmark of this condition); however, they are also at risk of other tumors such as cystic nephroma in the kidney (and to lower extent Wilms tumor and anaplastic renal sarcoma), sex cord-stromal tumors (especially Sertoli-Leydig cell tumor) in the ovaries, goiter and carcinoma in the thyroid, brain tumors (including pineoblastoma and pituitary blastoma), embryonal rhabdomyosarcoma, hepatic mesenchymal hamartoma, and a tumorlike condition known as nasal chondromesenchymal hamartoma.

Of note, the DICER1 syndrome is characterized by an incomplete penetrance, that is, not all subjects carrying DICER1 germline mutations develop cancer.

Pathology

PPB type I presents as a peripherally located, multicystic, and thin-walled structure. PPB type II is a mixed solid (nodule-like) and cystic tumor. PPB type III appears as a heterogeneous tumor composed of one or more of the following elements: (A) primitive blastema-like small cells with hyperchromatic nuclei, high nuclear-to-cytoplasm ratio, and numerous mitotic figures; (B) spindled and ovoid cells embedded in a myxoid stroma; (C) nodules of immature chondroid elements; and (D) large anaplastic cells with pleomorphic nuclei and atypical mitotic figures.

For PPB type I, **differential diagnosis** may be needed with bronchogenic cyst; for type III, differential diagnosis may be needed with the following: embryonal rhabdomyosarcoma, malignant peripheral nerve sheath tumor, malignant teratoma, mesothelioma, monophasic synovial sarcoma, PNET, and undifferentiated pleomorphic sarcoma.

Biomarkers

PPB tumor cells stain positive for vimentin (diffusely) and (focally) CD117 as well as alpha-1 antitrypsin; the surface epithelium expresses cytokeratins; rhabdomyoblasts and primitive cells stain positive for MSA[1] and desmin. PPB stains negative for EMA,[2] myogenin, S100, GFAP,[3] NSE,[4] TTF1,[5] alpha-fetoprotein, chromogranin, and synaptophysin.

---

[1] MSA: muscle-specific actin.

[2] EMA: epithelial membrane antigen.

[3] GFAP: glial fibrillary acidic protein.

[4] NSE: neuron-specific enolase.

[5] TTF1: thyroid transcription factor 1 (also known as NKX2–1, NK2 homeobox 1); it encodes a protein expressed in thyroid as well as lung carcinoma.

Prognosis

PPB classification into type I to III reflects tumor malignant potential: in particular, PPB types II and III can metastasize, usually to the brain, liver, and bones. The prognosis of PPB types II and III is poor.

Therapy

Current treatment of PPB is multimodal and includes surgery, chemotherapy, and radiotherapy.

Recommendations for surveillance strategies for DICER1 germline mutated subjects have been issued.

Suggested Readings

de Kock (2019) An update on the central nervous system manifestations of DICER1 syndrome. Acta Neuropathol [Epub ahead of print]

Dehner (2017) Type I pleuropulmonary blastoma versus congenital pulmonary airway malformation type IV. Neonatology 111(1):76

Grigoletto (2020) Inequalities in diagnosis and registration of pediatric very rare tumors: a European study on pleuropulmonary blastoma. Eur J Pediatr 179(5):749–756

Guillerman (2019) Imaging of DICER1 syndrome. Pediatr Radiol 49(11):1488–1505

Messinger (2015) Pleuropulmonary blastoma: a report on 350 central pathology-confirmed pleuropulmonary blastoma cases by the International Pleuropulmonary Blastoma Registry. Cancer 121(2):276–285

Schultz (2018) DICER1 and associated conditions: identification of at-risk individuals and recommended surveillance strategies. Clin Cancer Res 24(10):2251–2261

Stewart (2019) Neoplasm risk among individuals with a pathogenic germline variant in DICER1. J Clin Oncol 37(8):668–676

Zamora (2020) The effect of gross total resection on patients with pleuropulmonary blastoma. J Surg Res 253:115–120

Definition

Plexiform fibrohistiocytic tumor (PFHT) is a low-grade superficial sarcoma with intermediate malignant potential; it is classified among fibrohistiocytic tumors.

Epidemiology and Presentation

PFHT can affect any age, but it is most frequently observed in children and young adults. It is located in the dermis or subcutaneous tissue, mainly in the upper extremities or the head and neck region.

PFHT usually presents as a small, painless, slow-growing mass or plaque with a central depression. Overlying epidermis and dermis are usually normal.

Pathology

PFHT is composed of fibroblasts and histiocyte-like cells organized in a plexiform architecture (hence the name). Often, osteoclast-type multinucleate giant cells are also present. Cytological atypia and atypical mitoses are rare, mitotic count is generally low, and necrosis is absent.

Differential diagnosis may be needed with the following: benign fibrous histiocytoma (older patients, prominent foam cells, no plexiform extensions of fibrous tissue, no nodules of histiocyte-like cells, no multinucleated giant cells); cellular neurothekeoma (uniform population of epithelioid cells, no distinct nodules of histiocytoid cells or osteoclast-like giant cells, podoplanin positive); fibromatosis (centered in muscle, diffusely infiltrative, no nodules); fibrous hamartoma of infancy (immature cells present, also myxoid stroma); giant cell tumor of soft tissue (infiltrative nodules of mixed giant cells and spindle cells, frequent mitotic figures); and neurofibroma (no distinct nodules, S100 positive).

Biomarkers

PFHT is CD68 and vimentin positive in multinucleated giant cells and mononuclear histiocyte-like cells and SMA positive in fibroblast-like cells. Staining for S100 protein, desmin, and cytokeratins is negative.

Prognosis

PFHT locally recurs in up to 40% of cases; regional lymph node metastasis has been described in 6% of patients, whereas lung metastasis is rare.

Therapy

Surgical wide excision is the treatment of choice.

Suggested Readings

Fletcher. WHO classification of tumours of soft tissue and bone, 4th edition. 2020.

Ghuman. Plexiform fibrohistiocytic tumor: imaging features and clinical findings. Skeletal Radiol. 2019;48(3):437–43.

Gómez-Mateo M. Nonepithelial skin tumors with multinucleated giant cells. Semin Diagn Pathol. 2013;30(1):58–72.

Goh. Plexiform fibrohistiocytic tumor presenting as a central neck mass clinically mimicking a thyroglossal duct cyst: an unusual case reported with histo-cytopathologic correlation and a review of the cytopathology literature. Head Neck Pathol. 2020;14(1):262–7.

Valiga. Plexiform fibrohistiocytic tumor on the chest of a 5-year-old child and review of the literature. Pediatr Dermatol. 2019;36(4):490–6.

Definition

Plexiform fibromyxoma is a benign mesenchymal tumor specific to the stomach. It is also referred to as plexiform angiomyxoid myofibroblastic tumor and plexiform angiomyxoid tumor.

Epidemiology and Presentation

Plexiform fibromyxoma occurs over a broad age range (median: 46 years) without gender prevalence and generally presents as a multinodular mass involving the muscularis propria or submucosa of the antral/prepyloric region; very rare extra-gastric cases have been described. It has been estimated that plexiform fibromyxoma occurs at a rate of 1 case per 150 gastrointestinal stromal tumors (GISTs), although this figure should be probably higher.

The clinical presentation can range from incidental findings to nonspecific gastric symptoms (mild abdominal pain and abdominal discomfort) and further to gastric bleeding (with consequent anemia, melena, or hematemesis). Endoscopy reveals a pink to reddish tumor, elastic in texture, and covered with ulcerative, erosive, or smooth mucosa. Endoscopic ultrasonography can be helpful in defining the intramural location of the neoplasm, which appears hypoechoic.

Pathology

Macroscopically plexiform fibromyxoma presents as a mass of 1–17 cm in diameter (median size: 4 cm), lobulated tan white or grayish-whitish, gelatinous on the cut surface, cystic, with mucinous fluids, with multinodular or polypoidal growth pattern, unencapsulated, and with well-defined (but sometimes ill-defined) margins. Plexiform fibromyxoma originates from the submucosa and muscularis propria,

© The Editor(s) (if applicable) and The Author(s), under exclusive license to
Springer Nature Switzerland AG 2021
S. Mocellin, *Soft Tissue Tumors*, https://doi.org/10.1007/978-3-030-58710-9_210

with extension ranging from the mucosa to the serosa, causing ulceration that in turn can lead to hemorrhage.

Miscroscopically the tumor shows a multinodular proliferation of bland myofibroblastic cells and arborizing capillaries in a myxoid stroma. No mitoses are found.

Differential diagnosis may be needed with the following: GIST (CD117 and CD34 positive and is usually not multinodular and myxoid); inflammatory fibroid polyp (more inflammation is present and often demonstrates a concentric growth of the spindle cells around small blood vessels; in most cases, the spindle cells are CD34 positive); neurofibroma (S100 positive); sarcomatoid carcinoma (more malignant cytological feature, such as brisk mitotic or apoptotic activities, positive for epithelial biomarkers); and inflammatory myofibroblastic tumor (characterized by monotonous spindle cells arranged in fascicles or vague whorls in an inflammatory and edematous stroma full of neutrophils, eosinophils, or lymphoplasma cells; although the myofibroblastic nature of an inflammatory myofibroblastic tumor is similar to that of plexiform fibromyxoma by morphology and immunohistochemical studies, the lack of a plexiform growth pattern, a predominantly inflammatory cellular microenvironment, and positive ALK immunoreactivity should be sufficient to differentiate the two entities).

Biomarkers

Plexiform fibromyxoma is diffusely positive for SMA[1] and vimentin and focally for CD10 and caldesmon. It stains negative for EMA[2], cytokeratins, ALK, desmin, S100, CD34, c-Kit, and DOG1. Prominent arborizing capillaries are highlighted by CD34 staining.

Loss of the PTCH1 tumor suppressor (which leads to activation of the GLI1 oncogene and predisposes to sensitivity to hedgehog pathway inhibitors such as sonidegib) has been demonstrated in a subset of plexiform fibromyxomas.

Prognosis

Plexiform fibromyxoma is a benign tumor (neither metastasis nor local recurrence has been described after complete excision).

Therapy

Conservative management (endoscopic resection) is the best treatment, when feasible. Surgery should be reserved to cases unsuitable for endoscopic resection or when the diagnosis is uncertain.

---

[1] SMA: smooth muscle actin.

[2] EMA: epithelial membrane antigen.

Suggested Readings

Banerjee. Gastric plexiform fibromyxoma. J Gastrointest Surg. 2019;23(9):1936–9.

Banerjee. Loss of the PTCH1 tumor suppressor defines a new subset of plexiform fibromyxoma. J Transl Med. 2019;17(1):246.

Gan. A rare case of plexiform fibromyxoma in stomach: FNA diagnosis with histological correlation and differential diagnoses. Ann Diagn Pathol. 2020;44:151453.

Hong. Plexiform fibromyxoma of the stomach. J Gastrointest Surg. 2020;24(4):909–12.

Su. An update on clinicopathological and molecular features of plexiform fibromyxoma. Can J Gastroenterol Hepatol. 2019;2019:3960920.

Definition

Primitive myxoid mesenchymal tumor of infancy (PMMTI) is a myofibroblastic tumor with intermediate biological aggressiveness.

Epidemiology and Presentation

PMMTI is a recently described nosological entity. This tumor typically develops in infancy (usually within the first year of life).

Pathology

The lesion is composed of primitive spindled polygonal and round cells in a myxoid background. The tumor cells are arranged in a vaguely nodular pattern with peripheral collagenized stroma, higher cellularity at the periphery, and a delicate vascular network in the background.

Differential diagnosis may be needed with infantile fibrosarcoma (→ see dedicated section).

Biomarkers

Immunohistochemically, the tumor displays diffuse reactivity for vimentin and no reactivity for SMA, MSA, desmin, S100, or myogenin.

Identification of BCOR internal tandem duplication (the same genetic alteration detected in kidney clear cell sarcoma → see dedicated section) and/or nuclear immunoreactivity for BCOR or BCL6 can aid in the diagnosis of PMMTI and help to differentiate it from congenital infantile fibrosarcoma.

S. Mocellin, *Soft Tissue Tumors*, https://doi.org/10.1007/978-3-030-58710-9_211

Prognosis

PMMTI is an intermediate-grade malignancy with a high local recurrence rate but low metastatic potential.

Therapy

Surgical excision is the mainstay of treatment. Response to chemotherapy has been reported to be scarce.

Suggested Readings

Alaggio (2006) Primitive myxoid mesenchymal tumor of infancy: a clinicopathologic report of 6 cases. Am J Surg Pathol 30(3):388–394

Asaftei (2020) Management of unresectable metastatic primitive myxoid mesenchymal tumor of infancy: a case report and systematic review of the literature. J Pediatr Hematol Oncol 42(3):163–169

Astolfi (2019) BCOR involvement in cancer. Epigenomics 11(7):835–855

Cramer (2017) Successful treatment of recurrent primitive myxoid mesenchymal tumor of infancy with BCOR internal tandem duplication. J Natl Compr Canc Netw 15(7):868–871

Foster (2016) Primitive myxoid mesenchymal tumor of infancy involving chest wall in an infant: a case report and clinicopathologic correlation. Pediatr Dev Pathol 19(3):244–248

Hayes (2020) Primitive myxoid mesenchymal tumor of infancy in the orbit: a new location for a rare tumor. Ophthalmic Plast Reconstr Surg [Epub ahead of print]

Santiago (2017) Recurrent BCOR internal tandem duplication and BCOR or BCL6 expression distinguish primitive myxoid mesenchymal tumor of infancy from congenital infantile fibrosarcoma. Mod Pathol 30(6):884–891

Definition

Proliferative fasciitis is a mass-forming subcutaneous benign tumor made in part of fibroblastic/myofibroblastic cells similar to those found in nodular fasciitis.

Epidemiology and Presentation

Proliferative fasciitis is much less frequent than nodular fasciitis. It develops mainly in middle-aged or older adults (i.e., in people older than those affected with nodular fasciitis) within the subcutaneous tissue. The most frequent site involved is the upper extremity, followed by the lower extremity and trunk.

Due to rapid growth and pain, proliferative fasciitis is usually diagnosed early when it measures only a few centimeters.

Pathology

The mass is poorly circumscribed and is characterized by the proliferation of plump fibroblastic/myofibroblastic cells similar to those found in nodular fasciitis as well as large ganglion-like cells which can be multinucleated. Mitotic figures are found in both spindle cells and ganglion-like cells, without atypia.

Unlike nodular fasciitis, proliferative fasciitis shows ganglion-like cells. Proliferative myositis is histologically identical, but the location is intramuscular. Proliferative fasciitis differs from ganglioneuroma because ganglion cells and spindle cells are positive for neural markers (e.g., S100).

This benign neoplasm may also require differential diagnosis with malignant soft tissue tumors (it is considered a pseudosarcomatous lesion) which often display nuclear atypia, pleomorphism, atypical mitotic figures, and tumor necrosis and stain positive for specific types of cell differentiation (such as desmin and myogenin in rhabdomyosarcoma).

Biomarkers

The immunohistochemical pattern of this neoplasm resembles that of nodular fasciitis, with spindle cells usually staining positive for SMA[1] and MSA.[2] The ganglion-like cells usually stain positive for vimentin (and negative for actins). Staining for S100, desmin, and cytokeratins is negative.

Prognosis

Proliferative fasciitis is a benign neoplasm that rarely relapses after conservative surgical excision. It does not metastasize.

Therapy

Surgical excision is the mainstay of treatment (if needed for diagnostic purposes or desired by the patient).

Suggested Readings

Fletcher. WHO classification of tumours of soft tissue and bone, 5th edition. 2020.
Forcucci. Benign soft tissue lesions that may mimic malignancy. Semin Diagn Pathol. 2016;33(1):50–9.
Nishi. Proliferative fasciitis/myositis involving the facial muscles including the masseter muscle: a rare cause of trismus. Am J Case Rep. 2019;20:1411–7.
Preziosi. Proliferative fasciitis of the hand in a nine-year-old girl: a case report and review of the literature. Cureus. 2020;12(1):e6763.

---

[1] SMA: smooth muscle actin.

[2] MSA: muscle-specific actin.

Definition

Proliferative myositis is a mass-forming intramuscular benign tumor made in part of fibroblastic/myofibroblastic cells similar to those found in nodular fasciitis.

Epidemiology and Presentation

Proliferative myositis is much less frequent than nodular fasciitis. It develops mainly in middle-aged or older adults (i.e., in people older than those affected with nodular fasciitis) within skeletal muscles. The most frequent site involved is the upper extremity, followed by the lower extremity and trunk.

Due to rapid growth and pain, proliferative myositis is usually diagnosed early when it measures only a few centimeters.

Pathology

The mass is poorly circumscribed and is characterized by the proliferation of plump fibroblastic/myofibroblastic cells similar to those found in nodular fasciitis as well as large ganglion-like cells which can be multinucleated. Mitotic figures are found in both spindle cells and ganglion-like cells, without atypia.

Unlike nodular fasciitis, proliferative myositis shows ganglion-like cells. Proliferative fasciitis is histologically identical, but the location is subcutaneous. Proliferative myositis differs from ganglioneuroma because ganglion cells and spindle cells are positive for neural markers (e.g., S100).

This benign neoplasm may also require **differential diagnosis** with malignant soft tissue tumors (proliferative myositis is considered a pseudosarcomatous lesion) which often display nuclear atypia, pleomorphism, atypical mitotic figures, and

© The Editor(s) (if applicable) and The Author(s), under exclusive license to
Springer Nature Switzerland AG 2021
S. Mocellin, *Soft Tissue Tumors*, https://doi.org/10.1007/978-3-030-58710-9_213

tumor necrosis and stain positive for specific types of cell differentiation (such as desmin and myogenin in rhabdomyosarcoma).

Biomarkers

The immunohistochemical pattern of this neoplasm resembles that of nodular fasciitis, with spindle cells usually staining positive for SMA[1] and MSA.[2] The ganglion-like cells usually stain positive for vimentin (and negative for actins). Staining for S100, desmin, and cytokeratins is negative.

Prognosis

Proliferative myositis is a benign neoplasm that rarely relapses after conservative surgical excision. It does not metastasize.

Therapy

Surgical excision is the treatment of choice (if needed for diagnostic purposes or desired by the patient).

Suggested Readings

Fletcher (2020) WHO classification of tumours of soft tissue and bone, 5th edition
Forcucci (2016) Benign soft tissue lesions that may mimic malignancy. Semin Diagn Pathol 33(1):50–59
Gan (2019) Proliferative myositis and nodular fasciitis: a retrospective study with clinicopathologic and radiologic correlation. Int J Clin Exp Pathol 12(12):4319–4328

---

[1] SMA: smooth muscle actin.

[2] MSA: muscle-specific actin.

Definition

Prostate stromal tumor of uncertain malignant potential (pSTUMP) is a prostatic mesenchymal neoplasm with borderline malignancy. It is also known as prostatic STUMP.

Epidemiology and Presentation

pSTUMP is a rare prostatic tumor occurring in men with a broad age range (median age: 58 years). It usually presents with urinary obstruction, other signs/symptoms being hematuria, hematospermia, and rectal fullness. Along with prostatic stromal sarcoma (→ see dedicated section), prostatic STUMP belongs to the prostatic stromal tumor family.

Pathology

pSTUMP is characterized by atypical stromal cells that insinuate between benign acini, with rare to no mitotic activity and no necrosis. Four patterns of pSTUMP have been described, all sharing stromal degenerative atypia (featuring vacuolated nuclei with degenerative/smudged chromatin): (A) hypercellular stroma with scattered degenerative atypia (50% of cases); (B) hypercellular stroma with bland spindle stromal cells; (C) breast phyllodes tumor (benign subtype) resembling STUMP, with "leaf-like" growth of hypocellular fibrous stroma surfaced by benign prostate epithelium; and (D) myxoid stroma with bland cells, lacking the nodularity seen in benign prostatic hyperplasia.

Differential diagnosis may be needed with the following: carcinosarcoma (features both epithelial and stromal components and thus is cytokeratin positive); sarcomatoid carcinoma (malignant stroma cells; epithelial cells are cytokeratin and

© The Editor(s) (if applicable) and The Author(s), under exclusive license to
Springer Nature Switzerland AG 2021
S. Mocellin, *Soft Tissue Tumors*, https://doi.org/10.1007/978-3-030-58710-9_214

ERG positive); and stromal nodule of nodular hyperplasia/benign prostatic hyperplasia (hyperplastic, not atypical stromal cells).

Biomarkers

CD34 and vimentin are most often positive (CD34 positivity helps rule out smooth muscle proliferations). As pSTUMP arises from specialized, hormonally responsive prostatic stromal cells, hormonal receptor immunostains are usually positive (progesterone receptor and androgen receptor).

pSTUMP should be cytokeratin negative, ruling out sarcomatoid carcinoma.

Prognosis

pSTUMP has a variable and unpredictable clinical course. Many pSTUMPs are incidental findings and behave indolently; however, a minority recurs after surgery or (even more rarely) metastasizes; progression to stromal sarcoma has been rarely reported.

Therapy

Surgery is the mainstay of treatment (due to their unpredictable malignant potential, patients also need close follow-up).

Suggested Readings

Leong (2019) Prostatic stromal tumors of uncertain malignant potential. Urology 132:e3–e4
McKenney (2018) Mesenchymal tumors of the prostate. Mod Pathol 31(S1):S133–S142
Murer (2014) Stromal tumor of uncertain malignant potential of the prostate. Arch Pathol Lab Med 138(11):1542–1545
Yamazaki (2020) CT and MRI findings of a stromal tumour of uncertain malignant potential of the prostate. Eur J Radiol Open 7:100233

Soft tissue tumors account for less than 1% of the prostatic tumors. Although prostate sarcomatoid carcinoma and carcinosarcoma are classified among prostatic carcinomas, they should be considered for the differential diagnosis with prostatic soft tissue tumors: biomarkers such as cytokeratins and PSA are useful for this purpose. Unfortunately, the spindle cell component of sarcomatoid carcinoma may lose the expression of epithelial (e.g., cytokeratins) and prostatic (e.g., PSA) specific biomarkers: in these cases, the pathological distinction between a sarcomatoid carcinoma and a prostatic sarcoma may be difficult or even impossible.

In addition, gastrointestinal stromal tumor (GIST → see dedicated section) of the rectum infiltrating the prostate should be taken into consideration for the differential diagnosis with primary prostate soft tissue tumors (biomarkers such as CD117 and DOG1 are useful for this purpose).

Among prostate soft tissue tumors, stromal proliferations/neoplasms represent the most frequent lesions. The below table is the list of the prostatic soft tissue tumors according to the 2016 classification of the World Health Organization. Of note, this classification does not consider other prostate soft tissue tumors (e.g., schwannoma) that are covered in this book.

For details on each single tumor, → see dedicated sections.

Tumor	Notes
Prostate stromal tumor of uncertain malignant potential	Also known as prostatic STUMP
Prostate stromal sarcoma	–
Solitary fibrous tumor	It may have significant histological overlap with prostatic stromal neoplasia and florid stromal hyperplasia
Leiomyoma	The distinction from prostatic stromal hyperplasia may be particularly difficult
Leiomyosarcoma	Though in its rarity, it is one of the most frequent types of prostate sarcomas in adults

© The Editor(s) (if applicable) and The Author(s), under exclusive license to
Springer Nature Switzerland AG 2021
S. Mocellin, *Soft Tissue Tumors*, https://doi.org/10.1007/978-3-030-58710-9_215

Tumor	Notes
Hemangioma	–
Inflammatory myofibroblastic tumor	Myofibroblastic proliferations may occur in the prostate but are much less common than those observed in the urinary bladder
Rhabdomyosarcoma	Rhabdomyosarcoma involving the prostate is usually of the embryonal subtype and occurs predominantly in children (it is the most frequent type of prostate sarcoma in this population). Correct diagnosis is critical because pediatric rhabdomyosarcoma of the genitourinary tract is associated with high cure rates with appropriate standard therapy
Undifferentiated pleomorphic sarcoma	It can be a radiation-induced tumor
Osteosarcoma	It can be a radiation-induced tumor
Angiosarcoma	It can be a radiation-induced tumor
Granular cell tumor	–
Synovial sarcoma	–

Definition

Prostate stromal sarcoma (PSS) is a malignant tumor putatively derived from prostatic specialized stroma.

Epidemiology and Presentation

PSS is a very rare malignancy (likely 0.1% of all prostate cancers) occurring on average in men aged 60 years (range 30–80 years).

The majority of patients presents with lower urinary tract obstructive symptoms, with PSA[1] plasma levels being usually normal. Along with prostatic stromal tumor of uncertain malignant potential (prostatic STUMP, → see dedicated section), PSS belongs to the prostatic stromal tumor family.

Pathology

PSS is a spindle cell tumor that usually presents as a single mass extending outside the prostate. Tumor cells show pleomorphism and atypia; mitotic activity and necrosis are usually present.

A variant including an epithelial component is called prostate phyllodes tumor (the counterpart of breast phyllodes tumor; → see dedicated section).

Differential diagnosis may be needed with the following: prostatic STUMP (more common, no marked atypia or necrosis); leiomyosarcoma (much more common; consistently positive for smooth muscle markers); GIST (CD117 positive); and sarcomatoid carcinoma (cytokeratin positive).

---

[1] PSA: prostate-specific antigen.

Biomarkers

At immunohistochemistry stromal cells are positive for vimentin, CD34, and progesterone receptor, whereas they stain negative for S100, CD117, and estrogen receptor. The phyllodes variant is PSA (see Footnote 1) and PSAP[2] positive in the epithelial component.

Prognosis

PSS is a malignancy characterized by high recurrence rates and metastatic potential. Based on mitotic rate, necrosis, and degree of atypia, this tumor can be categorized into low-grade PSS (locally aggressive) and high-grade PSS (metastatic potential).

Therapy

Surgical excision is usually combined with radiotherapy and/or chemotherapy to improve disease control.

Suggested Readings

Henry (2019) Stromal sarcoma of the prostate. Can J Urol 26(1):9683–9685
Herawi (2006) Specialized stromal tumors of the prostate: a clinicopathologic study of 50 cases. Am J Surg Pathol 30(6):694–704
McKenney (2018) Mesenchymal tumors of the prostate. Mod Pathol 31(S1):S133–S142
Tavora (2013) Mesenchymal tumours of the bladder and prostate: an update. Pathology 45(2):104–115

---

[2] PSAP: prostatic acid phosphatase.

Definition

Pseudoangiomatous stromal hyperplasia (PASH) is a benign lesion of myofibroblastic origin classified by the World Health Organization among the mesenchymal tumors of the breast. It is also known as pseudoangiomatous hyperplasia of mammary stroma.

Epidemiology and Presentation

PASH usually occurs in women aged between 20 and 50 years. It can occur also in men with gynecomastia and rarely in children. Generally, it is an incidental finding, but it may present as a nodular (single or multiple) lesion with rapid growth. Usually unilateral and well circumscribed, the lesion size ranges between 2 and 15 cm.

Pathology

Macroscopically it may resemble fibroadenoma; no hemorrhage or necrosis is present. Microscopically, PASH is composed of stromal elements (fibroblastic/myofibroblastic) mixed with breast ducts. Dense keloid-like stroma has anastomosing pattern of slit-like clefts (empty spaces) lined by single layer of flat spindle cells simulating vascular spaces. Rarely, multinucleated giant cells can be observed. Mitotic figures, necrosis, and atypia are lacking.

Differential diagnosis may be needed with low-grade angiosarcoma (hemorrhagic, anastomosing vascular channels containing red blood cells with invasion into breast parenchyma; papillary endothelial growth and hyperchromatic endothelial cells; positive for CD31 and Factor VIII).

© The Editor(s) (if applicable) and The Author(s), under exclusive license to
Springer Nature Switzerland AG 2021
S. Mocellin, *Soft Tissue Tumors*, https://doi.org/10.1007/978-3-030-58710-9_217

Biomarkers

Spindle cells stains positive for progesterone receptor, estrogen receptor, and androgen receptor, vimentin, and CD34; they stain negative for Factor VIII, CD31, and cytokeratin.

Prognosis

Although benign, PASH recurs in 10–35% of cases.

Therapy

Surgery is the treatment of choice. Breast conserving resection is the goal, but mastectomy may be required for larger or diffuse lesions (also based on the disease/breast ratio). Axillary dissection is not recommended since no lymph node involvement is expected.

Suggested Readings

Lee (2016) Pseudoangiomatous stromal hyperplasia presenting as rapidly growing bilateral breast enlargement refractory to surgical excision. Arch Plast Surg 43(2):218–221

Maciolek (2019) Pseudoangiomatous stromal hyperplasia of the breast: a rare finding in a male patient. Cureus 11(6):e4923

Naso (2019) Benign spindle cell lesions of the breast: a diagnostic approach to solitary fibrous tumour, nodular pseudoangiomatous stromal hyperplasia and nodular fasciitis. J Clin Pathol 72(6):438–442

Rapp (2018) Pseudoangiomatous stromal hyperplasia of the prostate: report of an unprecedented entity in prostate pathology. Int J Clin Exp Pathol 11(11):5486–5490

Smilg (2018) Pseudoangiomatous stromal hyperplasia: presentation and management—a clinical perspective. SA J Radiol 22(2):1366

Surace (2020) Pseudoangiomatous stromal hyperplasia (PASH) of the breast: an uncommon finding in an uncommon patient. Am J Case Rep 21:e919856

Definition

Pseudomyogenic hemangioendothelioma (PHE) is a vascular tumor of vascular origin with an intermediate biological aggressiveness.

PHE is also known as epithelioid sarcoma-like hemangioendothelioma.

Epidemiology and Presentation

PHE is a very rare tumor that occurs more frequently in young (mean age: 60 years) adult males (M:F = 4:1). It predominantly affects the lower limbs and presents as painless (50%) or painful (50%) cutaneous and subcutaneous nodules (usually 1–3 cm in size) of short preoperative duration.

In two thirds of cases, the disease is multifocal and involves multiple tissue planes (half patients have intramuscular lesions, and 20% of patients have lytic bone lesions).

Upon positron emission tomography, PHE is highly emitting, which can be helpful to detect deep lesions in patients with superficial nodules.

Pathology

Histologically, PHE (which shows infiltrative margins) resembles a myxoid tumor or epithelioid sarcoma. In fact, the tumor is composed of sheets and fascicles of plump spindle cells resembling rhabdomyoblasts; at the same time, a minority of cells have epithelioid cytomorphology. Nuclear atypia is usually mild, mitotic activity is scarce, and pleomorphism is present in a minority of cases.

Biomarkers

PHE cells stain positive for cytokeratins; positivity for CD31 is demonstrated in half cases. Staining for EMA,[1] S100 protein, CD34, and desmin is consistently negative. As opposed to epithelioid sarcoma, INI1 expression is present in neoplastic cells.

The **chromosomal translocation** t(7;19)(q22;q13)—leading to the formation of the SERPINE1-FOSB fusion gene[2]—has been recently identified as a consistent genetic alteration in PHE; less frequently, ACTB-FOSB and WWTR1-FOSB fusion genes have been described.

Prognosis

PHE is a rarely metastasizing endothelial neoplasm which recurs in up to 60% of patients. The rare metastatic disease localizes to the lymph nodes, lung, bone, scalp, and soft tissues.

Therapy

Surgical excision is the treatment of choice.

Suggested Readings

Al-Qaderi. Pseudomyogenic hemangioendothelioma. Arch Pathol Lab Med. 2019;143(6):763–7.
Fletcher. WHO classification of tumours of soft tissue and bone, 5th edition. 2020.
Hung. FOSB is a useful diagnostic marker for pseudomyogenic hemangioendothelioma. Am J Surg Pathol. 2017;41(5):596–606.
Liu. Pseudomyogenic hemangioendothelioma: distinctive FDG PET/CT findings with numerous multilayer lesions in a single distal extremity. Clin Nucl Med. 2020;45(3):248–9.
Panagopoulos. Fusion of the Genes WWTR1 and FOSB in Pseudomyogenic Hemangioendothelioma. Cancer Genomics Proteomics. 2019;16(4):293–8.
Pradhan. Pseudomyogenic hemangioendothelioma of skin, bone and soft tissue-a clinicopathological, immunohistochemical, and fluorescence in situ hybridization study. Hum Pathol. 2018;71:126–34.
Shon. Epithelioid vascular tumors: a review. Adv Anat Pathol. 2019;26(3):186–97.

---

[1] EMA: epithelial membrane antigen.

[2] SERPINE1-FOSB fusion gene: SERPINE1 (serpin family E member 1) encodes a member of the serine proteinase inhibitor (serpin) superfamily; this member acts as an inhibitor of fibrinolysis, since it is the main inhibitor of tissue plasminogen activator (tPA) and urokinase (uPA). FOSB (FosB proto-oncogene, also known as AP-1 transcription factor subunit) encodes one of the four members of the Fos gene family (the others being FOS, FOSL1, and FOSL2): these genes encode leucine zipper proteins that can dimerize with proteins of the JUN family, thereby forming the transcription factor complex AP-1 (which in turn is implicated in cell proliferation, differentiation, and transformation).

Definition

Pulmonary myxoid sarcoma (PMS) is a mesenchymal malignancy of the lungs; the cells of origin might be primitive mesenchymal cells with myofibroblastic or fibroblastic differentiation. It is also known as primary pulmonary myxoid sarcoma and low-grade malignant myxoid endobronchial tumor.

Epidemiology and Presentation

PMS is a rare sarcoma arising inside or close to the large airways (i.e., bronchi) of middle-aged adults (mean age: 45 years), with a slight female preponderance. It mainly presents with cough and hemoptysis, but it can be an incidental finding at radiological imaging of the chest.

Etiology and Predisposition

A smoking history is present in 80% of cases.

Pathology

PMS is composed of spindle and stellate cells arranged in clusters and cords embedded in a prominent myxoid stroma.

Differential diagnosis may be needed with the following: metastatic extraskeletal myxoid chondrosarcoma (history of primary soft tissue sarcoma; S100 positive; it carries EWSR1-NR4A3 fusion gene); angiomatoid fibrous histiocytoma (peripheral lymphoid cuff; it carries EWSR1-ATF1 fusion gene); inflammatory myofibroblastic tumor (often positive for ALK rearrangements); and myoepithelioma (clear

S. Mocellin, *Soft Tissue Tumors*, https://doi.org/10.1007/978-3-030-58710-9_219

and plasmacytoid cells; positive for myoepithelial biomarkers such as cytokeratins, S100, calponin).

Biomarkers

PMS stains positive for EMA[1] and vimentin. It stains negative for most other biomarkers such as S100, cytokeratins, CD34, CD31, SMA,[2] MSA,[3] desmin, TTF1, and calretinin.

PMS is characterized (about 85% of cases) by the **chromosomal translocation** t(2;22)(q33;q12), which leads to the formation of the EWSR1-CREB1 fusion gene.[4]

Prognosis

PMS is a low-grade malignancy, although distant metastases have been described in some cases.

Therapy

Surgery is the mainstay of treatment.

Suggested Readings

Chen (2020) Primary pulmonary myxoid sarcoma with EWSR1-CREB1 fusion: a case report and review of the literature. Diagn Pathol 15(1):15
Koelsche (2019) Primary pulmonary myxoid sarcoma with an unusual gene fusion between exon 7 of EWSR1 and exon 5 of CREB1. Virchows Arch. https://doi.org/10.1007/s00428-019-02716-4 [Epub ahead of print]

---

[1] EMA: epithelial membrane antigen.

[2] SMA: smooth muscle actin.

[3] MSA: muscle-specific actin.

[4] EWSR1-CREB1 fusion gene: EWSR1 encodes for an RNA-binding protein and is involved in the recurrent translocations associated with a number of soft tissue tumors other than angiomatoid fibrous histiocytoma such as the Ewing family of tumors, desmoplastic small round cell tumor, extraskeletal myxoid chondrosarcoma, myxoid liposarcoma (rarely), and clear cell sarcoma. CREB1 (cyclic AMP responsive-binding protein) encodes a basic leucine zipper transcription factor that is involved in cAMP and calcium-induced transcriptional activation. The EWSR1-CREB1 chimeric protein is believed to play a key role in oncogenesis. In particular, the formation of the EWSR1-CREB1 fusion gene leads to continuous activation of CREB1 and IL-6 production, because the promoter region of IL-6 has a CREB-binding site. IL-6 might be responsible of both paraneoplastic syndrome and tumor growth (by means of an autocrine loop).

Prieto-Granada (2017) Primary pulmonary myxoid sarcoma: a newly described entity-report of a case and review of the literature. Int J Surg Pathol 25(6):518–525

Thway (2012) Tumors with EWSR1-CREB1 and EWSR1-ATF1 fusions: the current status. Am J Surg Pathol 36(7):e1–e11

Yanagida (2017) Primary pulmonary myxoid sarcoma, a potential mimic of metastatic extraskeletal myxoid chondrosarcoma. Pathology 49(7):792–794

Definition

Pyogenic granuloma is a benign vascular tumor. It is also known as lobular capillary hemangioma and granuloma pyogenicum.

Epidemiology and Presentation

This is a common cutaneous lesion that usually presents as a rapidly growing polypoid red nodule surrounded by thickened epidermis, often in the fingers. It affects more often children and young adults and may be associated with keratinous cyst. Pyogenic granuloma can arise spontaneously, in sites of injury, as a result of chemotherapy, or within capillary malformations (e.g., port-wine stains).

Several variants have been described: classic polypoid, dermal, subcutaneous, intravenous, eruptive, or with multiple satellites. Pyogenic granuloma can also occur in mucous membranes (such as those of lips, oral cavity, and more rarely gastrointestinal tract).

Pathology

The lesion presents with a lobular pattern of vascular proliferation with inflammation and edema mimicking granulation tissue. The overlying epidermis is thin and can ulcerate; acanthosis and hyperkeratosis can be present at sides. The central branching vessel is called capillary or vascular lobule, with no/rare red blood cells, surrounded by endothelial cells. Mitotic activity is variable.

Differential diagnosis may be needed with the following: acrodermatitis, bacillary angiomatosis, benign (infantile) hemangioendothelioma, and reactive angioendotheliomatosis.

Biomarkers

Pyogenic granuloma stains positive for CD34 and usually positive for WT1 (which has been reported to be helpful in differentiating vascular neoplasms from vascular malformations). It stains negative for GLUT1 (positive in infantile hemangioma) and lymphatic biomarkers (D2–40, Prox-1, and LYVE-1).

Prognosis

Pyogenic granuloma is a benign lesion; spontaneous regression has been observed. It may recur as multiple satellites.

Therapy

Even though it is a benign tumor, treatment is often required due to associated risk of ulceration and bleeding, cosmetic concerns, and the low likelihood of spontaneous regression. Treatment options include excisional surgery, cryotherapy, electrocautery, laser ablation, and topical medical therapy with silver nitrate, phenol, podophyllin, imiquimod, and oral and topical beta-blockers (such as timolol, propranolol, and betaxolol). However, recurrence is a major problem.

Suggested Readings

Dany (2019) Beta-blockers for pyogenic granuloma: a systematic review of case reports, case series, and clinical trials. J Drugs Dermatol 18(10):1006–1010

Hayashi (2019) Clinical and endoscopic characteristics of pyogenic granuloma in the small intestine: a case series with literature review. Intern Med 59:501–505. https://doi.org/10.2169/internalmedicine.3745-19 [Epub ahead of print]

Johnson (2018) Vascular tumors in infants: case report and review of clinical, histopathologic, and immunohistochemical characteristics of infantile hemangioma, pyogenic granuloma, noninvoluting congenital hemangioma, tufted angioma, and kaposiform hemangioendothelioma. Am J Dermatopathol 40(4):231–239

Plachouri (2019) Therapeutic approaches to pyogenic granuloma: an updated review. Int J Dermatol 58(6):642–648

Definition

Retiform hemangioendothelioma (RHE) is a vascular tumor of intermediate aggressiveness.

It is also known as hobnail hemangioendothelioma.

Epidemiology and Presentation

RHE is a very rare neoplasm. It most commonly affects children or young adults, with no gender predilection.

RHE usually arises in the skin of the extremities, mainly the lower limbs. It appears as a red or blue slow-growing plaque or nodule, generally less than 3 cm in diameter.

Pathology

Microscopically it presents with distinctive arborizing blood vessels (which mimic the normal rete testis) lined by endothelial cells with typical hobnail morphology. Mitotic figures are rare, and pleomorphism is absent. RHE can be one of the components of composite hemangioendothelioma (→ see dedicated section).

Biomarkers

Tumor cells in RHE stain positive for vascular biomarkers (e.g., CD31 and CD34). CLDN5 has been proposed as a reliable biomarker for RHE (along with other vascular tumors). As regards lymphatic biomarkers, RHE stains positive for PROX1 but negative for podoplanin and VEGFR3. RHE is negative for HHV8.

S. Mocellin, *Soft Tissue Tumors*, https://doi.org/10.1007/978-3-030-58710-9_221

Prognosis

RHE is a locally aggressive, rarely metastasizing tumor. Local recurrence occurs in up to 60% of cases. The rare metastatic disease (mainly located in the lymph nodes) has not been associated with death.

Therapy

Surgical excision is the treatment of choice.

Suggested Readings

Fletcher. WHO classification of tumours of soft tissue and bone, 5th edition. 2020.
Nobeyama. Retiform hemangioendothelioma treated with conservative therapy: report of a case and review of the literature. Int J Dermatol. 2016;55(2):238–43.
Ranga. Retiform hemangioendothelioma: an uncommon pediatric vascular neoplasm. Indian J Dermatol. 2014;59(6):633.

Definition

Rhabdoid tumor is a malignant neoplasm first described as a rhabdoid variant of Wilms tumor in the kidney. Although the term rhabdoid is derived from the histologic resemblance of tumor cells to rhabdomyoblasts, the cell of origin is still undefined. Rhabdoid tumor is characterized by loss of expression of SMARC proteins ($\rightarrow$ see also Chap. 229).

It is also known as atypical teratoid rhabdoid tumor (ATRT, when localized in the central nervous system), rhabdoid tumor of the kidney (RTK), extra-central nervous system rhabdoid tumor, extracranial extrarenal rhabdoid tumor, and malignant rhabdoid tumor (MRT). Extracranial extrarenal rhabdoid tumor is also known as rhabdoid tumor of soft tissue ($\rightarrow$ see Chap. 89).

Epidemiology and Presentation

Rhabdoid tumor is a rare malignancy occurring mainly in infants and children younger than age 3 years (although adult cases have been reported). The age-standardized annual incidence rate is between 5 (extracranial rhabdoid tumors) and 8 per million (atypical teratoid/rhabdoid tumor) in children younger than age 1 year and decreases to between 0.6 and 2.2 per million at ages 1–4 years. Rhabdoid tumor can arise in almost any anatomic location: commonly in the central nervous system (ATRT, more than 50% in the cerebellum) but also in the kidney (RTK) and in extra-cranial extrarenal sites (e.g., head and neck, paravertebral muscles, liver, bladder, mediastinum, retroperitoneum, pelvis, and heart).

Clinical presentation is dominated by the signs and symptoms related to the tumor mass effect on adjacent structures. The tumor may occur as a single disease or as a multifocal disease (synchronous or metachronous): distinguishing primary multifocal disease in the setting of SMARCB1 germline mutations from oligometastatic disease is basically arbitrary or impossible.

© The Editor(s) (if applicable) and The Author(s), under exclusive license to
Springer Nature Switzerland AG 2021
S. Mocellin, *Soft Tissue Tumors*, https://doi.org/10.1007/978-3-030-58710-9_222

Etiology and Predisposition

Rhabdoid tumor can develop as sporadic neoplasms but also within the frame of a hereditary condition known as **rhabdoid tumor predisposition syndrome** (RTPS). In both cases, biallelic inactivation of tumor suppressor gene SMARCB1[1] (most frequently) or SMARCA4[2] (sometimes) is typically found in tumor cells. Individuals with RTPS typically present before age 12 months with synchronous tumors that exhibit aggressive clinical behavior. RTPS predisposes also to the development of small cell carcinoma of the ovary hypercalcemic type (SCCOHT), an entity related to rhabdoid tumors and characterized by loss of SMARCA4 (not SMARCB1) expression. The diagnosis of RTPS is established in a proband with a rhabdoid tumor and/or a family history of rhabdoid tumor and/or multiple SMARCA4- or SMARCB1-deficient tumors (synchronous or metachronous) and identification of a germline heterozygous pathogenic variant in SMARCA4 or SMARCB1 by molecular genetic testing. Among newly diagnosed individuals with a rhabdoid tumor, 25–35% have a germline pathogenic variant in SMARCB1. RTPS is inherited in an autosomal dominant manner: the vast majority of individuals diagnosed with RTPS have the disorder as the result of a de novo germline SMARCB1 pathogenic variant. Most individuals diagnosed with RTPS inherited a pathogenic variant from an unaffected parent. Each child of an individual with a germline SMARCA4 or SMARCB1 pathogenic variant has a 50% chance of inheriting the pathogenic variant. However, penetrance appears to be incomplete, and the types of RTPS-related tumors can vary among different members of the same family. Prenatal diagnosis for pregnancies at increased risk is possible if the pathogenic variant in the family is known.

Individuals diagnosed with RTPS should be carefully followed up for secondary prevention purposes (i.e., tumor surveillance programs are necessary for early diagnosis of neoplasms).

---

[1] SMARCB1: SWI/SNF-related matrix-associated actin-dependent regulator of chromatin, subfamily B, member 1 (also known as INI1) encodes a protein which is part of the BAF (hSWI/SNF) complex that relieves repressive chromatin structures, allowing the transcriptional machinery to access its targets more effectively. This ATP-dependent chromatin-remodeling complex plays an important role in different cell activities including cell differentiation; in particular, regulation of the stem cell-associated program, which is maintained by the repressive effect of the EZH2-dependent PRC2 (polycomb repressive complex 2), is disrupted by SMARCB1. Overall, SMARCB1 has been found to act as a tumor suppressor, and its mutations have been associated with a variety of malignancies including sarcomas.

[2] SMARCA4, located at 19p13, encodes the protein BRG1 and is part of the switch/sucrose-non-fermenting (SWI/SNF) chromatin remodeling complex that is also known as the BAF (BRG1-associated factors) complex. This complex is ATP-dependent and plays an important role in transcription, differentiation, and DNA repair and has been shown to behave as a tumor-suppressing complex. Each complex contains multiple subunits, each of which contains a mutually exclusive ATPase subunit, SMARCA4 (BRG1), or SMARCA2 (BRM).

Pathology

Microscopically, rhabdoid tumor usually presents as solid sheets of large cells with deep eosinophilic cytoplasm, possible laterally displaced nucleus, prominent nucleoli (rhabdoid cells, hence the name). Myxoid, hyalinized, pseudoalveolar areas may be present. Some cases display large anaplastic cells with similar nuclear morphology but frequently with more conspicuous macronucleoli; other less common patterns include small round cell and spindled morphologies that may represent focal findings in an otherwise conventional appearance or predominate, which represents a diagnostic challenge.

As morphologic rhabdoid features may not be present in all rhabdoid tumor biopsies because of inter- and intratumoral heterogeneity, any small blue round cell tumor in infants and young children should be evaluated for absence of nuclear SMARCB1/SMARCA4 staining.

Distinguishing rhabdoid tumor of soft tissue from proximal-type (large cell) epithelioid sarcoma on morphologic grounds alone is rather arbitrary as the extent of the rhabdoid differentiation might be the only feature that helps their distinction.

The theory of pure extrarenal rhabdoid tumors as a single nosological entity has been challenged by the observation of similarly rhabdoid cells as a component in otherwise differentiated neoplasms occurring at a wider age range, leading to the concept of composite extrarenal rhabdoid tumors as a common final pathway of dedifferentiation in a variety of neoplasms; recent studies from different organs confirmed the occurrence of true composite neoplasms composed of a differentiated (organ-specific, SWI/SNF intact) and an SWI/SNF-deficient undifferentiated variably rhabdoid component driven by secondary SWI/SNF gene deletions/inactivation.

Biomarkers

Immunohistochemically rhabdoid tumor cells may express vimentin, EMA, and cytokeratins. However, rhabdoid tumors are characterized by biallelic loss of SMARCB1 (see Footnote 1) or SMARCA4 (see Footnote 2): this feature can be demonstrated both at immunohistochemistry (absence of SMARCB1 or SMARCA4 expression) and at the molecular level (presence of somatic inactivating gene mutations). In subjects with RTPS, heterozygous loss of one of these genes can be found at the germline level (e.g., in the peripheral blood mononucleated cells).

Prognosis

Rhabdoid tumor is a highly aggressive neoplasm featuring early metastases (generally to lung, liver, and lymph nodes) and poor responsiveness to therapy. It is usually fatal within 1–2 years.

Therapy

Due to the rarity and recent identification of this nosological entity, standards for management are evolving. Most patients are treated by intensive multimodal therapeutic strategies combining surgery, radiotherapy, and chemotherapy. High-dose chemotherapy (with peripheral blood stem cell rescue) combined with radiotherapy has been recently reported to provide promising results.

Theoretically, SDTS might benefit from target therapy with inhibitors of enhancer of zeste homolog (EZH2) due to their activity against tumors with abnormalities in the SWI/SNF complex proteins: of note, one such drug called tazemetostat has been recently approved by the Food and Drug Administration for the treatment of epithelioid sarcoma (→ see dedicated section), a SMARCB1 deficient tumor.

As RTPS predisposes to the development of SCCOHT, prophylactic bilateral oophorectomy may be discussed after childbearing.

Suggested Readings

Agaimy. SWI/SNF complex-deficient soft tissue neoplasms: a pattern-based approach to diagnosis and differential diagnosis. Surg Pathol Clin. 2019;12(1):149–63.

Carugo. p53 is a master regulator of proteostasis in smarcb1-deficient malignant rhabdoid tumors. Cancer Cell. 2019;35(2):204–220.e9.

Chan. A systematic review of atypical teratoid rhabdoid tumor in adults. Front Oncol. 2018;8:567.

Ma. Overall survival of primary intracranial atypical teratoid rhabdoid tumor following multimodal treatment: a pooled analysis of individual patient data. Neurosurg Rev. 2020;43(1):281–92.

Nemes. Emerging therapeutic targets for the treatment of malignant rhabdoid tumors. Expert Opin Ther Targets. 2018;22(4):365–79.

Pawel. SMARCB1-deficient tumors of childhood: a practical guide. Pediatr Dev Pathol. 2018;21(1):6–28.

Pinto. Malignant rhabdoid tumors originating within and outside the central nervous system are clinically and molecularly heterogeneous. Acta Neuropathol. 2018;136(2):315–26.

Reddy. Efficacy of high-dose chemotherapy and three-dimensional conformal radiation for atypical teratoid/rhabdoid tumor: a report from the Children's Oncology Group Trial ACNS0333. J Clin Oncol. 2020;38(11):1175–85. https://doi.org/10.1200/JCO.19.01776. [Epub ahead of print]

Voisin. Atypical teratoid/rhabdoid sellar tumor in an adult with a familial history of a germline smarcb1 mutation: case report and review of the literature. World Neurosurg. 2019;127:336–45.

The rhabdomyoma family includes the following:

(A)	Cardiac rhabdomyoma
(B)	Extra-cardiac rhabdomyoma
	(1) Adult rhabdomyoma
	(2) Fetal rhabdomyoma
	(3) Genital rhabdomyoma

For details → see sections dedicated to each subtype.

Definition

Rhabdomyosarcoma (RMS) is a high-grade malignant soft tissue tumor with phenotypical and biological features of skeletal muscle cells. It includes four subtypes: embryonal (ERMS), alveolar (ARMS), pleomorphic (PRMS), and spindle cell/sclerosing (SRMS) (for more details → see dedicated sections).

Epidemiology and Presentation

Rhabdomyosarcomas comprise the single largest category of soft tissue sarcomas in children and adolescents accounting for 5–8% of all childhood cancers (the vast majority of cases occur under the age of 18 years). RMS is the third most common pediatric extracranial solid tumor after neuroblastoma and Wilms tumor; it accounts for about 50% of all soft tissue sarcomas in the pediatric population (which include about 7% of all malignancies in this age group). In the USA, RMS annual incidence is 4.5 cases per 1,000,000 individuals aged <20 years.

More than one third (35%) of RMS occurs in the head and neck, but RMS can occur in almost any soft tissue site in the body: genitourinary (24%), parameningeal (16%), extremity (19%), orbit (9%), other head and neck (10%), and miscellaneous other sites (22%). Site involvement depends on histotype: ERMS (which represents up to 80% of all RMS cases) most commonly arises in the head and neck or in genitourinary sites, whereas ARMS (which represents up to 20% of all RMS cases) typically arises at extremity sites (with a smaller fraction arising in the head and/or neck or torso).

Symptoms of RMS depend on the location and size of the primary disease. For instance, genitourinary tumors may present with hematuria, urinary tract obstruction, and/or a scrotal or vaginal mass; lesions arising in the retroperitoneum and mediastinum can become quite large before producing signs and symptoms; parameningeal tumors may present with cranial nerve dysfunction, symptoms of

© The Editor(s) (if applicable) and The Author(s), under exclusive license to
Springer Nature Switzerland AG 2021
S. Mocellin, *Soft Tissue Tumors*, https://doi.org/10.1007/978-3-030-58710-9_224

sinusitis, ear discharge, headaches, and facial pain. Orbital tumors often present with orbital swelling and proptosis. Extremity tumors generally present as a rapidly enlarging, firm mass in the relevant tissue. However, patients can also present with an asymptomatic mass.

Etiology and Predisposition

The majority of cases of RMS are sporadic. However, RMS has been associated with some familial syndromes, including the following:

1. **Beckwith-Wiedemann syndrome**: overgrowth disorder usually present at birth, characterized by an increased risk of childhood cancer and certain congenital features such as macrosomia, macroglossia, omphalocele, and predisposition to embryonal tumors such as Wilms tumor, hepatoblastoma, neuroblastoma, and rhabdomyosarcoma.
2. **Li-Fraumeni syndrome**: rare, autosomal dominant, hereditary cancer predisposition disease due to germline mutations of the p53 tumor suppressor gene; it is also known as the sarcoma breast leukemia and adrenal gland (SBLA) syndrome due to the increased risk especially of these tumors.
3. **Neurofibromatosis type 1**: autosomal dominant complex multi-system disorder caused by inactivating germline mutations of chromosome 17 gene NF1 that is responsible for production of a protein called neurofibromin; it is characterized by the formation of neurofibromas along the nervous system
4. **Noonan syndrome**: autosomal dominant disease characterized by short height, congenital heart disease, bleeding problems, and skeletal malformations; germline mutations in the RAS/MAPK (mitogen activated protein kinase) signaling pathways genes are known to be responsible for about 70% of this cases; it belongs to the RASopathy family of disorders.
5. **Costello syndrome**: also called faciocutaneoskeletal syndrome or FCS syndrome, is a rare autosomal dominant genetic disorder and is characterized by delayed development and intellectual disabilities, distinctive facial features, unusually flexible joints, and loose folds of extra skin, especially on the hands and feet; it increases the risk of rhabdomyosarcoma and to lower extent neuroblastoma and bladder carcinoma; it is due to germline activating mutations of the mutations HRAS oncogene; it belongs to the RASopathy family of disorders.
6. **Hereditary retinoblastoma**: due to germline inactivating mutations of the RB1 tumor suppressor gene, this autosomal dominant cancer predisposition syndrome causes about one third of all retinoblastomas; as opposed to those with sporadic retinoblastoma, subjects with this hereditary syndrome typically develop retinoblastoma in both eyes and also have an increased risk of other tumors such as pineoblastoma, bone and soft tissue sarcomas, and skin melanoma; the development of retinoblastoma can be explained by the two-hit model, where one inactivated allele is inherited and the other is inactivated in somatic cells.

7. **DICER1 syndrome**: is a rare pleiotropic tumor predisposition syndrome characterized by a distinctive set of neoplasms which are generally rare and affect children and young adults. The syndrome is caused by germline pathogenic variants in the DICER1 gene which encodes the DICER1 protein, a key component of the microRNA processing pathway. Variants are typically inherited in an autosomal dominant pattern but may arise de novo in the germline or in a somatic mosaic distribution. The tumors associated with this syndrome are the following: anaplastic sarcoma of the kidney, ciliary body medulloepithelioma, central nervous system sarcoma, thyroid carcinoma, embryonal RMS, mullerian adenosarcoma, pleuropulmonary blastoma, Sertoli-Leydig cell tumor, and Wilms tumor.
8. **Gorlin syndrome**: very rarely, RMS has been associated with this condition (also known as nevoid basal cell carcinoma syndrome, NBCCS), which is due to germline PATCHED1 (PTCH1) mutations which activate the hedgehog signaling pathway.

Pathology

RMS is a malignant tumor of mesenchymal origin and is part of the group of small round blue cell tumors of childhood which include neuroblastoma, primitive mesenchymal tumors (e.g., Ewing sarcoma), and lymphoma. Open biopsy is generally recommended to obtain enough tissue for biology and chromosomal analyses. If core needle biopsies are performed, multiple passes are needed to avoid sampling error and ensuring enough tissue is available for biologic studies.

Besides the four classical subtypes (ERMS, ARMS, PRMS, and SRMS), a rare epithelioid variant (known as epithelioid rhabdomyosarcoma) has been more recently described, mainly in adults: the cohesive aggregates of large polygonal cells and the absence of rhabdomyoblastic differentiation may represent a diagnostic challenge, mimicking carcinoma or melanoma (immunohistochemical findings confirm the myogenic lineage with a diffuse positivity for desmin, a nuclear expression of myogenin in scattered cells and no S100 or cytokeratin expression).

Biomarkers

RMS usually stains positive for myogenin, muscle-specific actin (MSA), MYOD1, and desmin.

About 80% of all ARMS cases are characterized by the **chromosomal translocation** t(1;13)(p36;q14) or, less commonly, t(1;13)(p36,q15) which lead to the formation of fusion genes between PAX3 or PAX7 and FOXO1 (previously known as FKHR) ($\rightarrow$ see "Alveolar Rhabdomyosarcoma").

ERMS usually carries a loss of heterozygosity (LOH) in the short arm of chromosome 11 (p11,15.5).

For more details $\rightarrow$ see sections dedicated to each specific type of RMS.

Prognosis

Metastases arise by both lymphatic and hematogenous routes, and spreading to the lung, bone, and bone marrow is fairly common. Based upon radiological studies, distant metastatic disease is present in about 20% of children at diagnosis; however, it is generally agreed that most (if not all) patients harbor microscopic disseminated disease at presentation.

Favorable **prognostic factors** include age <10 years at diagnosis, tumor size less 5 cm, ERMS subtype, fusion-negative ARMS (about 20% of all ARMS cases), orbit and non-parameningeal head/neck primary, tumor completely excised prior to initiation of chemotherapy, and the lack of metastatic disease at diagnosis. Although the cure rates of localized disease are generally >70%, the prognosis for children with disseminated disease is poor (metastatic disease is associated with a 5-year survival rate under 20%).

All investigators agree on the fact that adult RMS is associated on average with a poorer outcome than in children (only in part because adults develop RMS with worse prognostic factors), with overall survival ranging between 20 and 50%.

RMS disease status can be described in terms of both stage (→ see Table 224.1) and clinical group (→see Table 224.2). Based on these risk stratification categories, patients can be grouped into low, intermediate, and high risk (→ see Table 224.3): accordingly, a risk-tailored therapy (also known as risk-adapted therapy) can be devised.

Recurrent RMS has a very poor prognosis, and a standard of care has not been widely accepted.

For most patients, **disease staging** generally includes bone marrow biopsy, whole-body bone scan, total body computed tomography scan, and lumbar puncture for cerebrospinal fluid evaluation. Since lymph nodal disease is present in up to 25% of all RMS, the sentinel node biopsy is recommended in all patients without clinically evident lymph node metastasis (as a staging procedure); in contrast, completion lymph node dissection in patients with positive sentinel lymph node is unnecessary as it does not improve survival.

Table 224.1 Stage grouping for rhabdomyosarcoma

Stage	Sites	Invasiveness	Size	Nodes	Metastasis
1	Orbit, head and neck (no parameningeal), genitourinary (no bladder/prostate), biliary	T1, T2	Any	N0, N1, Nx	No
2	Bladder/prostate, extremity, parameningeal, other	T1, T2	<5 cm	N0, Nx	No
3	Bladder/prostate, extremity, parameningeal, other	T1, T2	<5 cm	N1	No
			>5 cm	N0, N1, Nx	
4	Any	T1, T2		N0, N1, Nx	Yes[a]

T1 Primary tumor confined to the site of origin, *T2* Primary tumor infiltrates surrounding structures
[a]Includes positive cytology of cerebrospinal, pleural, or peritoneal fluid

Table 224.2 Clinical grouping for rhabdomyosarcoma

Clinical group	Clinical subgroup	Definition
I	NA	Localized disease, completely resected
II	NA	Total gross resection with evidence for regional disease spread
	A	Grossly resected tumor with microscopic residual
	B	Involved regional lymph nodes, completely resected without microscopic residual
	C	Involved regional lymph nodes, grossly resected with microscopic residual
III	NA	Biopsy only or partial resection with gross residual
IV	NA	Distant metastatic disease

NA Not applicable

Table 224.3 Risk grouping for rhabdomyosarcoma

Risk group	Stage	Clinical group	Histology
Low, subset 1	1	I or II	ERMS
	1	III[a]	
	2	I or II	
Low, subset 2	1	III[b]	ERMS
	3	I or II	
Intermediate	2 or 3	III	ERMS
	1, 2 or 3	I, II or III	ARMS
High	4	IV	ERMS or ARMS

[a]Site of primary tumor: orbit
[b]Site of primary tumor: non-orbit

Therapy

Usually it is a combination of surgery, chemotherapy, and radiotherapy, based on stage, histological subtype, and residual disease after surgery (this approach is called risk-adapted therapy).

Surgery is considered the initial treatment for patients with non-metastatic disease that can be removed without compromising function; unfortunately, fewer than 20% of RMS are fully resected with negative margins.

Radiotherapy is utilized after radical surgery (adjuvant setting) in case of high-risk disease or microscopic residual disease or as a primary treatment when surgery is contraindicated (e.g., it would imply loss of important organs such as eye or bladder). Adjuvant radiotherapy usually follows chemotherapy: the exception to this schedule is the presence of parameningeal tumors that have invaded the brain, spinal cord, or skull; in these cases, radiation treatment is started immediately.

Chemotherapy is utilized both in the neoadjuvant, adjuvant, and metastatic setting. In North America the standard combination is the so-called VAC regimen (vincristine + actinomycin-D + cyclophosphamide). In Europe, the standard combination is the so-called IVA regimen (ifosfamide + vincristine + actinomycin-D). In a series of randomized trials carried out in the past few decades, attempts to intensify these chemotherapy regimens have not been successful in improving outcomes. Notably, a randomized comparison of either VAC or IVA as the initial therapy (followed by VAC for all patients) showed similar outcomes.

In a recent randomized controlled trial, maintenance chemotherapy (after standard VAC regimen) with vinorelbine and continuous low-dose cyclophosphamide has shown to improve overall survival of patients with non-metastatic high-risk RMS.

Before the use of chemotherapy, treatment of non-metastatic RMS based exclusively on surgery was associated with survival rates lower than 20%; in contrast, current survival rates following multimodality treatment are approximately 70%.

Suggested Readings

Bisogno. Addition of dose-intensified doxorubicin to standard chemotherapy for rhabdomyosarcoma (EpSSG RMS 2005): a multicentre, open-label, randomised controlled, phase 3 trial. Lancet Oncol. 2018;19(8):1061–71.

Bisogno. Vinorelbine and continuous low-dose cyclophosphamide as maintenance chemotherapy in patients with high-risk rhabdomyosarcoma (RMS 2005): a multicentre, openlabel, randomised, phase 3 trial. Lancet Oncol. 2019;20(11):1566–75.

Bompas. Outcome of 449 adult patients with rhabdomyosarcoma: an observational ambispective nationwide study. Cancer Med. 2018;7(8):4023–35.

Chen. Current and future treatment strategies for rhabdomyosarcoma. Front Oncol. 2019;9:1458.

de Kock. Ten years of DICER1 mutations: provenance, distribution, and associated phenotypes. Hum Mutat. 2019;40(11):1939–53.

Garren. NRAS associated RASopathy and embryonal rhabdomyosarcoma. Am J Med Genet A. 2020;182:195–299. [Epub ahead of print].

Hettmer. Myogenic tumors in nevoid Basal cell carcinoma syndrome. J Pediatr Hematol Oncol. 2015;37(2):147–9.

Jo. Epithelioid rhabdomyosarcoma: clinicopathologic analysis of 16 cases of a morphologically distinct variant of rhabdomyosarcoma. Am J Surg Pathol. 2011;35(10):1523–30.

Leiner. The current landscape of rhabdomyosarcomas: an update. Virchows Arch. 2020;476(1):97–108.

Pappo. Rhabdomyosarcoma, ewing sarcoma, and other round cell sarcomas. J Clin Oncol. 2018;36(2):168–79.

Ramadan. Signaling pathways in rhabdomyosarcoma invasion and metastasis. Cancer Metastasis Rev. 2020;39(1):287–301.

Skapek. Rhabdomyosarcoma. Nat Rev Dis Primers. 2019;5(1):1.

Definition

Schwannoma is a tumor originating from Schwann cells and is classified among benign soft tissue tumors, although one of its variants (i.e., melanotic Schwannoma → see dedicated section) is potentially malignant.

The benign version is also known as conventional Schwannoma, neurilemmoma, neurinoma, and neuroma.

Epidemiology and Presentation

Schwannoma is a relatively common tumor affecting all ages (peak incidence in the fourth to sixth decades of life) without gender prevalence. Along with neurofibroma (→ see dedicated section), it is the most common type of benign peripheral nerve tumor in adults. It most frequently arises along the peripheral nerves of the skin and subcutis, with special regard to the extremities (mainly flexor surfaces) and head and neck. Paraspinal extramedullary lesions (e.g., mediastinal or retroperitoneal lesions of the paravertebral space) can grow through neural foramina (known as dumbbell tumor or hourglass tumor), compress adjacent structures (e.g., vessels, nerve roots, ureters), and cause bone erosion.

Although less frequently, the tumor can locate intracranially: 85% of these schwannomas develop in the cerebellopontine angle as they originate from the vestibular component of the eighth cranial nerve (acoustic nerve neurinoma or acoustic neuroma or vestibular neuroma; for more details → see section entitled "Acoustic Neuroma"). Schwannomas of other sites (e.g., spinal intramedullary, central nervous system, bone, gastrointestinal lesions) are rare.

The tumor presents as a solitary slow-growing encapsulated well-circumscribed lesion (<10 cm in size), often asymptomatic (incidentaloma on imaging studies) as pain is more frequent in schwannomatosis (→ see next paragraph). At surgery, the lesion is attached to a (usually small) nerve in about 50% of cases. Paraspinal and intraspinal lesions can cause symptoms due to the compression of nerve roots or spinal cord; hearing loss and vertigo frequently precede the diagnosis of a vestibular schwannoma. Magnetic resonance imaging is considered the best imaging technique for this type of tumor.

Etiology and Predisposition

More than 90% of schwannomas are solitary and sporadic. Multiple schwannomas are a feature of three well-defined clinical conditions:

(a) **Neurofibromatosis type 2** is caused by inactivating mutations of the NF2 tumor suppressor gene, which encodes a protein called merlin (also known as schwannomin), which is expressed particularly in Schwann cells. This condition has an estimated incidence of 1 in 33,000 people and is considered to have an autosomal dominant pattern of inheritance. Patients with neurofibromatosis type 2 carry a germline mutation of a copy of NF2: in about 50% of cases, the altered gene is inherited from an affected parent, while the remaining cases result from new mutations in the NF2 gene (i.e., occur in patients without a family history of the disease). The biallelic inactivation of the NF2 gene is then acquired through a somatic mutation. Of note, up to 33% of individuals with a de novo pathogenic NF2 variant have somatic mosaicism for the variant (somatic mosaicism refers to the occurrence of two genetically distinct populations of cells within an individual, derived from a postzygotic mutation; in contrast to inherited mutations, somatic mosaic mutations may affect only a portion of the body and are not transmitted to progeny): these individuals may have normal molecular genetic testing of NF2 in unaffected tissue (e.g., peripheral blood lymphocytes), and thus molecular genetic testing of tumor tissue may be necessary to establish the presence of somatic mosaicism. Patients with neurofibromatosis type 2 usually develop multiple schwannomas before the age of 30 years: in particular, bilateral vestibular schwannoma is the hallmark of neurofibromatosis type 2 (which is also known as bilateral acoustic neuroma, BAN). Patients may also develop meningioma (50% of patients; often multiple) and glioma (most frequently ependymoma of the cervical spinal cord). For criteria to diagnose neurofibromatosis type 2, → see Table 225.1.

(b) **Schwannomatosis** is the rarest form of neurofibromatosis (which includes neurofibromatosis type 1 and neurofibromatosis type 2). The features of schwannomatosis resemble those of neurofibromatosis type 2: however, schwannomatosis almost never includes vestibular schwannomas (a hallmark of neurofibromatosis type 2); moreover, unlike the other forms of neurofibromatosis, schwannomatosis is not associated with the development of other tumor types. Schwannomatosis usually becomes clinically apparent in early adulthood, the most common symptom being pain, which ranges from mild to severe. Other signs and symptoms depend on the location of the tumors and which nerves are affected (e.g., numbness, weakness, tingling). The life

Table 225.1 Criteria for diagnosis of neurofibromatosis type 2 (NF2)

1	Bilateral vestibular schwannoma <70 years	**Or**
2	First-degree relative family history of NF2 **and** unilateral vestibular schwannoma <70 years	**Or**
3	First-degree relative family history of NF2 **or** unilateral vestibular schwannoma **and** 2 of meningioma, cataract, glioma, neurofibroma, schwannoma, cerebral calcification (if unilateral vestibular schwannoma plus =/> 2 non-intradermal schwannomas, negative LZTR1 test is needed[a])	**Or**
4	Multiple meningiomas (2 or more) **and** 2 of unilateral vestibular schwannoma, cataract, glioma, neurofibroma, schwannoma, cerebral calcification	**Or**
5	Constitutional or mosaic pathogenic NF2 gene mutation in blood **or** identical mutations in 2 distinct tumors	

[a]Ideally the LZTR1 test should be performed in the tumor, but blood test is still useful to rule out a germline schwannomatosis condition

expectancy of people with schwannomatosis is normal. Mutations in SMARCB1 and LZTR1 tumor suppressor genes are believed to cause schwannomatosis, although other genetic changes are likely needed to trigger the development of schwannomas. In this regard, the most common somatic aberrations in schwannomas are mutations in the NF2 gene and loss of chromosome 22 (where both SMARCB1, LZTR1, and NF2 are located). Most cases of schwannomatosis are sporadic, whereas only 15% of cases run in families. The familial cases have an autosomal dominant pattern of inheritance, which means a germline mutation in one copy of the SMARCB1 or LZTR1 gene greatly increases the risk of developing schwannomas (although the penetrance is not complete). Of note, germline inactivating mutations of SMARCB1 are also the cause of rhabdoid tumor predisposition syndrome (→ see section entitled "Rhabdoid Tumor").

(c) **Gorlin syndrome**: also known as Gorlin-Koutlas syndrome and nevoid basal cell carcinoma syndrome (NBCC), this cancer predisposition syndrome is characterized by the development of multiple cutaneous basal cell carcinomas (starting from adolescence or early adulthood) and keratocystic odontogenic tumors (which may cause painful facial swelling and tooth displacement). Other tumors associated with this syndrome are schwannomas, medulloblastoma, cardiac fibroma (10% of patients), and ovarian fibroma. The estimated prevalence of Gorlin syndrome is 1 in 30,000 people: of note, while more than 1 million new cases of basal cell carcinoma are diagnosed each year in the USA, fewer than 1% of these tumors are related with this syndrome. The causal gene is PTCH1 (located in chromosome 9), a tumor suppressor gene encoding patched-1 (a receptor for the ligand sonic hedgehog). The Gorlin syndrome is inherited in an autosomal dominant pattern: in most cases, the patient inherits a PTCH1 inactivating germline mutation from one affected parent (other cases result from new mutations in the PTCH1 gene and occur in people with no history of the disorder in their family). For the tumor to develop, a somatic mutation in the second copy of the PTCH1 gene must occur during the patient lifetime (according to the classical two-hit theory proposed for hereditary retinoblastoma).

Pathology

Conventional schwannoma is a nerve sheath tumor composed of well-differentiated Schwann cells. Most lesions are encapsulated biphasic tumors with compact areas of spindle cells (Antoni A tissue) with occasional palisading (parallel rows of Schwann cell nuclei; Verocay bodies are formed by a highly ordered arrangement of Schwann cell nuclei in rows separated by fibrillary processes), alternated with loosely arranged foci (Antoni B tissue). Cytoplasmic nuclear inclusions, nuclear pleomorphism, and mitotic figures may be observed. In a minority of cases, this biphasic pattern cannot be recognized, with some tumors showing predominantly Antoni B tissue, while others lacking it.

A neurinoma with degenerative nuclear atypia or extensive hyalinization is referred to as "ancient" schwannoma. Cellular schwannoma is composed almost exclusively of Antoni A tissue without Verocay bodies: these tumors most commonly locate in paravertebral space, mediastinum, retroperitoneum, and pelvis. Plexiform schwannoma, either biphasic or cellular, involves multiple nerve fascicles or a nerve plexus: this tumor usually is diagnosed earlier in life (e.g., childhood) and arises in the skin or subcutis. Microcystic/reticular schwannoma is the rarest variant of schwannoma and is characterized by a microcyst-rich network of interconnected bland spindle cells with scant eosinophilic cytoplasm and a myxoid, fibrillary, and/or hyalinized collagenous stroma. A variant called neurofibroma/schwannoma hybrid nerve sheath tumor has also been described, which is associated with larger nerves and occurs either sporadically or in the context of schwannomatosis or neurofibromatosis type 1 or 2 ($\rightarrow$ see Chap. 128).

Due to occasional increased cellularity, hyperchromasia, presence of pleomorphic nuclei, and frequent mitotic figures, some cases of schwannoma can be misinterpreted as malignant tumors.

Differential diagnosis may be needed with the following: neurofibroma ($\rightarrow$ see Table 225.2); leiomyoma and leiomyosarcoma (negative for S100, positive for

Table 225.2 Differential diagnosis between schwannoma and neurofibroma: clinicopathological features

	Schwannoma	Neurofibroma
Epidemiology	Age: 20–50 years Gender: M = F	Age: 20–40 years Gender: M = F
Etiology	Sporadic but may occur in NF2 > NF1	Sporadic, some in NF1
Pathology	Typically encapsulated; Antoni A and Antoni B areas (alternating hypercellular and hypocellular areas)	Usually no capsule; spindle cells, shredded carrot collagen, mast cells; hypocellular, myxoid areas without hypercellular areas
Plexiform variant	Less common	More common
Biomarkers	S100: strong and diffuse Calretinin: stronger CD34: scattered Factor XIIIa: negative/focal	S100: weaker Calretinin: focal CD34: stronger Factor XIIIa: stronger
Malignant potential	Malignant transformation: extremely rare	Malignant transformation occurs in 5–15% of patients with neurofibromatosis type 1

SMA and desmin); malignant peripheral nerve sheath tumor (infiltrative growth, hypercellular, pleomorphic nuclei, and high mitotic activity; areas of geographic necrosis can show divergent differentiation; staining for S100 is weak or negative); pleomorphic hyalinizing angiectatic tumor (no capsule, infiltrative border, large ectatic vascular spaces with perivascular hyalinization, fibrin within and around vessels; negative for S100 and CD31, positive for CD34); and solitary circumscribed neuroma (palisaded encapsulated neuroma; encapsulated dermal or subcutaneous tumor which may show nuclear palisading; silver stains show the axons traversing the Schwann cells: however, they are near the capsule in schwannomas; peripheral weak EMA positivity).

Biomarkers

Schwannoma typically stains diffusely positive for S100, whereas expression of GFAP (glial fibrillary acidic protein) is less common. Collagen IV and laminin are often diffusely positive. Staining for neurofilament protein is helpful to detect entrapped intratumoral axons (found in one third of sporadic schwannomas). Cytokeratins may be positive especially in retroperitoneal and mediastinal lesions. CD34 is often positive in subcapsular areas. Schwannoma stains negative for desmin and SMA (smooth muscle actin).

Complete or partial loss of chromosome 22 is the most common cytogenetic anomaly in schwannoma, and the loss of expression of merlin (also called neurofibromin 2 or schwannomin), the protein product of the NF2 tumor suppressor gene located at 22q12, is considered a key event in schwannoma tumorigenesis. Moreover, NF2 inactivating somatic mutations have been reported in about 60% of sporadic schwannomas.

Prognosis

Conventional schwannoma is a benign tumor which does not usually relapse after complete resection. Cellular and especially plexiform variants (which involve several nerve bundles) are less amenable to complete removal without nerve damage and sometimes can only be debulked: in these cases, disease recurrence is possible. Importantly, schwannoma is not considered a precursor of malignant peripheral nerve sheath tumor (MPNST), although exceptionally rare cases of malignant transformation have been reported.

Therapy

Surgical excision is the treatment of choice. Schwannoma usually does not infiltrate the associated nerve (typically originates from a single bundle within the main nerve and grows eccentrically displacing the rest of the nerve) so it can usually be separated from it without nerve damage during surgical treatment; as the schwannoma grows larger, more fascicles are affected, making nerve damage more difficult to be avoided (of note, neurofibroma tends to form more centrally within the nerve). Stereotactic radiotherapy is being increasingly utilized for deep lesions difficult to reach/treat with surgery.

Asymptomatic deep schwannomas (e.g., retroperitoneal lesions) can be managed by image-based follow-up.

For patients with neurofibromatosis type 2 and progressive bilateral acoustic neurinomas, bevacizumab (a monoclonal antibody blocking VEGFA) is associated with hearing improvement and tumor shrinkage in 30–60% of cases.

Suggested Readings

Ahlawat. Current status and recommendations for imaging in neurofibromatosis type 1, neurofibromatosis type 2, and schwannomatosis. Skeletal Radiol. 2020;49(2):199–219.

Fletcher. WHO classification of tumours of soft tissue and bone, 5th edition. 2020.

Kehrer-Sawatzki (2017). The molecular pathogenesis of schwannomatosis, a paradigm for the co-involvement of multiple tumour suppressor genes in tumorigenesis. Hum Genet. 2017;136(2):129–48.

Lu. Efficacy and safety of bevacizumab for vestibular schwannoma in neurofibromatosis type 2: a systematic review and meta-analysis of treatment outcomes. J Neurooncol. 2019;144(2):239–48.

Ogose. The natural history of incidental retroperitoneal schwannomas. PLoS One. 2019;14(4):e0215336.

Plotkin. Neurofibromatosis and Schwannomatosis. Semin Neurol. 2018;38(1):73–85.

Plotkin. Multicenter, prospective, phase ii and biomarker study of high-dose bevacizumab as induction therapy in patients with neurofibromatosis type 2 and progressive vestibular schwannoma. J Clin Oncol. 2019;37(35):3446–54.

Ronellenfitsch. Targetable ERBB2 mutations identified in neurofibroma/schwannoma hybrid nerve sheath tumors. J Clin Invest. 2020;130(5):2488–95.

Definition

Sclerosing epithelioid fibrosarcoma (SEF) is a malignant neoplasm classified among fibroblastic-myofibroblastic tumors.

Epidemiology and Presentation

SEF occurs most frequently in middle-aged and elderly patients, without significant difference in gender distribution. This tumor is located in deep tissues, most commonly involving the lower extremity or limb girdle, followed by the upper extremity, shoulder, trunk, and head and neck body sites. Rarely, SEF has been described in the pelvis, retroperitoneum, viscera, or bone.

The lesion usually presents. Most patients present with a mass of variable dimension (most tumors are <10 cm in diameter, but some greater than 20 cm have been described), well circumscribed, lobular, or multinodular which involves deep muscles with frequent periosteal erosion. Upon plain X-rays, areas of calcification are often observed.

Pathology

SEF features epithelioid fibroblasts arranged in distinct cords and nests in a densely sclerotic, hyalinized stroma. At least a subset of SEF appears to be related to low-grade fibromyxoid sarcoma (→ see dedicated section). The lesion lacks encapsulation and frequently shows areas with infiltration of muscle or periosteum. SEF may show rare areas with more prominent pleomorphism, focal necrosis, and higher mitotic rate, but most cases display very low mitotic counts.

S. Mocellin, *Soft Tissue Tumors*, https://doi.org/10.1007/978-3-030-58710-9_226

Some SEF contain areas of conventional low-grade fibrosarcoma or areas mimicking low-grade fibromyxoid sarcoma, with transition to higher-grade fibrosarcoma especially in recurrent cases.

Differential diagnosis may be needed with the following: hyalinizing spindle cell tumor with giant rosettes (histologic subtype of low-grade fibromyxoid sarcoma with similar features plus collagen rosettes); lobular breast carcinoma (single file pattern, but cells are low grade; usually estrogen and progesterone receptor positive, cytokeratin positive); low-grade fibromyxoid sarcoma (monotonous bland nuclei, alternating hypercellular and hypocellular areas, with alternating myxoid and collagenous stroma, only focal epithelioid cells; most cases harbor FUS-CREB3L2 fusion gene); poorly differentiated carcinoma (positive for cytokeratins); sclerosing lymphoma (positive for lymphocytic biomarkers such as CD45); and synovial sarcoma (more cellular, lacks large areas of hypocellular sclerotic collagen; harbors chromosomal translocation t(X;18)).

Biomarkers

SEF stains positive for MUC4 in up to 80% of cases, whereas it stains negative for cytokeratins, CD34, SMA[1], CD68, CD45, and desmin.

The **chromosomal translocation** t(7;16)(q33;p11), resulting in the FUS-CREB3L2 fusion gene[2] (characteristic of low-grade fibromyxoid sarcoma), has been reported also in SEF (which has led to the hypothesis that the two entities are related). Other chromosomal rearrangements described in SEF lead to the formation of either EWSR1-CREB3L1 fusion gene (from t(11;22)(p11;q12)) or EWSR1-CREB3L2 fusion gene[3]. Another recently described fusion gene is that between YAP1 and KMT2A[4].

---

[1] SMA: smooth muscle actin.

[2] FUS-CREB3L2 fusion gene: it derives from the fusion of FUS (fused in sarcoma, also known as TLS: translocated in liposarcoma) located on chromosome 16p11 and CREB3L2 (cAMP-responsive element-binding protein 3-like 2) located on chromosome 17q33. FUS encodes a multifunctional protein component of the heterogeneous nuclear ribonucleoprotein (hnRNP) complex, which is involved in pre-mRNA splicing and the export of fully processed mRNA to the cytoplasm: this protein belongs to the FET family of RNA-binding proteins which are involved in regulation of gene expression, maintenance of genomic integrity, and mRNA/microRNA processing. CREB3L2 encodes a member of the oasis bZIP transcription factor family.

[3] EWSR1: EWSR1 (Ewing sarcoma breakpoint region 1) encodes a multifunctional protein that is involved in various cellular processes, including gene expression, cell signaling, and RNA processing and transport. Of note, EWSR1 is a "promiscuous" gene because it can fuse with different partner genes in phenotypically similar neoplasms or with the same genes in morphologically and behaviorally different tumors. In fact, EWSR1-based chimeric genes can be found not only in Ewing and Ewing-like sarcomas but also in other tumors such as angiomatoid fibrous histiocytoma, clear cell sarcoma, low-grade fibromyxoid sarcoma, sclerosing epithelioid fibrosarcoma, hemangioma of bone, desmoplastic small round cell tumor, extraskeletal myxoid chondrosarcoma, myoepithelial tumor of soft tissue, and myxoid liposarcoma. It must be underscored that fluorescence in situ hybridization (FISH) analysis has a significant risk of false-negative results, making next-generation sequencing (NGS)-based diagnostic tools more sensitive for detecting EWSR1 rearrangements.

[4] YAP1-KMT2A fusion gene: YAP1 encodes yes-associated protein 1, a downstream nuclear effector of the Hippo signaling pathway (which is involved in development, growth, repair, and homeo-

Prognosis

SEF is an aggressive malignant tumor with high rates of local disease recurrence (>50% of cases) as well as distant metastasis (40–80% of cases; mainly in lung, pleura, bone, and brain). Poor prognostic factors are large tumor size and proximal location.

Therapy

Surgical exeresis is the mainstay of treatment. SEF is considered a chemoresistant malignancy.

Suggested Readings

Arbajian. Recurrent EWSR1-CREB3L1 gene fusions in sclerosing epithelioid fibrosarcoma. Am J Surg Pathol. 2014;38(6):801–8.

Chew. Clinical characteristics and efficacy of chemotherapy in sclerosing epithelioid fibrosarcoma. Med Oncol. 2018;35(11):138.

Doyle. MUC4 is a sensitive and extremely useful marker for sclerosing epithelioid fibrosarcoma: association with FUS gene rearrangement. Am J Surg Pathol. 2012;36(10):1444–51.

Fletcher. WHO classification of tumours of soft tissue and bone. 5th edition.

Kao. Recurrent YAP1 and KMT2A gene rearrangements in a subset of MUC4-negative sclerosing epithelioid fibrosarcoma. Am J Surg Pathol. 2020;44(3):368–77.

Prieto-Granada. A genetic dichotomy between pure sclerosing epithelioid fibrosarcoma (SEF) and hybrid SEF/low-grade fibromyxoid sarcoma: a pathologic and molecular study of 18 cases. Genes Chromosomes Cancer. 2015;54(1):28–38.

Puls. Recurrent fusions between YAP1 and KMT2A in morphologically distinct neoplasms within the spectrum of low-grade fibromyxoid sarcoma and sclerosing epithelioid fibrosarcoma. Am J Surg Pathol. 2020;44(5):594–606.

Tsuda. Clinical and molecular characterization of primary sclerosing epithelioid fibrosarcoma of bone and review of the literature. Genes Chromosomes Cancer. 2020;59:217–24. [Epub ahead of print]

---

stasis); YAP1 is known to play a role in the development and progression of multiple cancers as a transcriptional regulator of this signaling pathway. KMT2A encodes lysine methyltransferase 2A, a transcriptional coactivator that plays an essential role in regulating gene expression during early development and hematopoiesis. The SET domain of KMT2A is responsible for its histone H3 lysine 4 (H3K4) methyltransferase activity which mediates chromatin modifications associated with epigenetic transcriptional activation. Multiple chromosomal translocations involving KMT2A are believed to play a key role in the pathogenesis of different tumors including some types of acute lymphoid and myeloid leukemias.

Definition

Sclerotic fibroma is a benign skin tumor also known as storiform collagenoma, solitary sclerotic fibroma, collagenous fibroma, and plywood fibroma.

Epidemiology and Presentation

Sclerotic fibroma is an uncommon skin tumor that occurs either sporadically (in this case the lesion is typically solitary) or, when multiple, in association with Cowden syndrome (→ see below paragraph). The average patient age is 40 years, but the age range is wide, without gender prevalence.

Clinical presentation is not specific as the lesion mostly presents as a well-circumscribed flesh-colored waxy papule or nodule. The lesion is usually asymptomatic and may arise in any cutaneous localization, although the head and neck region is more frequently affected.

Etiology and Predisposition

Sclerotic fibroma can occur in association with **Cowden syndrome**, a cancer predisposition disorder characterized by multiple hamartomas and an increased risk of developing certain types of cancer. Almost all patients develop hamartomas, most commonly found on the skin and mucous membranes (e.g., oral, nasal, and gastrointestinal). Other benign lesions associated with this disease are trichilemmomas, acral keratosis, lipomas, neuromas, and orofacial papules. The syndrome is associated with an increased risk of developing several types of cancer, particularly cancers of the breast, thyroid, and endometrium. Other cancers that have been identified in these patients include colorectal cancer, kidney cancer, and melanoma. The estimated prevalence of Cowden syndrome is about 1 in 200,000 people.

S. Mocellin, *Soft Tissue Tumors*, https://doi.org/10.1007/978-3-030-58710-9_227

Mutations of at least four genes (PTEN, SDHB, SDHD, and KLLN) have been identified in people with Cowden syndrome or Cowden-like syndromes. Most cases of Cowden syndrome and a small percentage of cases of Cowden-like syndromes result from inactivating germline mutations in the PTEN tumor suppressor gene. Both Cowden syndrome and Cowden-like syndromes are inherited in an autosomal dominant pattern.

The presence of multiple sclerotic fibromas of the skin is considered an important clue for the diagnosis of Cowden syndrome.

Pathology

Sclerotic fibroma presents as a sharply circumscribed hypocellular dermal nodule with hyalinized dense collagen arranged in whorled or plywood pattern.

Biomarkers

CD34 and vimentin are usually expressed; scattered positivity for Factor XIII may be observed. EMA, cytokeratins, S100, and NSE (neuron-specific enolase) are usually negative.

Prognosis

Sclerotic fibroma is a benign tumor. The prognosis is dictated by the development of malignant tumors in cases associated with Cowden syndrome.

Therapy

Surgical excision is the treatment of choice.

Suggested Readings

Abdaljaleel. Sclerosing dermatofibrosarcoma protuberans shows significant overlap with sclerotic fibroma in both routine and immunohistochemical analysis: a potential diagnostic pitfall. Am J Dermatopathol. 2017;39(2):83–8.

Bhambri. Solitary sclerotic fibroma. J Clin Aesthet Dermatol. 2009;2(6):36–8.

Kieselova. Multiple sclerotic fibromas of the skin: an important clue for the diagnosis of Cowden syndrome. BMJ Case Rep. 2017;2017:bcr2017221695.

Pernet. Solitary sclerotic fibroma of the skin: a possible clue for Cowden syndrome. Eur J Dermatol. 2012;22(2):278–9.

Shi. Late-stage nodular erythema elevatum diutinum mimicking sclerotic fibroma. J Cutan Pathol. 2018;45(1):94–6.

Many primary benign and malignant soft tissue tumors can affect the skin: these neoplasms arise in the dermis or in the subcutis. The most common cutaneous soft tissue sarcomas are dermatofibrosarcoma protuberans (DFSP), atypical fibroxanthoma, pleomorphic dermal sarcoma, leiomyosarcoma, Kaposi sarcoma, and angiosarcoma.

The following is the list of primary soft tissue tumors of the skin, according to the World Health Organization classification published in 2018.

For details → see sections dedicated to each single tumor.

Tumor	Notes
Acral fibromyxoma	Also known as superficial acral fibromyxoma
Aneurismal fibrous histiocytoma	–
Angiokeratoma	–
Angioleiomyoma	–
Angiolipoma	–
Angiomatoid fibrous histiocytoma	–
Angiosarcoma	–
Atypical fibrous histiocytoma	–
Atypical fibroxanthoma	–
Atypical vascular lesion	–
Benign fibrous histiocytoma (dermatofibroma)	Along with its variants
Calcifying aponeurotic fibroma	–
Cellular fibrous histiocytoma	–
Cherry hemangioma	–
Composite hemangioendothelioma	–
Congenital hemangioma	Including variants
Cutaneous epithelioid angiomatous nodule	–
Cutaneous leiomyoma	Including variants

Tumor	Notes
Cutaneous leiomyosarcoma	Including variants
Dermal nerve sheath myxoma	–
Dermatofibrosarcoma protuberans	Along with its variants
Dermatomyofibroma	Also known as cutaneous myofibroma
Desmoplastic fibroblastoma	Also known as collagenous fibroma
Elastofibroma	–
Epithelioid fibrous histiocytoma	–
Epithelioid hemangioendothelioma	–
Epithelioid hemangioma	–
Epithelioid sarcoma	–
Fibroma of tendon sheath	–
Gardner fibroma	–
Glomeruloid hemangioma	–
Glomus tumor	Including variants
Granular cell tumor	–
Hobnail hemangioma	–
Infantile hemangioma	–
Kaposi sarcoma	–
Kaposiform hemangioendothelioma	–
Lipoma	–
Lymphangioma	Also known as superficial lymphatic malformation
Malignant peripheral nerve sheath tumor	–
Microvenular hemangioma	–
Myofibroma	Including myofibromatosis
Myopericytoma	Including variants
Myxofibrosarcoma	–
Myxoinflammatory fibroblastic sarcoma	–
Neurothekeoma	–
Nevus lipomatosus superficialis	–
Nodular fasciitis	–
Neurofibroma	–
Nuchal-type fibroma	–
Perineurioma	–
Pleomorphic dermal sarcoma	Also known as cutaneous undifferentiated pleomorphic sarcoma
Pleomorphic fibroma	–
Pleomorphic lipoma	–
Pleomorphic liposarcoma	Very rare in the skin
Plexiform fibrohistiocytic tumor	–
Pseudomyogenic hemangioendothelioma	–
Pyogenic granuloma	Also known as lobular capillary hemangioma
Retiform hemangioendothelioma	–
Schwannoma	–

Tumor	Notes
Sclerotic fibroma	Also known as storiform collagenoma
Solitary circumscribed neuroma	–
Spindle cell hemangioma	–
Spindle cell lipoma	–
Superficial angiomyxoma	Also known as cutaneous myxoma
Superficial fibromatosis	Along with its variants
Tufted hemangioma	–
Well differentiated liposarcoma	Very rare in the skin

Definition

SMARC-deficient soft tissue tumors are a group of neoplasms with varying histological appearance which share the loss of SMARC genes. For a list of such neoplasms, → see Table 229.1.

For details on single tumors, → see dedicated sections.

Table 229.1 Soft tissue tumors with SMARC deficiency

Tumor	Molecular features
Rhabdoid/large cell	
Epithelioid sarcoma, proximal type	SMARCB1 loss (very rarely SMARCA4 loss)
Rhabdoid tumor, pediatric	SMARCB1 loss (98%); SMARCA4 loss (2%)
Epithelioid malignant peripheral nerve sheath tumor (MPNST)	SMARCB1 loss (50%)
SMARC-deficient thoracic sarcoma	SMARCA4 and SMARCA2 loss
SMARC-deficient uterine sarcoma	SMARCA4 or SMARCB1 loss
Epithelioid/bland histiocytoid cell	
Epithelioid sarcoma, distal type	SMARCB1 loss
Undifferentiated round cell	
Chordoma, poorly differentiated, pediatric	SMARCB1 loss
Small cell synovial sarcoma	SS18-SSX fusion + frequent SMARCB1 loss
Myxoid/chordoid	
Extraskeletal myxoid chondrosarcoma	EWSR1-NR4A3 fusion; SMARCB1 loss (20%)
Myoepithelial carcinoma (also known as myoepithelioma)	Diverse gene fusions; SMARCB1 loss (40% pediatric; 10% adults cases)
Chordoma, poorly differentiated, pediatric	SMARCB1 loss
Myxoid epithelioid sarcoma (rare)	SMARCB1 loss

Epidemiology and Presentation

For details → see sections dedicated to each single tumor.

Etiology and Predisposition

The switch/sucrose nonfermentable (SWI/SNF) complex (also called BAF complex) is a multi-subunit system composed of a large set of genes mapping to different chromosomal regions. The complex is involved in the process of chromatin remodeling and thus in transcriptional regulation: in particular, the complex relieves repressive chromatin structures (supercoiling), allowing the transcriptional machinery to access its targets more effectively. Through its enrichment at promoters and enhancers of target genes, the SWI/SNF complex determines which genes are to be expressed and, ultimately, contributes to the regulation of cell processes such as cell differentiation and proliferation. Loss of different components of the switch/sucrose nonfermentable (SWI/SNF) chromatin remodeling complex (including SMARC genes) has been increasingly recognized as a central molecular event driving the tumorigenesis of different neoplasms arising in different body sites, including some soft tissue tumors with distinctive cytoarchitectural morphology, which ranges from fully anaplastic to well-differentiated organotypical lesions.

SMARC protein family includes the following: SMARCA1 (SWI/SNF-related, matrix-associated, actin-dependent regulator of chromatin, subfamily A, member 1), SMARCA2, SMARCA4, SMARCA5, SMARCB1, SMARCC1, SMARCC2, SMARCD1, SMARCD2, SMARCD3, and SMARCE1.

Overall, the SWI/SNF complex acts as a tumor suppressor: therefore, the inactivation of any of its constituent components is frequently associated with tumor initiation and/or progression. Gene inactivation can occur somatically in sporadic SMARC-deficient tumors but has been described also as the result of germline mutations in hereditary syndromes such as the **rhabdoid tumor predisposition syndrome** (RTPS): for more details on this condition, → see Chap. 222.

Pathology

With a few exceptions, SMARCB1-deficient soft tissue tumors are characterized by the presence of a varying component of rhabdoid cells. The hallmark is the rhabdoid cell, which possesses one or two large vesicular nuclei containing a very thin rim of marginated chromatin, a centrally located eosinophilic macronucleolus, and a large paranuclear filamentous cytoplasmic inclusion (so-called rhabdoid body), which displaces the nucleus to the periphery of the cell. The term rhabdoid was first coined to indicate an aggressive variant of Wilms tumor composed of cells mimicking rhabdomyoblasts but lacking true rhabdomyosarcomatous differentiation. Subsequently, the term "malignant rhabdoid tumor" (MRT) of the kidney has been coined for this distinctive nosological entity.

The presence and extent of the rhabdoid cell component in SMARCB1-deficient neoplasms varies greatly within same tumor and among different neoplasms from being totally absent to uniformly present (100%) throughout.

SMARC-deficient neoplasms fall into one of five major morphologic (cytoarchitectural) categories: (1) prototypic rhabdoid, (2) anaplastic nondescript large cell, (3) small round cell, (4) myxoid chordoid, and (5) heterogeneous differentiated organotypical categories or variable combination thereof. For more details → see Table 229.1.

Biomarkers

SMARC gene deficiency can be detected both directly (demonstrating gene loss) but also through immunohistochemistry using staining for the protein products, such as SMARCB1 (which is also known as INI1).

Prognosis

For details → see sections dedicated to each single tumor.

Therapy

For details → see sections dedicated to each single tumor.

Suggested Readings

Agaimy. SWI/SNF complex-deficient soft tissue neoplasms: a pattern-based approach to diagnosis and differential diagnosis. Surg Pathol Clin. 2019;12(1):149–63.

Voisin. Atypical teratoid/rhabdoid sellar tumor in an adult with a familial history of a germline smarcb1 mutation: case report and review of the literature. World Neurosurg. 2019;127:336–45.

Definition

SMARC-deficient thoracic sarcoma (SDTS) is a recently defined nosological entity characterized by loss of SMARCA4 gene. It belongs to the family of SMARC-deficient sarcomas (→ see dedicated section). It is also known as SMARCA4-deficient thoracic sarcoma. A debate exists as to whether or not this entity is a true sarcoma or it represents the extreme end of an epithelial- to- mesenchymal transition of a carcinoma.

Epidemiology and Presentation

This is a rare type of sarcoma arising in the mediastinum and/or the lung. Patients tend to be young adults (median age: 48 years) with a heavy smoking history. There is a clear male predominance.

Pathology

SDTS is characterized by a rhabdoid or poorly differentiated phenotype. In addition, necrosis (typically of the geographic type), and brisk mitotic activity are observed in all cases. Additional histologic pictures are stromal myxoid changes and changes that resembled a desmoplastic small round cell tumor.

Biomarkers

SDTS is characterized by complete loss of reactivity for both SMARCA4[1] and SMARCA2[2], with the background lymphocytes serving as a positive internal control. In contrast, SMARCB1/INI1 is completely retained. SDTS features also focal or diffuse expression of at least two of the following biomarkers: SOX2, CD34, or SALL4.

Prognosis

SDTS has a poor prognosis with a median overall survival time of 6–7 months. The metastatic rate is 77%.

Therapy

Surgery should be perfomed whenever feasible. As regards **chemotherapy**, SDTS is considered a chemoresistant malignancy. Theoretically, SDTS might benefit from **target therapy** with inhibitors of enhancer of zeste homolog (EZH2) due to their activity against tumors with abnormalities in the SWI/SNF complex proteins: of note, one such drug called tazemetostat has been recently approved by the Food and Drug Administration for the treatment of epithelioid sarcoma (→ see dedicated section), a SMARCB1 deficient tumor. **Immunotherapy** with anti-PD1 blocking antibodies (i.e., pembrolizumab and nivolumab) is promising but is in its infancy of clinical evaluation.

Suggested Readings

Iijima. Notable response to nivolumab during the treatment of SMARCA4-deficient thoracic sarcoma: a case report. Immunotherapy. 2020;12:563–9. [Epub ahead of print]

Le Loarer. SMARCA4 inactivation defines a group of undifferentiated thoracic malignancies transcriptionally related to BAF-deficient sarcomas. Nat Genet. 2015;47:1200–5.

Perret. SMARCA4-deficient thoracic sarcomas: clinicopathologic study of 30 cases with an emphasis on their nosology and differential diagnoses. Am J Surg Pathol. 2019;43:455–65.

Stewart. SMARCA4-deficient thoracic sarcoma: a case report and review of literature. Int J Surg Pathol. 2020;28(1):102–8.

---

[1] SMARCA4, located at 19p13, encodes the protein BRG1 and is part of the switch/sucrose-nonfermenting (SWI/SNF) chromatin remodeling complex that is also known as the BAF (BRG1-associated factors) complex. This complex is ATP-dependent and plays an important role in transcription, differentiation, and DNA repair and has been shown to behave as a tumor suppressing complex. Each complex contains multiple subunits, each of which contains a mutually exclusive ATP-ase subunit, SMARCA4 (BRG1) or SMARCA2 (BRM).

[2] SMARCA2: this gene encodes another core component of the switch/sucrose-nonfermenting (SWI/SNF) chromatin remodeling complex.

Sauter. SMARCA4-deficient thoracic sarcoma: a distinctive clinicopathological entity with undifferentiated rhabdoid morphology and aggressive behavior. Mod Pathol. 2017;30:1422–32.

Takada. Exceptionally rapid response to pembrolizumab in a SMARCA4-deficient thoracic sarcoma overexpressing PD-L1: a case report. Thorac Cancer. 2019;10(12):2312–5.

Yoshida. Clinicopathological and molecular characterization of SMARCA4-deficient thoracic sarcomas with comparison to potentially related entities. Mod Pathol. 2017;30:797–809.

Definition

SMARC-deficient uterine sarcoma (SDUS) is a recently defined nosological entity characterized by loss of SMARCA4 gene. It belongs to the family of SMARC-deficient sarcomas (→ see dedicated section).

It is also known as SMARCA4-deficient uterine sarcoma, SMARCA4-deficient undifferentiated uterine sarcoma and malignant rhabdoid tumor of the uterus.

Epidemiology and Presentation

SDUS is a rare malignancy occurring in young women (mean age: 36 years). It develops at a younger age as compared to its main mimic undifferentiated and dedifferentiated endometrial carcinoma (UDEC, mean age: 61 years).

Etiology and Predisposition

In a few cases, SDUS has been described to develop within the frame of the so called rhabdoid tumor predisposition syndrome (RTPS), a hereditary condition characterized by a markedly increased risk of developing rhabdoid tumors (for details → see Chap 222) and ovarian small cell carcinoma hypercalcemic type (SCCOHT). The syndrome is inherited with an autosomal dominant pattern and is caused by germline heterozygous loss-of-function mutations in SMARCA4 or SMARCB1. Identification of carriers is important because it allows for testing of family members and appropriate screening.

Pathology

SDUS is an undifferentiated malignancy with a microscopic morphology (e.g., epithelioid to rhabdoid cells, high mitotic rate, stromal hyalinization, necrosis, lymphovascular space invasion) overlapping with that of undifferentiated and dedifferentiated endometrial carcinoma (UDEC): the differential diagnosis between two entities is often impossible based on the sole microscopic appearance.

As SDUS appears to be a distinct clinicopathologic entity, it should be distinguished from its potential mimics which include UDEC, undifferentiated uterine sarcoma (→ see dedicated section), and adenosarcoma.

Biomarkers

SDUS is consistently characterized by the inactivation of the SWI/SNF genes SMARCA4[1] or SMARCB1[2]; of note, UDEC inconsistently shows the same gene alterations. All SDUS cases with SMARCA4 inactivation also display SMARCA2 loss.

Prognosis

Both SDUS and UDEC are aggressive tumors with a dismal prognosis, but SDUS has a worse prognosis.

Therapy

Given the rarity and the recent identification of this nosological entity, no much experience has been gained on its treatment. Theoretically, SDUSS might benefit from target therapy with inhibitors of enhancer of zeste homolog (EZH2) due to

[1] SMARCA4: SWI/SNF Related, Matrix Associated, Actin Dependent Regulator of Chromatin, Subfamily A, Member 4 (also known as BRG1) encodes a member of the SWI/SNF family of proteins. Members of this family have helicase and ATPase activities and are thought to regulate transcription of certain genes by altering the chromatin structure around those genes. The encoded protein is part of the large ATP-dependent chromatin remodeling complex SNF/SWI, which is required for transcriptional activation of genes normally repressed by chromatin.

[2] SMARCB1: SWI/SNF-Related Matrix-Associated Actin-Dependent Regulator of Chromatin, Subfamily B, Member 1 (also known as INI1) encodes a protein which is part of the BAF (hSWI/SNF) complex that relieves repressive chromatin structures, allowing the transcriptional machinery to access its targets more effectively. This ATP-dependent chromatin-remodeling complex plays an important role in different cell activities including cell differentiation; in particular, regulation of the stem cell-associated program, which is maintained by the repressive effect of the EZH2-dependent PRC2 (polycomb repressive complex 2), is disrupted by SMARCB1. Overall, SMARCB1 has been found to act as a tumor suppressor, and its mutations have been associated with a variety of malignancies including sarcomas.

their activity against tumors with abnormalities in the SWI/SNF complex proteins: of note, one such drug called tazemetostat has been recently approved by the Food and Drug Administration for the treatment of epithelioid sarcoma (→ see dedicated section), a SMARCB1 deficient tumor.

Suggested Readings

Connor. Germline mutations of SMARCA4 in small cell carcinoma of the ovary, hypercalcemic type and in SMARCA4-deficient undifferentiated uterine sarcoma: clinical features of a single family and comparison of large cohorts. Gynecol Oncol. 2020;157(1):106–14.
Kolin. SMARCA4-deficient undifferentiated uterine sarcoma (malignant rhabdoid tumor of the uterus): a clinicopathologic entity distinct from undifferentiated carcinoma. Mod Pathol. 2018;31(9):1442–56.
Kolin. SMARCA4-deficient uterine sarcoma and undifferentiated endometrial carcinoma are distinct clinicopathologic entities. Am J Surg Pathol. 2020;44(2):263–70.

Definition

Smooth muscle tumor of uncertain malignant potential (STUMP) is a uterine neoplasm originating from smooth muscle cells. According to the World Health Organization, it is a tumor that cannot be histologically diagnosed as unequivocally benign or malignant.

It is also known as uterine STUMP.

Epidemiology and Presentation

STUMP is considered to be a rare uterine neoplasm. The presentation is similar to uterine leiomyoma ($\rightarrow$ see dedicated section).

Pathology

The criteria to diagnose STUMP are based on the following features:

- Tumor necrosis; presence or absence is a powerful predictor of outcome for patients with uterine smooth muscle tumors; one must distinguish coagulative tumor cell necrosis (not in leiomyoma) and hyalinizing necrosis (common in leiomyoma); in STUMP, tumor necrosis is absent or difficult to define.
- Diffuse or multifocal atypia (classified as none/moderate/severe, based on nuclear pleomorphism, nuclear size, nuclear membrane irregularities, chromatin density and nucleoli size/prominence), and mitotic counts close to the threshold for malignancy (e.g., nine mitoses per ten HPF).
- More than 15 mitoses per 10 HPF.
- Atypia or proliferative activity intermediate between their benign and malignant counterparts.

S. Mocellin, *Soft Tissue Tumors*, https://doi.org/10.1007/978-3-030-58710-9_232

– Myometrial invasion without usual features of malignancy.
– Atypical mitotic figures without other canonical features of malignancy.

Differential diagnosis may be needed with leiomyoma (no coagulative tumor cell necrosis, no significant atypia; any degree of mitotic activity: it is called "with significant mitotic activity" if 5 or more mitotic figures/10 HPF; benign behavior), atypical leiomyoma (moderate to severe atypia, <10 mitotic figures/10 HPF, no coagulative tumor cell necrosis), and leiomyosarcoma (usually hemorrhagic tissue; typically but not always marked pleomorphism; 15–30 mitotic figures/10 HPF with abundant abnormal mitotic figures; coagulative tumor cell necrosis is present).

Biomarkers

There is no specific pattern. For details → see Chap 249.

Prognosis

Uterine STUMPs are generally characterized by indolent behavior and long survival, but cases of patients with distant metastases and a rapid clinical course have also been reported (clearly, a correct histological diagnosis is crucial to properly classify these lesions and avoid confusion with clearly benign leiomyomas and clearly malignant leiomyosarcomas). The recurrence rate is about 10%. The likelihood of leiomyosarcomatous transformation is believed to be low. Overall, STUMP should probably be considered a low-grade malignancy.

Therapy

Hysterectomy is recommended as the treatment of choice for women who have no desire to maintain fertility; myomectomy is often preferred in premenopausal women with childbearing desires. For the latter group, imaging follow-up is needed.

Suggested Readings

Guntupalli. Uterine smooth muscle tumor of uncertain malignant potential: a retrospective analysis. Gynecol Oncol. 2009;113(3):324–6.
Kempson. Smooth muscle, endometrial stromal, and mixed müllerian tumors of the uterus. Mod Pathol. 2000;13(3):328–42.
Miettinen. Smooth muscle tumors of soft tissue and non-uterine viscera: biology and prognosis. Mod Pathol. 2014;27(Suppl 1):S17–29.
Rizzo. Recurrent uterine smooth-muscle tumors of uncertain malignant potential (stump): state of the art. Anticancer Res. 2020;40(3):1229–38.

Shapiro. Uterine smooth-muscle tumor of uncertain malignant potential metastasizing to the humerus as a high-grade leiomyosarcoma. Gynecol Oncol. 2004;94(3):818–20.

Shim. Clinical experience of uterine smooth muscle tumor of uncertain malignant potential in two gynecological centers: oncological and obstetrical aspects. Eur J Obstet Gynecol Reprod Biol. 2020;246:7–13.

Zheng. Smooth muscle tumor of uncertain malignant potential (stump): a clinicopathologic analysis of 26 cases. Int J Clin Exp Pathol. 2020;13(4):818–26.

Definition

Solitary circumscribed neuroma (SCN) is a benign peripheral nerve sheath tumor. It is also known as palisaded encapsulated neuroma.

Epidemiology and Presentation

SCN is a relatively common neoplasm affecting people at any age (but mainly adults) without gender prevalence. Typically, it involves the skin of the head and neck (face in particular) and the mucosa of the oral cavity; fewer than 10% of cases occur on the trunk, extremities, and glans penis. SCN presents as a dermis-centered, small, solitary (hence the name), painless, skin-colored, dome-shaped slow-growing nodule (usually <1 cm in size). Clinical diagnosis very difficult, and it can be mistaken for non-pigmented melanocytic nevus and basal cell carcinoma.

Pathology

SCN is a well-circumscribed (hence the name) lesion composed of Schwann cells, axons, and perineurial fibroblasts with a lobular growth pattern. The overlying epidermis lacks remarkable changes. The nerve of origin is apparent only in 50% of cases. In a minority of cases, SCN displays vascular, epithelioid, or myxoid features. Palisading may be present but is unusual (Verocay bodies are uncommon); no Antoni A and Antoni B zonation is present. Mitoses and nuclear pleomorphism are absent. As opposed to schwannoma and neurofibroma, SCN is rich of multiple neurofilament-positive axons.

© The Editor(s) (if applicable) and The Author(s), under exclusive license to   743
Springer Nature Switzerland AG 2021
S. Mocellin, *Soft Tissue Tumors*, https://doi.org/10.1007/978-3-030-58710-9_233

Biomarkers

Schwann cells are positive for S100 and are surrounded by type IV collagen. Axons are strongly positive for neurofilament protein. Perineurial fibroblasts are CD34 positive. The (incomplete) perineurial capsule is positive for EMA. SCN stains negative for GFAP.

Prognosis

SCN is a benign tumor which does not recur after exeresis.

Therapy

Surgery is the treatment of choice.

Suggested Readings

Fernández-Crehuet. Solitary circumscribed neuroma: a clinical and dermoscopic mimicker of basal cell carcinoma. Int J Dermatol. 2015;54(7):e275–7.
Fletcher. WHO classification of tumours of soft tissue and bone, 5th edition. 2020.
Leblebici. Palisaded encapsulated (solitary circumscribed) neuroma: a review of 30 cases. Int J Surg Pathol. 2019;27(5):506–14.

Definition

Solitary fibrous tumor (SFT) is a neoplasm with an intermediate biological aggressiveness and is classified among fibroblastic-myofibroblastic tumors.

It is also known as hemangiopericytoma, giant cell angiofibroma, and extrapleural solitary fibrous tumor.

Epidemiology and Presentation

SFT accounts for less than 2% of all soft tissue tumors and occurs most frequently in middle-aged adults, without gender differences.

Originally described in the pleura (pleural solitary fibrous tumor), SFT has been subsequently documented in almost every anatomic site (extrapleural solitary fibrous tumor).

Clinically, it usually presents as a solitary (hence the name), well-delineated, slow-growing, painless mass (which can be cystic and hemorrhagic if large) which measures between 1 and 25 cm (median: 5–8 cm) in diameter. Large lesions can compress adjacent structures and become variably symptomatic. Malignant SFT are locally infiltrative and can generate metastatic disease.

Rarely, large tumors may be associated with paraneoplastic syndromes: the association of paraneoplastic hypoglycemia with SFT is defined as Doege-Potter syndrome, where the hypoglycemia is due to the tumor production of IGF2.[1]

Pleural SFT is also called benign mesothelioma, localized mesothelioma, solitary fibrous mesothelioma, and localized fibrous tumor. It accounts for approximately 30% of all SFT cases. Confined to surface of the lung, usually it does not cause pleural effusion. It is of fibroblastic and not mesothelial in origin, as it arises

---

[1] IGF2: insulin-like growth factor 2 is a member of the insulin family of polypeptide growth factors, which are involved in development and growth.

from submesothelial mesenchyme. Unlike pleural mesothelioma, its pathogenesis is not associated with asbestos exposure.

Extrapleural SFT has been described virtually in any location. The head (approximately 30%; in particular meninges and orbit), thorax (about 30%; in particular lung parenchyma, mediastinum and diaphragm), and abdomen (about 20%) are the most frequent sites, but many other locations have been reported. Among extrapleural tumors, about 40% arise in subcutaneous tissue, with the remaining cases occurring in deep soft tissues, retroperitoneum, mediastinum, abdominal cavity, and meninges among other sites.

Pathology

SFT shows a patternless architecture characterized by the combination of hypocellular and hypercellular areas (made of oval to spindled fibroblastic cells) separated by thick bands of hyalinized collagen and a prominent thin-walled branching hemangiopericytoma-like vascular pattern. Tumor necrosis and infiltrative margins (about 10% of cases) are mostly observed in locally aggressive or malignant lesions.

Myxoid change and interstitial mast cells are often observed. Mitoses are generally scarce (rarely exceeding 3 per 10 HPF). Sometimes giant multinucleated stromal cells and pseudovascular spaces can be encountered (hence the former name "giant cell angiofibroma").

Malignant SFT is usually hypercellular, with higher number of mitoses (> 4 mitoses per 10 HPF), variable cytological atypia, tumor necrosis, and infiltrative margins: of these features, the number of mitoses appears to be the most important prognostic factor.

A variant known as fat-forming SFT is uncommon and is characterized by a variably prominent adipocytic component; a small subgroup of fat-forming SFT shows malignant histological features: of note, lipoblasts and/or atypical lipomatous tumor-like areas can be found in these lesions, closely resembling liposarcoma.

Differential diagnosis may be needed with the following: malignant peripheral nerve sheath tumor, sarcomatoid mesothelioma, desmoid-type fibromatosis, cellular schwannomas, monophasic synovial sarcoma, dermatofibrosarcoma protuberans, low-grade fibromyxoid sarcoma, perineurioma, deep fibrous histiocytoma, gastrointestinal stromal tumor (spindle cell type), dedifferentiated liposarcoma, spindle cell lipoma, and cellular angiofibroma.

Biomarkers

Tumor cells are typically CD34 positive (>90% of cases) and negative for desmin, cytokeratins, S100, CD117 (c-Kit), and CD31.

The **intra-chromosomal inversion** inv12(q13q13) has been found to be a consistent finding in SFT: it generates the NAB2-STAT6 fusion gene,[2] which in turn is responsible for the nuclear overexpression of STAT6, which can be routinely detected by immunohistochemistry (it is currently a key biomarker for both diagnosis and differential diagnosis of SFT).

Prognosis

The clinical behavior of SFT is quite unpredictable. Most cases (90%) are benign lesions, but 10% behave aggressively, with local recurrences and distant metastasis, which can occur many years after primary diagnosis. Malignant histological features (especially high mitotic rate) are the best prognostic indicator. However, some SFT classified as histologically benign behave as malignant SFT, and the behavior of SFT with atypia alone is basically unpredictable. Pleural SFT appears to be on average less aggressive than extrapleural SFT; moreover, among extrapleural SFT, lesions arising in the mediastinum, abdomen, pelvis, retroperitoneum, and/or meninges also appear to be more aggressive than those in other locations (e.g., limbs). Tumor size greater than 10 cm and positive surgical margins is associated with poorer outcome. Metastatic disease locates more frequently in the lungs, bone, and liver.

Long-term follow-up is necessary in order to detect disease relapse even many years after primary diagnosis.

Therapy

Surgical excision is the mainstay of treatment.

The role of adjuvant treatment is basically unknown, although recent retrospective evidence suggests that postoperative radiotherapy is associated with reduced risk of local relapse (especially in cases with less favorable resection margins and tumors with a high mitotic count).

For metastatic disease, systemic chemotherapy is associated with overall scarce results. Pazopanib[3] has been recently reported to be active against advanced SFT.

---

[2] NAB2-STAT6 fusion gene: NGFI-A-binding protein 2 encodes a member of the family of NGFI-A binding (NAB) proteins, which function in the nucleus to repress transcription induced by some members of the EGR (early growth response) family of transactivators. Signal transducer and activator of transcription 6 encodes a member of the STAT family of transcription factors: in response to cytokines and growth factors, STAT family members are phosphorylated by the receptor associated kinases and then form homo- or heterodimers that translocate to the cell nucleus where they act as transcription activators. STAT6 induces the expression of BCL2L1/BCL-X(L), which is responsible for the anti-apoptotic activity of IL-4. The generation of the NAB2-STAT6 fusion gene is considered the driving genetic event in solitary fibrous tumor.

[3] Pazopanib: tyrosine kinase inhibitor targeting the following: VEGFR, PDGFR, KIT

Suggested Readings

Davanzo (2018) Solitary fibrous tumor. Transl Gastroenterol Hepatol 3:94

Doyle (2014) Nuclear expression of STAT6 distinguishes solitary fibrous tumor from histologic mimics. Mod Pathol 27(3):390–395

Fletcher (2020). WHO classification of tumours of soft tissue and bone, 5th edition

Haas (2020) Extrameningeal solitary fibrous tumors-surgery alone or surgery plus perioperative radiotherapy: a retrospective study from the global solitary fibrous tumor initiative in collaboration with the sarcoma patients EuroNet. Cancer 2020 [Epub ahead of print]

Martin-Broto (2019) Pazopanib for treatment of advanced malignant and dedifferentiated solitary fibrous tumour: a multicentre, single-arm, phase 2 trial. Lancet Oncol 20(1):134–144

Ronchi (2018) Extrapleural solitary fibrous tumor: a distinct entity from pleural solitary fibrous tumor. An update on clinical, molecular and diagnostic features. Ann Diagn Pathol 34:142–150

Schöffski (2020) Clinical presentation, natural history, and therapeutic approach in patients with solitary fibrous tumor: a retrospective analysis. Sarcoma 2020:1385978

Definition

Spindle cell hemangioma (SCH) is a benign vascular tumor also known as spindle cell hemangioendothelioma.

Epidemiology and Presentation

SCH can occur at any age (although it is more common in children and young adults) with no gender predilection. It usually presents as a solitary nodule located in the skin or subcutaneous tissue of the distal extremities. Cases involving deep soft tissues or viscera have been very rarely reported.

Etiology and Predisposition

Maffucci syndrome is a rare disorder characterized by multiple enchondromas, skeletal deformities, and cutaneous vascular anomalies including SCH (when hemangiomas are not present, the condition is known as Ollier disease). This syndrome should be suspected when multifocal SCH appear along with multiple enchondromas.

Maffucci syndrome is caused by somatic (the syndrome is acquired, not hereditary) mutations of IDH1 or IDH2. It affects both genders equally and usually manifests around 5 years of age. SCH is the most common form of vascular anomaly in Maffucci syndrome with predilection to acral sites. Thrombosis within SCH can cause pain that severely affects patient's quality of life.

© The Editor(s) (if applicable) and The Author(s), under exclusive license to   749
Springer Nature Switzerland AG 2021
S. Mocellin, *Soft Tissue Tumors*, https://doi.org/10.1007/978-3-030-58710-9_235

Pathology

Histologically, SCH is composed of proliferating spindle cells (hence the name) and cavernous blood vessels.

Spindle cell proliferation between vascular lumina with extravasated erythrocytes is a feature similar to the microscopic appearance of Kaposi sarcoma, whereas vacuolated cells and epithelioid endothelial cells differentiate SCH from Kaposi sarcoma.

Prognosis

SCH is a benign tumor. Within the frame of Maffucci syndrome, pain associated with multiple SCH can impair quality of life.

Therapy

Surgery is the mainstay of treatment for SCH. However, local recurrence occurs in up to 50% of cases. Currently no medical treatment is approved for SCH; growing evidence suggests that mTOR inhibitors (e.g., sirolimus) might play a role in the management of this disease.

Suggested Readings

Adams (2016) Efficacy and safety of sirolimus in the treatment of complicated vascular anomalies. Pediatrics 137:e20153257

Duqing (2019) Multiple spindle cell hemangiomas in both lungs: a rare case report and review of the literature. J Cardiothorac Surg 14(1):86

Gao (2019) Spindle cell hemangioma of the spleen: a case report. Medicine (Baltimore) 98(9):e14555

Lekwuttikarn (2019) Successful treatment of spindle cell hemangiomas in a patient with Maffucci syndrome and review of literatures. Dermatol Ther 32(3):e12919

Definition

Spindle cell lipoma (SCL) is an adipocytic benign tumor. It is also called pleomorphic lipoma.

Epidemiology and Presentation

SCL typically develops in older men (up to 90% of cases). Most cases are located in the neck and upper trunk. It usually develops in the subcutaneous adipose tissue (superficial): in case of deep location, the diagnosis of well-differentiated liposarcoma ($\to$ see dedicated section) should be suspected.

Pathology

SCL is characterized by an admixture of mature fat and bland spindled cells, along with multinucleated floret giant cells (hyperchromatic, multinucleated, wreath-like nuclei). Neither lipoblasts nor prominent vascularity are usually present.

Differential diagnosis may be needed with the following: neurofibroma (different morphology, no prominent adipose tissue, strongly positive for S100; floret cells may be present); well-differentiated liposarcoma (deep location, more lipoblasts, variable thick collagen, variable floret giant cells, CD34 negative); cellular angiofibroma (tumor with vascular features); lipomatous hemangiopericytoma (staghorn vascular pattern); myxoid liposarcoma (lipoblasts and pleomorphic spindle cells, prominent plexiform vascular pattern, CD34 negative); schwannoma (different morphology, no prominent adipose, strongly S100 positive); and solitary fibrous tumor (patternless pattern, no prominent adipose tissue; positive for CD99, BCL2 and CD34).

© The Editor(s) (if applicable) and The Author(s), under exclusive license to Springer Nature Switzerland AG 2021
S. Mocellin, *Soft Tissue Tumors*, https://doi.org/10.1007/978-3-030-58710-9_236

Biomarkers

The spindle cells are strongly positive for CD34 and vimentin, while they are negative for cytokeratins, S100 (fat cells are S100 positive), CD68, desmin, RB1, and SMA (smooth muscle actin). This tumor typically shows unbalanced karyotypes (mainly hypodiploid).

Prognosis

SCL is a benign neoplasm, although local recurrence has been rarely reported.

Therapy

Surgical excision is the treatment of choice.

Suggested Readings

Fletcher (2020) WHO classification of tumours of soft tissue and bone, 5th edition

Jebastin (2019) Atypical lipomatous tumor/well-differentiated liposarcoma with features mimicking spindle cell lipoma. Int J Surg Pathol 2019 [Epub ahead of print]

Lincoln (2016) Uncommon tumor, uncommon location: a dermal-based spindle cell/pleomorphic lipoma. Am J Dermatopathol 38(8):e122-4

Panagopoulos (2018) Cytogenetics of spindle cell/pleomorphic lipomas: karyotyping and FISH analysis of 31 tumors. Cancer Genomics Proteomics 15(3):193–200

Persichetti (2004) Pleomorphic lipoma: a definite histopathological entity. Anticancer Res 24(5B):3157–3159

Definition

Spindle cell/sclerosing rhabdomyosarcoma (SRMS) is a malignancy classified among skeletal muscle tumors. It is also known as spindle cell rhabdomyosarcoma and sclerosing rhabdomyosarcoma.

It is one of the four subtypes of rhabdomyosarcoma (→ see Chap. 224 for further details) along with embryonal (ERMS), alveolar (ARMS), and pleomorphic (PRMS) rhabdomyosarcoma (→ see dedicated sections).

Epidemiology and Presentation

SRMS is a rare subtype of RMS (about 5–10% of all cases of RMS). It affects both children and adults, with a striking male preference (M:F = 6:1). In children, SRMS arises mainly in the paratesticular region, while in adults >50% of cases affect the deep soft tissues in the head and neck. Lesions with sclerosing morphology in both age groups are more common in the limbs. Other body sites are very rarely affected. The tumor most commonly presents as a painless mass that can range from 2 to 35 cm in diameter.

Pathology

SRMS is characterized by infiltrative edges and show a fascicular or storiform growth pattern. The spindle cell variant is composed of a predominant population of spindled cells. Nuclear atypia and mitotic figures are common. When a tumor with spindle cell morphology shows focal, subtotal, or total stromal hyalinization with tumor cells arranged in nests, microalveoli, or trabeculae (conferring a pseudovascular appearance), the lesion is defined as the sclerosing variant of rhabdomyosarcoma. The sclerosing pattern refers to rhabdomyosarcomas associated with a hyaline matrix so abundant that it may mimic an osteosarcoma or angiosarcoma.

Biomarkers

Spindle cell rhabdomyosarcoma is characterized by diffuse expression of desmin, with most cases also expressing SMA[1] and MSA.[2] Nuclear expression of myogenin is observed in almost all cases. Sclerosing rhabdomyosarcoma may show only very limited expression of desmin and myogenin but is often strongly positive for myoD1.

From the genomic viewpoint, three subgroups of SRMS have been defined:

1. Spindle cell rhabdomyosarcoma harboring either VGLL2-based fusion genes (more frequent) or NCOA2-based fusion genes (less frequent). This group of lesions has been reported almost exclusively in infants of less than 5 years of age. Of note, virtually all congenital spindle cell RMS are associated with fusions, VGLL2 and NCOA2 being the most frequently involved genes. These tumors (all located in soft tissues) are associated with an intermediate malignant potential, with tendency to local recurrence but no metastatic dissemination and a favorable outcome with conservative management.

2. MYOD1-mutant rhabdomyosarcoma commonly associated with sclerosing morphology. This subtype may occur at any age (age ranging from 2 to 94 years) with female predominance. This subtype is associated with poor outcome with a death rate of 68% at 28 months of follow-up, with worse prognosis in children. Tumor sites include the head and neck in one third of cases, the extremities, and the trunk. These tumors are caused by somatic activating MYOD1 mutations (mainly represented by the hot spot mutation p.L122R in exon 1): the mutated gene has a dominant negative function and binds to MYC sequences.

3. SRMS lacking recurrent genetic abnormalities. All rhabdomyosarcomas associated with a pure spindle cell phenotype should be tested for the presence of MYOD1 mutation and/or VGLL2/NCOA2 fusions: spindle cell rhabdomyosarcomas that lack these molecular alterations should be probably classified as spindle cell embryonal rhabdomyosarcomas. This subcategory has a predilection for the paratesticular and intra-abdominal areas.

Prognosis

In the pediatric population, SRMS is usually diagnosed at an early stage, and, in contrast to other types of rhabdomyosarcoma, lymph node metastasis is observed in a small subset of cases: these patients have a favorable prognosis (5-year survival

---

[1] SMA: smooth muscle actin

[2] MSA: muscle-specific actin

rate: 95%). The prognosis of adults with SRMS is significantly worse, with a rate of recurrence and metastasis of approximately 40–50%.

For general information on staging and prognosis of rhabdomyosarcoma, → see Chap. 224.

Therapy

For general information on treatment of rhabdomyosarcoma, → see Chap. 224.

Suggested Readings

Agaram (2019) MYOD1-mutant spindle cell and sclerosing rhabdomyosarcoma: an aggressive subtype irrespective of age. A reappraisal for molecular classification and risk stratification. Mod Pathol 32(1):27–36

Fletcher (2020) WHO classification of tumours of soft tissue and bone, 5th edition

Leiner (2019) The current landscape of rhabdomyosarcomas: an update. Virchows Arch 2019 [Epub ahead of print]

Pappo (2018) Rhabdomyosarcoma, Ewing sarcoma, and other round cell sarcomas. J Clin Oncol 36(2):168–179

Skapek (2019) Rhabdomyosarcoma. Nat Rev. Dis Primers 5(1):1

The spleen can be (rarely) affected by benign and primary malignant soft tissue tumors. From the clinical viewpoint, these lesions must be distinguished from other types of splenic neoplasms, such as lymphoid tumors (e.g., Hodgkin disease, non-Hodgkin lymphomas) and secondary tumors (metastatic disease from primary malignancies arising elsewhere).

Splenomegaly is the commonest finding. Upper quadrant discomfort, pain, or tenderness may also be complained by the patient, but some cases are asymptomatic and are diagnosed incidentally during imaging studies performed for other reasons (incidentaloma). Anemia, granulocytopenia, and thrombocytopenia are also possible (hypersplenism), depending on the size of the lesion. In case of malignancy, splenomegaly may be associated with fever, cachexia, and pleural effusion.

Computed tomography scan and magnetic resonance imaging are useful but can rarely identify the nature of the splenic lesion. Since the biopsy is usually contraindicated (due to the risk of bleeding) and imaging can rarely be pathognomonic, splenectomy is often needed to make a precise diagnosis.

The following is a list of the most frequent soft tissue tumors of the spleen reported in the literature:

Hemangioma	The most common benign neoplasm of the spleen (incidence: 0.02–0.16%); also known as splenic angioma For general details → see Chap. 117
Littoral cell angioma	This tumor can be found only in the spleen For details → see Chap. 156
Hemangioendothelioma	For general details → see Chap. 116
Angiosarcoma	Rare but still the most common non-lymphoid malignancy of the spleen. For general details → see Chap. 25
Inflammatory myofibroblastic tumor	For general details → see Chap. 133

© Springer Nature Switzerland AG 2021

757

S. Mocellin, *Soft Tissue Tumors*, https://doi.org/10.1007/978-3-030-58710-9_238

Definition

Superficial angiomyxoma (SAM) is a benign tumor of uncertain differentiation and represents the cutaneous version of deep angiomyxoma (→ see dedicated section). It is also known as cutaneous myxoma.

Epidemiology and Presentation

It has been reported to arise from virtually any skin region. It presents as single or multiple multilobular pink-colored masses of 0.5–2 cm in diameter.

Etiology and Predisposition

SAM can be sporadic or associated with the **Carney complex**, a rare multiple cancer predisposition syndrome inherited in an autosomal dominant manner and characterized by pigmented lesions of the skin (e.g., lentigines and blue nevi), multiple endocrine tumors, cardiac myxoma, and (usually multiple) superficial angiomyxoma (present in about 50% of cases).

Another typical manifestation is an ACTH-independent Cushing's syndrome due to the so-called primary pigmented nodular adrenocortical disease (PPNAD).

One of the putative causal genes is PRKAR1A located on 17q22–24, which encodes the regulatory subunit of PKA (protein kinase A). Heterozygous inactivating mutations of PRKAR1A have been reported in most index cases. PRKAR1A is a key component of the cAMP signaling pathway which has been implicated in endocrine tumorigenesis and might function as a tumor suppressor gene.

The treatment of Carney complex may require surgery for removal of cardiac myxomas as well as other tumors; bilateral adrenalectomy is the most common treatment for Cushing's syndrome due to PPNAD.

© The Editor(s) (if applicable) and The Author(s), under exclusive license to
Springer Nature Switzerland AG 2021
S. Mocellin, *Soft Tissue Tumors*, https://doi.org/10.1007/978-3-030-58710-9_239

Pathology

Macroscopically SAM presents as a gelatinous tumor. Microscopically it is composed of moderately to sparsely cellular angiomyxoid nodules centered in the dermis (sometimes involving the subcutis) with moderately cellular, bland, spindled, and stellate cells and a prominent proliferation of small blood vessels.

Biomarkers

At immunohistochemistry the tumor cells stain positively for vimentin and CD34; variably positive for Factor XIIIa, SMA, and S100; and negative for desmin and cytokeratins.

Differential diagnosis may be needed with the following: deep angiomyxoma (located in the subcutis or deep-seated, infiltrative diffuse growth pattern, mean diameter >5 cm, stains positive for desmin); low-grade myxofibrosarcoma ($\rightarrow$ see dedicated section); cellular angiofibroma (hyalinized round vessels, stromal lymphocytes); angiomyofibroblastoma (desmin positive); dermal nerve sheath myxoma (also known as myxoid neurothekeoma, no prominent vessel proliferation, S100 always negative, frequent epithelioid component); and myxoid neurofibroma (poorly circumscribed, always S100 positive, intralesional nerve).

Prognosis

SAM is a benign tumor.

Therapy

Surgical excision is the treatment of choice.

Suggested Readings

Abarzúa-Araya (2016) Superficial angiomyxoma of the skin. Dermatol Pract Concept 6(3):47–49

Allen (2000) Myxoma is not a single entity: a review of the concept of myxoma. Ann Diagn Pathol 4(2):99–123

Bembem (2017) Cyto-Histo correlation of a very rare tumor: superficial Angiomyxoma. J Cytol 34(4):230–232

Takahashi (2002) Carney complex: report of a Japanese case associated with cutaneous superficial angiomyxomas, labial lentigines, and a pituitary adenoma. J Dermatol 29(12):790–796

Superficial fibromatosis is a family of fibromatoses of superficial tissues and includes palmar/plantar fibromatosis, penile fibromatosis (also known as Peyronie disease and induratio penis plastica), knuckle pads (also known as Garrod's pads), pachydermodactyly, and infantile digital fibromatosis (also known as Reye's tumor, multiple hyaline fibromatosis).

For more details on palmar/plantar fibromatosis, → see dedicated section.

For fibromatosis of the deep tissues (deep fibromatosis), → see Chap. 69.

Definition

Synovial hemangioma (SH) is a benign neoplasm of vascular differentiation. It belongs to the hemangioma family ($\rightarrow$ see Chap. 117).

Epidemiology and Presentation

SH is a very rare tumor occurring in children or adolescents, with males being affected more often than females. It arises in a synovium-lined surface (intra-articular space or a bursa): the most common site is the knee; much less common sites are the elbow and hand.

SH presents as a slow-growing lesion, usually associated with joint swelling and effusion (including hemarthrosis). Pain is a frequent, but not constant symptom.

Magnetic resonance imaging is the best radiological technique to diagnose the lesion.

Pathology

Microscopically, most cases resemble a cavernous hemangioma with multiple dilated thin-walled vascular channels. The remaining cases have the appearance of either a capillary or arteriovenous malformation hemangioma. The vascular channels are located underneath the synovial membrane and are surrounded by myxoid or fibrotic stroma.

Differential diagnosis may be needed with diffuse tenosynovial giant cell tumor ($\rightarrow$ see dedicated section).

© The Editor(s) (if applicable) and The Author(s), under exclusive license to
Springer Nature Switzerland AG 2021
S. Mocellin, *Soft Tissue Tumors*, https://doi.org/10.1007/978-3-030-58710-9_241

Biomarkers

There is no specific panel.

Prognosis

SH is a benign tumor. Small lesions are easy to remove completely, whereas more diffuse lesions can be difficult to manage with complete excision, which may predispose to disease relapse.

Therapy

Surgical excision is the treatment of choice.

Suggested Readings

Arslan (2015) Synovial Hemangioma in the knee: MRI findings. J Clin Imaging Sci 5:23
Fletcher (2013) WHO classification of tumours of soft tissue and bone, 4th ed
Kalson (2011) Destructive synovial hemangioma of the hip resembling pigmented Villonodular Synovitis. J Arthroplast 26(2):339.e15-20
Muramatsu (2019) Synovial hemangioma of the knee joint in pediatrics: our case series and review of literature. Eur J Orthop Surg Traumatol 29(6):1291–1296

Definition

Synovial sarcoma (SyS) is a malignant tumor of uncertain differentiation (despite the name, the cells of origin are not synovial cells). In the past it has been named tenosynovial sarcoma, synoviosarcoma, synovial cell sarcoma, malignant synovioma, and synovioblastic sarcoma. As below described, two variants exist: biphasic synovial sarcoma and monophasic synovial sarcoma.

Epidemiology and Presentation

SyS may develop at any age (median: 35 years), but most patients are teenagers and young adults (15–30 years), without gender prevalence. Overall, this tumor accounts for 5–10% of all soft tissue sarcomas; however, the proportion of SyS among soft tissue sarcomas varies with age, ranging from 15% in subjects aged 10–18 years to 1.5% in patients older than 50 years. In the USA, its incidence is approximately 800 to 1000 cases per year.

SyS can locate virtually anywhere in the body. In most cases (70%), it arises in the deep soft tissues of the upper or lower extremity (frequently in a juxta-articular site); approximately 15% of cases develop in the trunk and 7% in the head and neck region. In the remaining cases (<10%), SyS locates in the male and female external and internal sex organs, kidney, adrenal gland, other viscera, retroperitoneum, mediastinum, bone, and central nervous system.

Clinically, SyS usually presents as a 3–10 cm in diameter well-circumscribed mass which is frequently painful. Minute lesions (less than 1 cm) may occur, especially in hands and feet. Cystic change and hematoma formation may contribute to delayed diagnosis along with misleadingly benign clinical appearance. Calcifications may be radiologically detectable; bone erosion and infiltration may occur.

Etiology and Predisposition

Unlike undifferentiated pleomorphic sarcoma, extraskeletal osteosarcoma, fibrosarcoma, malignant peripheral nerve sheath tumor, and angiosarcoma, SyS is exceptionally associated with radiation exposure.

Pathology

Macroscopically, the cut surface appearance depends upon cellularity, myxoid change, or hemorrhage; the tumor is frequently multinodular and can be multicystic; calcification, metaplastic ossification, and necrosis may be observed.

Microscopically, SyS is characterized by monotonous spindle cells with vesicular plump and overlapping nuclei, a variable degree of epithelial differentiation (including gland formation), and "hemangiopericytic" staghorn branching vessels.

Histologically, two main types of SyS can be distinguished:

1. In **biphasic synovial sarcoma**, epithelial and spindle cell components are present in varying proportions. The epithelial cells are arranged in solid nests or cords or in glands with a tubular or sometimes alveolar or papillary architecture. The glandular component can predominate and may be confused with an adenocarcinoma: however, a scant spindle cell component is virtually always found.
2. In **monophasic synovial sarcoma**, the spindle cells predominate and mimic those in biphasic SyS: they are fairly uniform and relatively small with a high nuclear-to-cytoplasmic ratio and are arranged in cellular sheets or fascicles. The amount of collagen is variable and usually scarce, but areas of dense fibrosis may be observed. Many cases focally show a staghorn-shaped vascular pattern similar to solitary fibrous tumor. Many mast cells are frequently found.

In both biphasic and monophasic SyS, poorly differentiated areas with hypercellularity, rounded or spindled cells showing severe nuclear atypia, and high mitotic activity (>15 per 10 HPFs) may be observed; these areas may be composed of small round hyperchromatic tumor cells (similar to Ewing sarcoma), fascicular spindle cells (similar to MPNST), or epithelioid cells. Poorly differentiated areas are much more frequent in elderly patients. The term **poorly differentiated synovial sarcoma** can be used to refer to a SyS with a consistent proportion of poorly differentiated component.

Differential diagnosis may be needed with the following (SSX translocation is always helpful, see below paragraph on biomarkers):

A. **Biphasic SyS**: adenocarcinoma (lack spindle cell areas and are typically TLE1 negative); biphasic mesothelioma (can show sarcomatoid features and cytokeratin positivity, but is WT1 positive); nerve sheath tumors (very rarely malignant peripheral nerve sheath tumor and schwannoma show glandular features); ectopic hamartomatous thymoma (composed of spindle cells and epithelial tissue, mature adipose tissue should be present, myoepithelial component with positivity for cytokeratins, SMA, CD10, and calponin).

B. **Monophasic SyS**: malignant peripheral nerve sheath tumor (hypocelluler and hypercellular areas; SOX10 positive, often shows focal cytokeratin positivity and TLE1 positivity in up to 30%; it displays loss of H3K27me3 in 33% of cases); cellular schwannoma (dilated vessels with hyalinized walls, S100 and SOX10 are positive, TLE1 positivity can cause confusion); solitary fibrous tumor (CD34 positive with characteristic "patternless" pattern; STAT6 positive; TLE1 can be positive in up to 40% of cases); leiomyosarcoma (often shows more nuclear pleomorphism; may be desmin, SMA, calponin, and h-caldesmon positive); spindle cell rhabdomyosarcoma (desmin, myogenin, and myoD1 positive); adult fibrosarcoma (diagnosis of exclusion when other spindle cell sarcomas have been ruled out); dermatofibrosarcoma protuberans with fibrosarcomatous transformation (usually CD34 positive and has an area with more classic histology); epithelioid sarcoma (it can be cytokeratin positive, TLE1 positive in 30%; it can have spindle cell morphology; CD34 positive in half cases and INI1 lost in most cases); biphenotypic sinonasal sarcoma (it has neural and myogenic biomarkers including S100 and SMA, calponin, desmin or myogenin; PAX3 rearrangements); sarcomatoid carcinoma (cytokeratin positive; look for overlying epithelium involved by carcinoma; TLE1 negative).

C. **Poorly differentiated SyS**: small round blue cell tumors (SS18-SSX translocation studies and lineage specific biomarkers such as myogenin, myoD1, desmin, FLI1 are useful); molecular studies for PAX3/PAX7 rearrangements, EWSR rearrangements, and CIC-DUX4 and BCOR rearrangements help rule out alveolar rhabdomyosarcoma, Ewing sarcoma, and undifferentiated round cell sarcoma (Ewing-like sarcomas; → see dedicated section).

Biomarkers

Among epithelial biomarkers, EMA[1] is expressed more often than cytokeratins, especially in monophasic SyS and poorly differentiated areas. Epithelial cells in biphasic SyS consistently express EMA and cytokeratins. The spindle cells of monophasic SyS display focal expression of EMA in nearly all cases, whereas focal expression of cytokeratins is found in 70–80% of cases. Poorly differentiated areas of SyS almost always show focal staining for EMA, whereas cytokeratin expression is found in about half cases. Focal expression of S100 may be detectable in up to 40% of cases. Staining for CD34, desmin, h-caldesmon, myogenin, MyoD1, FLI1, and WT1 is virtually always negative. Most SyS are positive for CD99, mimicking the staining of Ewing sarcoma. Moderate or strong nuclear staining for the transcriptional corepressor TLE1 is found in 80% of biphasic SyS, monophasic SyS, and SyS with poorly differentiated areas; of note, TLE1 positivity is not specific for SyS since it may also be observed in mimics of SyS such as MPNST and solitary fibrous tumor.

---

[1] EMA: epithelial membrane antigen

The **chromosomal translocation** t(X;18)(p11;q11) is found exclusively in this neoplasm and occurs in more than 95% of cases. This genetic abnormality leads to the formation of the SS18-SSX1 fusion gene[2] (about 66% of cases) or SS18-SSX2 fusion gene[3] (about 33%). Both FISH[4] and RT-PCR[5] of fusion transcripts are routinely utilized to make an accurate diagnosis of SyS. Of note, most biphasic SyS carry SS18-SSX1, whereas monophasic SyS may carry either fusion gene. This translocation—which affects multiple oncogenic pathways (including the SWI/SNF chromatin remodeling complex, polycomb repressor complex, and canonical Wnt pathway)—is believed to drive the oncogenesis of SyS.

Prognosis

SyS is a malignant tumor with variable prognosis. Distant metastasis affects most frequently the lungs and bone. Although most distant relapses occur within a few years after the initial diagnosis, late recurrences can occur even after 10 years. Poor prognostic factors are higher tumor stage at presentation, larger tumor size (>5 cm in diameter), more than 20% of poorly differentiated areas, higher FNCCLC[6] grade (> 10 mitoses per 1.7 mm^2, necrosis), older age (adults versus children), and axial site (trunk or head and neck versus extremities). The 5- and 10-year disease-specific survival is 83% and 75% in children/adolescents (age < 19 years) and 62% and 52% in adults. On average, metastatic SyS has better overall survival and progression-free survival as compared to other metastatic soft tissue sarcomas.

Therapy

Surgery is the mainstay of treatment and should preserve function whenever feasible (combined with medical treatments if needed, see below). Patients with low-risk SyS (defined as grade II tumor of any size or grade III tumor <5 cm) probably can be safely treated with surgery alone if adequately (R0) resected (avoiding adjuvant chemotherapy and radiotherapy). Isolated limb perfusion can be utilized to

---

[2] SS18-SSX1 fusion gene: SS18 (SS18 subunit of BAF chromatin remodeling complex) encodes a protein that functions synergistically with RBM14 as a transcriptional coactivator: in particular, it is a component of the SWI/SNF chromatin remodeling subcomplex GBAF that changes chromatin structure by altering DNA-histone contacts within a nucleosome in an ATP-dependent manner. SSX1 (SSX family member 1) encodes a protein that belongs to the family of highly homologous synovial sarcoma X (SSX) breakpoint proteins: these proteins may function as transcriptional repressors. The encoded hybrid proteins are likely responsible for transforming activity (likely through the Wnt pathway).

[3] SS18-SSX2 fusion gene: SSX2 (SSX family member 2) encodes a protein that belongs to the family of highly homologous synovial sarcoma X (SSX) breakpoint proteins: these proteins may function as transcriptional repressors.

[4] FISH: fluorescence in situ hybridization

[5] RT-PCR: reverse transcriptase polymerase chain reaction

[6] FNCCLC: Fédération Nationale des Centres de Lutte Contre Le Cancer

avoid amputation in limb-threatening SyS. Although lymph node metastasis rate ranges from 5% to 20%, the role of sentinel node biopsy in SyS staging is debated.

Radiotherapy. Neoadjuvant or adjuvant radiotherapy for high-risk SyS of extremities/trunk wall is recommended to reduce local disease recurrence.

Chemotherapy. The role of neoadjuvant/adjuvant chemotherapy for high-risk SyS is still debated. On average, metastatic SyS shows better response rates as compared to other metastatic soft tissue sarcomas; nevertheless, metastatic SyS is virtually incurable. Anthracycline-based regimen remains the gold standard chemotherapy. The combination doxorubicin plus ifosfamide is associated with tumor response rates ($\approx$40%) higher that those obtained with doxorubicin alone ($\approx$20%), but this advantage does not translate into survival benefit, and the combination is burdened by an increased toxicity rate. Although SyS is deemed to be somewhat more sensitive to ifosfamide, high-dose ifosfamide (which is associated with response rates $\approx$40%) resulted inferior to epirubicin plus ifosfamide in terms of disease-free survival in a randomized trial of neoadjuvant chemotherapy for soft tissue sarcomas including SyS (ISG-STS 1001). For second-line chemotherapy, ifosfamide is often chosen; otherwise, trabectedin might be effective (although results are from a randomized trial including different types of translocation-positive soft tissue sarcomas); in contrast, gemcitabine plus docetaxel do not appear to be useful.

Immunotherapy. In a single trial, immunotherapy with pembrolizumab (an anti-PD1 antibody) led to a 10% tumor response rate in patients with advanced/metastatic SyS refractory to standard chemotherapy. In another trial conducted in the same type of patient population, adoptive immunotherapy (with autologous T cells expressing NY-ESO-1c259, an affinity-enhanced T-cell receptor TCR recognizing an HLA-A2-restricted NY-ESO-1/LAGE1a-derived peptide) has been associated with a 50% tumor response rate.

Target therapy. For second-line chemotherapy, pazopanib[7] might be effective (although results are from a randomized trial including different types of soft tissue sarcomas).

In a randomized trial, regorafenib[8] significantly improves progression-free survival (as compared to placebo) in patients with metastatic SyS refractory to standard chemotherapy.

Suggested Readings

Andreou (2013) Sentinel node biopsy in soft tissue sarcoma subtypes with a high propensity for regional lymphatic spread—results of a large prospective trial. Ann Oncol 24(5):1400–1405

Brodowicz (2018) Efficacy and safety of regorafenib compared to placebo and to post-cross-over regorafenib in advanced non-adipocytic soft tissue sarcoma. Eur J Cancer 99:28–36

---

[7] Pazopanib: tyrosine kinase inhibitor targeting the following: VEGFR, PDGFR, KIT

[8] Regorafenib: tyrosine kinase inhibitor targeting the following: RET, VEGFR1, VEGFR2, VEGFR3, KIT, PDGFRA, PDGFRB, FGFR1, FGFR2

Cironi (2016) The fusion protein SS18-SSX1 employs core Wnt pathway transcription factors to induce a partial Wnt signature in synovial sarcoma. Sci Rep 6:22113

D'Adamo (2019) A phase II trial of Sorafenib and Dacarbazine for Leiomyosarcoma, synovial sarcoma, and malignant peripheral nerve sheath Tumors. Oncologist 24(6):857–863

D'Angelo (2018) Antitumor activity associated with prolonged persistence of adoptively transferred NY-ESO-1 c259T cells in synovial sarcoma. Cancer Discov 8(8):944–957

Desar (2018) Systemic treatment for adults with synovial sarcoma. Curr Treat Options in Oncol 19(2):13

Edmonson (1993) Randomized comparison of doxorubicin alone versus ifosfamide plus doxorubicin or mitomycin, doxorubicin, and cisplatin against advanced soft tissue sarcomas. J Clin Oncol 11(7):1269–1275

Edmonson (2003) Phase II study of Ifosfamide+doxorubicin in patients with advanced synovial sarcomas (E1793): a trial of the eastern cooperative oncology group. Sarcoma 7(1):9–11

Egger (2002) Radiation-associated synovial sarcoma: clinicopathologic and molecular analysis of two cases. Mod Pathol 15(9):998–1004

Ferrari (2017) Surgery alone is sufficient therapy for children and adolescents with low-risk synovial sarcoma: a joint analysis from the European paediatric soft tissue sarcoma Study Group and the Children's Oncology Group. Eur J Cancer 78:1–6

Fletcher (2020) WHO classification of tumours of soft tissue and bone, 5th edition

Gronchi (2017) Histotype-tailored neoadjuvant chemotherapy versus standard chemotherapy in patients with high-risk soft-tissue sarcomas (ISG-STS 1001): an international, open-label, randomised, controlled, phase 3, multicentre trial. Lancet Oncol 18(6):812–822

Italiano (2009) Neo/adjuvant chemotherapy does not improve outcome in resected primary synovial sarcoma: a study of the French Sarcoma Group. Ann Oncol 20(3):425–430

Kawai (2015) Trabectedin monotherapy after standard chemotherapy versus best supportive care in patients with advanced, translocation-related sarcoma: a randomised, open-label, phase 2 study. Lancet Oncol 16(4):406–416

Khan (2019) Surgical excision and not chemotherapy is the most powerful modality in treating synovial sarcoma: the UK's North East experience. Arch Orthop Trauma Surg 139(4):443–449

Maduekwe (2009) Role of sentinel lymph node biopsy in the staging of synovial, epithelioid, and clear cell sarcomas. Ann Surg Oncol 16(5):1356–1363

Minami (2020) The role of neoadjuvant chemotherapy in resectable primary synovial sarcoma. Anticancer Res 40(2):1029–1034

Nielsen (2000) Effect of high-dose ifosfamide in advanced soft tissue sarcomas. A multicentre phase II study of the EORTC Soft Tissue and Bone Sarcoma Group. Eur J Cancer 36(1):61–67

Nielsen (2015) Synovial sarcoma: recent discoveries as a roadmap to new avenues for therapy. Cancer Discov 5(2):124–134

Pender (2018) Poor treatment outcomes with palliative gemcitabine and docetaxel chemotherapy in advanced and metastatic synovial sarcoma. Med Oncol 35(10):131

Pollack (2017) First-in-human treatment with a dendritic cell-targeting Lentiviral vector-expressing NY-ESO-1, LV305, induces deep, durable response in refractory metastatic synovial sarcoma patient. J Immunother 40(8):302–306

Pollack (2020) Clinical outcomes of patients with advanced synovial sarcoma or myxoid/round cell liposarcoma treated at major cancer centers in the United States. Cancer Med [Epub ahead of print]

Pukhalskaya (2020) TLE1 expression fails to distinguish between synovial sarcoma, atypical fibroxanthoma, and dermatofibrosarcoma protuberans. J Cutan Pathol 47(2):135–138

Stacchiotti (2018) Synovial sarcoma: current concepts and future perspectives. J Clin Oncol 36(2):180–187

Tawbi (2017) Pembrolizumab in advanced soft-tissue sarcoma and bone sarcoma (SARC028): a multicentre, two-cohort, single-arm, open-label, phase 2 trial. Lancet Oncol 18(11):1493–1501 van der Graaf (2012) Pazopanib for metastatic soft-tissue sarcoma (PALETTE): a randomised, double-blind, placebo-controlled phase 3 trial. Lancet 379(9829):1879–1886

Vlenterie (2016) Outcome of chemotherapy in advanced synovial sarcoma patients: review of 15 clinical trials from the European Organisation for Research and Treatment of Cancer soft tissue and bone sarcoma group; setting a new landmark for studies in this entity. Eur J Cancer 58:62–72

Tenosynovial giant cell tumors (TGCT) actually are a family of neoplasms most often arising from the synovium of joints, bursae, and tendon sheaths. There are two subtypes:

- Localized tenosynovial giant cell tumor (LTGCT)
- Diffuse tenosynovial giant cell tumor (DTGCT)

These two subtypes have different clinical behavior: → see dedicated sections for more details.

This term includes two entities: benign triton tumor and malignant triton tumor. For details → see dedicated Chaps. 36 and 168.

Definition

Tufted hemangioma is a benign tumor of the blood vessels. It is also known as tufted angioma and angioblastoma of Nakagawa.

A related neoplasm, called kaposiform hemangioendothelioma (→ see dedicated section), presents similarly but is more likely to lead to Kasabach-Merritt syndrome (→ see below): although still often classified as separate nosological entities, they are becoming increasingly recognized as a spectrum of the same pathology.

Epidemiology and Presentation

This rare tumor mainly affects the skin and subcutaneous tissue of infants (about half cases are congenital) and young children, although cases have been reported in older children and adults. The upper trunk and neck are the most common sites of development. Tufted hemangioma eventually stabilizes and stops growing, and only in rare cases it regresses.

Tufted hemangioma—whose diameter cancer range from 1 to over 10 cm—often looks like a faint area of pink or brown discoloration of the skin. With time the lesion may become thicker and turn reddish or purplish in color. If Kasabach-Merritt phenomenon develops, the first sign is a rapid growth of the tumor, which becomes painful; moreover, the tumor gets a purple or brownish-red spotty appearance caused by bleeding underneath the skin.

Pathology

Tufted hemangioma derives its name from the characteristic "tufts" of capillaries observed microscopically. Multiple, scattered lobules of small capillary-type vessels are observed throughout the dermis and subcutaneous tissue conferring a

S. Mocellin, *Soft Tissue Tumors*, https://doi.org/10.1007/978-3-030-58710-9_245

"cannonball" or glomerular appearance. Some mitoses (without nuclear atypia) may be present.

Differential diagnosis may be needed with the following: pyogenic granuloma (inflammation cells are typically present); Kaposi sarcoma (slit-like vascular spaces and plasma cells, positive for HHV8); and kaposiform hemangioendothelioma (not confined to skin and more infiltrative).

Biomarkers

Tufted hemangioma stains positive for endothelial biomarkers CD31 and CD34, whereas it stains negative for GLUT1 and HHV8 (human herpes virus 8).

Prognosis

Tufted hemangioma is a benign tumor; nevertheless, a serious complication called Kasabach-Merritt syndrome develops in about 10% of cases. This phenomenon—which is associated with a mortality rate of 30%—is characterized by thrombocytopenia and coagulopathy. The risk of developing the Kasabach-Merritt syndrome is higher when the tumor is larger and when present at birth.

Therapy

Small asymptomatic tumors may not need treatment (except for esthetic reasons). If the tumor has not penetrated into the deeper layers of the skin, laser treatment may be taken into consideration for esthetic purposes. If the tumor involves a large skin area, treatment is suggested even if asymptomatic: for these cases, both medications (aspirin, sirolimus) and surgical excision have been advocated.

In case of Kasabach-Merritt syndrome, the patient should be hospitalized and treated with the above therapeutic options or with others such as chemotherapy (usually vincristine) and corticosteroids; furthermore, infusion of clotting factors may be needed in case of severe coagulopathy.

Suggested Readings

Papke (2020) What is new in endothelial neoplasia? Virchows Arch 476(1):17–28

Yao (2018) Comparison of corticosteroid and vincristine in treating kaposiform hemangioendothelioma and tufted angioma: a systematic review and meta-analysis. Eur J Pediatr Surg [Epub ahead of print]

Liu (2016) Treatment of kaposiform hemangioendothelioma and tufted angioma. Int J Cancer 139(7):1658–1666

Croteau (2016) The clinical spectrum of kaposiform hemangioendothelioma and tufted angioma. Semin Cutan Med Surg 35(3):147–152

Undifferentiated Pleomorphic Sarcoma

Definition

Undifferentiated pleomorphic sarcoma (UPS) is a soft tissue sarcoma without identifiable line of differentiation. It belongs to a heterogeneous subgroup of sarcomas known as undifferentiated/unclassified sarcomas, which includes also undifferentiated spindle cell sarcoma, undifferentiated round cell sarcoma, undifferentiated epithelioid sarcoma, and undifferentiated sarcoma NOS (not otherwise specified). Not included are dedifferentiated types of specific soft tissue sarcomas (e.g., dedifferentiated liposarcoma), where the dedifferentiated component is frequently undifferentiated.

The obsolete term malignant fibrous histiocytoma (MFH) has been utilized in the past to identify sarcomas currently classified (in most cases) as UPS.

A subgroup of undifferentiated round cell sarcomas is characterized by specific chromosomal translocations and corresponding fusion genes and is now considered a separate nosological entity: for more details, → see Chap. 88.

Epidemiology and Presentation

Undifferentiated soft tissue sarcomas account for approximately 20% of all soft tissue sarcomas that occur at any age anywhere in the body, without gender differences. Undifferentiated round cell sarcoma is more frequent in young patients. UPS occurs most frequently in older adults. Although undifferentiated soft tissue sarcomas may arise anywhere, these tumors are more frequently located in somatic soft tissues. Clinically, the lesion usually presents as a rapidly growing mass with possible compression signs/symptoms.

The etiology of most undifferentiated soft tissue sarcomas is unknown: however, approximately 25% of radiation-induced soft tissue sarcomas are undifferentiated.

S. Mocellin, *Soft Tissue Tumors*, https://doi.org/10.1007/978-3-030-58710-9_246

UPS accounts for about 15% of all adult soft tissue sarcomas and represents one of the most common soft tissue sarcomas of older adults, most lesions occurring in patients aged between 50 and 70 years. Most UPS are deep-seated lesions most frequently located in the limbs followed by the trunk; rarely, it can be found also in retroperitoneum, head and neck, subcutis, dermis (where it is known also as pleomorphic dermal sarcoma, → see dedicated section), breast, viscera, and bone.

Etiology and Predisposition

As extraskeletal osteosarcoma, fibrosarcoma, malignant peripheral nerve sheath tumor (MPNST), and angiosarcoma, UPS is one of the sarcomas most frequently associated with radiation exposure.

Moreover, like other soft tissue tumors (i.e., leiomyosarcoma, fibrosarcoma, MPNST, rhabdomyosarcoma, and synovial sarcoma), UPS has been linked to an inherited cancer predisposition condition called **Werner syndrome** (also known as adult progeria), a disease with a prevalence of around 1/200,000 inhabitants. The syndrome presents between 20 and 30 years with early onset bilateral cataracts, graying of the hair, short stature, and skin changes (e.g., ankle ulceration, hyperkeratosis, age spots). In most cases, additional age-related disorders occur (e.g., osteoporosis, diabetes mellitus, and atherosclerosis). These patients carry a high risk of developing cancer, with special regard to soft tissue sarcomas and melanoma. Life expectancy is shortened as compared to the general population, death being usually due to either malignancies or myocardial infarction (following extensive atherosclerosis). The syndrome is caused by a mutation in the WRN gene (chromosome 8p11–12), which codes for one of the five RecQ helicases; ultimately these mutations lead to genome instability. Mutations in the WRN gene are found in about 90% of cases. The Werner syndrome is inherited in an autosomal recessive manner. Once a patient is diagnosed with this disorder, the patient and the family should receive genetic counseling to identify persons who could develop the disease and those who are carriers.

Pathology

Importantly, the diagnosis of undifferentiated soft tissue sarcoma is a diagnosis of exclusion on the basis of the absence of a specific line of differentiation.

Macroscopically, necrosis is frequently found. Microscopically, undifferentiated soft tissue sarcomas are classically divided into five types: pleomorphic, spindle cell, round cell, epithelioid, and not otherwise specified. However, all of them lack specific features, and the common denominator is just the lack of an identifiable line of differentiation. UPS closely mimics other specific types of pleomorphic sarcoma and is often patternless, with frequent bizarre multinucleate giant tumor cells with variation in cytoplasmic and nuclear size throughout the tumor. Spindle cell lesions frequently display a fascicular architecture. Round cell tumors have relatively uniform rounded to ovoid cells with a high nucleus to cytoplasm ratio and frequently mimic other specific types of round cell sarcomas (e.g., Ewing sarcoma). Epithelioid tumors closely resemble metastatic carcinoma or melanoma but generally lack nesting.

Differential diagnosis may be needed with the following: poorly differentiated carcinoma (expression of epithelial biomarkers such as cytokeratins, EMA, p63, p40); melanoma (positive for S100, HBM45, Melan-A); dedifferentiated liposarcoma (most often presence of a well differentiated lipogenic component; MDM2 and CDK4 staining and amplification); pleomorphic liposarcoma (presence of pleomorphic lipoblasts; S100 positivity); pleomorphic leiomyosarcoma (histology of smooth muscle differentiation; positivity for h-caldesmon and desmin); pleomorphic rhabdomyosarcoma (positivity for desmin and myogenin); malignant peripheral nerve sheath tumor (fascicles of alternating cellularity, whorls, palisades or rosette-like arrangements, perineural/intraneural spread when associated with nerve, large areas of geographic-like necrosis); high-grade myxofibrosarcoma (prominent myxoid stroma, often lower histological grading, averagely less aggressive and thus better prognosis); atypical fibroxanthoma (difficult differential diagnosis for the rare cases of skin UPS); dermatofibrosarcoma protuberans (typical chromosomal translocation with COL1A1-PDGFB fusion gene; for the rare cases of skin UPS); anaplastic large cell lymphoma (CD30 positivity); and metastatic renal cell carcinoma (cytokeratin positivity).

Biomarkers

By definition, undifferentiated soft tissue sarcomas have no immunophenotype pattern allowing for the definition of a specific cell differentiation. These tumors may express—at least in subgroups of their composing cells—proteins such as cytokeratins, SMA,[1] desmin, EMA,[2] CD99, vimentin, and CD34; however, their diagnostic value is scarce. The lesions stain negative for melanocytic markers, CD45, and S100. By definition, no ultrastructure feature (as defined by electron microscopy) is helpful to characterize the cell differentiation of these malignancies.

UPS is characterized by highly complex karyotypes. Wide intercellular variation and coexistence of several ploidy levels demonstrate that UPS is genetically highly unstable, without specific recurrent aberrations being identified. The consequence of these genetic alterations lead to complex combinations of chromosomal gains and losses, with virtually all chromosomes being involved. Potential target genes in frequently deleted regions include RB1 (chromosome 13q), TP53 (17p), CDKN2A and CDKN2B (9p), and PTEN (10q).

PRDM10-bases fusion genes have been reported in around 5% of UPS.

---

[1] SMA: smooth muscle actin

[2] EMA: epithelial membrane antigen

The Cancer Genome Atlas (TCGA) research network has shown that UPS and myxofibrosarcoma (MFS) share a high level of genomic similarities and fall into a single spectrum of tumor.

Prognosis

Undifferentiated soft tissue sarcomas are high-grade malignancies. The 5-year survival of all patients with UPS is 50–60% with a local and distant disease recurrence rates of 40% and 25%, respectively. On average, patients with advanced UPS have the worse outcomes compared with patients affected with other soft tissue sarcomas.

Therapy

Surgery (wide excision) is the treatment of choice for localized primary tumors. **Radiotherapy** (adjuvant or neoadjuvant) is utilized for improving local disease control, although the role of adjuvant/neoadjuvant treatments is unclear in patients with USP.

For patients with locally advanced/unresectable or metastatic disease, anthracycline-based **chemotherapy** remains the standard first-line treatment. Other drugs such as trabectedin, gemcitabine and docetaxel, and pazopanib also have shown activity in the advanced setting and are utilized as second-line treatment.

Although UPS is deemed to be somewhat more sensitive to gemcitabine plus docetaxel, this drug combination resulted inferior to epirubicin plus ifosfamide in terms of disease-free survival in a randomized trial of neoadjuvant chemotherapy for soft tissue sarcomas including UPS (ISG-STS 1001).

Immunotherapy (e.g., pembrolizumab, an anti-PD1 monoclonal antibody) is also being tested in the clinical setting with some promising results.

Genomic profiling (looking for druggable molecular derangements) is being explored for patients with metastatic disease, although the rate of targetable genetic alterations appears to be low.

Suggested Readings

Ali (2019) Genomic and transcriptomic characterisation of undifferentiated pleomorphic sarcoma of bone. J Pathol 247(2):166–176

Cancer Genome Atlas Research Network (2017) Comprehensive and integrated genomic characterization of adult soft tissue sarcomas. Cell 171(4):950–965

Chen (2018) Primary undifferentiated pleomorphic sarcoma of the thyroid: a case report and review of the literature. Medicine (Baltimore) 97(7):e9927

Chen (2019) Undifferentiated pleomorphic sarcoma: long-term follow-up from a large institution. Cancer Manag Res 11:10001–10009

Fletcher (2020) WHO classification of tumours of soft tissue and bone, 5th edition

Gronchi (2017) Histotype-tailored neoadjuvant chemotherapy versus standard chemotherapy in patients with high-risk soft-tissue sarcomas (ISG-STS 1001): an international, open-label, randomised, controlled, phase 3, multicentre trial. Lancet Oncol 18(6):812–822

Guram (2018) Radiation therapy combined with checkpoint blockade immunotherapy for metastatic undifferentiated pleomorphic sarcoma of the maxillary sinus with a complete response. Front Oncol 8:435

Hofvander (2015) Recurrent PRDM10 gene fusions in undifferentiated pleomorphic sarcoma. Clin Cancer Res 21(4):864–869

Kamat (2019) The outcome of patients with localized undifferentiated pleomorphic sarcoma of the lower extremity treated at Stanford University. Am J Clin Oncol 42(2):166–171

Keung (2018) Phase II study of neoadjuvant checkpoint blockade in patients with surgically resectable undifferentiated pleomorphic sarcoma and dedifferentiated liposarcoma. BMC Cancer 18(1):913

Kong (2020) Radiation-induced undifferentiated pleomorphic sarcoma of the breast. BMJ Case Rep 13(2):e232616

Lauper (2013) Spectrum and risk of Neoplasia in Werner syndrome: a systematic review. PLoS One 8(4):e59709

Lee (2020) The clinical outcomes of undifferentiated pleomorphic sarcoma (UPS): a single-centre experience of two decades with the assessment of PD-L1 expressions. Eur J Surg Oncol S0748-7983(20)30131-1

Lewin (2018) Identifying actionable variants using next generation sequencing in patients with a historical diagnosis of undifferentiated pleomorphic sarcoma. Int J Cancer 142(1):57–65

Mass (2018) Undifferentiated pleomorphic sarcoma of liver: case report and review of the literature. Case Rep Pathol 2018:8031253

Matushansky (2009) MFH classification: differentiating undifferentiated pleomorphic sarcoma in the twenty-first century. Expert Rev. Anticancer Ther 9(8):1135–1144

Mukherjee (2018) Werner syndrome protein and DNA replication. Int J Mol Sci 19(11):3442

Qorbani (2019) Primary pulmonary undifferentiated pleomorphic sarcoma (PPUPS). Autops Case Rep 9(3):e2019110

Roland (2016) Analysis of clinical and molecular factors impacting oncologic outcomes in undifferentiated pleomorphic sarcoma. Ann Surg Oncol 23(7):2220–2228

Savina (2017) Patterns of care and outcomes of patients with METAstatic soft tissue SARComa in a real-life setting: the METASARC observational study. BMC Med 15:78

Soleymani (2017) Conception and management of a poorly understood spectrum of dermatologic neoplasms: atypical fibroxanthoma, pleomorphic dermal sarcoma, and undifferentiated pleomorphic sarcoma. Curr Treat Options in Oncol 18(8):50

Tawbi (2017) Pembrolizumab in advanced soft-tissue sarcoma and bone sarcoma (SARC028): a multicentre, two-cohort, single-arm, open-label, phase 2 trial. Lancet Oncol 18(11):1493–1501

Tsai (2018) Radiation-induced undifferentiated pleomorphic sarcoma of the heart: a case report. Pract Radiat Oncol 8(2):136–139

Vallés-Torres (2019) Cardiac undifferentiated pleomorphic sarcoma mimicking left atrial Myxoma. J Cardiothorac Vasc Anesth 33(2):493–496

Widemann (2018) Biology and management of undifferentiated pleomorphic sarcoma, myxofibrosarcoma, and malignant peripheral nerve sheath Tumors: state of the art and perspectives. J Clin Oncol 36(2):160–167

Winchester (2018) Undifferentiated pleomorphic sarcoma: factors predictive of adverse outcomes. J Am Acad Dermatol 79(5):853–859

Yamazaki (2018) A case of undifferentiated pleomorphic sarcoma of the breast with lung and bone metastases. Int J Surg Case Rep 51:143–146

Yoshimoto (2020) Comparative study of Myxofibrosarcoma with undifferentiated pleomorphic sarcoma: histopathologic and clinicopathologic review. Am J Surg Pathol 44(1):87–97

Zhou (2018) A primary undifferentiated pleomorphic sarcoma of the lumbosacral region harboring a LMNA-NTRK1 gene fusion with durable clinical response to crizotinib: a case report. BMC Cancer 18(1):842

Undifferentiated/unclassified sarcomas are a group of soft tissue sarcomas which includes the following:

- Undifferentiated pleomorphic sarcoma (UPS).
- Undifferentiated spindle cell sarcoma.
- Undifferentiated round cell sarcoma.
- Undifferentiated epithelioid sarcoma.
- Undifferentiated sarcoma NOS (not otherwise specified).

For more details → see the Chap. 246.

S. Mocellin, *Soft Tissue Tumors*, https://doi.org/10.1007/978-3-030-58710-9_247

Definition

Adenosarcoma of the uterus is a malignant tumor characterized by benign epithelial elements and a malignant mesenchymal component.

It is also known as Mullerian adenosarcoma.

Epidemiology and Presentation

Uterine adenosarcoma represents about 5% of all uterine sarcomas and usually presents with vaginal bleeding. It often affects young women.

Pathology

Adenosarcoma is characterized by epithelial and stromal elements with stromal hypercellularity. The epithelium is usually endometrioid and also ciliated, mucinous, and even squamous. The stroma has polypoid or leaf-like projections into glandular lumina, resembling phyllodes tumor of breast; stromal elements have mild or occasionally moderate atypia and resemble low-grade endometrial stroma sarcoma (LGESS) but are less bizarre and less undifferentiated. On average, 33% of cases show sarcomatous overgrowth.

Biomarkers

The most common immunohistochemical markers for adenosarcoma are CD10 and WT1, but they are not specific. Cytokeratins and muscle markers can be positive in the epithelial and mesenchymal component, respectively. Hormone receptors may be positive.

Prognosis

The majority of patients present with early stage disease, with a 5-year overall survival of 60–80%. Survival is influenced by the presence of sarcomatous overgrowth, myometrial invasion, lymphovascular invasion, necrosis, and the presence of heterologous elements including rhabdomyoblastic differentiation.

The risk of relapse is especially linked to the presence of sarcomatous overgrowth. The reported prevalence of sarcomatous overgrowth in patients with uterine adenosarcoma varies greatly, from 8% to 65%. Patients with sarcomatous overgrowth have significantly increased risk of recurrence 23% versus 77% and decreased 5-year overall survival 50–60%.

Therapy

Surgery is the cornerstone of treatment (total hysterectomy plus bilateral salpingo-oophorectomy without lymphadenectomy, as the incidence of lymph node metastasis is rare). Fertility preservation is an emerging field of investigation in gynecological oncology, and it is particularly relevant in uterine adenosarcoma, where patients are diagnosed as young as 15-year-old.

No studies are available for the adjuvant therapy of uterine adenosarcoma.

For advanced/metastatic disease, evidence is scant. Where there is hormone receptor expression, then an endocrine therapy may be considered. As regards chemotherapy, the approach is that for soft tissue sarcomas.

Suggested Readings

Desar (2018) Systemic treatment in adult uterine sarcomas. Crit Rev. Oncol Hematol 122:10–20
L'Heveder (2019) Conservative management of uterine adenosarcoma: lessons learned from 20 years of follow-up. Arch Gynecol Obstet 300(5):1383–1389
Nathenson (2016) Uterine adenosarcoma: a review. Curr Oncol Rep 18(11):68
Nathenson (2018) Prognostic factors for uterine adenosarcoma: a review. Expert Rev. Anticancer Ther 18(11):1093–1100
Pinto (2016) Uterine adenosarcoma. Arch Pathol Lab Med 140(3):286–290
Yuan (2019) Uterine adenosarcoma: a retrospective 12-year single-center study. Front Oncol 9:237

Definition

Uterine leiomyoma (ULM) is a benign tumor originating from the smooth muscle cells of the myometrium.

It is also known as uterine fibroma, uterine fibroid, uterine myofibroma, uterine fibromyoma, uterine leiomyofibroma, uterine leiomyomata, and uterine myoma.

It belongs to the family of leiomyomas ($\rightarrow$ see Chap. 146).

Epidemiology and Presentation

ULM is an extremely common neoplasm, as it is found in up to 70% of adult women. Often asymptomatic (ULM can be found as an incidentaloma in about 70% of cases), ULM can cause abnormal uterine bleeding (metrorrhagia, menorrhagia, or a combination of the two) and/or pelvic pain at least 30% of affected women. Large ULM can interfere with pregnancy (infertility) or block ureters. Rarely, it is associated with polycythemia (which regresses upon tumor removal). Pedunculated subserosal ULM may undergo torsion and thus cause acute abdominal pain. As an estrogen responsive neoplasm, ULM may regress after menopause or upon castration and enlarge during pregnancy. Transvaginal ultrasound is the gold-standard imaging method. Magnetic resonance imaging provides a better overall picture of the number, size, vascular supply, and boundaries of the ULMs, but it is unnecessary for a routine diagnosis and cannot differentiate ULM from leiomyosarcoma.

Many other diseases share the chief ULM complication (i.e., bleeding); they can be remembered using the mnemonic PALM-COEIN, which groups structural and nonstructural causes of abnormal uterine bleeding: polyps, adenomyosis, leiomyoma, malignancy, coagulopathy, ovulatory dysfunction, endometrial, iatrogenic, and those not yet classified.

It is important to realize that leiomyosarcoma can present similar to ULM and that there is no reliable way to clinically or radiologically differentiate the two

S. Mocellin, *Soft Tissue Tumors*, https://doi.org/10.1007/978-3-030-58710-9_249

entities: therefore, a biopsy is necessary but is not always sufficient (due to limitations in representativeness of the specimen), and exeresis of the entire lesion is often required for a definitive diagnosis.

Etiology and Predisposition

Both naturally occurring (e.g., genistein) and synthetic (e.g., diethylstilbestrol) xenoestrogens have been linked to a higher risk of developing ULM. In contrast, oral contraceptives and progestin-only compounds are associated with a reduced risk. No clear association between overall dairy consumption and uterine leiomyoma risk has been observed.

ULM is most often sporadic; however, women with an autosomal dominant genetic syndrome called **multiple cutaneous and uterine leiomyomatosis** (MCUL) are at higher risk of developing both skin and uterine leiomyomas. This condition, also known as Reed syndrome and hereditary leiomyomatosis with renal cell carcinoma (HLRCC), typically occurs as a result of a heterozygous germline mutation of the fumarate hydratase (FH) gene, which is involved in the Krebs's cycle and could act as a tumor suppressor gene. Approximately 90% of patients with multiple cutaneous leiomyomas harbor a heterozygous germline mutation in the FH gene. Female patients with FH mutations commonly display both piloleiomyomas (85%) and symptomatic uterine leiomyomas (>90%). Uterine leiomyomas associated with FH mutation tend to be larger (up to 10 cm), more numerous, develop at a younger age, and more frequently require hysterectomy in comparison to non-hereditary uterine leiomyomas. However, the most concerning feature of an FH mutation is the association with an aggressive variant of renal cell carcinoma (type II papillary renal cell carcinoma) which develops in approximately 15% of patients: of note, in this subgroup of patients developing renal cell carcinoma the malignancy is metastatic at presentation in about 50% of cases.

Pathology

Macroscopically, ULM is sharply circumscribed, round, firm, and grayish white in color; it usually develops within the myometrium (intramural), but it may be submucosal or subserosal; of note, only 8% of ULMs occur in the uterine cervix. It can grow up to several centimeters in diameter and often is multicentric.

Microscopically, ULM is characterized by a fascicular pattern of smooth muscle bundles separated by well-vascularized connective tissue. Larger lesions may develop areas of degeneration including hyaline or mucoid change, calcification, and cystic change. Typically, it grows in a non-infiltrative manner. Mitotic figures are usually fewer than 5 per 10 HPF in the most mitotically active area, without significant atypia.

The following ULM variants have been described:

- Lipoleiomyoma: a rare variant of ULM that combines leiomyoma with mature adipocytes; it accounts for 2% of all ULMs; it might transform into a primary liposarcoma of the uterus, an (extremely rare) malignant uterine neoplasm.
- Mitotically active leiomyoma: it typically occurs in young women as a submucous lesion; it is characterized by 5–15 mitoses per 10 HPF; it lacks nuclear atypia, abnormal mitotic figures, and tumor cell necrosis; although the behavior is usually benign, recurrence as leiomyosarcoma has been reported, which calls for adequate follow-up.
- Cellular leiomyoma: it is characterized by increased cellularity, but it lacks atypia and mitotic figures; generally it has large, thick-walled blood vessels; its behavior is benign.
- Leiomyoma with bizarre nuclei: it is characterized by bizarre multinucleated tumor cells (moderate to severe atypia), but mitotic figures are fewer than 10 per 10 HPF, and there is no tumor cell necrosis; it has been associated with progestin use; its behavior is generally benign although leiomyosarcoma may rarely arise from this lesion; it was formerly called symplastic leiomyoma or atypical leiomyoma.
- Myxoid leiomyoma: it is composed of islands of smooth muscle cells in myxoid connective tissue containing large vessels, without infiltrative growth; it lacks both atypia and mitotic activity; its behavior is generally benign, although myxoid leiomyosarcoma may rarely arise from this lesion.
- Epithelioid leiomyoma: it is composed of round epithelioid, rhabdoid, and large vacuolated cells intermingled with spindled cells; nuclear atypia is not prominent; tumor cell necrosis and mitotic figures are lacking; it stains positive for desmin and SMA but also for cytokeratins, while it is negative for CD1a and HMB45; it should be differentiated from PEComa (positive for HMB45 and CD1a) and endometrial carcinoma (atypia, mitotic figures, and tumor cell necrosis are present); it is also known as clear cell leiomyoma and leiomyoblastoma.
- Intravenous leiomyomatosis: this very rare condition occurring when mature smooth muscle grows inside the lumen of uterine and pelvic veins and can reach the heart chambers (usually right heart); it has an excellent prognosis as distant metastases are exceptional; however, it may recur or embolize.

Differential diagnosis is needed with leiomyosarcoma and (less often) endometrial stroma sarcoma (h-caldesmon negative). In typical cases, ULM can be easily distinguished because of the low/absent mitotic activity, lack of cytologic atypia, lack of necrosis, lack of pleomorphism, and non-infiltrative growth. However, low-grade leiomyosarcoma may resemble ULM, with special regard to some of its variants (e.g., mitotically active leiomyoma).

As regards the differential diagnosis with smooth muscle tumor of uncertain malignant potential (STUMP) and benign metastasizing leiomyoma → see dedicated sections.

Biomarkers

ULM stains positive for SMA,[1] MSA,[2] desmin, h-caldesmon, and vimentin. It is generally (but not always) negative for cytokeratins and EMA.[3]

About 40% of ULMs have nonrandom tumor-specific chromosomal rearrangements, the most common being chromosomal translocation t(12;14)(q15;q23-q24), which leads to dysregulated expression of HMGA2.[4]

Prognosis

ULM is a benign tumor.

Therapy

Surveillance is the method of choice to manage women with asymptomatic ULM; current guidelines do not recommend serial imaging for these patients.

Medical therapy is utilized to decrease the severity of bleeding and pain symptoms. Hormonal contraceptives (i.e., oral contraceptive pills and the levonorgestrel intrauterine device) are common options, although there is only limited data showing their effectiveness; the levonorgestrel intrauterine device (IUD) is currently the recommended hormonal therapy for symptomatic ULMs due to the low side effect profile. GnRH agonist leuprolide acts on the pituitary gland to decrease gonadal hormone production, thus decreasing the hormone-stimulated growth of the neoplasm; however, as GnRH agonist has a short-term effect and is associated with significant bone loss (in the long run), its use should be limited to 6 months and is considered mainly as pre-surgical therapy for symptomatic ULM. Nonsteroidal anti-inflammatory drugs (NSAIDs) are utilized to palliate pain and bleeding, but they have no impact on ULM size. Other potential medical treatments include aromatase inhibitors and selective estrogen receptor modulators (SERM), such as raloxifene or tamoxifen: however, there is little evidence supporting the use of these medications. Tranexamic acid has been approved for the treatment of abnormal and heavy uterine bleeding, but it does not decrease the disease burden.

---

[1] SMA: smooth muscle actin

[2] MSA: muscle specific actin

[3] EMA: epithelial membrane antigen

[4] HMGA2: High-mobility group AT-hook 2 encodes a protein that belongs to the non-histone chromosomal high-mobility group (HMG) protein family. HMG proteins function as architectural factors and are essential components of the enhanceosome; HMGA2 contains structural DNA-binding domains and may act as a transcriptional regulating factor; rearrangements of this gene that have been associated with myxoid liposarcoma suggest a role in adipogenesis and mesenchymal differentiation.

As regards operative treatments, **endometrial ablation** offers an alternative to more radical surgery in patients whose primary complaint is heavy bleeding. **Uterine artery embolization** is a minimally invasive approach for women who wish to preserve fertility: this technique decreases the total blood supply to the uterus, thereby minimizing bleeding symptoms. Surgery includes myomectomy and hysterectomy. **Myomectomy** is an invasive surgical option for women who desire fertility preservation (although there is no definitive evidence showing that myomectomy can improve fertility, which is highly dependent on the location and size of the lesion). **Hysterectomy** remains the definitive treatment for ULM and continues to be the leading indication for hysterectomy. The laparoscopic approach is largely diffuse for this type of surgery: nevertheless, the use of intraoperative morcellation is highly debated due to the risk of tumor cell dissemination in the (rare) case where the pathological examination reveals the unexpected presence of a leiomyosarcoma.

Suggested Readings

Cohen (2016) Updates in uterine fibroid tissue extraction. Curr Opin Obstet Gynecol 28(4):277–282

Dubuisson (2019) The current place of mini-invasive surgery in uterine leiomyoma management. J Gynecol Obstet Hum Reprod 48(2):77–81

Emoto (2018) Power morcellation-induced dissemination of sarcomatous component arising in leiomyoma. J Obstet Gynaecol Res 44(9):1843–1849

Lewis (2018) A comprehensive review of the pharmacologic management of uterine leiomyoma. Biomed Res Int 2018:2414609

McDonald (2011) Liposarcoma arising in uterine lipoleiomyoma: a report of 3 cases and review of the literature. Am J Surg Pathol 35(2):221–227

Orta (2020) Dairy and related nutrient intake and risk of uterine leiomyoma: a prospective cohort study. Hum Reprod 35(2):453–463

Seidman (2012) Peritoneal dissemination complicating morcellation of uterine mesenchymal neoplasms. PLoS One 7(11):e50058

Wang (2020) MED12 exon 2 mutation is uncommon in intravenous leiomyomatosis: clinicopathologic features and molecular study. Hum Pathol 99:36–42

Definition

Uterine leiomyosarcoma (ULMS) is a malignant neoplasm originating from smooth muscle cells. For general information on uterine sarcomas, → see dedicated section.

Epidemiology and Presentation

ULMS is the most common uterine sarcoma. It usually presents as a bulky tumor in women >40 years (it peaks at ages 40–69 years; mean age is 54 years) with complaints of vaginal bleeding (56%), a palpable pelvic mass (54%) and/or pelvic pain (22%).

Magnetic resonance imaging (MRI) is the optimal imaging modality to characterize masses originating from the uterus: however, although certain features may raise the suspicion of ULMS, it remains difficult to definitively distinguish a leiomyosarcoma from a leiomyoma with a complex appearance. Tumor biopsy is burdened by a non-negligible rate of false negativity (a negative biopsy does not rule out the diagnosis until the hysterectomy specimen is pathologically examined). Overall, in many patients, the diagnosis is made postoperatively, in place of the expected benign leiomyoma.

Pathology

ULMS shows hypercellularity with spindle cells resembling smooth muscle with moderate to severe pleomorphism; the infiltrative border is the most helpful feature for diagnosis. There are usually >10 mitotic figures per 10 HPF with abundant abnormal mitotic figures.

Differential diagnosis may be needed with the following: endometrial stromal sarcoma with smooth muscle metaplasia, mitotically active leiomyoma, cellular

© The Editor(s) (if applicable) and The Author(s), under exclusive license to
Springer Nature Switzerland AG 2021
S. Mocellin, *Soft Tissue Tumors*, https://doi.org/10.1007/978-3-030-58710-9_250

leiomyoma, hemorrhagic leiomyoma, atypical leiomyoma (leiomyoma with bizarre nuclei), myxoid leiomyoma, epithelioid leiomyoma, and leiomyoma with massive lymphoid infiltration.

Differential diagnosis: distinction between leiomyoma and leiomyosarcoma is made with conventional morphological criteria (mitosis, atypia, and necrosis).

The term STUMP (smooth muscle tumors of undefined malignant potential) is used in a setting when both leiomyoma as well as leiomyosarcoma cannot be diagnosed with certainty (→ see dedicated section).

Biomarkers

It stains positive for smooth muscle actin (SMA) and desmin. Estrogen and progesterone receptors are expressed in 45% and 65% of ULMS, respectively.

Prognosis

ULMS is usually a high-grade tumor with a mitotic rate > 15 per 10 HPF. The prognosis of leiomyosarcoma is poor, even when confined to the uterus at the time of diagnosis. Recurrence rates are high (between 53% and 71%), and the 5-year overall survival rate is poor (overall: 42%; advanced stage: 15%). The most common site of first recurrence is in the lungs (40%). Lymph node metastasis occurs in 3–11% of cases.

Although ULMS is associated with a poor prognosis when considering all cases, the following are considered independent prognostic factors: grade, tumor size, mitotic rate, presence of cervical invasion, presence of locoregional metastases, and presence of distant metastases.

ULMS is generally staged according to the staging system proposed by the Federation of Gynecology and Obstetrics (FIGO) (→ see Table 251.1 in the Chap. 251).

Therapy

For early stage disease, **surgery** (total hysterectomy + bilateral salpingo-oophorectomy) is the cornerstone of treatment for localized disease. In the absence of clinically evident lymph node metastasis, lymphadenectomy is not recommended. For locally recurrent disease, complete cytoreductive surgery (if feasible) is considered an option, although it usually requires complex procedures (burdened by a non-negligible rate of postoperative complications).

Based on the findings of a randomized controlled trial, adjuvant **radiotherapy** does not provide any significant survival advantage (unlike carcinosarcoma of the uterus). Similarly, there is no evidence of a survival benefit associated with adjuvant **chemotherapy**: the only randomized controlled trial of gemcitabine plus docetaxel showed no benefit, although the study was closed prematurely due to accrual issues. Analogously, adjuvant **hormonal therapy** appears to play no role in the management of these patients. Nonetheless, adjuvant chemotherapy (e.g., four to six cycles of doxorubicin or gemcitabine-docetaxel) might be advised in young and otherwise healthy women with a high risk of recurrence (e.g. high-grade, tumor spillage, or morcellation).

For locally advanced but unresectable disease or in the metastatic setting, hormonal therapy (mainly aromatase inhibitors) can be an option for receptor positive lesions; otherwise (or upon failure of endocrine therapy), systemic chemotherapy is the standard treatment. For the first-line treatment, doxorubicin (with or without ifosfamide) is the first choice; after first-line failure, gemcitabine plus docetaxel or trabectedin can be utilized.

As regards **target therapy**, pazopanib has a place in the treatment of uterine sarcoma after failure of anthracycline-based first-line therapy.

Although the experience is still limited, **immunotherapy** with anti-PD1 monoclonal antibodies does not appear to be active against ULMS.

Suggested Readings

Ben-Ami (2017) Immunotherapy with single agent nivolumab for advanced leiomyosarcoma of the uterus: results of a phase 2 study. Cancer 123(17):3285–3290

Benson (2016) Outcome of uterine sarcoma patients treated with pazopanib: a retrospective analysis based on two European Organisation for Research and Treatment of Cancer (EORTC) Soft Tissue and Bone Sarcoma Group (STBSG) clinical trials 62,043 and 62,072. Gynecol Oncol 142(1):89–94

Bizzarri (2019) Secondary cytoreductive surgery in recurrent uterine leiomyosarcoma: a multi-institutional study. Int J Gynecol Cancer 29(7):1134–1140

Cybulska (2019) Secondary surgical resection for patients with recurrent uterine leiomyosarcoma. Gynecol Oncol 154(2):333–337

Demetri (2016) Efficacy and safety of trabectedin or dacarbazine for metastatic liposarcoma or leiomyosarcoma after failure of conventional chemotherapy: results of a phase III randomized multicenter clinical trial. J Clin Oncol 34(8):786–793

Friedman (2018) Options for adjuvant therapy for uterine leiomyosarcoma. Curr Treat Options in Oncol 19(2):7

Gadducci (2018) A phase II randomised (calibrated design) study on the activity of the single-agent trabectedin in metastatic or locally relapsed uterine leiomyosarcoma. Br J Cancer 119(5):565–571

George (2017) Loss of PTEN is associated with resistance to anti-PD-1 checkpoint blockade therapy in metastatic uterine leiomyosarcoma. Immunity 46(2):197–204

Hensley (2017) Efficacy and safety of trabectedin or dacarbazine in patients with advanced uterine leiomyosarcoma after failure of anthracycline-based chemotherapy: subgroup analysis of a phase 3, randomized clinical trial. Gynecol Oncol 146(3):531–537

Hensley (2018) Adjuvant gemcitabine plus docetaxel followed by doxorubicin versus observation for high-grade uterine leiomyosarcoma: a phase III NRG oncology/Gynecologic Oncology Group Study. J Clin Oncol [Epub ahead of print]

Meng (2020) Construction and validation of nomograms for predicting the prognosis of uterine leiomyosarcoma: a population-based study. Med Sci Monit 26:e922739

Reed (2008) Phase III randomised study to evaluate the role of adjuvant pelvic radiotherapy in the treatment of uterine sarcomas stages I and II: an European organisation for research and treatment of cancer gynaecological cancer group study (protocol 55,874). Eur J Cancer 44(6):808–818

Roberts (2018) Uterine leiomyosarcoma: a review of the literature and update on management options. Gynecol Oncol 151(3):562–572

Sun (2019) How to differentiate uterine leiomyosarcoma from leiomyoma with imaging. Diagn Interv Imaging 100(10):619–634

Yuan (2019) Outcome of adjuvant radiotherapy after total hysterectomy in patients with uterine leiomyosarcoma or carcinosarcoma: a SEER-based study. BMC Cancer 19(1):697

Zang (2019) Hormonal therapy in uterine sarcomas. Cancer Med 8:1339–1349

Definition

Uterine sarcomas are malignant neoplasms and are classified into mesenchymal tumors or mixed (epithelial plus mesenchymal) tumors.

Mesenchymal tumors are further classified as follows:

- Uterine leiomyosarcoma (ULMS, 63%).
- Endometrial stromal sarcoma (ESS, 21%), which is usually divided into low-grade ESS (LGESS) and high-grade ESS (HGESS).
- Undifferentiated uterine sarcoma (UUS, 5%).
- Other rarer subtypes, such as rhabdomyosarcoma (RMS), inflammatory myofibroblastic tumor (IMF), perivascular epithelioid cell tumor (PEComa), and the recently described SMARC-deficient uterine sarcoma.

HGESS and UUS are also known as high-grade uterine sarcomas (HGUS).

Mixed epithelial and mesenchymal tumors include the following:

- Uterine adenosarcoma, which is a mixed tumor with a combination of a benign epithelial component and malignant mesenchymal cells.
- Uterine carcinosarcoma, also called malignant mixed Mullerian tumor, is generally regarded and treated as a neoplasm of epithelial origin, and therefore is not covered here.

→ See sections dedicated to single uterine sarcomas for more details.

Epidemiology and Presentation

Uterine sarcomas account for 3–9% of all uterine cancers, 1% of female genital tract malignancies, and 7% of all sarcomas. The annual incidence is estimated to be 0.3–0.8/100.000 women. Notably, uterine leiomyoma (also known as fibroid, fibroma, or simply myoma)—a benign soft tissue tumor arising from smooth muscle cells—is very frequent (with a prevalence from 5% to 20%, it is the most common benign tumor in women and the leading indication for hysterectomy).

Since the incidence of sarcomatous features within a suspected leiomyoma increases with age (especially in the perimenopausal state), preoperative diagnosis is strongly recommended in women with a rapidly enlarging fibroid in the post- or perimenopausal state with other suspicious features such as postmenopausal bleeding.

For further details → see sections dedicated to single uterine sarcomas.

Prognosis

Uterine sarcomas are often associated with poor prognosis; the median overall survival for patients with advanced/metastatic disease is approximately 10 months.

Uterine sarcomas are traditionally staged according to the Federation of Gynecology and Obstetrics (FIGO) staging system (→ see the below Table 251.1).

For details on single uterine sarcomas → see dedicated sections.

Therapy

Surgery (total hysterectomy plus bilateral salpingo-oophorectomy) is the standard of care for early stage disease treatment. The risk of lymph node and omental metastases is negligible, which rules out the need for bilateral pelvic lymphadenectomy and omentectomy.

With the advent of minimally invasive techniques to remove benign uterine tumors, it is of pivotal importance to make sure that these techniques are not utilized to treat a uterine sarcoma: in fact, simple myomectomy and morcellation have been reported to be a poor prognostic factor for survival of woman with uterine sarcoma.

Table 251.1 FIGO staging for uterine sarcomas

Stage		Definition
I		Tumor limited to uterus
	IA	<5 cm in greatest dimension
	IB	>5 cm in greatest dimension
II		Tumor extends beyond the uterus, within the pelvis
	IIA	Adnexal involvement
	IIB	Involvement of other pelvic tissues
III	IIIA	1 site
	IIIB	> 1 site
	IIIC	Involves pelvic and/or Para-aortic lymph nodes
IV		Tumor invades pelvic organs and/or distant metastasis
	IVA	Invasion of bladder or rectum
	IVB	Distant metastasis

Currently, there is no evidence to support the role of adjuvant **chemotherapy** or adjuvant **radiotherapy** in all uterine sarcoma subtypes. The combination of adjuvant chemotherapy plus radiotherapy slightly improves disease-free survival but has no impact on overall survival.

There are no randomized controlled trials of **hormonal therapy** in uterine sarcomas, either in the adjuvant or in the metastatic setting, but endocrine therapy (aromatase inhibitors, progestins, GnRH analogs) is often utilized for tumors expressing estrogen and/or progesterone receptors (mainly LGESS and ULMS); of note, tamoxifen is contraindicated due to its known stimulating effect on cell proliferation in the uterus (as opposed to its anti-proliferative effect in breast tissues).

In the metastatic setting, systemic chemotherapy is associated with low response rates. For the first-line treatment, doxorubicin (with or without ifosfamide) is the first choice; after first-line failure, gemcitabine plus docetaxel or trabectedin can be utilized. As regards target therapy, pazopanib has a place in the treatment of uterine sarcoma after failure of anthracycline-based first-line therapy.

For more details → see sections dedicated to single uterine sarcomas.

Suggested Readings

Benson (2016) Outcome of uterine sarcoma patients treated with pazopanib: a retrospective analysis based on two European Organisation for Research and Treatment of Cancer (EORTC) Soft Tissue and Bone Sarcoma Group (STBSG) clinical trials 62,043 and 62,072. Gynecol Oncol 142(1):89–94

Benson (2017) Uterine sarcoma—current perspectives. Int J Women's Health 9:597–606

Demetri (2016) Efficacy and safety of trabectedin or dacarbazine for metastatic liposarcoma or leiomyosarcoma after failure of conventional chemotherapy: results of a phase III randomized Multicenter clinical trial. J Clin Oncol 34(8):786–793

Gantzer (2018) Gynecological sarcomas: what's new in 2018, a brief review of published literature. Curr Opin Oncol 30(4):246–251

Mandato (2017) Uterine inflammatory myofibroblastic tumor: more common than expected. Case report and review. Medicine (Baltimore) 96(48):e8974

Pannier (2019) Hormonal therapies in uterine sarcomas, aggressive angiomyxoma, and desmoid-type fibromatosis. Crit Rev. Oncol Hematol 143:62–66

Pautier (2013) A randomized clinical trial of adjuvant chemotherapy with doxorubicin, ifosfamide, and cisplatin followed by radiotherapy versus radiotherapy alone in patients with localized uterine sarcomas (SARCGYN study). A study of the French Sarcoma Group. Ann Oncol 24(4):1099–1104

Ray-Coquard (2016) Impact of chemotherapy in uterine sarcoma (UtS): review of 13 clinical trials from the EORTC Soft Tissue and Bone Sarcoma Group (STBSG) involving advanced/metastatic UtS compared to other soft tissue sarcoma (STS) patients treated with first line chemotherapy. Gynecol Oncol 142(1):95–101

Reed (2008) Phase III randomised study to evaluate the role of adjuvant pelvic radiotherapy in the treatment of uterine sarcomas stages I and II: an European Organisation for Research and Treatment of Cancer Gynaecological Cancer Group Study (protocol 55,874). Eur J Cancer 44(6):808–818

Si (2017) Role of lymphadenectomy for uterine sarcoma: a meta-analysis. Int J Gynecol Cancer 27(1):109–116

Zimmermann (2012) Prevalence, symptoms and management of uterine fibroids: an international internet-based survey of 21,746 women. BMC Womens Health 12:6

The following is the 2014 World Health Organization classification of uterine soft tissue tumors.

For details on each single tumor → see dedicated sections.

Of note, other entities have been described to affect the uterus, such as inflammatory myofibroblastic tumor and SMARC-deficient uterine sarcoma: for details, → see dedicated sections.

Tumor	Variants
Leiomyoma	Cellular leiomyoma
	Leiomyoma with bizarre nuclei
	Mitotically active leiomyoma
	Hydropic leiomyoma
	Apoplectic leiomyoma
	Lipomatous leiomyoma (lipoleiomyoma)
	Epithelioid leiomyoma
	Myxoid leiomyoma
	Dissecting (cotyledonoid) leiomyoma
	Diffuse leiomyomatosis
	Intravenous leiomyomatosis
	Metastasizing leiomyoma
Smooth muscle tumor of uncertain malignant potential (STUMP)	–
Leiomyosarcoma	Epithelioid leiomyosarcoma
	Myxoid leiomyosarcoma
Endometrial stromal and related tumors	Endometrial stromal nodule
	Low-grade endometrial stromal sarcoma
	High-grade endometrial stromal sarcoma
	Undifferentiated uterine sarcoma
	Uterine tumor resembling ovarian sex cord tumor

803

S. Mocellin, *Soft Tissue Tumors*, https://doi.org/10.1007/978-3-030-58710-9_252

Tumor	Variants
Rhabdomyosarcoma	–
Perivascular epithelioid cell tumor (PEComa)	Benign
	Malignant
Mixed epithelial and mesenchymal tumors	Adenomyoma (uncovered)
	Adenofibroma (uncovered)
	Adenosarcoma
	Carcinosarcoma (uncovered)

Definition

Uterine undifferentiated sarcoma (UUS) is a high-grade malignancy. It is also known as undifferentiated uterine sarcoma.

Epidemiology and Presentation

UUS is a very rare malignancy of the uterus affecting women at a mean age of 45 years. It usually presents with vaginal bleeding.

Pathology

UUS is a poorly differentiated sarcoma composed of cells that do not resemble those of the proliferative-phase endometrial stroma. Two UUS subtypes are recognized: uniform UUS and pleomorphic UUS.

Uniform-type UUS shows extensive myometrial involvement with lymphovascular embolism and no destructive involvement of the myometrium in contrast to high-grade endometrial stroma sarcoma (HGESS). Uniform-type UUS shows fusiform spindle cells or round cells.

Pleomorphic-type UUS shows high-grade cytological atypia with pronounced nuclear pleomorphism associated with a high mitotic rate (almost always >10 MF/10 HPF and up to 50 MF/10 HPF) and the presence of tumor necrosis. UUS is often heterogeneous and composed of different components, such as HGESS, dedifferentiated leiomyosarcoma, sarcomatous component of adenosarcoma, and carcinosarcoma.

Some investigators believe that at least some UUS are actually HGESS (as confirmed by detection of YWHAE-NUTM2 fusion gene).

S. Mocellin, *Soft Tissue Tumors*, https://doi.org/10.1007/978-3-030-58710-9_253

Biomarkers

No specific panel exists. UUS stains negative for cytokeratins.

Prognosis

Approximately 60% of the patients present with stage III or IV disease. Overall, the prognosis is very poor.

Therapy

Surgery is the mainstay of treatment for localized disease.

For advanced/metastatic disease, evidence is scant and the approach is that for soft tissue sarcomas.

Given the lack of hormonal receptor expression, endocrine therapy has no rational in UUS, either in the adjuvant or metastatic setting.

Given the low response rates to conventional chemotherapy, these patients should be considered for clinical trials of novel agents.

For the general approach to systemic chemotherapy for uterine sarcomas → see Chap. 251.

Suggested Readings

Benson (2017) Uterine sarcoma—current perspectives. Int J Women's Health 9:597–606
Cotzia (2019) Undifferentiated uterine sarcomas represent under-recognized high-grade endometrial stromal sarcomas. Am J Surg Pathol 43(5):662–669
Desar (2018) Systemic treatment in adult uterine sarcomas. Crit Rev. Oncol Hematol 122:10–20
Gantzer (2018) Gynecological sarcomas: what's new in 2018, a brief review of published literature. Curr Opin Oncol 30(4):246–251

Definition

VHA is a benign lesion of vascular differentiation. For general information on hemangioma → see dedicated section. It is still debated if VHA should be considered a tumor or a malformation.

Epidemiology and Presentation

This is a rare disease generally occurring in adults. It generally develops in subcutaneous or deeper soft tissues of the limbs. Other soft tissue and visceral sites have been rarely reported.

VHA typically presents as a long-standing slow-growing mass. Radiological imaging can demonstrate calcification due to presence of phleboliths.

Pathology

VHA is composed of thick-walled veins of variable size. Dilated vessels can show attenuation of their walls, mimicking a cavernous hemangioma. Intramuscular hemangioma and angiomatosis (→ see dedicated sections) are also composed of veins but are usually intermixed with other vessel types.

Biomarkers

No specific panel exists.

© The Editor(s) (if applicable) and The Author(s), under exclusive license to
Springer Nature Switzerland AG 2021
S. Mocellin, *Soft Tissue Tumors*, https://doi.org/10.1007/978-3-030-58710-9_254

Prognosis

This is a benign disease.

Therapy

Deep-seated lesions can be difficult to surgically excise and can recur locally.

Suggested Reading

Fletcher (2013) WHO classification of tumours of soft tissue and bone

Definition

Well differentiated liposarcoma (WDLS)is a malignant neoplasm with adipocytic differentiation.

Sometimes WDLS is named atypical lipomatous tumor (ALT) or atypical lipoma, which can generate some confusion. The term ALT should be used only for tumors arising in "somatic" adipose tissue (such as that of extremities or thoraco-abdominal wall, as opposed to "visceral" adipose tissue—such as that of retroperitoneum or mediastinum), since their surgical complete excision is usually curative and thus the term "sarcoma" may be excessively prognostically negative for a lesion with a favorable behavior. The term atypical lipoma should be probably abandoned.

For general information on liposarcomas, → see Chap. 156. As regards the other types of liposarcomas (i.e., dedifferentiated liposarcoma, myxoid/round cell liposarcoma, pleomorphic liposarcoma) → see dedicated sections.

Epidemiology and Presentation

WDLS accounts for about 40–50% of all liposarcomas and therefore represent the most frequent type of malignant adipocytic tumor. It occurs mainly in middle-aged adults (incidence peak: 50–60 years), with no significant difference in terms of gender. Childhood cases are extremely rare.

WDLS occurs most frequently in deep soft tissue of the limbs (under the muscle fascia), especially the thigh, followed by the retroperitoneum; more rarely the paratesticular area (spermatic cord) and the mediastinum can be affected; the head and neck, skin, and viscera are very rare locations for this tumor.

WDLS is a slow-growing tumor usually painless; it can reach very large dimensions (>20 cm, especially in the retroperitoneal space) before it becomes clinically evident and is diagnosed.

S. Mocellin, *Soft Tissue Tumors*, https://doi.org/10.1007/978-3-030-58710-9_255

Both computed tomography and magnetic resonance imaging show a high diagnostic accuracy.

Lipoma is at least 100-folds more frequent than WDLS: however, lesions that are >5 cm in diameter, rapidly growing, and/or deep to the superficial fascia warrant evaluation to exclude malignancy.

Pathology

WDLS is composed completely or in part of mature adipocytes displaying significant variation in cell size (pleomorphic adipocytes) and at least focal nuclear atypia (which is a consistent finding). Scattered hyperchromatic (often multinucleated) stromal cells and a varying number of lipoblasts may be present (but do not necessarily ease the diagnosis of liposarcoma).

WDLS usually consists of a well-circumscribed often lobulated mass which varies in color (from yellow to white) and firmness depending on the proportion of adipocytic, fibrous, and myxoid components. An infiltrative growth pattern is rarely encountered. Areas of fat necrosis can be found in larger lesions.

WDLS can be morphologically subdivided into four subtypes: adipocytic liposarcoma (also known as lipoma-like liposarcoma), sclerosing liposarcoma, inflammatory liposarcoma, and spindle cell liposarcoma; the coexistence of more patterns in the same tumor is frequent, especially in the retroperitoneal space.

Differential diagnosis may be needed with the following: lipoma (no retroperitoneum, often above muscle fascia, no nuclear atypia, MDM2 negative); Hodgkin lymphoma (MDM2 negative); inflammatory myofibroblastic tumor (highly cellular proliferation of SMA positive myofibroblasts, MDM2 negative, half cases are ALK positive); idiopathic retroperitoneal fibrosis (no well-differentiated liposarcomatous component, MDM2 negative); IgG4-related disease (IgG4 positive plasma cells, MDM2 negative); lipoblastoma (usually age 3 or younger, MDM2 negative); angiomyolipoma (HMB45-positive epithelioid cells, MDM2 negative); myxoid liposarcoma (MDM2 negative, positive for FUS-DDIT3 fusion gene); dedifferentiated liposarcoma (non lipogenic high-grade sarcoma; typically shows abrupt transition between well-differentiated and dedifferentiated components; low-grade dedifferentiation: cellularity between WDLS and DDLS); and lipomatous hemangiopericytoma (solitary fibrous tumor with fatty differentiation: patternless type of growth, round to spindle cell morphology, characteristic hemangiopericytomatous vasculature; positive for NAB2-STAT6 fusion gene with diffuse STAT6 and CD34 positivity, and negative for MDM2).

Biomarkers

Adipocytic cells are usually S100 positive. MDM2 and/or CDK4 nuclear immunopositivity is present in most (if not all) cases, which is in line with the consistently present **gene amplification** of the DNA region spanning these two genes.

This positivity is important when the differential diagnosis between WDLS and lipoma is needed. MDM2 is frequently negative in spindle cell liposarcoma. Other genes located in the 12q14–15 region, including HMGA2, YEATS4, CPM, and FRS2 are frequently co-amplified with MDM2 and/or CDK4.

Prognosis

WDLS has no metastatic potential unless it undergoes dedifferentiation ($\rightarrow$ see section dedicated to dedifferentiated liposarcoma).

The prognosis varies according to the site of origin. In fact, unlike cases originating from somatic adipose tissues (which can be generally completely extirpated with surgery), lesions arising in the retroperitoneum and mediastinum can only rarely be treated with a wide excision, which leads to the high rate of local recurrence; these local relapses can lead to death due to compression of adjacent organs or due to dedifferentiation (and thus metastatization). WDLS of the spermatic cord can relapse into the retroperitoneum, thus presenting the abovementioned potentially lethal behavior.

Transformation of WDLS into dedifferentiated liposarcoma is estimated to occur in 20% of cases.

Overall, the prognosis of WDLS is better than that of other types of liposarcoma ($\rightarrow$ see dedicated sections): for instance, 5-year disease-specific survival in patients with WDLS and dedifferentiated liposarcoma is about 90% and 45%, respectively; however, long follow-up data show that mortality is about 80% for WDLS arising in the retroperitoneum, the median time to death ranging from 6 to 12 years.

Therapy

Surgery is the mainstay of treatment. As abovementioned, this therapeutic option is almost always curative for cases originating from the extremities, but more rarely for retroperitoneal tumors.

There is some retrospective evidence that resection of retroperitoneal sarcomas along with adjacent organs (e.g., kidney, colon) might be beneficial in terms of survival (even when the organs are not infiltrated), probably because of the higher chance to be oncologically radical. In contrast, WDLS of the extremities (or the thoraco-abdominal wall) can be treated conservatively with 1 cm margin of healthy tissue, when feasible (narrower margins are acceptable to preserve function or cosmesis); moreover, no vascular resection is necessary for lesions encasing a neurovascular bundle because the prognosis is favorable even after local disease recurrence (which can be treated with redo surgery).

No adjuvant treatment (either chemotherapy or radiotherapy) is currently recommended, either in retroperitoneal or extremity WDLS.

The only randomized controlled trial (STRASS) so far available on neoadjuvant **radiotherapy** for retroperitoneal sarcomas has not demonstrated an abdominal recurrence-free survival advantage over surgery alone in patients with histologically proven localized and resectable primary soft tissue malignancies (although subgroup analysis shows a significant benefit for the liposarcoma subset).

For locally recurrent disease, surgery remains the best option (when feasible).

WDLS is considered a chemoresistant neoplasm. For patients with locally advanced unresectable disease, anthracycline-based **chemotherapy** remains the standard first-line treatment, although WDLS is poorly chemosensitive. As second-line treatment, gemcitabine plus docetaxel and high-dose ifosfamide monotherapy can be used. More recently, trabectedin and eribulin have been approved for the treatment of patients with metastatic liposarcoma who failed anthracycline-based first-line chemotherapy. As regards **target therapy**, based on the characteristic CDK4/MDM2 amplification, both CDK inhibitors (e.g., palbociclib, which is currently approved for the treatment of other malignancies such as breast cancer) and MDM2 inhibitors are under investigation.

Suggested Readings

Bonvalot (2009) Primary retroperitoneal sarcomas: a multivariate analysis of surgical factors associated with local control. J Clin Oncol 27:31–37

Bonvalot (2019) STRASS (EORTC 62092): a phase III randomized study of preoperative radiotherapy plus surgery versus surgery alone for patients with retroperitoneal sarcoma. J Clin Oncol 37(15_suppl):11001

Choi (2020) Surgical management of truncal and extremities atypical lipomatous tumors/well-differentiated liposarcoma: a systematic review of the literature. Am J Surg 219(5):823–827

Crago (2016) Liposarcoma: multimodality management and future targeted therapies. Surg Oncol Clin N Am 25(4):761–773

Demetri (2016) Efficacy and safety of trabectedin or dacarbazine for metastatic liposarcoma or leiomyosarcoma after failure of conventional chemotherapy: results of a phase III randomized multicenter clinical trial. J Clin Oncol 34(8):786–793

Dickson (2016) Progression-free survival among patients with well-differentiated or dedifferentiated liposarcoma treated with CDK4 inhibitor palbociclib: a phase 2 clinical trial. JAMA Oncol 2(7):937–940

Fletcher (2020) WHO classification of tumours of soft tissue and bone, 5th edition

Gronchi (2009) Aggressive surgical policies in a retrospectively reviewed single-institution case series of retroperitoneal soft tissue sarcoma patients. J Clin Oncol 27:24–30

Keung (2020) Evaluating the impact of surveillance follow-up intervals in patients following resection of primary well-differentiated Liposarcoma of the Retroperitoneum. Ann Surg Oncol [Epub ahead of print]

Lee (2017) Clinical and molecular spectrum of liposarcoma. J Clin Oncol 36:151–159

Miura (2018) Primary mediastinal dedifferentiated liposarcoma: five case reports and a review. Thorac Cancer 9(12):1733–1740

Schöffski (2016) Eribulin versus dacarbazine in previously treated patients with advanced liposarcoma or leiomyosarcoma: a randomised, open-label, multicentre, phase 3 trial. Lancet 387(10,028):1629–1637

Shim (2020) An MRI-based decision tree to distinguish lipomas and lipoma variants from well-differentiated liposarcoma of the extremity and superficial trunk: classification and regression tree (CART) analysis. Eur J Radiol 127:109012

Thway (2019) Well-differentiated liposarcoma and dedifferentiated liposarcoma: an updated review. Semin Diagn Pathol 36(2):112–121

Index

© The Editor(s) (if applicable) and The Author(s), under exclusive license to
Springer Nature Switzerland AG 2021
S. Mocellin, *Soft Tissue Tumors*, https://doi.org/10.1007/978-3-030-58710-9